Textbook of Disorders and Injuries of the Musculoskeletal System

Second Edition

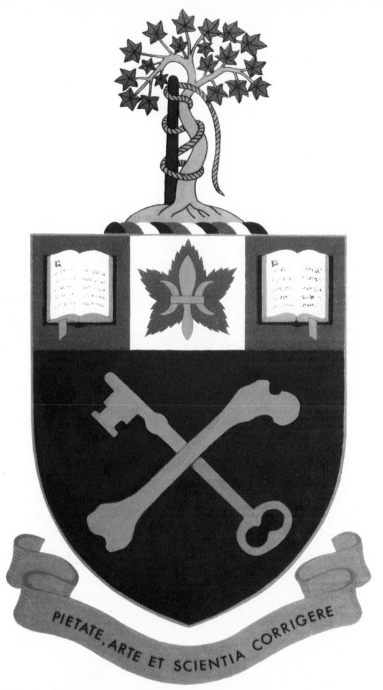

The Coat of Arms of the Canadian Orthopaedic Association

The presentation of a coat of arms, or armorial bearings, to an Association carries both symbolic and historic significance.

During his presidency of the Canadian Orthopaedic Association (1981–82), Dr. Robert B. Salter conceived and designed the above coat of arms and presented it as a personal gift to the Association at its 1982 annual meeting.

At the time of writing the second edition of this textbook, Dr. Salter, whose hobbies include heraldry, is the President of the Heraldry Society of Canada (1981–83).

Description and Symbolism of the Coat of Arms

The coat of arms of the Canadian Orthopaedic Association reflects the Association's tradition, philosophy, and goals, as well as the nature of orthopaedics.

The Crest

The crest atop the shield depicts the "orthopaedic tree" from Nicolas Andry's 18th century book entitled *Orthopaedia, or the Art of Preventing and Correcting Deformities in Children*. This crooked tree, which, like a deformed child, can be helped to grow straight by the application of appropriate forces, has become the international symbol of orthopaedic surgery. For the *Canadian Orthopaedic Association* the tree is a Canadian maple, the leaves of which have turned red as they do in the late autumn.

The Shield

Appearing in the middle section of the upper part of the shield is a red maple leaf with a superimposed gold *fleur-de-lis* from the Canadian Orthopaedic Association's original "seal" which had been designed by the late Dr. Alexander Gibson, a distinguished anatomist and orthopaedic surgeon. The maple leaf represents the Association's English-speaking members while the *fleur-de-lis* represents the French-speaking members and the common stock symbolizes the concept of national unity.

Since one of the goals of the Canadian Orthopaedic Association is *education*, the two open books in the upper part of the shield have been chosen as heraldic symbols of teaching.

In the lower part of the shield the femur represents the skeletal tissues with which orthopaedic surgeons work and hence symbolizes orthopaedic *patient care*.

The key is an ancient symbol of a closed mystery and a way by which to unlock it. Thus, the key has been chosen to represent *research* which the Association fosters. Because orthopaedic research involves skeletal tissues, a "skeleton key" has been depicted.

The Latin motto, "*Pietate, Arte et Scientia Corrigere*" is a statement of orthopaedic philosophy.

Pietate means "with compassion," which is so important in the art of patient care.

Arte is "skill," and refers to the combination of surgical dexterity and precision required in orthopaedic surgery.

Scientia is "knowledge," specifically scientific knowledge, which forms the basis for orthopaedic judgment.

Corrigere is a verb meaning to "correct, straighten, or set things right." For the sake of brevity, what we correct, namely musculoskeletal disorders and injuries, is unstated but implied.

Thus, the complete motto means: "With compassion, skill and knowledge we correct, straighten or set right [musculoskeletal disorders and injuries]."

Textbook of
Disorders and Injuries of

1353 ILLUSTRATIONS ON 805 FIGURES
577 REFERENCES

Of Books and Patients

"To study the phenomenon of disease without books is to sail an uncharted sea, while to study books without patients is not to go to sea at all."

—Sir William Osler

An Introduction to Orthopaedics, Fractures and Joint Injuries, Rheumatology, Metabolic Bone Disease and Rehabilitation

the Musculoskeletal System

Second Edition

Robert Bruce Salter

O.C., M.D., M.S. (Tor), F.R.S.C., F.R.C.S.(C), F.A.C.S.
Hon. Dr. Med. (Uppsala), Hon. D.Sc. (Memorial),
Hon. LL.D. (Dalhousie), Hon. F.R.C.P.S. Glasg.,
Hon. F.R.C.S. Edin., Hon. F.C.S.S.A., Hon. F.R.C.S. Eng.,
Hon. F.R.A.C.S., Hon. F.R.C.S. Ire., Hon. M.C.F.P.C.

University Professor of the University of Toronto

Professor and Chairman of Orthopaedic Surgery, University of Toronto

Faculty, Institute of Medical Science and School of Graduate Studies

Senior Orthopaedic Surgeon, The Hospital for Sick Children, Toronto

Research Project Director, Research Institute, The Hospital for Sick Children

Orthopaedic Surgeon, Orthopaedic and Arthritic Hospital, Toronto

Orthopaedic Consultant, The Easter Seal Society of Ontario

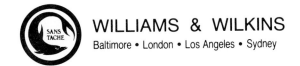

WILLIAMS & WILKINS
Baltimore • London • Los Angeles • Sydney

First Edition, 1970
Reprinted, 1971, 1972, 1974, 1975, 1977, 1978, 1979, 1980, 1981, 1982
Second Edition, 1983
Reprinted 1984

Library of Congress Cataloging in Publication Data

Salter, Robert Bruce.
    Textbook of disorders and injuries of the musculoskeletal system.

    Includes index.
    1. Musculoskeletal system—Diseases. 2. Musculoskeletal system—Wound and
injuries. I. Title. [DNLM: 1. Bone diseases. 2. Joint diseases. 3. Muscular diseases.
4. Orthopedics. 5. Rehabilitation. WE 140 S177t]
RC925.S2 1983   616.7   82-21728
ISBN 0-683-07500-4

Composed and printed at the
WAVERLY PRESS, INC.
Mt. Royal and Guilford Aves.
Baltimore, Md. 21202, U.S.A.

		86	87	88	89	
10	9	8	7	6	5	4

Foreword to the Second Edition

by PAUL H. CURTISS, Jr, M.D.

The appearance of the first edition of Dr. Salter's *Textbook of Disorders and Injuries of the Musculoskeletal System* in 1970 was a benchmark in the teaching of the principles of orthopaedics. Written by a master educator and directed to the inquiring minds of medical students and orthopaedic residents, it's scope and authority immediately made it the premier textbook in this area. Also unique was the fact that pertinent knowledge in the basic sciences as well as of the clinical problems of the musculoskeletal system were presented together. Its organization by "body systems" is as logical an approach to undergraduate teaching now as it was then. This still remains the best means of teaching the histology, pathology, physiology and principles of diagnosis and treatment of the musculoskeletal system. Of equal importance, however, is the clear sense of underlying concern for the patient which permeates all of the text. A feeling for the art of medicine as well as its science is clearly evident in Dr. Salter's approach. This is completely consistent with his standing as one of the leading pediatric orthopaedic surgeons in the world today.

In the thirteen years since publication of the first edition, however there have been many scientific and technical advances relevant to the basic knowledge, diagnosis, and treatment of orthopaedic problems. This second edition, therefore contains much new material as well as updating of the information retained from the first edition. Space does not permit a complete listing of all of the new and relevant information which have been included in this second edition, but particular mention should be made of Dr. Salter's studies on the healing and regeneration of articular cartilage through continuous passive motion, the new concepts of chemonucleolysis in spinal disc problems, the great advances which have taken place in the care of malignant tumors of the musculoskeletal system and the potential of restoring growth following epiphyseal plate injuries. Most fascinating however is the completely new chapter entitled "The Philosophy and Nature of Medical Research." This unique and inspiring chapter was written by Dr. Salter to stimulate both undergraduate and graduate students to participate in the exciting and unlimited field of research. This has long been a primary interest of Dr. Salter's, and considering his important research contributions, there is no one who can speak more inspiringly and eloquently on this subject. The respect in which Dr. Salter is held throughout the world as a leading orthopaedic educator has again been reconfirmed by this second edition. It is the fortunate student indeed who has the opportunity to learn from him.

Paul H. Curtiss, Jr., M.D.
Editor
The Journal of Bone and Joint Surgery

Foreword to the First Edition of Salter's Textbook of Disorders and Injuries of the Musculoskeletal System (1970)*

Medical education, with its traditional three-fold commitment to patient care, research, and continuing education, presents a difficult challenge. The complexity of medical education requires a new set of values to be placed upon the selection of subjects which are considered essential for all physicians. The term "core curriculum" has been used widely, but seldom has it been defined. It would now appear that the problems in definition and implementation have come from an awkwardness in selecting and integrating the essential information into an appropriate and effective method of study of the various body systems, their physiology and pathology, and the overall impact of their disorders upon the patient as a unit in society. A doctrinaire or discipline-oriented experience for the student falls short of the objective if emphasis is upon the discipline rather than the subject material. It is with the prospect of solving these problems that Dr. Salter's new textbook on the musculoskeletal system has been written.

Medical students, for whom this book is created, have come to their schools superbly endowed with intellect, a proven capability of assimilating large amounts of information, and a willingness to serve mankind. Today's student expects his institution and its teachers to provide a basis for study and experience, and he understands that he must continue to study to keep up with new developments. While there are no simple answers to the problems of medical education, there is no question that an excellent medical textbook remains one of the essentials required by the student.

A good medical textbook provides not only information but also a philosophy or approach which makes the knowledge relevant. Ask the student and he will tell you that he is not interested in brief handbooks which summarize the favorite prejudices of a traditional discipline. He shuns the textbook which fails to provide a link between the body of scientific information and the bedside of the patient. The task of producing a new and forceful text for medical students in these times is formidable indeed. The author must have experience, ability, empathy, and dedication to the mission of teaching. He should be scientifically accurate and capable of projecting his personalized approach.

An exciting example of the new approach in medical textbook writing is Dr. Robert Salter's *Disorders and Injuries of the Musculoskeletal System*. In a superbly organized manner a vast amount of information is presented on the basic nature of the musculoskeletal system as well as on its disorders and injuries from infancy through old age. The biologic and physiologic relationships are fully developed and presented in a pattern which makes for coherence; the illustrations are both abundant and clear. The interesting and graphic manner of presentation, a native gift possessed by the author, comes through in clear style. Throughout, there shines through the scientific and clinical details a wholesome reassertion of the human element in medicine, an essence which ranks in importance with the most elegant molecular concept.

This book may mark a turning point in textbook writing for clinical subjects, and we

* This Foreword, which was written by the late Dr. J. William Hillman shortly before his untimely death, is retained in the textbook out of profound respect for this outstanding academic orthopaedic surgeon.

would hope that other areas of medical education may follow with the production of books which will be equally effective in meeting the needs of medical students today. Although the text is addressed to medical students specifically, there is little question that it will be studied extensively by residents and their teachers. It may also prove to be of great value in the education of paramedical personnel who will be involved in the care of patients with disabilities of the musculoskeletal system.

Dr. Salter is respected throughout the world as one of the leaders in medical education and as a major contributor to orthopaedic surgery. He has been recognized internationally for his fundamental scientific investigations of musculoskeletal disorders and injuries in his laboratories, and he has advanced the orthopaedic care of children through the development of new and imaginative methods of treatment. He is an exemplary physician, and his patients as well as his students have come from all continents. His ability to inspire students whatever their age or setting, has become legendary. It was natural that many of his colleagues urged him to undertake the production of this book. The writing of the text, which is his work alone, has been carried on with the same attention to detail that has distinguished all his scientific efforts.

I join Dr. Salter's host of admiring colleagues in expressing appreciation for a service to patients through tomorrow's physicians—a task in which he has no peer.

J. William Hillman, M.D.
Professor of Orthopaedic Surgery
Vanderbilt University
Nashville, Tennessee.

Dedication

To You—
a medical student of today,
a medical doctor of tomorrow,
this textbook is cheerfully and respectfully dedicated.

An Open Letter to a Medical Student

Dear student:

I have written this textbook expressly for a select group, namely *you and your fellow medical students.* A textbook that attempts to meet the combined and varied needs of medical students, internes, residents, family physicians and specialists may fail to meet the specific needs of any group and in particular, the specific needs of the medical student. By writing this book solely for *you*, I have endeavoured to fulfill *your* specific needs as a medical student in relation to the exciting and fascinating subject of clinical disorders and injuries of the musculoskeletal system.

Your specific needs in relation to the musculoskeletal system are to acquire the following: First, knowledge of the normal structure and function of musculoskeletal tissues as well as their cellular reactions to disorders and injuries in order that you may *understand* the natural course and clinical manifestations of the more common conditions; second, skill in eliciting, interpreting and co-relating clinical information including the pertinent physical signs, radiographic features and laboratory data in order that you may recognize or *diagnose* accurately the various clinical conditions when you encounter them in your patients; third, judgement concerning the clinical application of the general principles and specific methods of musculoskeletal *treatment* to the care of patients.

An explanation of the title of this book may help to clarify its purpose and its scope. It is generally understood among teachers and publishers that a "textbook" or "text" is a book written for undergraduate students. A "textbook" as defined by Webster is "a book containing the principles of a subject, used as a basis for instruction." A textbook is, therefore, quite different from a reference book which must be encyclopaedic in nature; it is different from a monograph which must include virtually all available knowledge in a very limited field; it is different from an atlas of operative technique; it is even different from a synopsis, an outline, a manual, or a handbook. Thus, a textbook, as suggested by its definition, should serve as the broad base and framework upon which you may build the additional knowledge that you will gain from your own clinical teachers as well as from the patients whom you will be privileged to see in the outpatient clinics and on the wards of your own teaching hospitals.

The *purpose* of this Second Edition, like that of its predecessor, is to introduce you to the basic sciences pertaining to the musculoskeletal tissues as well as to the clinical practice, i.e., diagnosis and treatment of the wide variety of disorders and injuries from which these tissues may suffer. Accordingly, its *scope* includes the "surgical" subjects of orthopaedics and fractures as well as the "medical" subjects of rheumatology, metabolic bone disease and rehabilitation. Woven throughout the fabric of this book you will find the thread of emphasis on kindness and compassion which are the hallmarks of total care for the total patient as an individual person.

In this Second Edition I have included a final chapter entitled "The Nature and Philosophy of Medical Research" in the fervent hope of stimulating, and perhaps even inspiring *you* to consider the possibility of your own personal involvement, either part-time or full-time, in this essential and rewarding component of our profession's responsibilities.

While the teacher of medical students carries the responsibility for *teaching*, the responsibility for *learning* rests with *you*—the student. I urge you therefore, to learn from this textbook, from your own clinical teachers and from the observation of patients so that you may be better prepared to serve the needs of patients who will seek your advice in the years to come. As Amiel has written. "The highest function of the teacher is not so much in imparting knowledge as in stimulating the pupil in its love and pursuit."

I wish you well in your pursuit of knowledge not only as a medical student of today but also as a medical doctor of tomorrow, and equally importantly, as a continuing student throughout your entire professional life!

Yours sincerely,

Robert B. Salter

Acknowledgments

The philosophy of teaching embraces the tradition of sharing knowledge—through teaching of present and future generations of students in a given discipline—in return for what has been shared with the teacher by his or her own teachers. Accordingly, I am indebted to those persons, both living and dead, from whom I have learned and especially to those who have stimulated and encouraged me, in turn, to teach others.

The teacher who undertakes to write a textbook covering such a broad field as disorders and injuries of the musculoskeletal system must, of necessity, add to his own personal knowledge from that of colleagues in the same discipline as well as in related disciplines. Then the teacher sifts and synthesizes this accumulated knowlege and offers it to students as food for their minds in a manner that is palatable, digestible, satisfying and nourishing.

I am particularly grateful to Dr. Paul H. Curtiss, Jr., the Editor and Chairman of the Board of Editors of the American Volume of The Journal of Bone and Joint Surgery, for his typically gracious and elegant Foreword to this Second Edition. My gratitude to the late Dr. J. William Hillman continues "in perpetuity" for his contribution of the Foreword for the First Edition—a Foreword that has been retained in the Second Edition.

I have appreciated the comments and suggestions concerning the First Edition offered by both students and teachers from numerous countries and have endeavoured to respond to them in the preparation of the Second Edition. Since orthopaedic surgery is a rapidly developing specialty, updating of a textbook such as this necessitates an extensive review of the relevant literature that has been published during the intervening years. In addition to the various journals of orthopaedic surgery and related fields, one particular source of new knowledge merits special mention, namely the annual Year Books of Orthopaedic Surgery (from 1970 to 1982) thoughtfully edited prior to 1976 by the late Dr. H. Herman Young and subsequently by Dr. Mark B. Coventry, both of the Mayo Clinic. I am indebted to both of them for their most helpful reviews of the orthopaedic literature.

In the University of Toronto, many friends and colleagues have read specific sections of the manuscript and have offered constructive criticisms. Accordingly, I wish to record their names with grateful thanks.

Those whose discipline is other than orthopaedic surgery include the following: Dr. Dianne Wilson Cox (genetics), Dr. Donald Fraser (metabolic bone disease), Dr. David L. Gilday (nuclear medicine), Dr. Duncan A. Gordon (rheumatology), Dr. Derek Harwood-Nash (radiology), Dr. Harold J. Hoffman (neurosurgery), Dr. Robin P. Humphreys (neurosurgery), Dr. Sang Whay Kooh (metabolic bone disease), Dr. Charles G. Prober (infectious diseases), Dr. Abraham Shore (rheumatology), Dr. William C. Sturtridge (metabolic bone disease), Dr. Alvin Zipursky (hematology) and Dr. Ronald M. Zuker (plastic surgery).

University of Toronto orthopaedic colleagues who have so helped include Drs. Walter P. Bobechko, Norris C. Carroll, Robert Gillespie, Allan Gross, J. Hamilton Hall, David E. Hastings, Robert W. Jackson, John C. McCulloch, Colin F. Moseley, Mercer Rang and Joseph Schatzker.

Many of the clinical photographs from the First Edition have been retained in the Second Edition because Dr. Judith Wunderly Walker (who at that time was a medical illustrator) has painstakingly prepared these illustrations in such a way as to provide uncluttered uniformity in the background of the final prints. In addition, she had done most of the line drawings. Consequently, I continue to appreciate her industry and ingenuity.

The work of providing prints of the illustrations for the Second Edition has been cheerfully accomplished by the following members of the Department of Visual Education of The Hospital for Sick Children under the direction of Mr. Alex Wright; Mr. William Bryson, Mr. Louis Scaglione and Mrs. Eva Struthers. To them I express my sincere thanks.

For the typing and retyping and re-retyping of the manuscript I am indebted to Mrs. Carol Robinson, whose skill as a typist is exceeded only by her dedication to this textbook.

To the staff of Williams & Wilkins in general and to Barbara Tansill, Senior Editor, in particular, I am most grateful for bringing my manuscript to publication.

As a science writer and a novelist, my wife, Robbie, has carefully read each portion of the manuscript as it has been written and has made many valuable editorial suggestions; in addition, Robbie has assisted with the time-consuming and exacting task of reading page proofs, as well as with the preparation of the index. More importantly, however, in her role as my wife and as the mother of our five children, Robbie has been a constant source of inspiration. For her unselfish understanding and for her abiding love I am, and always will be, most thankful.

Robert B. Salter

About the Author

Robert B. Salter, a sixth generation Canadian, is a graduate in Medicine of the University of Toronto. After serving for two years with the Grenfell Medical Mission in Northern Newfoundland and Labrador, he took his postgraduate orthopaedic training in Toronto and an additional year on a McLaughlin Fellowship in London, England with the late Sir Reginald Watson-Jones and Sir Henry Osmond-Clarke.

On his return to Canada in 1955, Dr. Salter was appointed to the Staff of The Hospital for Sick Children, Toronto and two years later he was appointed Chief of Orthopaedic Surgery. After nine years in this position he became Surgeon-in-Chief of the Hospital and a Professor of Surgery. Following the completion of his ten-year term in this role he was appointed to his present position of Professor and Head of Orthopaedic Surgery in the University of Toronto.

A world renowned orthopaedic surgeon, teacher and researcher, Dr. Salter has developed a number of innovative methods of orthopaedic treatment including the innominate osteotomy (the "Salter operation") for children and young adults with certain abnormalities of the hip joint. The Salter-Harris classification of epiphyseal plate injuries, which he created with Dr. W. R. Harris, is widely accepted.

As an orthopaedic teacher, he has written over 100 articles in the scientific literature as well as two editions of the *Textbook of Disorders and Injuries of the Musculoskeletal System* and chapters in numerous other books. He has taught as a Visiting Professor at 120 universities. As an orthopaedic statesman, he has served as President of the Canadian Orthopaedic Association and also as President of the Royal College of Physicians and Surgeons of Canada.

In his capacity as an orthopaedic scientist, Dr. Salter has conducted imaginative and original basic research on numerous problems including avascular necrosis of the femoral head, the harmful effects of immobilization of joints—with, and without, compression—and currently, the beneficial effects of his exciting new concept of "continuous passive motion" on the healing and regeneration of articular cartilage and peri-articular tissues.

For his contributions to orthopaedic surgery Dr. Salter has received many honours including the Gairdner International Award for Medical Science, the Nicolas Andry Award, and the Lawrence Chute Award for Undergraduate Teaching. He has been appointed a Fellow of the Royal Society of Canada, an Officer of the Order of Canada (O.C.) and also a University Professor of the University of Toronto, the university's highest honour to a member of its faculty, "for excellence in research and teaching."

Contents

PART 1 Basic Musculoskeletal Science and Its Application

PART 2 Musculoskeletal Disorders—General and Specific

PART 3 Musculoskeletal Injuries—General

PART 4 Musculoskeletal Injuries—Specific

PART 5 Research

Part 1

Basic Musculoskeletal Science and Its Application

"We see so far because we stand on the shoulders of giants."
—SIR ISAAC NEWTON

CHAPTER 1

Introduction: The Past and the Present

BRIEF HISTORICAL BACKGROUND

As a medical student in the second half of the twentieth century, you live in a tremendously exciting era. As you pursue your studies of the basic sciences and of modern clinical medicine and surgery, you will come to realize how much of what you are currently learning has been developed since *you* were born. This is simply an indication of the recently accelerated acquisition of scientific knowledge. However, as Cicero has said: "Not to know what happened before one was born is to remain a child." The history of medicine and surgery deserves your attention, not only because it is fascinating and inspiring, but also because it places your present knowledge in perspective and may even stimulate original thought concerning possible developments of the future. Following graduation, if you should choose to study one particular field of medicine or surgery in depth, you should delve into the history of that particular field in order that you may avoid repeating the errors of the past.

The bones of prehistoric men provide mute testimony of disorders and injuries of the musculoskeletal system, and from the beginning, man has sought ways to alleviate the crippling conditions of his fellow man. As early as 9000 B.C., in the paleolithic age, superstitions were being replaced by ra-

tional thinking and man was beginning to use splints for weak limbs and broken bones. In the neolithic age, around 5000 B.C., man had already begun to perform crude amputations of diseased or damaged limbs. The Egyptians had developed the concept of the crutch by 2000 B.C. Greece replaced Egypt as the center of culture by the fifth century B.C. and Hippocrates, through his teaching and through his students, had become the "father of medicine." In the second century A.D. Galen, a Greek physician who moved to Rome, became the founder of experimental investigation.

The first eighteen centuries A.D. saw the slow but progressive advance of knowledge in medicine and surgery, culminating in the significant contributions of England's John Hunter (1828–93), who has been revered ever since as the "father of surgical research." Understandably, however, the development and performance of major surgical operations had to await the nineteenth-century revolutionary discoveries of general anesthesia by Long and Morton (USA), of the bacterial basis of disease by Pasteur (France), of antisepsis by Lister (Scotland) and of X-rays by Roentgen (Germany).

Progress in the science of medicine and surgery in the twentieth century, and more particularly in its second half, has been staggering in its rapidity. Happily, there is no end in sight for such escalating progression. Indeed this is but one of the factors that make the study and practice of medicine in general and of orthopaedic surgery in particular so tremendously exciting and challenging.

In the current century the care of patients with disorders and injuries of the musculoskeletal system has evolved through three phases. First was the "strap and buckle" phase in which various orthopaedic splints, braces and other types of appliance constituted the predominant form of management. Next came the phase of excessive orthopaedic operations, many of which were based more upon clinical empiricism than upon scientific investigation. In the third and current phase, science is rapidly replacing empiricism, as evidenced by the combination of increased *experimental research* aimed at understanding the physiology and pathology of the musculoskeletal system more completely, and *clinical investigation*, both retrospective and prospective, to study the natural course of disorders as well as to evaluate critically the results of various forms of treatment.

In this scientific phase the study of clinical problems of the musculoskeletal system has become increasingly stimulating and challenging. The care of patients remains as *art*—but the art must be based on *science*.

You will gain much knowledge from those who have gone before you, both recently and in the distant past, but you may be assured that there is very much more that remains to be discovered and to be understood.

THE SCOPE OF ORTHOPAEDICS

While the history of disorders and injuries of the musculoskeletal system dates back to antiquity, the specialty of orthopaedics, as a branch of medicine and surgery, is relatively young. In 1741, Nicolas Andry, then Professor of Medicine in Paris, published a book, the English translation of which is *Orthopaedia, or the Art of Preventing and Correcting Deformities in Children*. He coined the term "orthopaedia" from the words "orthos" (straight, or free from de-

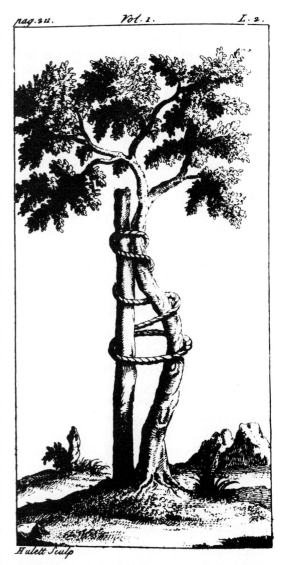

Figure 1.1. This "orthopaedic tree" from Nicolas Andry's eighteenth-century book has become the international symbol of orthopaedic surgery. It illustrates the concept that a crooked young tree—like a deformed young child—can be helped to grow straight by the application of appropriate forces.

formity) and "pais" (child), and expressed the view that most deformities in adults have their origin in childhood (Fig. 1.1). While the term "orthopaedics" is not entirely satisfactory, it has persisted for over two centuries and is unlikely to be replaced in your academic lifetime.

The present scope of orthopaedics has

come to include all ages and is considered to consist of the art and science of the prevention, investigation, diagnosis and treatment of disorders and injuries of the musculoskeletal system by medical, surgical and physical means and, in addition, the study of musculoskeletal physiology, pathology and other related basic sciences.

Thus, the modern and sophisticated orthopaedic surgeon serves as both physician and surgeon (as implied by the American synonym "orthopaedist"). To provide exemplary total care for patients with certain musculoskeletal disorders or injuries the orthopaedic specialist must work in close collaboration with medical specialists including rheumatologists, metabolic bone physicians and rehabilitation physicians (physiatrists) or other surgical specialists, particularly plastic surgeons and neurosurgeons.

Musculoskeletal disorders and injuries as a group are remarkably common. Indeed, it has been ascertained from numerous surveys in North America that of the total number of patients seen by a primary care or family physician, at least 15% suffer from either a disorder or injury of the musculoskeletal system either with or without some coexistent condition.

CURRENT TRENDS IN CLINICAL CONDITIONS OF THE MUSCULOSKELETAL SYSTEM

Our environment is the scene of continual change and from decade to decade we see many changes in the nature and the frequency of the musculoskeletal disorders and injuries that confront us. While certain musculoskeletal conditions, such as congenital deformities and bone neoplasms, have remained with us always, others have gradually become less common; in their place have arisen new problems which must receive increasing attention. Thus if you had been a medical student in the early decades of the present century, you would have been taught much about bone and joint tuberculosis, vitamin deficiencies of bone and paralytic poliomyelitis. Today, these conditions have been largely brought under control by

prevention and therefore they merit less emphasis in your teaching. Other conditions, such as acute bone and joint infections, have been partially controlled, but only by the application of intensive modern treatment at the very onset of the disease. Thus, the current emphasis in teaching of these conditions must be on early recognition, or diagnosis, of the clinical picture, and on early treatment.

Severe cerebral palsy and extensive spina bifida with their associated paralytic problems are even more common than before because some infants with these conditions, who previously died in early life, now survive and grow up with their problems. The age span of man has become progressively longer and, as a result, the various degenerative conditions, such as degenerative arthritis, are assuming greater clinical importance. Likewise, senile weakening of bone, osteoporosis, with its complication of fractures in the elderly, has become an increasingly important problem. Certain conditions, such as rheumatoid arthritis, which in previous decades were treated by medical means alone, have become partially amenable to surgical treatment. The increase in the number of automobiles combined with their increasing speed has been responsible in part for the great increase in the number and severity of musculoskeletal injuries—fractures and associated trauma—and in particular the increasing number of patients who sustain multiple serious injuries involving several major systems of the body.

RECENT ADVANCES

During the past two decades the dynamism of orthopaedics has been demonstrated by many important developments that have had a significant impact on the prevention, diagnosis and treatment of musculoskeletal disorders and injuries. *Preventive* orthopaedics has become a reality through more precise counseling as well as through intrauterine detection of certain disorders by means of amniocentesis. Earlier *diagnosis* of potentially serious orthopaedic disorders such as congenital dislocation of the hip through the routine examination of all newborn infants and also of scoliosis (curvature of the spine) through school screening programs have proven to be effective. Non-invasive diagnostic "imaging" of musculoskeletal disorders and injuries has been remarkably enhanced by radioactive isotope bone scans, ultrasound scans and especially by computed tomographic (CT) scans. Endoscopic examination of the interior of large joints such as the knee is now possible with an arthroscope and even certain intra-articular operations can be performed thereby (arthroscopic surgery.)

Recent advances in orthopaedic *treatment* include: total prosthetic joint replacements and osteochondral allograft for irreversible arthritis; more effective mechanical and electrical spinal instrumentation for scoliosis; back education units; chemonucleolysis for intervertebral disc protrusion; hyperbaric oxygenation for impaired peripheral circulation; detection and monitoring of increased pressure in various "compartment syndromes"; more effective methods of non-operative treatment of fractures (cast bracing), for operative treatment (AO system of rigid internal fixation), for stimulation of delayed fracture healing or even non-union (electricity) and for stimulation of the repair and regeneration of articular cartilage (continuous passive motion—CPM); systemic chemotherapy for malignant diseases; steroid injection for simple bone cysts; resection of a bony bridge across an epiphyseal plate; more appropriate materials for splints and braces (orthoses) and for artificial limbs (prostheses).

The development of surgery performed under the magnificent magnification of the operating microscope (microsurgery) has made possible the replantation of completely severed digits and limbs, the transfer of free vascularized bone grafts and even vascularized and re-innervated autogenous muscle grafts.

These recent advances which have greatly enhanced the prevention, diagnosis and treatment of musculoskeletal disorders and injuries are discussed in appropriate chapters in this textbook.

Suggested Additional Reading

Andry, N.: *Orthopaedia: or the art of Correcting and Preventing Deformities in Children* (facsimile reproduction of first edition in English, London, 1743). Philadelphia, J. B. Lippincott, 1961, vols. 1 and 2.

Bick, E. M.: *Source Book of Orthopaedics*, 2nd ed. Baltimore, Williams & Wilkins, 1948. (Facsimile reprint of 1948 edition by Hafner Publishing Co., Inc., New York, 1968).

Bick, E. M.: *Classics of Orthopaedics*. Philadelphia, J. B. Lippincott, 1976.

Howorth, M. B.: *A Textbook of Orthopaedics*. Philadelphia, W. B. Saunders, 1952.

Keith, A.: *Menders of the Maimed*. London, Froude (1919 limited edition); Philadelphia, J. B. Lippincott, 1951.

Lister, J.: On the antiseptic principles in the practice of surgery. Lancet 2: 253, 1867.

Mayer, L.: Orthopaedic surgery in the United States of America. J. Bone Joint Surg. 32B: 461, 1950.

Osmond-Clarke, H.: Half a century of orthopaedic progress in orthopaedic surgery. J. Bone Joint Surg. 32B: 620, 1950.

Platt, H.: The evolution and scope of orthopaedics. In *Modern Trends in Orthopaedics*. London, Butterworth, 1950, vol. 1.

Raney, R. B.: Andry and the orthopaedics. J. Bone Joint Surg. 31A: 675–682, 1949.

Rang, M.: *Anthology of Orthopaedics*. Edinburgh and London, E. & S. Livingstone, 1966 (Williams & Wilkins, U.S. Agents).

Roentgen, W. K.: On a new kind of ray. Nature 53: 274, 377, 1896.

"Anatomy is to physiology as geography is to history; it describes the theatre of events."
—JEAN FERNE (1497–1558)
On the Natural Part of Medicine (Ch. I)

CHAPTER 2

Normal Structure and Function of Musculoskeletal Tissues

Having completed the preclinical phase of your undergraduate course in medicine, you will have learned much about the embryology, anatomy, histology, biochemistry and physiology of the musculoskeletal tissues in man. This is extremely important, because in order to understand the abnormal, you must have an understanding of the normal; indeed, your knowledge of the normal will serve as a broad base upon which you can build a knowledge of the abnormal. Some of the more important aspects of this broad base will now be reviewed to refresh your memory and to prepare you for subsequent study of the abnormal clinical conditions of the musculoskeletal system (also known as the locomotor system).

BONES AS STRUCTURES AND BONE AS AN ORGAN

You should consider the tissue bone from two entirely different points of view: individual bones as *anatomical structures* and bone of the entire skeleton collectively as a *physiological organ*.

Since the non-living intercellular matrix of bone is calcified, or stonelike, it is one of the hard tissues. Indeed, its very hardness provides strength to individual bones as *structures* that enables them to serve three functions: (1) to provide the rigid framework for the trunk and extremities; (2) to serve as levers for the locomotor function of skeletal muscles; (3) to afford protection for vulnerable viscera, e.g. skull for the brain, spine for the spinal cord and thoracic cage for the heart and lungs. Bone of the entire skeleton as an *organ* serves two additional functions: (4) it contains hemopoietic tissue of the myeloid type for the production of erythrocytes, granular leucocytes and platelets; and (5) it is the organ of storage or reservoir for calcium, phosphorus, magnesium and sodium that helps to maintain the "milieu intérieur" by storing or releasing them as the need arises.

Embryonic Development of Bones

In the initial stages of development, the tube-shaped embryo contains three primary germ layers of cells: the *ectoderm* or covering layer, the *endoderm* or lining layer and the *mesoderm* or middle layer. From the mesoderm is derived the *mesenchyme*, a diffuse cellular tissue which is pluripotential in the sense that its undifferentiated cells are capable of differentiating into any one of several types of connective tissue such as bone, cartilage, ligaments, muscle, tendon and fascia. Bone and cartilage, being able to support weight though their non-living intercellular substances, may be thought of as *supporting connective tissues.*

During the 5th week of embryonic development, the ectodermal covered limb buds appear and in the central axis of each limb bud the mesenchymal cells become condensed in the form of a short cylinder. This cylinder is segmented by less densely cellular areas at the sites of future joints and each segment represents a tiny *mesenchymal model* of the future long bone that will develop from it (Fig. 2.1). By the 6th week, the undifferentiated mesenchymal cells of each model begin to differentiate by manufacturing cartilage matrix thereby forming a *cartilaginous model* of the future bone. The cartilaginous model grows partly from within (*interstitial growth*) and partly by the apposition of new cells on its surface (*appositional growth*) from the deeper layers of the *perichondrium* (Fig. 2.1).

After the 7th week the cartilage cells in the center of the model hypertrophy and form longitudinal rows, following which the intercellular substance, or matrix, calcifies with resultant death of the cells. Vascular connective tissue then grows into the central area of dead cartilage bringing *osteoblasts* which secrete collagen and proteoglycans in the matrix; the matrix is then impregnated with calcium salts and becomes immature

bone on the calcified cartilage matrix thereby forming the *primary center of ossification.* This process of replacement of cartilage by bone is called *endochondral ossification* and it occurs only in the presence of capillaries. The endochondral ossification advances toward each end of the cartilage model which, in turn, is continuing to grow in length at its carilaginous ends by interstitial growth. The perichondrium by this time has become periosteum and in its deeper layer, the mesenchymal cells, which have differentiated into osteoblasts, lay down bone directly by the process of *intramembranous ossification*, there being no intermediate cartilaginous phase (Fig. 2.1).

By the 6th month resorption of the central part of the long bone results in the formation of a medullary cavity—the process of *tubulation.* At the time of birth the largest epiphysis in the body (distal femoral epiphysis) has developed a *secondary center of ossification* by the process of endochondral ossification within it (Fig. 2.2). Secondary centers of ossification appear in the other cartilaginous epiphyses at varying ages after birth. Each such center, or ossific nucleus, is separated from the metaphysis by a special plate of growing cartilage—the *epiphyseal plate*—which provides growth in length of the bone by interstitial growth of cartilage cells.

The short bones (such as the carpal bones) are developed by endochondral ossification in the same manner as the epiphyses. By contrast, the clavicle and most of the skull develop bone directly in the mesenchymal model by the process of intra-

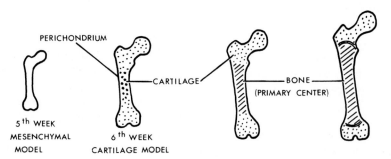

Figure 2.1.   Embryonic development of a long bone during the first six months.

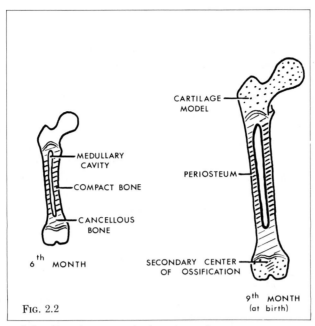

CARTILAGE
MODEL

MEDULLARY
CAVITY

PERIOSTEUM

COMPACT BONE

CANCELLOUS
BONE

6th MONTH

SECONDARY CENTER
OF OSSIFICATION

9th MONTH
(at birth)

FIG. 2.2

Figure 2.2. Development of a long bone from six to nine months.

membraneous ossification from the periosteum without going through a cartilaginous phase.

During the early weeks of intrauterine life, the developing embryo is particularly susceptible to noxious environmental factors that arrive via the placental circulation. For example, if the mother develops a Rubella infection or takes a harmful drug such as thalidomide during this critical period, the embryonic development is likely to be seriously affected. The extent of the resultant abnormality will depend on the *exact* phase of embryonic development at the time; in general, the earlier the stage of development, the more extensive will be the resultant abnormality. When you consider the remarkable speed and complexity of the embryonic development of the human, it is hardly surprising that some children are born with an obvious congenital abnormality; indeed, what is surprising is that the vast majority of children are completely normal at birth.

Bone Growth and Remodeling

Bones grow in *length* by one process (involving endochondral ossification) while they grow in *width* by another process (involving intramembranous ossification).

GROWTH IN LENGTH

Since interstitial growth within *bone* is not possible, a bone can grow in length only by the process of interstitial growth within *cartilage* followed by endochondral ossification. Thus, there are two possible sites for cartilaginous growth in a long bone—articular cartilage and epiphyseal plate cartilage (Fig. 2.3).

Articular Cartilage

In a long bone the articular cartilage is the only growth plate for growth of its *epiphysis.* In a short bone the articular cartilage provides the only growth plate for the whole bone.

Epiphyseal Plate Cartilage

The epiphyseal plate provides growth in length of the *metaphysis* and *diaphysis* of a long bone. In this site of growth a constant balance is maintained between two separate processes; (1) interstitial growth of the cartilage cells of the plate which are making it thicker, thereby moving the epiphysis farther away from the metaphysis and (2) calcification, death and replacement of cartilage on the metaphyseal surface by bone through the process of endochondral ossification.

Four zones of the epiphyseal plate can be distinguished (Fig. 2.4): (1) *The zone of resting cartilage* anchors the epiphyseal plate to the epiphysis and contains immature chon-

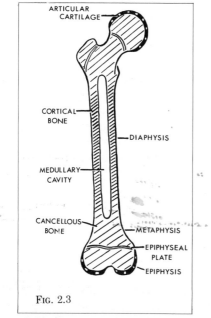

FIG. 2.3

Figure 2.3.   Bone growth during childhood.

drocytes, as well as delicate vessels which penetrate it from the epiphysis and which bring nourishment to the entire plate.

(2) *The zone of young proliferating cartilage* is the site of most active interstitial growth of the cartilage cells which are arranged in vertical columns.

(3) *The zone of maturing cartilage* reveals a progressive enlargement and maturation of the cartilage cells as they approach the metaphysis. These chondrocytes accumulate glycogen in their cytoplasm and produce phosphatase which may be involved in the calcification of their surrounding matrix.

(4) *The zone of calcifying cartilage* is thin and its chondrocytes have died as a result of calcification of the matrix. This is structurally the weakest zone of the epiphyseal plate. Bone deposition is very active on the metaphyseal side of this zone and as new bone is added to the calcified cores of cartilage matrix, the metaphysis becomes correspondingly longer.

The Hormonal Control of Longitudinal Bone Growth

Throughout the world, and especially in developing countries, malnutrition remains the most common cause of retardation of

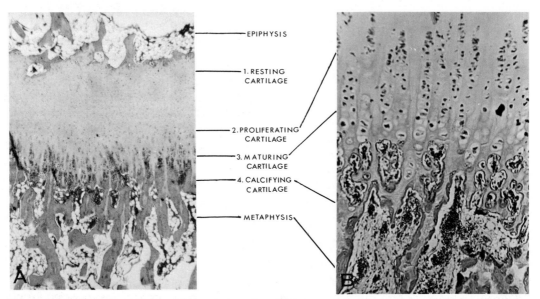

Figure 2.4.   Histology of an epiphyseal plate (from the upper end of tibia of a child). *A*, low power; *B*, high power.

longitudinal bone growth. Nevertheless, such malnutrition is also accompanied by disturbances of endocrine function.

Human growth hormone, which is synthesized in the anterior pituitary gland, exerts its growth-promoting effect through the production of somatomedin in the liver. Thyroxine is also essential for normal longitudinal growth. Sex hormones are involved in the characteristic post-pubertal "growth spurt" in adolescent boys and girls. Glucocorticoids (cortisones) have an inhibitory effect on growth as seen in Cushing's syndrome, whether naturally occurring or secondary to prolonged therapeutic administration of cortisone to children.

GROWTH IN WIDTH

Bones grow in width by means of appositional growth from the osteoblasts in the deep, or inner (cambium) layer of the *periosteum*, the process being one of intramembranous ossification. Simultaneously, the medullary cavity becomes larger by osteoclastic resorption of bone on the inner surface of the cortex which is lined by endosteum.

REMODELING OF BONE

During longitudinal growth of bone, the flared metaphyseal regions of bone must be continually remodeled as the epiphysis moves progressively farther away from the shaft. This is accomplished by simultaneous osteoblastic deposition of bone on one surface and osteoclastic resorption on the opposite surface.

However, remodeling of bone continues throughout life, since some Haversian systems, or osteons, are being eroded continually through cell death as well as through factors that demand removal of calcium from bone; therefore, deposition of bone must also continue in order to maintain *bone balance.* During the growing years, bone deposition exceeds bone resorption and the child is in a state of *positive* bone balance. By contrast, in old age, bone deposition cannot keep pace with bone resorption and the elderly person is in a state of *negative* bone balance.

Remodeling of bone also occurs in response to physical stresses—or to the lack of them—in that bone is deposited in sites subjected to stress and is resorbed from sites where there is little stress. This phenomenon is generally referred to as *Wolff's law*, and is exemplified by marked cortical thickening on the concave side of a curved bone (Fig. 2.5) as well as by the alignment of trabecular systems along the lines of weight-bearing stress in the internal architecture of the upper end of the femur (Fig. 2.6).

It is quite likely that the phenomenon of Wolff's law is mediated by induced electrical potentials. For example, in a bowed tubular bone—or a curved trabeculum of cancellous bone—a negative electrical charge or potential exists on the concave side (compression force) and a positive charge on the convex side (tension force). Furthermore, it would seem that a negative charge induces bone deposition whereas a positive charge in-

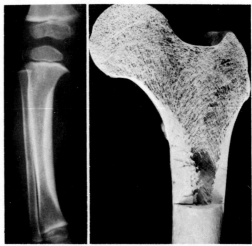

Figure 2.5 (left). An example of Wolff's law is seen in the tibia of a 2-year-old child with a bow leg deformity. Note the marked thickening of the medial cortex which is on the concave side of the deformity and which is subjected to the most stress on weight bearing.

Figure 2.6 (right). An example of Wolff's law is see in the internal architecture of this dried specimen of the upper end of a femur of an adult. Note the alignment of the trabecular systems of cancellous bone along the lines of weight-bearing stresses.

duces bone resorption. (During the past decade this concept of electrical stimulation of osteogenesis has been increasingly applied to the healing of delayed union of fractures in patients, as discussed in Chapters 6 and 15).

Anatomy and Histology of Bones as Structures

ANATOMICAL STRUCTURE

Bones, from the viewpoint of their gross structure, are classified as (1) long bones, or tubular bones (e.g. femur), (2) short bones or cuboidal bones (e.g. carpal bones) and (3) flat bones (e.g. scapula). Furthermore, each bone consists of dense cortical bone (*compacta*) on the outside and a sponge-like arrangement of trabecular bone (*spongiosa*) on the inside (Fig. 2.7). In children the covering periosteum is thick, loosely attached to the cortex and produces new bone readily; in adults, by contrast, the periosteum becomes progressively thinner, more adherent to the cortex and produces new bone less readily. This fundamental difference explains, in part, why fractures heal more rapidly in young children than in adults.

THE BLOOD SUPPLY TO LONG BONES

Three distinct vascular systems exist in long bones: (1) an *afferent* vascular system comprising nutrient and metaphyseal arteries that together supply the inner two-thirds of the cortex and periosteal arteries that supply the outer one-third; (2) an *efferent* vascular system that conveys venous blood; (3) an *intermediate* vascular system of capillaries within the cortex. The direction of blood flow through a long bone is normally centrifugal, i.e. from the medullary cavity to the periosteal surface.

HISTOLOGICAL STRUCTURE

From the viewpoint of its microscopic structure, bone is classified in the following way (the commonly used synonyms are included in parentheses):

(1) *Immature bone* (non-lamellar bone, woven bone, fiber bone).

(2) *Mature bone* (lamellar bone). (a), cortical bone (dense bone, compacta). (b), cancellous bone (trabecular bone, spongiosa).

The two major histological types of bone demonstrate significant differences in their relative content of cells, collagen and proteoglycans.

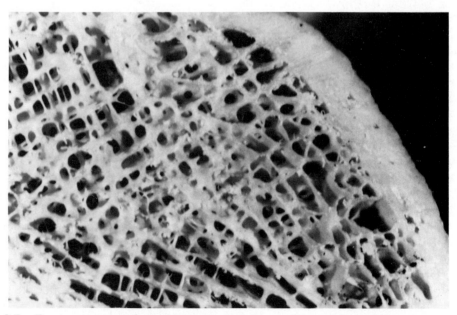

Figure 2.7.   Transverse cut surface of the innominate bone of the pelvis exhibiting an outer shell of dense cortical bone, or compacta (*right*) covering cancellous, trabecular bone or spongiosa.

Immature Bone

The first bone that is formed by endochondral ossification during embryonic development is of the immature type; subsequently, it is gradually replaced by mature bone so that by the age of one year, immature bone is no longer seen under normal conditions. Nevertheless, throughout life, under any abnormal condition in which new bone is formed rapidly (such as in the healing of a fracture or the reaction to infection), the *first* bone that is formed is of the immature type. Here again, the rapidly formed immature bone is subsequently replaced by mature bone.

Immature bone, also called fiber bone, or woven bone, because of its large proportion of irregularly "woven" collagen fibers in a haphazard arrangement, is very cellular and contains more proteoglycan but less cement substance as well as less mineral than mature bone (Fig. 2.8).

Mature Bone

In the dense cortex, mature bone is characterized by the concentric arrangement of its microscopic layers or lamellae and also by the complex formation of *Haversian systems* or *osteons* which are well designed to permit circulation of blood within the thick mass of cortical bone (Fig. 2.9). As in the structure of plywood, the collagen fibrils in any given concentric layer of a Haversian system course in a different direction from those of adjoining layers—an arrangement which adds strength to bone.

In cancellous bone the arrangement of lamellae is somewhat less complex because the trabeculae are thin and can therefore be nourished by surrounding vessels in the marrow spaces (Fig. 2.10).

Mature bone is less cellular and contains more cement substance as well as more mineral than immature bone.

The interstices of cancellous bone contain blood vessels, nerve fibers, fat and hemopoietic tissue. Although during childhood hemopoietic tissue is found in cancellous bone throughout the skeleton, it is limited in adult life to the cancellous bone of the spine, shoulder and pelvic girdle.

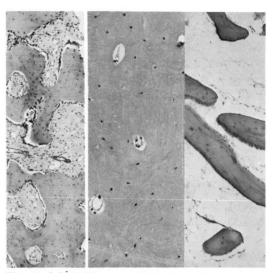

Figure 2.8 *(left).* Immature bone (fiber bone, woven bone) in the human. This very cellular type of bone is laid down in an irregular, "woven" pattern.

Figure 2.9 *(middle).* Cross-section of the dense cortex of mature bone in the human. Note the concentric arrangement of the layers, or lamellae, around a central vessel thereby forming Haversian systems, or osteons.

Figure 2.10 *(right).* Trabeculae of mature cancellous bone in the human. The thin trabeculae are nourished by surrounding vessels in the marrow spaces.

Bone Cells and Their Function

The *osteoblasts*, which represent one type of differentiated mesenchymal cell, are essential for the process of *osteogenesis* or *ossification*, since they alone can produce the organic intercellular substance, or *matrix*, in which *calcification* can occur later. The uncalcified tissue, because of its microscopic similarity to bone (in decalcified preparations), is called *osteoid*; once calcification occurs in the matrix, the tissue is *bone*. Thus, you will appreciate that ossification and calcification are not synonymous. As soon as an osteoblast has surrounded itself by organic intercellular substance, it lies in a *lacuna* and is henceforth known as an *osteocyte*.

Each osteocyte, imprisoned in its own lacuna, extends cytoplasmic processes via *canuliculi* to connect with similar processes from neighboring osteocytes. It is through these tiny channels that the osteocytes receive their nutrition from tissue fluid derived from regional blood vessels (in horizontal Volkmann's canals and in longitudinal Haversian canals).

Unlike cartilage, bone cannot enlarge by interstitial growth because its matrix is calcified. Thus a given bone can enlarge only by appositional growth on an existing surface.

Urist has discovered a non-collagenous glycoprotein, a small polypeptide in bone called bone morphogenic protein, (BMP) which is responsible for the differentiation of mesenchymal cells to osteoblasts.

The large, multinucleated cells which lie on the naked or uncovered bone surfaces and which are capable of resorbing or removing bone are called *osteoclasts.* Ham believes that osteoclasts are derived from the fusion of many stem cells—monocytes or macrophages—that cover or line bone surfaces and that the osteoclasts are, in effect, a type of foreign body giant cell. Calcium can be removed from bone only by osteoclastic activity (*osteoclasis*), which removes the organic matrix and the calcium simultaneously, a process that is more accurately described as *deossification* than as "decalcification."

Biochemistry and Physiology of Bone as an Organ

While the *gross appearance* of bones as structures changes only slowly, particularly after the period of skeletal growth, there is much *microscopic change* taking place within the bones as a result of the very active physiology of bone as an organ. The main biochemical function of bone concerns calcium and phosphorus metabolism.

BIOCHEMISTRY OF BONE

The biochemical composition of bone is as follows: organic substances, 35%; inorganic substances, 45%; water, 20%.

Organic Substances

The organic component of bone includes the bone cells as well as the organic intercellular substance, or matrix. Collagen fibrils constitute over 90% of the organic matrix

which contains, in addition, small quantities of reticular fibrils and amorphous substances (including hyaluronic acid and chondroitin sulphuric acid).

Inorganic Substances

The most important inorganic substances in bone are calcium and phosphorus, but other ions present include magnesium, sodium, hydroxyl, carbonate, and fluoride. Although the actual chemical composition of the bone crystal is known to vary during life, it is generally considered to be an hydroxyapatite crystal with the possible formula of $Ca_{10}(PO_4)_6(OH)_2$; the first deposit of mineral is probably amorphous $Ca_3(PO_4)_2$.

Enzymes. *Bone alkaline phosphatase*, which is produced by osteoblasts, may play a role in the osteoblastic production of organic matrix before calcification, i.e., osteoid, and may also play a role in its subsequent calcification. The metabolism of the living bone cells—and indeed of all cells—is dependent upon a multiplicity of enzyme systems.

CALCIUM AND PHOSPHORUS METABOLISM

The metabolisms of calcium (Ca) and phosphorus are so closely interdependent that they are best considered together. Indeed, the normal plasma levels of both calcium and inorganic phosphate are regulated by three hormones: the active metabolites of vitamin D (now considered to be hormones rather than vitamins), parathyroid hormone (PTH) and calcitonin. The metabolically active tissues on which these three hormones act are bones, kidneys and intestine. Bone as a physiological organ is the reservoir for 99% of the total body calcium (1000 g) and 90% of the total body phosphorus, the calcium and phosphate of bone being bound to each other as hydroxyapatite, $CA_{10}(PO_4)_6(OH)_2$. Thus, only 1% (1000 mg) of calcium is in the extracellular fluid (ECF) and only a minute—but critically important—amount (50 mg) is intracellular, mostly in mitochondria.

Maintenance of a narrow normal range of total plasma calcium is vital (9.0 to 10.4 mg/

100 ml or 2.25 to 2.60 mM). Of the total plasma calcium, approximately one-half is ionized (Ca++) and the other half is protein-bound (mainly to albumin). Less critical is maintenance of a normal plasma inorganic phosphate concentration (P_i) of approximately 3 mg/100 ml or 1 mM in adults and 5 mg/ml or 1.6 mM in children.

Calcium has a large number and wide variety of functions in the body including the following: (1) internal regulation of function of all cells. Calmodulin and actin have prime functions in modulating the intracellular effects of calcium. (2) Cell membrane permeability, nerve excitability, muscle contraction and gland secretion. (3) Extracellular calcium ion concentration regulates synthetic and secretory functions of the parathyroid gland (for PTH) and thyroid C-cells (for calcitonin). (4) Adhesiveness between cells. (5) The hardness and rigidity of bones and teeth through hydroxyapatite ($Ca_{10}(PO_4)_6(OH)_2$.

Calcium Homeostasis

Calcium in the diet is absorbed through the small intestine into the bloodstream, and this process is dependent upon normal integrity of the intestinal mucosa, normal gastric acidity, the presence of the active metabolites of vitamin D as well as the presence of bile salts and pancreatic enzymes (to digest fatty acids which would otherwise combine with calcium in the small bowel to form insoluble calcium soaps). Calcium is excreted both in the urine and in the feces. The calcium homeostasis in a normal adult is depicted in Figure 2.11.

Phosphate Homeostasis

Inorganic phosphate (P_i) in the diet is also absorbed through the small intestine both by diffusion and by active transport mechanisms stimulated in part by the active metabolites of vitamin D, especially the hormone $1,25(OH)_2D$. The precise mechanisms

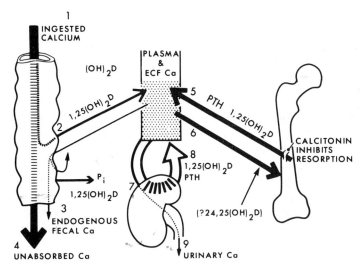

Figure 2.11. Processes that determine plasma and ECF calcium concentrations. *1*, ingested calcium: normally 500 to 1000 mg/day (500 to 1000 ml of milk provides ~1000 mg of calcium). *2*, intestinal absorption: normally ~300 mg/day; most absorption occurs in duodenum and proximal ileum. *3*, endogenous fecal calcium: this represents an obligatory calcium loss. The calcium is excreted in bile, intestinal juices and desquamated cells. It amounts to ~150 mg/day. *4*, unabsorbed calcium (*3 + 4*) = total fecal calcium. *5*, resorption from bone. *6*, accretion into bone. In the normal adult, resorption = accretion. The exact mechanism that couples these processes is not understood. Between 500 and 1000 mg of Ca are exchanged per day. In growth, accretion > resorption. *7*, glomerular filtration. A passive process depending on glomerular filtration rate (GFR) and concentration of ultrafiltrable Ca, amounting to ~10 g/day. *8*, renal tubular reabsorption, an active, 99% efficient process. *9*, urinary calcium, 50 to 300 mg/day. Net calcium balance = intake (*1*) minus (total fecal (*3 + 4*) Ca + urine Ca (*9*). 1.0 g calcium is equivalent to 25 mmoles. (Courtesy of Dr. Donald Fraser)

governing the transport of phosphate in and out of cells are not well understood. It is clear, however, that the kidney plays a pivotal role in regulating the level of plasma P_i as shown schematically (Fig. 2.12).

Actions of Parathyroid Hormone

The secretion of PTH is stimulated by hypocalcemia (but not directly by hypophosphatemia). The main effect of PTH is stimulation of bone resorption but it also increases renal tubular reabsorption of calcium and phosphate both of which increase the plasma Ca, thereby correcting the hypocalcemia and decreasing the secretion of PTH. In addition, PTH stimulates the synthesis of $1,25(OH)_2D$ (Figs. 2.11 and 2.12).

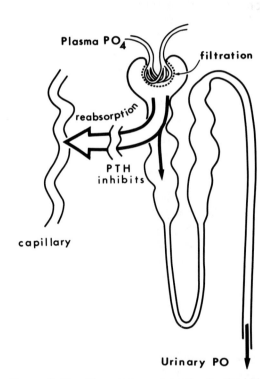

Figure 2.12. Phosphate reclamation by the kidney. Plasma inorganic phosphate (P_i) exists in almost completely ultrafiltrable state. Glomerular filtrate phosphate (GFP), a passive process. Calculated from GFR × plasma P_i. Renal tubular reabsorption of phosphate (TRP) is normally very efficient, 70 to 90% of GFP. It is an active process, occurring mainly at the proximal convoluted tubule. TRP = GFP minus UP. Urinary phosphate (UP). (Courtesy of Dr. Donald Fraser)

Actions of Calcitonin

This hormone, discovered by Copp in 1962, is secreted by the C-cells in the thyroid. Its secretion is stimulated by hypercalcemia and inhibited by hypocalcemia. The clinical significance of calcitonin in the homeostasis of calcium and phosphate in man is not yet clear. It is known, however, that calcitonin decreases bone resorption by suppressing osteoclastic activity (this effect is of clinical significance in the treatment of Paget's disease as discussed in Chapter 9). Both salmon and porcine calcitonin have an effect in the human.

Actions of Vitamin D Metabolites

It is now known that vitamin D *per se* is metabolically inactive. Of its active metabolites, however, the most significant is 1,25-dihydroxycalciferol (1,25-dihydroxy vitamin D) ($1,25(OH)_2D$) which acts like a steroid hormone as shown by DeLuca, Kodicek, Norman and others.

The major effect of the active normal metabolites of vitamin D (principally 1,25 $(OH)_2D$) is to increase absorption of both calcium and phosphate from the intestine; 1,25-dihydroxyvitamin D also increases the mobilization of Ca (and secondarily P_i) from bone. Additional actions of less apparent significance are increased renal tubular reabsorption of calcium and stimulation of synthesis of calcium-binding protein in intestinal mucosa cells. The net effect of all of these phenomena is to elevate the plasma levels of calcium. Recent evidence suggests that $24,25(OH)_2D$ may participate in the deposition of mineral in the uncalcified matrix of bone, i.e. in osteoid.

As for all hormones, the synthesis of $1,25(OH)_2D$ and $24,25(OH)_2D$ is under feedback regulation. The main factors for stimulating the most active metabolite of vitamin D, namely $1,25(OH)_2D$, are hypocalcemia, hypophosphatemia and parathyroid hormone.

JOINTS AND ARTICULAR CARTILAGE

A joint is simply a junction between two or more bones. Joints provide segmentation of the skeleton of man and allow for varying degrees of motion between the segments, as well as for varying amounts of segmental growth.

Classification of the Types of Joints

Five distinct types of joints exist in the body, each with its particular characteristics.

(1) *Syndesmosis*—a joint in which the two bones are bound together by fibrous tissue only, as in the suture joints between the skull bones.

(2) *Synchrondrosis*—a joint in which the two bones are bound together by cartilage. An epiphyseal plate is, in effect, a temporary synchrondrosis which binds the epiphysis to the metaphysis and which permits longitudinal growth. The cartilaginous joints between some of the endochrondral bones in the base of the skull are also synchondroses.

(3) *Synostosis*—a joint which, at some stage, has become obliterated by bony union. Some syndesmoses and all synchrondroses eventually fuse and thereby become synostoses.

(4) *Symphysis*—a joint in which the two opposing surfaces are covered by hyaline cartilage and joined by fibrocartilage and strong fibrous tissue. There may be a small central cleft (as in the symphysis pubis) but not a true joint cavity. Symphyses allow little movement but provide much stability. Intervertebral joints (usually called intervertebral discs) are a specialized form of symphysis in which the opposing cartilage-covered surface of adjacent vertebrae bodies are joined together by a ring of dense fibrous tissue and fibrocartilage (the annulus fibrosus). The central cleft or space is filled with a semifluid substance (the nucleus pulposus).

(5) *Synovial Joint*—one in which the two opposing surfaces are covered by hyaline articular cartilage and joined peripherally by a fibrous tissue capsule enclosing a joint cavity which contains synovial fluid. Synovial joints, which are present throughout the limbs, allow free movement, but at the expense of providing less stability than the other four types of joints.

Embryonic Development of Synovial Joints

At the site of future synovial joints in the central condensation of mesenchyme of the limb bud, an articular disc of mesenchyme appears (*the primitive joint plate*). A dense tissue, which is the counterpart of perichondrium of the cartilaginous model, surrounds the primitive joint plate and is the forerunner of the joint capsule. By the 10th week of embryonic life, clefts or spaces, which are filled with tissue fluid, appear in the primitive joint plate and gradually coalesce to form a single joint cavity. The synovial fluid may be considered a mucin (hyaluronic acid) diluted by tissue fluid. The outer layer of the joint capsule differentiates into fibrous tissue while the inner layer becomes specialized to form the synovial membrane.

It is known from scientific studies that from the 6th week of embryonic life active intrauterine movement of the limbs is essential to the normal embryonic development of synovial joints (This is but one example of the critical importance of motion in the maintenance of healthy joints).

Anatomy and Histology of Synovial Joints

ANATOMICAL STRUCTURE

The various anatomical structures of a typical synovial joint are best depicted diagrammatically (Fig. 2.13). The joint surface that is convex is always larger than the opposing joint surface that is concave—an arrangement that allows gliding motion. Articular cartilage has the consistency of firm rubber, and like rubber, it is resilient. It is also called *hyaline* cartilage (Gr. *hyalos*, glass) because like "frosted" glass, articular cartilage is pearly white and partially translucent, an appearance that is due to its distinctive intercellular matrix.

Articular cartilage is a viscoelastic tissue which is a mixture of an elastic solid and a viscous liquid; as such it is admirably suited to withstand the intermittent shear and compression forces of normal joint function. Through tribology (the science of friction, wear and lubrication of interacting surfaces

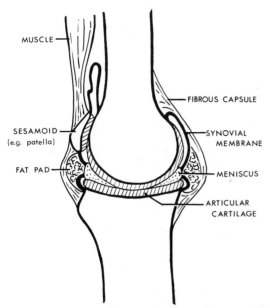

Figure 2.13. Diagrammatic representation of the various anatomical structures of a typical synovial joint in the human (a sagittal section of the knee viewed from the side).

in relative motion) we learn that the coefficient of friction between the two surfaces of a normal joint is extremely small, in fact only one-fifth that between two pieces of ice! A form of "boundary lubrication" or "weeping lubrication" is made possible by a mucin (hyaluronate) in the synovial fluid so that motion occurs between two thin layers of fluid rather than directly between two surfaces of articular cartilage.

The macroscopically smooth articular surface is provided by a tough skin-like limiting membrane that exhibits lines of tension (comparable to Langer's lines of the skin). Indeed, intact cartilage *in vivo* has been likened to an inflated air tent, or a tire in that much water is imbibed by the hydrophilic matrix and this "inflates" the cartilage, which is therefore pressurized; the intracartilage pressure is contained by the intact surface membrane. The thickness of articular cartilage varies from one joint to another and even from one area to another within a given joint.

Within the substance of the cartilage the bundles of collagen fibers form arcades like the curved ribs of an umbrella (Benninghoff's arcades). Thus, they rise vertically from their deep attachment to the subchondral bone, gradually become horizontal as they reach the joint surface and then descend in a vertical configuration again to the bone (Fig. 2.14).

The synovial membrane lines the entire joint cavity except over the surfaces of articular cartilage and menisci. It has the ability to secrete as well as to absorb. Synovial covered fat pads, which are quite mobile, project into peripheral spaces in the joint, thereby preventing a vacuum from developing in the cavity. The outer fibrous capsule becomes greatly thickened in some areas to form strong ligaments which help to provide some degree of joint stability.

HISTOLOGICAL STRUCTURE OF ARTICULAR CARTILAGE

Hyaline articular cartilage is characterized by a paucity of sparsely scattered chondrocytes in a vast matrix of intercellular substance. Unlike most other tissues, such cartilage is completely devoid of blood vessels, lymphatic vessels or nerve fibers. Indeed the chondrocytes in normal cartilage live in immunological isolation from the cells of the rest of the body, which explains the success of cartilage allografts.

The chondrocytes in their lacunae are arranged in three rather indistinct layers or zones (Fig. 2.15). In the superficial zone the limiting membrane, known as the lamina splendans, is characterized by a plethora of collagen fibers that are parallel to the surface and small oval cells similarly aligned. Unlike bone that is clothed in periosteum, the articular surface is not covered by perichondrium. In the middle zone the chondrocytes are younger and somewhat more active than in the other two zones. Mitotic figures may be seen in this zone during childhood, but in adulthood they are not normally seen. In the deep zone the collagen fibers are vertical and the chondrocytes are mature. During the growing years this layer functions as the growth cartilage of the underlying epiphysis, allowing it to increase in both height and

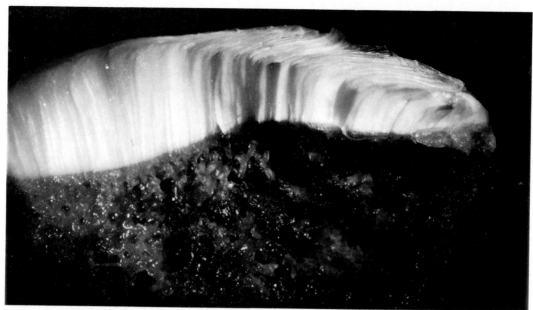

Figure 2.14. Fracture surface of a fresh fracture involving the articular cartilage (*above*) and underlying cancellous bone of the patella in a young man. Note the vertical alignment of the bundles of collagen fibers in the deep zone of the cartilage and the horizontal alignment in the superficial zone from which they will then descend vertically to the deep zone thereby forming arcades. (Courtesy of Dr. Roby Thompson)

width. In adult life, however, the matrix of the deepest part of this zone becomes calcified and the border between the calcified zone and the uncalcified remainder of the articular cartilage is known as the tide mark.

The distinctive matrix is composed of water (70 to 80%), collagen (10 to 15%) and proteoglycans (10 to 15%). Although the water can move in and out of the matrix, cartilage is hydrophilic and the water gives this tissue its turgidity. The collagen of hyaline articular cartilage is Type II collagen (in contrast to that of the fibrocartilage of menisci which is Type I). Like the rods in reinforced concrete, the collagen fibers provide cartilage with its strength, especially in tension. It is the hydrophilic proteoglycans that bind or "glue" the collagen fibers together and provide the articular cartilage with its resilience and elasticity so necessary in resisting intermittent shear and compressive forces and in providing the rigid subchondral bone with a protective "shock absorber."

Rosenberg has made extensive studies of the remarkable macromolecules of proteo-glycan aggregates with their central cores of hyaluronic acid, their link proteins and multiple subunits composed of a central core and bristle-like rods of three glycosaminoglycans: chondroitin-4-sulfate, chondroitin-6-sulfate and keratan sulfate (the obsolete term for glycosaminoglycans is mucopolysaccharides). These glycosaminoglycans in the subunits resemble the bristles of a test-tube brush; since each "bristle" carries a negative electrical charge they repel one another, and this is what gives articular cartilage its characteristic resilience. The complex structures of proteoglycan aggregates and their subunits are best appreciated schematically (Figs. 2.16 and 2.17).

Both the collagen and the proteoglycans are synthesized by the chondrocytes which therefore carry the responsibility for maintaining the physical properties of the cartilage. Indeed these cells, once thought to be somewhat dormant, are metabolically quite active—more so during childhood, of course, than during adult life. Chondrocytes require very little oxygen for their metabo-

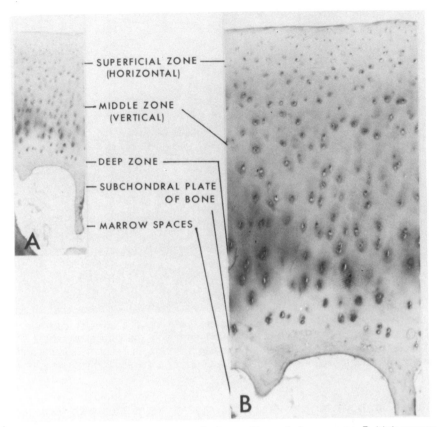

SUPERFICIAL ZONE
(HORIZONTAL)

MIDDLE ZONE
(VERTICAL)

DEEP ZONE

SUBCHONDRAL PLATE
OF BONE

MARROW SPACES

Figure 2.15.   Histology of human articular cartilage. *A*, low power; *B*, high power.

lism, but they are dependent for their nutrition on the diffusion of nutrients from the synovial fluid which is essentially a modified type of tissue fluid. Therefore the two most important factors in the optimal nutrition of articular cartilage are a healthy synovial membrane to produce the synovial fluid and adequate "circulation" or diffusion of this nourishing fluid through the matrix to reach the chondrocytes. Understandably, nutrition of the cartilage is enhanced by joint motion which squeezes synovial fluid in and out of the sponge-like matrix. By contrast, immobilization of a synovial joint, especially if prolonged, leads to stasis of synovial fluid and to disuse atrophy of the cartilage.

STRUCTURE AND FUNCTIONS OF THE SYNOVIAL MEMBRANE

The synovial membrane is composed of two distinct layers—an inner and an outer.

Not a true membrane, the inner synovial lining is a thin syncitium of only a few layers of loosely connected cells supported by an outer layer of fibrous and fatty tissue that, in contrast to cartilage, has a rich supply of blood vessels, lymphatic vessels and nerve fibers. Of the cells in the inner layer there are two types. The predominant Type A synoviocytes, which have many features of macrophages, serve to clear the joint of waste materials while the Type B synoviocytes synthesize hyaluronate, a mucin that provides synovial fluid with its viscosity and its remarkable lubricating qualities. Because of the countless villi in the synovial membrane its functional surface area is enormous; for example, as much as 100 square meters in a human knee joint.

Crystalloids, including most antibiotics, diffuse across the synovial membrane readily in both directions via the capillaries, but

PROTEOGLYCAN   AGGREGATE

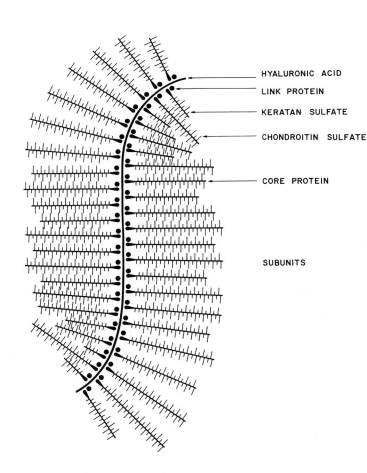

HYALURONIC ACID

LINK PROTEIN

KERATAN SULFATE

CHONDROITIN SULFATE

CORE PROTEIN

SUBUNITS

Figure 2.16. Tentative model of the molecular architecture of the proteoglycan aggregate. (Courtesy of Dr. Lawrence Rosenberg)

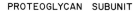

PROTEOGLYCAN   SUBUNIT

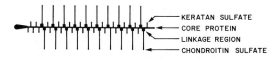

KERATAN SULFATE
CORE PROTEIN
LINKAGE REGION
CHONDROITIN SULFATE

Figure 2.17. Diagram of the proposed structure of the proteoglycan subunit. (Courtesy of Dr. Lawrence Rosenberg)

proteins with their large colloidal molecules leave the joint cavity via the lymphatics. Particulate matter (such as hemosiderin from a joint hemorrhage) is removed from the synovial cavity through phagocytosis by the macrophage-like Type A synoviocytes, but then may remain in the synovial membrane and subsynovial tissues for many months, leading to synovial hypertrophy.

SYNOVIAL FLUID

A viscous, pale yellow, clear fluid resembling the white of an egg (L. *ovum*, egg), synovial fluid is a dialysate of plasma, a type of tissue fluid to which the lubricant hyaluronate has been added. Thus, synovial fluid serves the dual function of nourishing the articular cartilage and lubricating the joint surfaces. A normal joint contains relatively little synovial fluid; for example, the normal adult knee, which is the largest joint in the body, contains less than 5 cc (ml). Thus, the true joint space is virtually a potential space. (The so-called "joint space" seen between the bony surfaces of a joint in a radiograph is more appropriately designated the cartilage space.) Synovial fluid is present not only in synovial joints but also in synovial tendon sheaths and synovial bursae.

In a normal joint the total cell count of synovial fluid is less than 200 per ml; monocytic macrophages and lymphocytes predominate with only a small percentage of polymorphonuclear leukocytes. Synovial fluid contains albumin and globulin but no fibrinogen. The absence of fibrinogen may explain why normal synovial fluid does not clot. Blood, mixed with synovial fluid in a joint, likewise does not clot.

SKELETAL MUSCLES

The skeletal muscles, of which there are over 400 in the human body, are the "living motors" which provide *active movement* of the articulated skeleton as well as *maintenance of its posture*. The basic property of skeletal muscle is *contractility* of its protoplasm (*sarcoplasm*) which enables the individual muscle either to shorten and thereby provide movement (*isotonic contraction*), or to resist lengthening without allowing movement (*isometric contraction*).

Anatomy and Histology of Skeletal Muscle

The size, shape and gross structure of muscles vary tremendously in accordance with their particular function and workload, but the basic cellular structure is the individual *muscle cell*, which, because of its long, thin, thread-like shape is called a *muscle fiber*. Skeletal muscle is designated *voluntary* muscle because it is under the individual's will, and *striated* because of its characteristic microscopic cross-striations (Fig. 2.18). Each individual muscle cell, or fiber, is innervated by a single anterior horn cell of the spinal cord through a single axon within a peripheral nerve fiber (although a given anterior horn cell innervates more than one muscle cell, or fiber, in a muscle). The anterior horn cell, its axon, the myoneural junctions and the individual muscle fibers supplied by the single anterior horn cell constitute a *single motor unit*. The connective tissue components of a skeletal muscle serve as a medium through which course the rich nerve and blood supply to the muscle fibers; in addition, they provide a non-contractile framework or "harness" through which the contraction of muscle fibers is transmitted to bone. The connective tissue surrounding the entire muscle is termed *epimysium*, that surrounding bundles of muscle fibers is termed *perimysium* and that surrounding each individual muscle fiber is termed *endomysium* (Fig. 2.19).

Each muscle fiber is, in fact, a thin, markedly elongated, multinucleated cell which varies tremendously in length depending upon the muscle in which it is situated. In a unipennate muscle (such as the sartorius) there is evidence to suggest that each muscle cell, or fiber, probably extends the full length of the muscle. The protoplasm, or *sarcoplasm*, of each muscle fiber is contained by a thin membrane, the *sarcolemma*, under which lie the eccentrically placed cell nuclei, about 40 for each millimeter length of the fiber. Of these nuclei, a small percentage represent *satellite cells* (*dormant myoblasts*) which may be important sources of muscle regeneration after injury. Each muscle fiber contains many *myofibrils*, each of which, in turn, is transversely divided into thousands of tiny cylindrical areas (*sarcomeres*) by the cross-striations (a muscle fiber 5 mm long would have about 20,000 such divisions) (Fig. 2.20). Electron microscopy reveals that each sarcomere, in turn, contains about three million *thick myofilaments* consisting of molecules of the muscle protein, *myosin*, and thin myofilaments consisting of molecules of another muscle protein, *actin* (Fig. 2.21). The sarcomeres are, in fact, the functional units of muscle contraction.

Biochemistry and Physiology of Muscle

The processes by which skeletal muscle converts stored chemical energy into mechanical energy to perform work are very complex indeed. Acetylcholine is the chemical mediator of the nerve impulses at the myoneural junction and it is believed that the energy for muscle action is derived from the breakdown of adenosine triphosphate (ATP) by adenosine triphosphatase (ATPase) with the liberation of adenosine diphosphate (ADP). Current thinking is that muscle con-

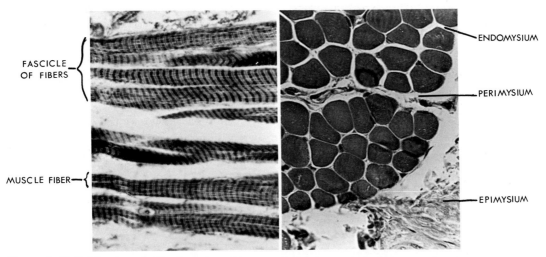

FASCICLE OF FIBERS

MUSCLE FIBER

ENDOMYSIUM

PERIMYSIUM

EPIMYSIUM

Figure 2.18 (*left*).   Longitudinal section of human skeletal muscle (voluntary, striated muscle). Note the characteristic cross-striations in each muscle fiber.
Figure 2.19 (*right*).   Cross-section of human skeletal muscle showing the connective tissue components which provide a non-contractile harness through which the contraction of the muscle fibers is transmitted to bone.

traction, which occurs within the individual sarcomeres, takes place as a result of the sliding of the thin myofilaments (actin) of the I bands in between the thick myofilaments (myosin) of the A bands. As a result of this sliding, which may be likened to the bristles of two hair brushes that are being pushed together, the thousands of cross striations move closer together and the entire fiber shortens (contracts). During relaxation the thin myofilaments slide out again from between the thick myofilaments and the sarcomeres lengthen as does the entire muscle fiber.

The most important practical consideration of skeletal muscle is its ability to develop *tension*, part of which is due to its *contractile force* and part of which is due to the *resistance of its connective tissue components to stretch*. Each individual muscle fiber obeys the *"all-or-none law"* in that it either contracts maximally, or not at all. Thus, in a given muscle, the difference between a powerful contraction and a weak contraction lies in the number of individual fibers that are contracting within the muscle at that time. For each muscle there is definite relationship between its "starting length" and the

amount of tension it can develop. When the muscle is passively shortened by approximating its origin and insertion, it can develop very little contractile force. The greatest contractile force is developed when the muscle is at its *"resting length"* (about halfway between its extremes of length). As the muscle is passively stretched beyond its resting length, the contractile force gradually diminishes, but the passive resistance of the connective tissue components gradually develops more tension so that the *total tension* in the muscle increases. This muscle length-tension relationship can be depicted graphically by what is known as the *Blix curve* (Fig. 2.22). You can demonstrate this phenomenon readily in your own hand. With your fingers and wrist in the position of complete flexion, your finger flexor muscles are shortened, and they can develop very little contractile force during any attempt to squeeze an object such as the index finger of your opposite hand; furthermore, there is no tension from passive resistance of the connective tissue components. With your wrist in the neutral position and your fingers slightly flexed, your finger flexors are at their "resting length" and you can demonstrate

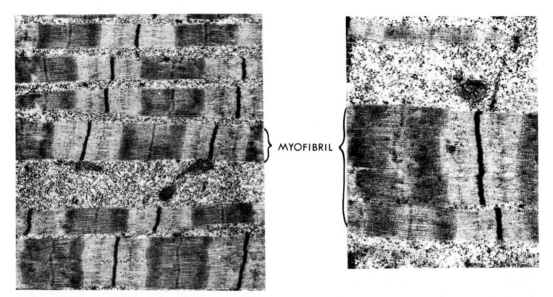

Figure 2.20. Longitudinal section of a human skeletal muscle fiber which consists of many myofibrils each of which is divided into sarcomeres by cross-striations. Note the various "bands" in each sarcomere. Magnification left is 12,000×; right, 20,000×. Note the dark A bands alternating with the light I bands and the clearer H zone within each of the A bands.

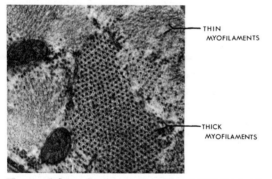

Figure 2.21. Cross-section of a sarcomere of human skeletal muscle showing thick myofilaments (myosin) and thin myofilaments (actin). Magnification 60,000×.

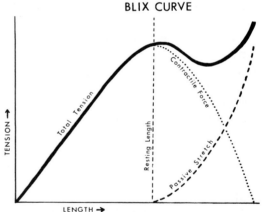

Figure 2.22. The Blix curve depicting muscle length-tension relationship. Note that the greatest contractile force is developed when the muscle is at its resting length, about halfway between its extremes of length. As the muscle is passively stretched beyond its resting length, its contractile force gradually diminishes, but the passive resistance of the connective tissue components gradually develop more tension so that the total tension in the muscle increases.

that they have much greater contractile force. When your wrist and fingers are completely extended, there is little contractile force but much passive resistance to further stretch. Thus, the normal "resting length" of a given muscle is of great importance in musculoskeletal function and any undesirable alteration in this "resting length" by disorders or injuries (including surgical operations) will result in loss of power.

TENDONS AND LIGAMENTS

Tendons and ligaments, in contrast to muscle, are composed chiefly of inert intercellular substance or matrix in the form of

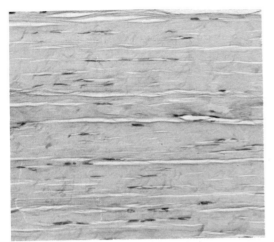

Figure 2.23. Longitudinal section of human tendon showing rows of flattened fibroblasts scattered between collagen fibers longitudinally aligned in the line of tension. Note that this tissue contains relatively few cells but an abundance of intercellular substance.

collagen fibers longitudinally aligned (in the line of tension) with rows of flattened *fibroblasts* scattered between them (Fig. 2.23). It is this regular internal arrangement of tendons and ligaments that provides them with their remarkable tensile strength. In adult life the fibroblasts become relatively dormant *fibrocytes,* and since the intercellular substance requires no nutrition, the blood supply is minimal. At sites of friction, a tendon is enveloped by a *synovial sheath* consisting of a visceral and a parietal layer of synovial membrane and lubricated by a synovial-like fluid containing hyaluronate. The synovial sheath, in turn, is covered by a dense fibrous tissue sheath. Both tendons and ligaments gain an extremely firm attachment to bone at their sites of insertion by a continuation of their collagen fibers which penetrate deeply into the solid substance of cortical bone and fan out within it as Sharpey's fibers. So strong is this attachment that even with severe traction injuries neither ligaments nor tendons "pull out" of bone; instead the ligament or tendon either tears within its substance or a fragment of bone is avulsed along with the inserted tendon or ligament.

Suggested Additional Reading

Albright, J. A. and Brand, R. A. (eds.): *The Scientific Basis of Orthopaedics.* New York, Appleton-Century-Crofts, 1979.

Boyd, W. and Sheldon, H.: *Introduction to the Study of Disease.* Philadelphia, Lea and Febiger, 1980.

Bourne, G. H. *The Biochemistry and Physiology of Bone.* New York, Academic Press, 1976.

Bullough, P. G.: Bone. In *Scientific Foundations of Orthopaedics and Traumatology,* edited by Owen, R., Goodfellow, J. and Bullough, P. G. London, William Heinemann Medical Books, 1980.

Bullough, P. G.: Cartilage. In *Scientific Foundations of Orthopaedics and Traumatology,* edited by Owen, R., Goodfellow, J. and Bullough, P. G. London, William Heinemann Medical Books, 1980.

Buxton, P. H.: Skeletal muscle structure and development. In *Scientific Foundations of Orthopaedics and Traumatology,* edited by Owen, R., Goodfellow, J. and Bullough, P. G. London, William Heinemann Medical Books, 1980.

Copp, D. H.: Calcitonin—recent advances and clinical implications. Mod. Med. Can. 28: 41–44, 1973.

Cruess, R. L. (Ed): *The Musculoskeletal System. Embryology, Biochemistry and Physiology.* New York, Edinburgh, London and Melbourne. Churchill-Livingstone, 1982.

DeLuca, H. F.: Calcium metabolism. Acta Orthop. Scand. 46: 286–314, 1975.

Fraser, D., Kind, H. P., Kooh, S. W.: Disturbances of parathyroid hormone and calcitonin. In *Textbook of Pediatrics,* 2nd ed., edited by Arneil, G. C. and Forfar, J. O. Edinburgh & London, Churchill-Livingstone, 1001–1014, pp. 1978,

Freeman, M. A. R. (ed.) *Adult Articular Cartilage,* 2nd ed. Kent, U. K., Pitman Medical, 1979.

Ghadially, F. H.: Structure and function of articular cartilage. Clin. Rheum. Dis. 7: 3–27, 1981.

Hall, F. M. and Wyshak, G.: Thickness of articular cartilage in the normal knee. J. Bone Joint Surg. 62A: 408–413, 1980.

Ham, A. W. and Cormack, D. H.: Histophysiology of cartilage, bone and joints. In *Histology,* ed. 8. Philadelphia and Toronto, J. B. Lippincott, 1979.

Hughes, S. and Sweetman, R.: *The Basis and Practice of Orthopaedics.* London, William Heinemann Medical Books Ltd., 1980.

Jowsey, J.: Metabolic diseases of bone. In *Saunders Monographs in Clinical Orthopaedics.* Philadelphia, W. B. Saunders, 1977, vol. 1.

Malemud, C. J. and Moskowitz, R. W.: Physiology of articular cartilage. Clin. Rheumatol. Dis. 7: 29–55, 1981.

Paget, S. A. and Bullough, P. G.: Synovium and synovial fluid. In *Scientific Foundations of Orthopaedics and Traumatology,* edited by Owen, R., Goodfellow, J. and Bullough, P. G. London, William Heinemann Medical Books Ltd., 1980.

Posner, A. S.: Bone mineral. In *Scientific Foundations of Orthopaedics and Traumatology,* edited by Owen, R., Goodfellow, J. and Bullough, P. G. London, William Heinemann Medical Books Ltd., 1980.

Rosenberg, L. C.: Proteoglycans. In *Scientific Foundations of Orthopaedics and Traumatology,* edited by Owen, R., Goodfellow, J. and Bullough, P. G. London, William Heinemann Medical Books Ltd., 1980.

Rosenberg, L.: Structure of cartilage proteoglycans. In *Dynamics of Connective Tissue Macromolecules*, edited by Burleigh, P. M. C. and Poole, A. R. North Holland Publishing, 1975.

Simmons, D. J. and Kumin, A. S.: *Skeletal Research: An Experimental Approach.* New York, Academic Press, 1979.

Sledge, C. B.: Structure, development and function of joints. Orthop. Clin. North Am. 6: 619–628, 1975.

Smith, R.: Calcium, phosphorus and magnesium metabolism. In *Scientific Foundations of Orthopaedics and Traumatology*, edited by Owen, R., Goodfellow, J. and Bullough, P. G. London, William Heinemann Medical Books Ltd., 1980.

Sokoloff, L. (ed.): *The Joints and Synovial Fluid. A Two Volume Treatise.* New York, Academic Press, 1978.

Thompson, R. C. and Robinson, H. J.: Current concepts review. Articular cartilage matrix metabolism. J. Bone Joint Surg. 1981.

Turek, S. L.: *Orthopaedics. Principles and Their Application*, 3rd ed. Philadelphia, J. B. Lippincott, 1977.

Urist, M. R.: Biochemistry of calcification. In Bourne, G. H. (ed.): *The Biochemistry and Physiology of Bone*, ed. 2. New York, Academic Press, 1976, vol. 4, p. 2.

Urist, M. R.: Solubilized and insolubilized bone morphogenetic protein. Proc. Nat. Acad. Sci. U.S.A. 76: 1828–1832, 1979.

Wolf, A. W., Benson, D. R., Shoji, H., Riggins, R., Shapiro, R. F., Castles, J. J. and Wild, J.: Current concepts in synovial fluid analysis. Clin. Orthop. 134: 262–265, 1978.

Wyke, B.: The neurology of joints: a review of general principles. Clin. Rheumatol. Dis. 7: 223–239, 1981.

CHAPTER 3

Reactions of Musculoskeletal Tissues to Disorders and Injuries

BONE

Having reviewed the *normal* structure and function of the various musculoskeletal tissues, you are now ready to review the *abnormal* structure and function caused by the *biological reactions* of these tissues to disorders and injuries. As a medical student and as a medical doctor you must always remember that your patient is a *person*— with all that this implies. Nevertheless you will find it helpful to think about his tissue reactions, or pathological processes, not only in terms of the resultant *gross lesions* but also in terms of the dynamic biological activity of his *cells*, acting and reacting as living populations both in time and in specific *sites*, i.e. the pathogenesis of various pathological states. Enlightened by a knowledge of these reactions, or pathological processes, you will be better prepared to *understand* the clinical, radiographic and laboratory *manifestations* of the many abnormal clinical conditions of the musculoskeletal system that you will encounter in your patients. Indeed, these manifestations will enable you make an intelligent diagnosis as discussed in Chapter 5. In addition, you will be better able to appreciate the *reason*, or rationale, for the general principles and specific methods of their treatment as outlined in Chapter 6.

Reactions of Bone

Bone, which is a highly specialized type of connective tissue, is capable of only a very limited number of reactions to a large number of abnormal conditions. While the results of these reactions may be manifest by marked changes in the gross structure of a bone or bones, the basic nature of the reactions is best considered at a *microscopic, or cellular level*, since the reactions are those of living bone and the cells are the only living components.

There are but three basic ways in which bone can react to abnormal conditions (1) *local death*, (2) *an alteration of bone depo-*

25

sition, and (3) *an alteration of bone resorp-tion.* When an area of bone is completely deprived of blood supply, its reaction is local death (*avascular necrosis of bone*). The resultant segment of dead bone, however, then becomes an abnormal condition in itself and incites further reactions from the surrounding living tissues, as discussed in Chapter 13. Bone that remains *alive* can react to abnormal conditions either by an alteration of deposition or by an alteration of resorption (or both). Bone deposition, however, involves a combination of two major processes, namely, osteoblastic formation of organic matrix (osteoid) and calcification of this matrix to form bone; calcification of matrix may be less than normal (hypocalcification) but it is seldom more than normal. Thus the reactions of living bone may be outlined as follows:

1. Altered deposition of bone
    (a) Increased deposition (increased formation of matrix with normal calcification)
    (b) Decreased deposition (either decreased formation of matrix or hypocalcification)
2. Altered resorption of bone
    (a) Increased resorption
    (b) Decreased resorption
3. Combinations of altered deposition and altered resorption

The abnormal condition may incite one or more reactions in a given bone or part of a bone (*a localized reaction of bone as a structure*), or it may incite one or more reactions in all bones (*a generalized reaction of all bone as an organ*). These reactions in bone are of more than academic interest; indeed, they are of great *practical significance* because they cause changes in *bone density* and therefore can be detected and studied by ordinary *radiographic examination* as well as by *computed tomography* (CT scan). Thus, either increased deposition or decreased resorption (or a combination of the two) results in *more bone* and is detected by *increased radiographic density (sclerosis)* (Fig. 3.1), whereas the opposite reactions result in *less bone* and are detected by

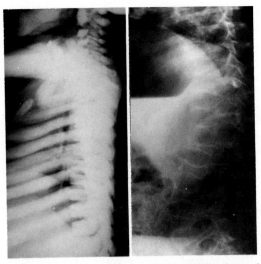

Figure 3.1 (*left*).   Osteopetrosis (marble bones). An example of generalized increase in bone. The spine of this child with "marble bones" reveals increased radiographic density of all the bones.
Figure 3.2 (*right*).   Osteoporosis (osteopenia). An example of generalized decrease in bone. The spine of this child with osteogenesis imperfecta ("fragile bones") reveals decreased radiographic density of all the bones.

decreased radiographic density (rarefaction) (Fig. 3.2).

Examples of Reactions of Living Bone

The various reactions of living bone may be incited by a wide variety of clinical disorders and injuries, some of which arise within the musculoskeletal system and some of which arise within other systems of the body. Examples of these abnormal clinical conditions are only mentioned here but each is discussed in subsequent chapters. In each of these clinical conditions there is an alteration in the normal *equilibrium* or *balance* between bone deposition and bone resorption.

GENERALIZED REACTIONS OF ALL BONE AS AN ORGAN

1. Bone Deposition Greater Than Bone Resorption (Generalized Increase in Bone)

Osteopetrosis (marble bones) (Chapter 8). Bone deposition is probably normal but bone resorption is defective and therefore there is an increase in the total amount of bone (Fig. 3.1).

Acromegaly (Chapter 9). Bone deposition is increased by excessive intramembranous ossification from the periosteum.

2. Bone Deposition Less Than Bone Resorption (Generalized Decrease in Bone)

Osteoporosis (Osteopenia) (Chapter 9). Bone deposition is decreased because of decreased osteoblastic formation of matrix (osteoid) and, in addition, bone resorption is increased, with the result that there is a marked decrease in the total amount of bone. Examples of generalized osteoporosis are osteogenesis imperfecta ("fragile bones") and postmenopausal osteoporosis. (Fig. 3.2).

Rickets and Osteomalacia (Chapter 9). Although the osteoblastic formation of matrix is normal, there is decreased calcification (hypocalcification) of the matrix with resultant decrease in the amount of (calcified) bone.

LOCALIZED REACTIONS OF BONE AS A STRUCTURE

1. Bone Deposition Greater Than Bone Resorption. (Localized Increase in Bone)

Work Hypertrophy. The bone reacts to the extra stresses and strains of increased function by increased bone deposition—an example of Wolff's law. For example, in a rigid varus deformity of the foot in which most of the weight is being borne on the lateral edge of the foot, the fifth metatarsal hypertrophies (Fig. 3.3).

Degenerative Osteoarthritis (Chapter 11). The subchondral bone underlying that portion of the joint surface that is taking the greatest amount of excessive intermittent pressure reacts by increased bone deposition that is seen radiographically as subchondral sclerosis.

Fractures (Chapter 15). The periosteum and endosteum react to bony injury by a localized increase in bone deposition to form callus as part of the healing process.

Infection (Chapter 10). The periosteum elevated by pus, reacts to the infection by deposition of new bone.

Osteosclerotic Neoplasms (Chapter 14). The reaction of increased bone deposition to certain benign neoplasms and neoplasm-like lesions of bone (such as osteoid osteoma) is called "*reactive bone*" whereas the bone produced by certain malignant bone neoplasms (such as osteosarcoma and osteoblastic metastases) is called "*tumor bone.*"

2. Bone Deposition Less Than Bone Resorption (Localized Decrease in Bone)

Disuse Atrophy (Disuse Osteoporosis). The bone reacts to the diminished stresses and strains of decreased function (disuse) by decreased bone deposition, while the bone resorption continues unchanged; the result is a localized decrease in bone. Thus

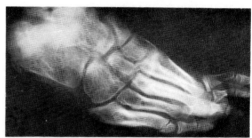

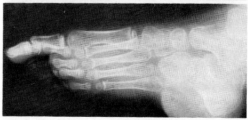

Figure 3.3 (*top*). Work hypertrophy of bone. An example of localized increase in bone. The hypertrophy of the fifth metatarsal of this boy's foot is a reaction to the increased stresses and strains of taking most of the weight on the lateral edge of this rigid and deformed foot.

Figure 3.4 (*bottom*). Disuse atrophy of bone (disuse osteoporosis). An example of localized decrease in bone. The atrophy of all the metatarsals of this boy's foot is a reaction to the decreased stress and strains of taking no weight on the forefoot due to paralysis of the calf muscles and resultant inability of the patient to push the forefoot down against the floor or the ground while walking.

in a lower limb, for example, prolonged immobilization, prolonged relief of weight bearing and severe paralysis of long duration, all cause disuse atrophy of bone (Fig. 3.4).

Rheumatoid Arthritis (Chapter 10). The bone reacts to the periarticular soft tissue inflammation by a decreased bone deposition and possibly an increased bone resorption as well. Of course, disuse atrophy may also be a factor because of the coexistent decrease in function of the involved joint.

Infection (Chapter 10). The inflammatory process within the bone results in destruction of existing bone by increased resorption locally ("*osteolysis*") even though the periosteum reacts by deposition of new bone on the outside of the bone.

Osteolytic Neoplasms (Chapter 14). Some benign bone neoplasms and most malignant bone neoplasms (both primary and secondary) cause a localized destruction of existing bone by increased resorption (*osteolysis*) even though the periosteum and endosteum may deposit "reactive bone."

EPIPHYSEAL PLATES

Reactions of Epiphyseal Plates

You will recall that each epiphyseal plate is a highly specialized cartilaginous structure through which longitudinal growth of bone occurs. Like bone, it is capable of only a very limited number of reactions to a large number of abnormal conditions. There are but three basic ways in which an epiphyseal plate can react: (1) *increased growth*, (2) *decreased growth*, and (3) *torsional growth*. Normal growth in each epiphyseal plate requires an intact structure of the plate, a normal blood supply (which comes in from the epiphyseal side of the plate), and the intermittent pressures associated with normal physical activity. An injury involving the epiphyseal plate may cause part or all of it to close, i.e. to ossify, and thereby stop growing. Prolonged hyperemia stimulates growth while relative ischemia retards it; indeed, complete ischemia of the epiphysis results in necrosis of the attached epiphyseal plate and therefore complete cessation of growth. Excessive *continuous* pressure

on an epiphyseal plate retards growth, and yet, a decrease in the normal *intermittent* pressure (as occurs with decreased function of a limb) also retards growth. If either stimulation or retardation occurs in one part of an epiphyseal plate while normal growth continues in the remainder, growth becomes *uneven*; under these circumstances, a progressive angulatory deformity develops in the bone during subsequent growth.

Examples of Reactions of Epiphyseal Plates

As with bone, the various reactions of epiphyseal plates may be incited by a wide variety of clinical disorders and injuries, some of which arise within the musculoskeletal system and some of which arise within other systems of the body. Examples of these abnormal clinical conditions are only mentioned here but each is discussed in subsequent chapters.

GENERALIZED REACTIONS OF ALL EPIPHYSEAL PLATES

1. Generalized Increase in Growth (Gigantism)

Arachnodactyly (Hyperchondroplasia) (Marfan's Syndrome) (Chapter 8). In this inborn error of development, there is excessive cartilaginous growth (hyperchondroplasia) in all epiphyseal plates (Fig. 3.5).

Pituitary Gigantism (Chapter 9). Excessive growth hormone from an eosinophil adenoma of the anteror pituitary gland *during childhood* stimulates growth in all epiphyseal plates.

2. Generalized Decrease in Growth (Dwarfism)

Achondroplasia (Chapter 8). In this inborn error of development, there is deficient cartilaginous growth (achondroplasia) in all epiphyseal plates (Fig. 3.6).

Pituitary Dwarfism (Lorain type) (Chapter 9). Deficient growth hormone from the anterior pituitary gland *during childhood* retards growth in all epiphyseal plates.

Rickets (Chapter 9). The deficient calcification (hypocalcification) of the pre-osseous cartilage of the epiphyseal plate in the zone of calcifying cartilage results in a retardation of growth in all epiphyseal plates.

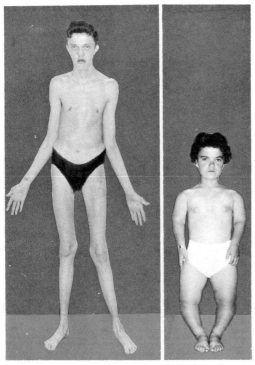

Congenital Arteriovenous Malformations. The continuing hyperemia associated with the various types of arteriovenous malformations provides a continuing stimulation of the epiphyseal plates in the involved limb and consequently an overgrowth of the limb.

2. Localized Decrease in Growth

Disuse Retardation. When a limb is not used normally over a long period, as with prolonged immobilization, prolonged relief of weight bearing or severe paralysis of long duration, the associated decrease in the normal intermittent pressures causes a retar-

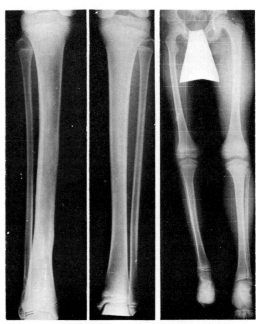

Figure 3.5 (*left*). Arachnodactyly (hyperchondroplasia, Marfan's syndrome). An example of generalized increase in growth. This 14-year-old boy's limbs are long and thin due to excessive cartilaginous growth (hyperchondroplasia) in all epiphyseal plates.
Figure 3.6 (*right*). Achondroplasia (achondroplastic dwarf). An example of generalized decrease in growth. This 13-year-old girl's limbs are short and deformed due to a defective growth (achondroplasia) in all epiphyseal plates.

LOCALIZED REACTIONS OF AN EPIPHYSEAL PLATE

1. Localized Increase in Growth

Chronic Inflammation (Chapter 10). The prolonged hyperemia associated with any chronic inflammatory condition *near* an epiphyseal plate stimulates local growth. This phenomenon is observed in such disorders as chronic osteomyelitis and rheumatoid arthritis (Fig. 3.7).

Displaced Fracture of the Shaft of a Long Bone (Chapter 15). When the nutrient artery to the shaft of a long bone is disrupted by a fracture there follows a temporary compensatory hyperemia at the epiphyseal ends of the long bone and the result is a temporary stimulation of local growth.

Figure 3.7 (*left*). Chronic inflammation of a long bone. An example of localized increase in longitudinal growth in the right tibia of a 14-year-old girl. Chronic osteomyelitis of the right tibia associated with prolonged hyperemia over the preceding 7 years has stimulated local epiphyseal plate growth thereby producing a limb length discrepancy.
Figure 3.8 (*right*). Disuse retardation of bone growth. An example of localized decrease in longitudinal growth in the right lower limb of a 12-year-old boy. Severe residual paralysis from poliomyelitis in early childhood has resulted in a decrease in normal intermittent pressures of muscle pull across the joints and of weight bearing on the long bones of the right lower limb and has thereby led to a local disuse retardation of epiphyseal plate growth and a resultant limb length discrepancy.

dation of growth in the involved limb (Fig. 3.8).

Physical Injury (Chapter 15). A fracture that either crosses the epiphyseal plate or crushes it, is frequently followed by bony union across the plate and therefore a local cessation of growth.

Thermal injury. The cartilage of the epiphyseal plate is sometimes destroyed by either local cold (frostbite) or local heat (burns).

Ischemia (Chapter 13). Total avascular necrosis of an epiphysis is always associated with necrosis of the cartilage of the underlying epiphyseal plate (and cessation of growth) since the epiphyseal vessels supply both structures.

Infection (Chapter 10). The cartilage of the epiphyseal plate is particularly susceptible to the chondrolytic action of the pus produced by some infections, especially those due to Staphylococcus. The cartilage destruction usually involves only part of an epiphyseal plate with the result that subsequent growth is uneven.

3. Localized Torsional Growth

When a growing long bone and its epiphyseal plate are subjected either to continual or to intermittent twisting (torsional) forces, as in certain postural habits of sitting on the floor the bone gradually becomes twisted (develops torsion) in the same direction as the applied force. The torsional deformity in the long bone occurs through torsional growth in the involved epiphyseal plate and it can usually be reversed by applying corrective torsional forces in the opposite direction. Clinical conditions caused by torsional deformities of growing long bones and their correction are discussed in Chapter 7.

SYNOVIAL JOINTS

In a normal synovial joint the smooth and reciprocally shaped cartilaginous opposing surfaces permit frictionless and painless movement. By contrast, any irregularity, or damage, of the articular surface leads inevitably to progressive degenerative changes

in the joint with resultant limitation of movement and pain. The joint capsule is particularly sensitive to stretching and increased fluid pressure within the joint, which helps to explain why abnormal conditions of joints are so distressingly painful. Indeed, disorders and injuries of joints constitute the greatest single physical cause of disability in civilized man.

Reactions of Articular Cartilage

Articular cartilage, which contains no blood vessels, lymphatics or nerves, is capable of reacting to abnormal conditions in only three ways: (1) *destruction*, (2) *degeneration* and (3) *peripheral proliferation*.

In this section on articular cartilage brief reference is made to four scientific investigations that we have conducted using rabbits in our laboratory in the Research Institute of The Hospital for Sick Children in Toronto. They are included here not only as research data relevant to the destruction, degeneration and possible regeneration of articular cartilage but also as examples of the importance of "the philosophy and nature of the medical research" which are presented in Chapter 18. These four investigations include: the harmful effects on articular cartilage of prolonged immobilization of a synovial joint; of continuous compression of joint surfaces; of repeated intra-articular injections of hydrocortisone; and the beneficial effects of a completely new concept, namely continuous passive motion of a synovial joint, on the healing and regeneration of articular cartilage.

The limitations of space in this textbook preclude the possibility of recording the many excellent scientific investigations of orthopaedic surgeon-scientist colleagues in other centers.

1. Destruction

The powers of regeneration of articular cartilage are so limited that destruction of cartilage is a serious and irreparable lesion. Articular cartilage is destroyed by any condition that interferes with its main source of nutrition from synovial fluid, and also by the chondrolytic enzymes present in certain types of pus. Although cartilage is radiolucent, destruction of the cartilage can be detected radiographically by a decrease in the normal width, or thickness, of the *cartilage space* between the radio-opaque bone ends (Fig. 3.9).

The following are examples of abnormal

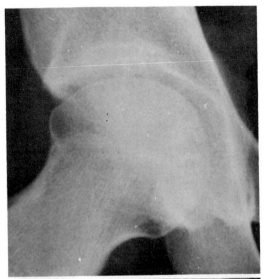

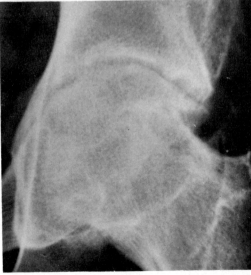

Figure 3.9. Destruction of articular cartilage due to infection. The left hip joint of this 14-year-old girl has been the site of pyogenic infection (septic arthritis). Note the decreased thickness of the cartilage space (a more accurate term than "joint space") of the left hip compared to that of the normal opposite hip (in the radiograph on top), indicating loss of articular cartilage.

conditions that cause destruction of articular cartilage:

Rheumatoid Arthritis (Chapter 10). The pannus, which adheres to cartilage, interferes with nutrition of the cartilage by synovial fluid.

Infections (Chapter 10). The pus of staphylococcal septic arthritis and tuberculous arthritis is particularly chondrolytic.

Ankylosing Spondylitis (Chapter 10). The joint gradually becomes completely obliterated by bony fusion (bony ankylosis).

Prolonged Immobilization of a Synovial Joint. With immobilization of a normal rabbit knee in flexion for as short a period as only three weeks—and more consistently for ten weeks or longer—the synovial membrane becomes adherent to the articular cartilage that is not in contact with the opposing joint surface. This phenomenon obliterates the fluid space between cartilage and synovial membrane thereby blocking the normal synovial fluid nutrition of the underlying cartilage and producing an irreparable lesion that we have called *obliterative degeneration of articular cartilage.* This lesion can also be seen in the cartilage of human patients secondary to prolonged limitation of joint motion associated with persistent joint deformity.

Continuous Compression of Articular Cartilage. When the two opposing joint surfaces of the rabbit knee are continuously compressed against one another (either by means of a skeletal pin compression device or by immobilizing the joint in an extreme, i.e. a forced position of compression) for as short a period as eight days the contact area of the two articular surfaces are completely deprived of their synovial fluid nutrition and the inevitable result is a "pressure sore" that we have designated *compression necrosis of articular cartilage.*

Intra-articular Injections of Hydrocortisone. After two or more weekly injections of hydrocortisone T.B.A. into the knee joint of the rabbit the following progressive degenerative changes are seen in the articular cartilage: thinning, fissuring, fibrillation, depletion of proteoglycans and cystic lesions containing calcium deposits within the matrix. We refer to these harmful effects as *hydrocortisone arthropathy.*

2. Degeneration

A slowly progressive type of degenerative change in articular cartilage is seen as part of the normal aging process; the cartilage becomes thinner and less cellular. These gradual changes of wear and tear render the cartilage less resilient and therefore more susceptible to injury; they are aggravated by excessive loads on joint surfaces (as with obesity), decrease in viscosity of the synovial fluid and local damage, or destruction, of cartilage.

Degeneration of articular cartilage is initiated by a change in the intercellular cement substance of the matrix (*chondromalacia*) and subsequent uncovering of the collagen fibrils (*fibrillation*). Finally the degenerated cartilage, which is primarily in the central or weight-bearing area, becomes eroded thereby exposing the subchondral bone which, with continued movement, becomes thickened, dense (*sclerotic*) and polished (*eburnated*) (Fig. 3.10).

The following abnormal conditions lead to degeneration of articular cartilage:

Premature Aging of Cartilage. This is due to an acceleration of the normal aging process in articular cartilage and is aggravated by excessive wear and tear.

Previous Destruction of Cartilage. All of the destructive lesions mentioned in the previous section (including obliterative degeneration, compression necrosis and hydrocortisone arthropathy) lead to progressive degeneration in the remaining cartilage as has been proven both experimentally and clinically.

Incongruity or Irregularity of joint surfaces. When, as a result of a previous disorder or injury, the two opposing joint surfaces are no longer smooth and congruous, the associated increase in localized areas of increased pressure and increased joint friction leads to excessive and uneven wearing of the articular cartilage with resultant degeneration.

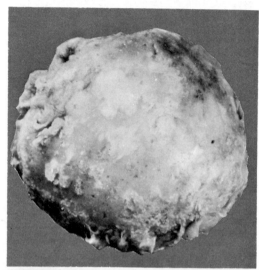

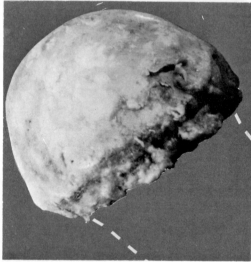

Figure 3.10. Degeneration of articular cartilage of the femoral head of a 70-year-old man with severe degenerative joint disease (osteoarthritis) of the hip. Note the exposed subchondral bone where the degenerated articular cartilage has almost disappeared over the weight-bearing surface. Small islands of thin, degenerated cartilage have persisted over part of the femoral head. The cartilage of the non-weight-bearing area is fibrillated.

3. Peripheral Proliferation

The peripheral articular rim of cartilage of a synovial joint, unlike the central area, is covered by a type of perichondrium which is continuous with the synovial membrane. In the presence of degeneration of the central area of cartilage and with continued movement, the peripheral perichondrium proliferates and gradually produces an almost complete peripheral ring of thickened cartilage. Thus, the peripheral ring (which in any single view resembles a lip) is initially composed of cartilage (*chondrophyte formation*) but it subsequently ossifies (*osteophyte formation*) (Fig. 3.11).

The Possibility of Healing and Regeneration of Articular Cartilage. As has been demonstrated by many investigators, damaged articular cartilage is extremely limited in its ability to either heal or regenerate; this accounts for the relentless progression of degenerative arthritis (osteoarthritis) as an inevitable sequel to such damage.

Despite the fact that *rest* and *motion* are the most commonly prescribed forms of treatment for musculoskeletal disorders and injuries, the relative importance, timing and duration of each remain controversial. Unfortunately, the majority of involved physicians and surgeons are "resters" rather than "movers"—based more on long established tradition and time-honored empiricism than on scientific investigations.

The aforementioned investigations on the deleterious effects of immobilization of joints, with or without compression (as well as the investigations of others) led us to consider the exact antithesis of continuous rest, namely continuous motion. It was obvious that because of the fatiguability of skeletal muscle, continuous motion would have to be passive rather than active. Con-

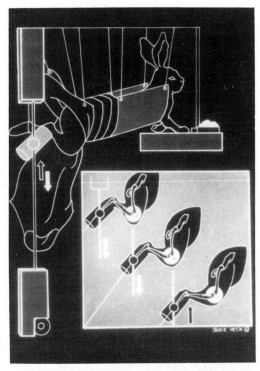

Figure 3.12. A rabbit's right hind limb in the continuous passive motion apparatus that is run by an electric motor. The range of motion used was an arc of 70° (from 40° to 110° of flexion).

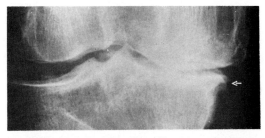

Figure 3.11. Peripheral proliferation of articular cartilage in the right knee joint of a 60-year-old man with degenerative joint disease (osteoarthritis). Note the bony "lip" or "spur" on the medial edge of the tibial joint surface (arrow) indicating osteophyte formation which was preceded by chondrophyte formation.

sequently, in 1970 we developed the new concept of *continuous passive motion* (CPM) of a synovial joint *in vivo* based on the hypothesis that such motion would stimulate the healing and regeneration of articular cartilage through differentiation of pluripotential mesenchymal cells in the subchondral bone. Since then a wide variety of scientific investigations in our Research Institute have proven that CPM stimulates and accelerates the healing of tendons and ligaments as well as the healing of cartilage in intra-articular fractures and the regeneration of articular cartilage in full-thickness defects much more than does either immobilization or intermittent active motion (Figs. 3.12 to 3.18). This new concept has now been applied to the post-operative management of various musculoskeletal disorders and injuries in human patients as is discussed in Chapters 6 and 15.

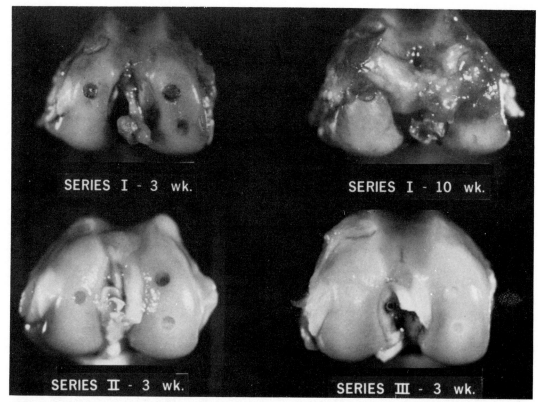

Figure 3.13. Gross appearances of typical defects in the three series of experiments (adolescent rabbits). *Series I* (immobilization for ten weeks): note the granulation-like tissue in the defects. *Series I* (immobilization for ten weeks: note the numerous extensive intra-articular synovial adhesions in the region of each of three defects in the femoral condyles; there are no adhesions in the region of the defects in the patellar groove. *Series II* (intermittent active motion for three weeks): healing of the defects is somewhat better in this series than in Series I at three weeks, but healing is still incomplete. *Series III* (continuous passive motion for three weeks): healing of the defects is by tissue grossly resembling articular cartilage. Healing in this series is considerably more complete than in either Series I or Series II.

Reactions of Synovial Membrane

The synovial membrane, which secretes synovial fluid, for both nutrition and lubrication of the articular cartilage, is capable of reacting to abnormal conditions in one or more of three ways: (1) by producing an excessive amount of fluid (*an effusion*), (2) by becoming thicker (*hypertrophy*) and (3) by forming *adhesions* between itself and the articular cartilage. A joint effusion may be *serous*, as with mild sprains; it may be an *inflammatory exudate*, as in synovitis and rheumatoid arthritis; it may be grossly *purulent*, as with septic arthritis, or it may be *hemorrhagic*, as with severe injury or in hemophilia. All but the transient serous effusions are accompanied by varying degrees of synovial hypertrophy and synovial adhesion formation. Synovial adhesions can also form as a result of prolonged limitation of joint movement from any cause, including immobilization in a cast or a rigid splint.

The synovial membranes of tendon sheaths and bursae are capable of the same reactions to abnormal conditions as are the synovial membranes of joints.

Reactions of Joint Capsule and Ligaments

The fibrous joint capsule and ligaments allow the *desired* range of movement but provide stability of the joint by preventing *undesired* movements. These structures

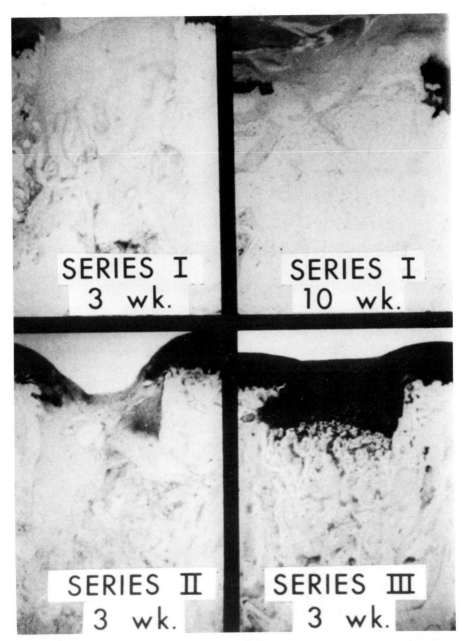

Figure 3.14. Appearances by light microscopy, depicting the degree of metachromasia of the matrix in typical defects of the three series in adolescent animals (toluidine blue, 27×). *Series I* (immobilization for three weeks): there is no metachromatic staining of the matrix. *Series I* (immobilization for ten weeks): there is still no metachromatic staining of the matrix. *Series II* (intermittent active motion for three weeks): the matrix of the reparative tissues exhibits only slight metachromatic staining. *Series III* (continuous passive motion for three weeks): the matrix of the reparative tissue exhibits near-normal metachromatic staining compared with that of the intact articular cartilage beyond the edges of the defect.

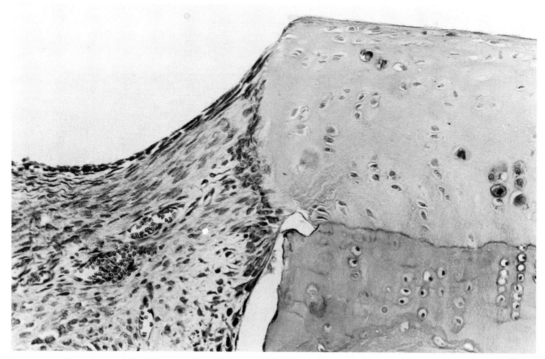

Figure 3.15. Series I (immobilization for three weeks). At three weeks, the defect at the left is filled with predominantly vascular fibrous tissue that is not well bonded to the subchondral bone (hematoxylin and eosin, 301×).

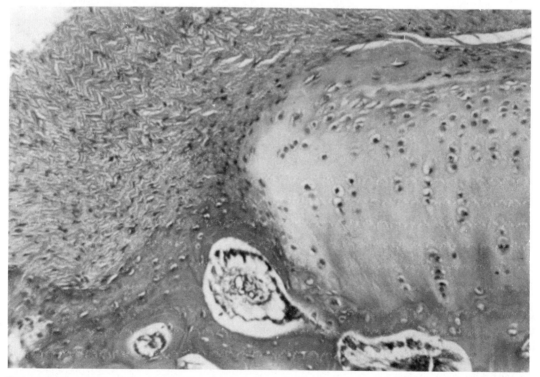

Figure 3.16. Series I (immobilization for ten weeks). At ten weeks, the superficial portion of the defect at the left has been filled with predominantly fibrous tissue that is continuous with the fibrous tissue of an extensive overlying intra-articular synovial adhesion. The deeper portion of the defect is filled with new bone hematoxyline and eosin, 301×).

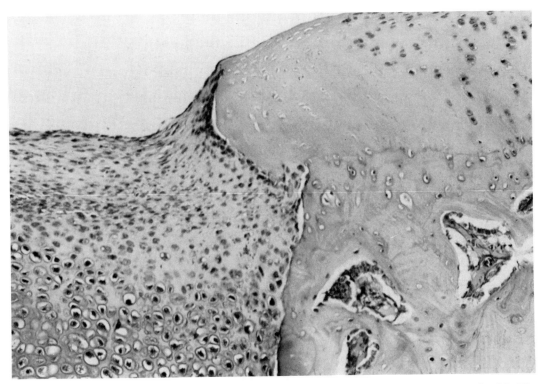

Figure 3.17. Series II (intermittent active motion for three weeks in adolescent animals). The depressed surface layers of the healing tissue at the left contain predominantly fibrous tissue. Immediately below the level of the tide mark the tissue is composed of incompletely differentiated mesenchymal cells. In the deeper layer the tissue is preosseous cartilage that will undergo endochondral ossification (hematoxyln and eosin, 200×).

react to abnormal conditions either (1) by becoming unduly stretched and elongated (*joint laxity*), thereby permitting instability of the joint, or (2) by becoming tight and shortened (*joint contracture*), thereby limiting the range of joint movement.

1. JOINT LAXITY

The following abnormal conditions result in undue joint laxity:

Generalized Congenital Laxity of Capsules and Ligaments (Chapter 7). This abnormality is probably determined genetically.

Injury (Chapters 15, 16, 17). Traumatic dislocation or subluxation with rupture of capsule or ligaments leads to instability of the joint.

Infection (Chapter 10). In septic arthritis the capsule may be destroyed by pus, thereby leading to a *pathological dislocation* of the joint.

2. JOINT CONTRACTURE

The following abnormal conditions may result in a joint contracture with limitation of joint motion.

Congenital Joint Contractures. These are seen in certain congenital deformities such as clubfeet.

Infection. Fibrosis and scar formation of the capsule following infection may lead to a fibrous contracture of the joint.

Chronic Arthritis. Rheumatoid arthritis and degenerative joint disease both lead to progressive fibrous contracture of the joint.

Muscle Contracture. Ischemic contracture, muscle imbalance and prolonged muscle spasm eventually result in muscle contracture with consequent limitation of motion of the joint that is normally moved by the involved muscle.

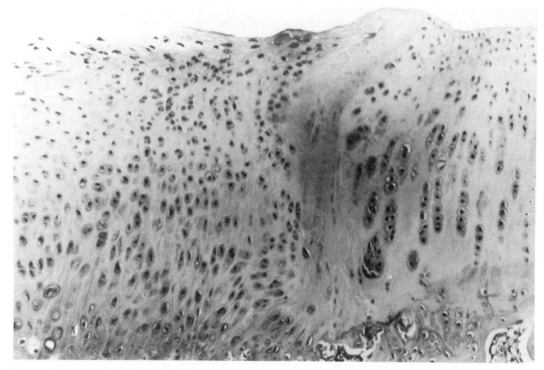

Figure 3.18. Series III (continuous passive motion for four weeks in adolescent animals). The cells of the reparative tissue at the the left are chondrocytes. This tissue is more cellular than the adjacent mature cartilage (hematoxylin and eosin, 200×).

SKELETAL MUSCLE

Reactions of Skeletal Muscle

The complex structure of skeletal muscle reacts to the many disorders and injuries of the musculoskeletal system in a limited number of ways including *atrophy, hypertrophy, necrosis, contracture* and *regeneration.* You will recall from the discussion of muscle in Chapter 2 that a *single motor unit* of skeletal muscle consists of the anterior horn cell, its axon within a peripheral nerve fiber, the myoneural junctions and the individual muscle fibers supplied by the single anterior horn cell. Thus, the reactions of skeletal muscle may be incited by a disorder or injury of any one of these components.

DISUSE ATROPHY

Skeletal muscle that is not being used normally, for whatever reason, invariably reacts by becoming weaker and smaller (*disuse atrophy*) (Fig. 3.19). A disorder of the anterior horn cell (such as poliomyelitis),

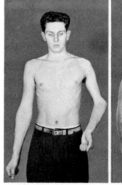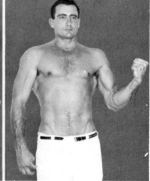

Figure 3.19. (*left*).   Disuse atrophy of muscle in the left arm of a 15-year-old boy due to prolonged stiffness of the left elbow from an old intra-articular fracture that had been treated by prolonged immobilization in a cast.

Figure 3.20 (*right*).   Work hypertrophy of muscle. This man vigorously exercises his muscles daily (by isometric contraction) to make them stronger and larger. The resultant hypertrophy of muscle, which is due to an enlargement of individual muscle fibers, is dependent upon continuation of the exercises.

of the peripheral nerve fiber (such as polyneuritis), of the myoneural junction (such as myasthenia gravis), or of the individual muscle fiber (such as muscular dystrophy) can all incite the reaction of disuse atrophy, as can injury to any of these components. In addition, disuse atrophy is caused by prolonged immobilzation of the associated joints, stiffness of the joints and chronic joint disease. Indeed, pain arising in an abnormal joint initiates a reflex inhibition of contraction in associated muscles, a phenomenon that results in additional atrophy of muscle.

WORK HYPERTROPHY

When a given muscle is repeatedly exercised against resistance, particularly by isometric contraction, it reacts by becoming stronger and larger (*work hypertrophy*) (Fig. 3.20). The hypertrophy is due to an enlargement of individual muscle fibers and not to an increased number of fibers; it is dependent upon continuation of the exercises.

ISCHEMIC NECROSIS (CHAPTER 15)

Occlusion of arteries supplying muscle, whether by persistent traumatic vascular spasm, thrombosis or embolism, results in *ischemic necrosis* of the muscle within six hours, a fact that is of great practical importance, particularly when you are dealing with injuries of the limbs.

CONTRACTURE

If a muscle remains in a shortened state for a prolonged period, it develops a persistent shortening that is resistant to stretching (*muscle contracture*). Such a contracture eventually becomes irreversible. Muscle contractures also develop in certain diseases of muscle such as polymyositis, muscular dystrophy and cerebral palsy. In addition, the muscle fibers of a necrotic muscle are subsequently replaced by dense fibrous scar tissue which undergoes progressive *fibrous contracture* with the production of progressive joint deformities (Fig. 3.21).

REGENERATION

Injured muscle fibers may regenerate, to some degree at least, from the sarcolemma and muscle cells and possibly from the activity of the satellite cells in each fiber. Following *partial* loss of innervation of a skeletal muscle, at least some of the paralyzed muscle fibers may gain a new motor nerve fiber from remaining intact nerve fibers, in which case there will be a corresponding recovery of muscle power.

MUSCULOSKELETAL DEFORMITIES

Many disorders and injuries of the musculoskeletal system are manifest by an abnormal form, or shape, of the affected limb or trunk (*musculoskeletal deformity*). Some of these deformities, such as clubfeet, are strikingly obvious on external inspection even to the casual observer, whereas others, such as a mild curvature of the spine, are more subtle and not immediately obvious; still others, such as an abnormal shape of a joint surface, are hidden by the skin and soft tissues and are apparent only on "*internal inspection*" by radiographic examination. Musculoskeletal deformities may arise in bones, in joints, or in soft tissues and a given deformity may involve one or more of these structures.

When confronted with a musculoskeletal deformity in one of your patients, you must consider first the *structure*, or *structures*, in which the deformity is taking place, and secondly, the likely *cause* of the deformity.

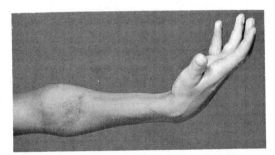

Figure 3.21. Fibrous contracture of muscle. This 10-year-old boy's forearm had been ischemic for a period of 12 hours as a result of vascular damage associated with a supracondylar fracture of the humerus. The resultant ischemic necrosis of the forearm muscles (Volkmann's ischemic necrosis) has resulted in replacement of muscle by dense fibrous scar tissue with production of a fibrous contracture of the muscles.

In addition, you must assess the *significance* of the deformity, not only concerning its *appearance*, but also concerning its present or future effect on *function*. A deformity may be *congenital* (present at the time birth) or it may be *acquired* during post-natal life. The many musculoskeletal deformities will be discussed individually in subsequent chapters, but at this stage, having studied the reactions of musculoskeletal tissues to disorders and injuries, you will find it helpful to consider, in a general way, the *types* and *causes* of deformity in the various musculoskeletal *structures*. Indeed, an *understanding* of these aspects of deformities will help you to think in terms of their diagnosis and their possible *prevention* as well as their *correction*.

Types of Bony Deformity

1. LOSS OF ALIGNMENT

A long bone may be out of alignment either because it is twisted in its long axis (*torsional deformity*), or because it is crooked (*angulatory deformity*) (Fig. 3.22). If the angulatory deformity is close to a joint, the deformity may *seem* on external inspection to be taking place in the joint, but "internal inspection" by radiographic examination will reveal the true site of the deformity. Angulatory deformity in a short bone, such as a vertebral body, is associated with a change in its entire shape, and since its upper and lower surface are no longer parallel, it resembles a wedge.

2. ABNORMAL LENGTH

A long bone may be abnormally short (or even absent), or it may be abnormally long. When the deformity involves only one of a pair of limbs, the results is a *limb length discrepancy* (Fig. 3.23).

3. BONY OUTGROWTH

A lesion, such as an osteochondroma, arising from the surface of a bone may change its configuration sufficiently to produce a bony deformity that is obvious clinically (Fig. 3.24).

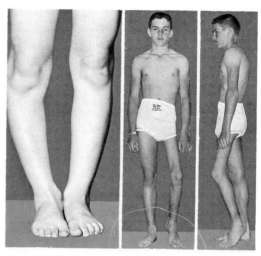

Figure 3.22 (*left*). Angulatory deformity in the upper part of the right tibia of a 9-year-old girl as a result of retarded growth on the medial side of the epiphyseal plate and continuing growth on the lateral side.

Figure 3.23 (*right*). Limb length discrepancy due to retardation of growth in the epiphyseal plates of the left lower limb of a 15-year-old boy following paralytic poliomyelitis in early childhood. Note also the marked atrophy of the limb and the knee flexion deformity.

Causes of Bony Deformity

1. CONGENITAL ABNORMALITIES OF BONY DEVELOPMENT (CHAPTER 8)

The bone may be absent, because of failure to develop (*aplasia*), may be underdeveloped (*hypoplasia*), or may be abnormally developed (*dysplasia*) or even doubly developed as in extra digits (*duplication*).

2. FRACTURES (CHAPTERS 15, 16 and 17)

Loss of alignment may occur at the time of fracture and if it is not corrected by adequate reduction, the bone will heal with residual bony deformity (*malunion*). When a fracture fails to unite (*non-union*), there is usually residual deformity at the site. Fractures through abnormal bone (*pathological fractures*) may be gross and produce deformities similar to those of fractures through normal bone, or they may be microscopic and repeated, in which case, they produce progressive bony deformities as in osteoporotic vertebral bodies.

3. DISTURBANCES OF EPIPHYSEAL PLATE GROWTH (CHAPTERS 7, 8, 13 AND 16)

The deformities arising from the various reactions of epiphyseal plates to disorders and injuries have already been considered in a general way in this chapter.

4. BENDING OF ABNORMALLY SOFT BONE (CHAPTER 9)

In certain generalized metabolic bone diseases, such as rickets and osteomalacia, the bone matrix (osteoid) is not normally calcified so that the bones are abnormally "soft" and will gradually bend or twist without an obvious fracture.

5. OVERGROWTH OF ADULT BONE (CHAPTERS 9 AND 14)

In certain disseminated bone disorders, such as osteitis deformans (Paget's disease), the adult bone becomes thickened and crooked. Furthermore, certain bone lesions, such as an osteochondroma, growing outward from the surface of bone produce a localized bony deformity which, if large and superficial, results in an obvious clinical deformity (Fig. 3.24).

Types of Joint Deformity

1. DISPLACEMENT OF THE JOINT

When the normal reciprocal relationship between the two joint surfaces is lost, the joint is said to be displaced. The joint may be completely displaced (*dislocated, luxated*) or it may be only partially displaced (*subluxated*). In either case the joint is unstable and is associated with deformity (Fig. 3.25).

2. EXCESSIVE MOBILITY (HYPERMOBILITY) OF THE JOINT

The fibrous joint capsule and ligaments normally serve as "check-reins" preventing excessive mobility (hypermobility) of the joint. If they are congenitally lax, stretched, or torn, the resultant hypermobility causes a deformity to appear when stress, such as

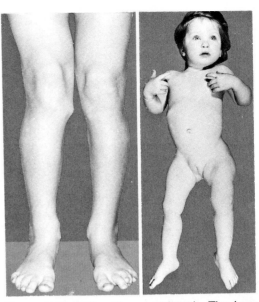

Figure 3.24 (*left*).   Bony outgrowth. The bony deformity on the medial side of this woman's right knee is due to an osteochondroma (osteocartilaginous exostosis), a type of benign bone lesion arising from the medial surface of the upper end of the tibia.

Figure 3.25 (*right*).   Displacement of a joint. This 2-year-old girl's left hip joint has been completely displaced (dislocated) since birth and is therefore unstable. Note the associated deformity of adduction and shortening of the left lower limb.

bearing weight, is transmitted to that joint (Fig. 3.26).

3. RESTRICTED MOBILITY OF THE JOINT

When for any reason, mobility of a joint is restricted, a type of joint deformity is present. For example, if a knee joint lacks the last 30° of extension, the condition is described as a 30° knee-flexion deformity (Fig. 3.27).

Causes of Joint Deformity

1. CONGENITAL ABNORMALITIES OF JOINT DEVELOPMENT (CHAPTER 8)

The joint may be unstable at birth and become dislocated, as in congenital dislocation of the hip; it may develop with restricted mobility and contractures, as in a congenital clubfoot; or it may fail to develop (*failure of segmentation*), as in congenital

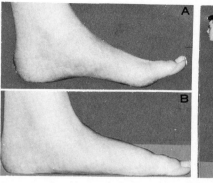
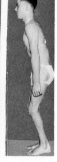

Figure 3.26 (*left*).   Excessive mobility (hypermobility) of joints. *A*, this 10-year-old boy's foot is hypermobile due to generalized joint laxity but it looks normal when not weight bearing. *B*, On bearing weight, the hypermobile joints in the foot allow the foot to appear flat and therefore deformed.
Figure 3.27 (*right*).   Restricted mobility of a joint. This 12-year-old boy demonstrates a bilateral knee flexion deformity in that he is unable to extend his knee joints completely. The cause of this boy's deformity is muscle imbalance due to persistent spasticity and contracture of the hamstring muscles from cerebral palsy, an upper motor neuron lesion.

radioulnar synostosis. All joints of the body may be hypermobile due to congenital generalized laxity of ligaments. Any of these congenital abnormalities can produce joint deformity (Fig. 3.18)

2. ACQUIRED DISLOCATIONS

When a joint is dislocated, either as a result of injury (traumatic dislocation), or infection (pathological dislocation), an unstable joint deformity occurs.

3. MECHANICAL BLOCKS

In degenerative joint disorders, such as osteoarthritis, and displaced intra-articular fractures, the opposing surfaces of the joint become irregular and since they no longer fit well, they are said to be *incongruous*; as a result, joint mobility is restricted by a mechanical bony block. Internal derangements of a joint, such as a displaced torn meniscus and a loose body, can likewise restrict joint mobility by a mechanical block within the joint.

4. JOINT ADHESIONS

In certain inflammatory joint disorders, such as rheumatoid arthritis and septic arthritis, the articular cartilage is partially or completely destroyed with the result that adhesions may form within the joints, either between the joint surfaces or between synovial membrane and a joint surface. Likewise, following either injury or infection, muscles or their tendons may become tethered to bone by adhesions thereby preventing normal muscle action and tendon gliding. Whether the adhesions are in the joint (intra-articular) or outside the joint (extra-articular), the associated restriction of joint motion results in joint deformity.

5. MUSCLE CONTRACTURES

In a given muscle, persistent shortening which is resistant to stretching (muscle contracture), may result from prolonged muscle spasm (due to pain), prolonged immobilization, muscle diseases and ischemic necrosis of muscle. The result of the muscle contracture is deformity in the joint, or joints, normally controlled by that muscle.

6. MUSCLE IMBALANCE

Persistent imbalance of power between the various muscles that control movement of a given joint may be due to *flaccid* paralysis, as in poliomyelitis, or *spastic* paralysis, as in the spastic type of cerebral palsy. In either case the continuing unequal muscle pull gradually produces a progressive joint deformity, particularly during childhood because of the added factor of skeletal growth. (Fig. 3.20).

7. FIBROUS CONTRACTURES OF FASCIA AND SKIN

Persistent shortening of fibrous scar tissue (fibrous contracture) in skin, as seen in severe burns, and of deep fascia, as seen in Dupuytren's contracture of the palmar aponeurosis, produces restriction of joint mobility with resultant deformity in the underlying and nearby joints.

8. EXTERNAL PRESSURES

When external pressures repeatedly force a joint into a deformed position, the ligaments on the convex side of the deformity become stretched while those on the concave side become contracted. As a result the deformity eventually becomes permanent. Common examples are the various toe deformities such as hallux valgus with a bunion produced or aggravated by the pressure effects of tight, pointed shoes in girls and women, the victims of fashion.

9. JOINT DEFORMITIES OF UNKNOWN ETIOLOGY (IDIOPATHIC)

Certain joint deformities, such as the *idiopathic* type of lateral curvature of the spine (scoliosis), develop in otherwise healthy children for no apparent reason. Secondary bony deformities and secondary soft tissue contractures develop eventually in idiopathic scoliosis but the primary cause of the scoliosis has eluded detection to date and remains a challenging mystery.

Suggested Additional Reading

Albright, J. A. and Brand, R. A. (ed.): *The Scientific Basis of Orthopaedics*. New York, Appleton-Century Crofts, 1979.

Bentley, G.: Repair of articular cartilage. In *Scientific Foundations of Orthopaedics and Traumatology*, edited by Owen, R., Goodfellow, J. and Bullough, P. G. London, William Heinemann Medical Books Ltd., 1980.

Boyd, W. and Sheldon H.: *Introduction to the Study of Disease*. Philadelphia, Lea and Febiger, 1980.

Freeman, M. A. R. (ed.): *Adult Articular Cartilage*, 2nd ed. Kent, U.K., Pitman Medical, 1979

Ham, A. W. and Cormak, D. H.: Histophysiology of cartilage, bone and joints. In *Histology*, 8th ed. Philadelphia, J.B. Lippincott, Co., 1979.

Hughes, S. and Sweetnam, R.: *The Basis and Practice of Orthopaedics*. London, William Heinemann Medical Books Ltd., 1980.

Main, B. J.: Effects of immobilization on the skeleton. In *Scientific Foundations of Orthopaedics and Traumatology*, edited by Owen, R., Goodfellow, J. and Bullough, P.G. London. William Heinemann Medical Books Ltd., 1980.

Mankin, H. J.: The response of articular cartilage to mechanical injury. J. Bone Joint Surg. 64A: 460–466, 1982.

Salter, R. B., Gross, A. and Hall, J. H.: Hydrocortisone arthropathy—an experimental investigation. Can. Med. Assoc. 97: 374–377, 1967.

Salter, R. B. and Field, P.: The effects of continuous compression on living articular cartilage. An experimental investigation. J. Bone Joint Surg. 42A: 31–49, 1960.

Salter, R. B., McNeill, O. R. and Carbin, R.: The pathological changes in articular cartilage associated with persistent joint deformity. An experimental investigation. In *Studies of Rheumatoid Disease: Proceedings of the Third Canadian Conference on the Rheumatic Diseases*, University of Toronto Press, Toronto, 1965.

Salter, R. B. and Ogilvie-Harris, D. J.: Healing of intra-articular fractures with continuous passive motion. American Academy of Orthopaedic Surgeons, Instructional Course Lectures, vol. 28, chap. 6, pp. 102–117, St Louis, C. V. Mosby 1979.

Salter, R. B., Simmonds, D. F., Malcolm, B. W., Rumble, E. J., Macmichael, D. and Clements, N. G.: The biological effects of continuous passive motion on the healing of full thickness defects in articular cartilage: an experimental investigation in the rabbit. J. Bone Joint Surg. 62A: 1232–1251, 1980.

Sokoloff, L. (ed.): *The Joints and Synovial Fluid. A Two Volume Treatise*. New York, Academic Press, 1978.

Turek, S. L.: *Orthopaedics, Principles and Their Application*, 3rd ed. Philadelphia, J.B. Lippincott, 1977.

Uhthoff, H. K. and Jaworski, Z. F. G.: Bone loss in response to long-term immobilization. J. Bone Joint Surg. 60B: 420–429, 1978.

Woo, S. L. Y., Kuei, S. C., Amiel, D., Gomez, M. A., Hayes, W. C., White F. C. and Akeson, W. H.: The effect of prolonged physical training on the properties of long bone: a study of Wolff's law. J. Bone Joint Surg. 63A: 780–787, 1981.

"If you wish to converse
with me, define your terms."
—Voltaire

CHAPTER 4

Some Important Pairs of Clinical Terms

Terms Describing Movements of Joints
   Active and Passive Movement
   Abduction and Adduction
   Dorsiflexion and Plantar (or Palmar) Flexion
   Eversion and Inversion
   Internal Rotation and External Rotation
   Pronation and Supination
Terms Describing Deformities in Limbs
   Calcaneus and Equinus
   Cavus and Planus
   Internal Torsion and External Torsion
   Anteversion and Retroversion
   Angulation or Bowing Deformities
   Varus and Valgus

Before introducing you to the various clinical conditions of the musculoskeletal system, it would seem only fair to explain the meaning of several important pairs of clinical terms in the musculoskeletal language in order to avoid confusion from the start. The terms of each pair have opposite meanings and, as such, are frequently confused in the minds of medical students (occasionally even in the minds of medical doctors). All of the terms describe either movements of joints or deformities in limbs and, therefore, they are used very frequently in discussions of clinical conditions of the musculoskeletal system. Once you have learned these terms thoroughly, they will become as much a part of your vocabulary as "right" and "left" and you will no longer have to stop and figure out which is which in any given pair.

TERMS DESCRIBING MOVEMENTS OF JOINTS

Active and Passive Movement

Movement of a joint may be either *active* or *passive*. *Active movement* occurs as a result of the individual's own muscular activity. *Passive movement* occurs as a result of an external force, such as movement of the joint by another individual (such as a physiotherapist), gravity, or even—in the case of continuous passive motion (CPM)—by a motorized device, a "CPM mobilimb" (as discussed in Chapter 6).

Abduction and Adduction

The movements of abduction and adduction occur at the shoulder, hip, metacarpophalangeal and metatarsophalangeal joints.

Abduction: the movement of a part *away from* the midline of the body (Fig. 4.1).

Adduction: the movement of a part *toward* the midline of the body (Fig. 4.2).

In the hand and in the foot, the midline

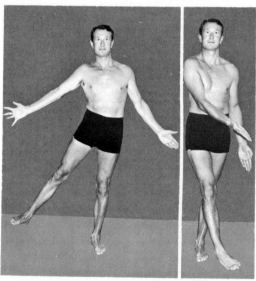

Figure 4.1 (*left*).   Abduction at right shoulder, right hip and metacarpophalangeal joints of right hand.

Figure 4.2 (*right*).   Adduction at right shoulder, right hip and metacarpophalangeal joints of right hand.

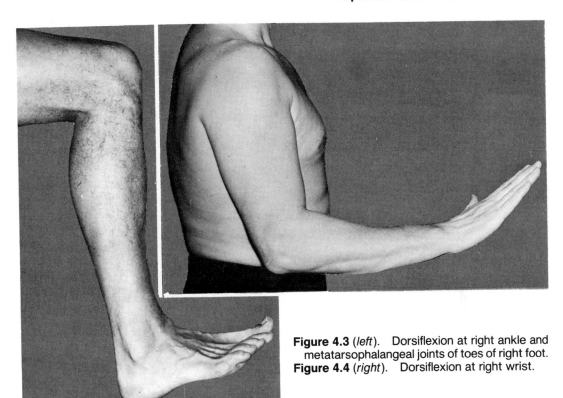

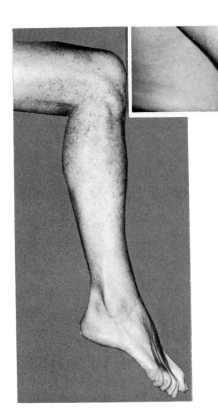

Figure 4.3 (*left*). Dorsiflexion at right ankle and metatarsophalangeal joints of toes of right foot.
Figure 4.4 (*right*). Dorsiflexion at right wrist.

Figure 4.5. Plantar flexion at right ankle and metatarsophalangeal joints of toes of right foot.
Figure 4.6. Palmar flexion at right wrist, metacarpophalangeal joints and interphalangeal joints of fingers of right hand.

used as a reference for the digits is a line along the middle finger and middle toe respectively.

Dorsiflexion and Plantar (or Palmar) Flexion

The movements of dorsiflexion and plantar flexion occur at the ankle and toe joints. The movements of dorsiflexion and palmar flexion occur at the wrist and finger joints.

Dorsiflexion: the movement of the foot or toes in the direction of the *dorsal* surface (Fig. 4.3). Also movement of the hand or fingers in the direction of the *dorsal* surface (Fig. 4.4).

Plantar flexion: the movement of the foot or toes in the direction of the *plantar* surface (Fig. 4.5).

Palmar flexion: the movement of the hand or fingers in the direction of the *palmar* surface (Fig. 4.6).

Eversion and Inversion

The movements of eversion and inversion occur by simultaneous motion at the subtalar and midtarsal joints of the foot.

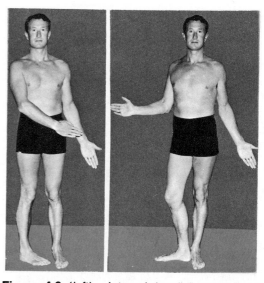

Figure 4.9 (*left*). Internal (medial) rotation at right shoulder and right hip.
Figure 4.10 (*right*). External (lateral) rotation of right shoulder and right hip.

Eversion: the turning of the plantar surface of the foot *outward* in relation to the leg (Fig. 4.7).

Inversion: the turning of the plantar surface of foot *inward* in relation to the leg (Fig. 4.8).

Internal Rotation and External Rotation

The movements of internal rotation (medial rotation) and external rotation (lateral rotation) occur at the shoulder, the hip and to a slight degree at the knee.

Internal (medial) rotation: the turning of the anterior surface of the limb *inward or medially* (Fig. 4.9).

External (lateral) rotation: the turning of the anterior surface of the limb *outward or laterally* (Fig. 4.10).

Pronation and Supination

The movements of pronation and supination occur in the forearm through the elbow and wrist joint, and in the forefoot through the midtarsal joint.

Pronation of the forearm: the turning of the palmar surface of the hand *downwards* or toward the *posterior* surface of the body (Fig. 4.11).

Pronation of the forefoot usually refers to

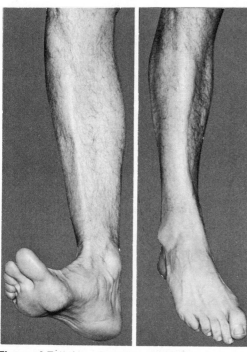

Figure 4.7 (*left*). Eversion of right foot at subtalar and midtarsal joints.
Figure 4.8 (*right*). Inversion of right foot at subtalar and midtarsal joints.

a deformity in which the forefoot is maintained in a position of *eversion* (Fig. 4.7).

Supination of the forearm: the turning of the palmar surface of the hand *upward* or toward the *anterior* surface of the body (Fig. 4.12).

Supination of the forefoot usually refers to a deformity in which the forefoot is maintained in a position of *inversion* (Fig. 4.8).

TERMS DESCRIBING DEFORMITIES IN LIMBS

The types and causes of musculoskeletal deformities are discussed in a general way in Chapter 3, but the descriptive terminology of such deformities merits discussion here. The following terms are used clinically in describing joint deformities:

Postural deformity: one associated with,

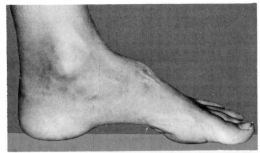
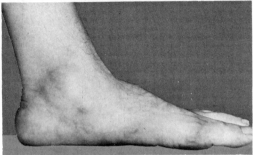

Figure 4.15 (*upper*). Cavus deformity of left foot (pes cavus).
Figure 4.16 (*lower*). Planus deformity of left foot (pes planus) (flat foot).

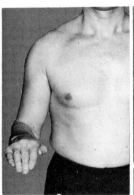
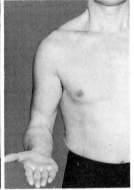

Figure 4.11 (*left*). Pronation of the right forearm at proximal and distal radioulnar joints.
Figure 4.12 (*right*). Supination of the right forearm at proximal and distal radioulnar joints.

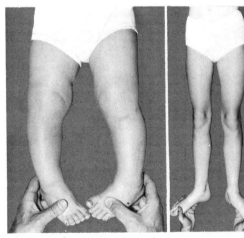

Figure 4.17 (*left*). Internal torsion of the tibia (bilateral).
Figure 4.18 (*right*). External torsion of the tibia (bilateral).

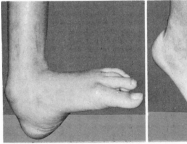
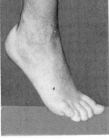

Figure 4.13 (*left*). Calcaneus deformity (ankle calcaneus).
Figure 4.14 (*right*). Equinus deformity (ankle equinus)

or the result of, a given posture. This type of deformity can be corrected by the patient's own muscle action.

Static deformity: one associated with the role of gravity when the body is not in motion.

Dynamic deformity: one which occurs as

a result of the patient's own muscle action. Such a deformity is usually the result of muscle imbalance and is not resistant to passive correction; it is a mobile deformity.

Fixed or structural deformity: one which is relatively resistant to passive correction.

Calcaneus and Equinus

These deformities occur at the ankle only (ankle calcaneus, ankle equinus).

Calcaneus: a deformity in which the foot is maintained in a position of *dorsiflexion* so that on weight bearing, only the *heel* touches the floor (Fig. 4.13).

Equinus: a deformity in which the foot is maintained in a position of *plantar flexion* so that on weight bearing only the *forefoot* touches the floor (Fig. 4.14).

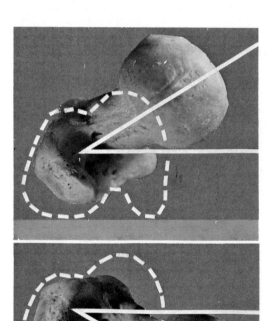

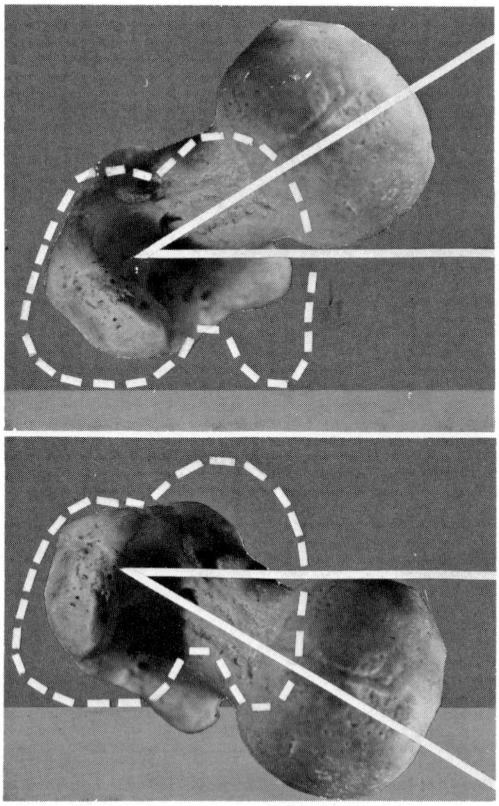

Figure 4.19 (*upper*).   Anteversion of the femoral neck (femoral anteversion).
Figure 4.20 (*lower*).   Retroversion of the femoral neck (femoral retroversion).

Cavus and Planus

These deformities occur only in the foot (pes cavus and pes planus).

(Pes) cavus: an *exaggeration* of the normal longitudinal arch of the foot, an unduly *high* arch (Fig. 4.15). The combined deformity of calcaneus of the hind foot and equinus, or plantar flexion, of the forefoot is called *calcaneocavus.*

(Pes) planus: a diminution of the normal longitudinal arch of the foot, an unduly *low* arch, or flat foot (Fig. 4.16).

Internal Torsion and External Torsion

These deformities represent a twist in the longitudinal axis of a long bone, usually the tibia or the femur.

Internal torsion: the anterior aspect of the distal end of the long bone is twisted *inward* or *medially* in relation to the anterior aspect of its proximal end, e.g. internal tibial torsion (Fig. 4.17) and internal femoral torsion.

External torsion: the anterior aspect of the distal end of the long bone is twisted *outward* or *laterally* in relation to the anterior aspect of its proximal end, e.g. external tibial torsion (Fig. 4.18) and external femoral torsion.

Anteversion and Retroversion

These deformities refer to the relationship between the neck of the femur and the femoral shaft.

(Femoral) anteversion: when the knee is directed anteriorly, the femoral neck is directed *anteriorly* to some degree (Fig. 4.19).

(Femoral) retroversion: when the knee is directed anteriorly, the femoral neck is directed *posteriorly* to some degree (Fig. 4.20).

Angulation or Bowing Deformities

An angulation deformity occurs most frequently at the site of a fracture in the shaft of a long bone but may also occur as a bowing deformity within an intact bone. Considerable confusion exists concerning the description of such angulation or bowing deformities. (Anterior or posterior? Medial or lateral?) The adjective describing an angu-

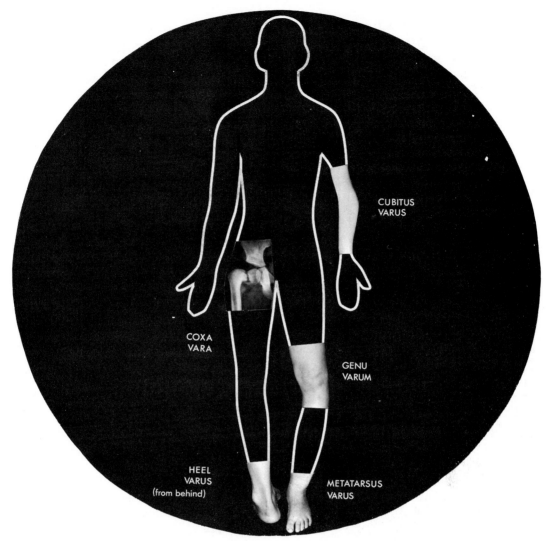

Figure 4.21. Varus deformities. The angulation of the deformity conforms to imaginary circle in which the patient is placed.

lation or bowing deformity refers to the direction in which the *apex of the angle* points (rather than the direction in which the distal fragment points).

Varus and Valgus

The deformities of varus and valgus refer to *abnormal angulation* within a limb. The angulation deformity is usually in a joint, or in a bone near a joint, but it may also take place through the shaft of a long bone. This particular pair of terms has probably caused more confusion than any other pair, partly because the original Latin terms had the opposite meaning to that which is now universally accepted. You will find it easy to remember which is which by thinking of the patient, in the anatomical position, *within an imaginary circle.*

VARUS

An angulation that *conforms* to an imaginary circle in which the patient is placed (Fig. 4.21).

Cubitus varus: a decrease in the normal carrying angle at the elbow.

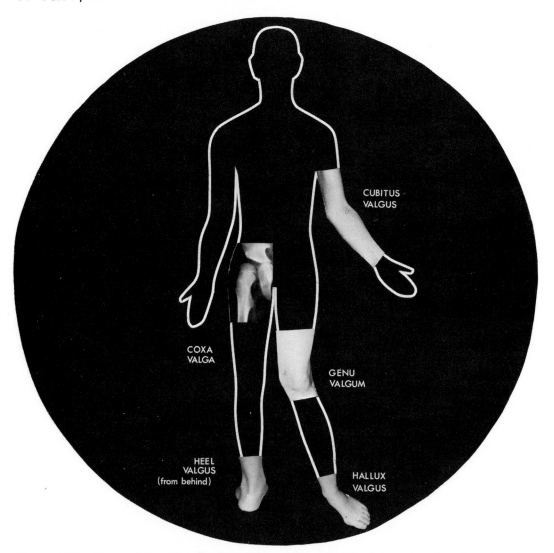

Figure 4.22. Valgus deformities. The angulation of the deformity does *not* conform to an imaginary circle in which the patient is placed.

Coxa vara: a *decrease* in the femoral neck-shaft angle (less than 130°), e.g. an angle of 90° conforms more to a circle than the normal angle of 130°.

Genu varum: "bow leg" the knees are apart when the feet are together.

Heel varus: a decrease in the normal angle between the axis of the leg and that of the heel, as in the position of inversion.

Talipes equinovarus: an inversion deformity of the foot combined with an equinus or plantar flexion deformity of the ankle. This combination is seen in a congenital clubfoot.

Metatarsus varus: more properly called "metatarsus adductus"; an adduction deformity of the forefoot in relation to the hind foot.

Hallux varus: an adduction deformity of the great toe through the metatarsophalangeal joint.

VALGUS

An angulation that does *not* conform to an imaginary circle in which the patient is placed (Fig. 4.22).

Cubitus valgus: an *increase* in the femoral

neck-shaft angle (more than 130°), e.g. an angle of 170° conforms less to a circle than the normal angle of 130°.

Genu valgum: "knock-knee," the feet are apart when the knees are together.

Heel valgus: an *increase* in the normal angle between the axis of the leg and that of the heel, as in the position of eversion.

Talipes calcaneovalgus: an eversion deformity of the foot combined with a calcaneus or dorsiflexion deformity of the ankle.

Hallux valgus: an abduction deformity of the great toe through the metatarsophalangeal joint.

Suggested Additional Reading

American Academy of Orthopaedic Surgeons: *Joint Motion: Method of Measuring and Recording*, 1965.

American Orthopaedic Association: *Manual of Orthopaedic Surgery, 5th ed*, 1979.

Blawvel, C. T. and Nelson, F. R. T.: *A Manual of Orthopaedic Terminology.* St. Louis, C.V. Mosby, 1977.

Houston, C. S.: Varus and valgus—no wonder they are confused. N. Engl. J. Med. 302: 471–472, 1980.

"Ad sanitatem gradus est movisse morbum."
(The first step toward cure is to know what the disease is.)
—LATIN PROVERB

CHAPTER 5

The Diagnosis of Musculoskeletal Disorders and Injuries

As a medical doctor of the future, your *first responsibility* to each of your patients will be to determine just what the problem or disease is (the *diagnosis*). This you must determine with great care and accuracy in order that you may make the correct start toward the *goal of helping your patient* because, of course, he will have come to you— a medical doctor—*primarily to seek help with a problem*.

Problem solving holds a certain fascination for us all—and who among us is not stimulated by a mystery? The field of medicine will afford you daily opportunity to solve mysteries and other problems, not only in diagnosis and in treatment, but also in the many types of medical research. Solving the mystery of a diagnosis is the "detective work of medicine," and to be consistently accurate, you must emulate that greatest of all detectives, Sherlock Holmes, who constantly demanded: "Data, give me data!" (Fig. 5.1). In the investigation of a diagnostic mystery, you, like Sherlock Holmes, must be keenly interested, inquiring, attentive, alert, observant, perceptive, skillful in correlating data, or clues, as well as in making logical deductions and conclusions from them.*

METHODS OF OBTAINING DATA (CLUES)—THE INVESTIGATION

Certain musculoskeletal conditions, such as a typical congenital clubfoot, are so obvious that their diagnosis presents little dif-

---

* It is of interest that both the literary creator of Sherlock Holmes, as well as his "model," were members of the medical profession. Sir Arthur Conan Doyle was inspired to create the fictional figure of the master detective in 1880 as a result of his close association as a postgraduate medical student with Joseph Bell, a brilliant Edinburgh surgeon who was renowned for his remarkable powers of observation and deduction in relation to diagnosis.

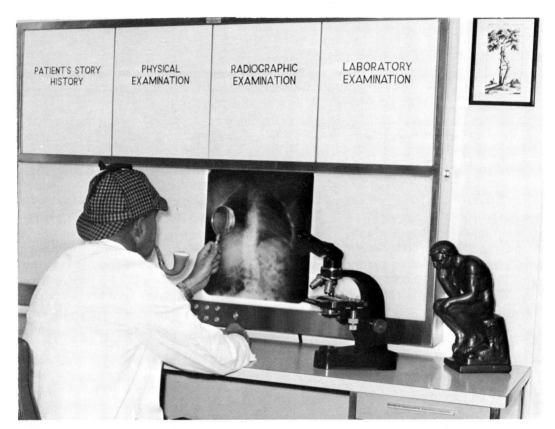

| PATIENT'S STORY HISTORY | PHYSICAL EXAMINATION | RADIOGRAPHIC EXAMINATION | LABORATORY EXAMINATION |

Figure 5.1. The medical doctor, like Sherlock Holmes, must search out and correlate all available data in order to solve the mystery of a diagnosis.

ficulty (as Holmes would say: "Elementary, my dear Watson"). However, other conditions, such as a malignant bone neoplasm in its earliest stages, or symptoms such as progressive weakness in a limb, present diagnostic problems that may require extensive investigation. Thus, not all of the methods of obtaining data, or clues, are essential to making every diagnosis, but you must be prepared to use as many as necessary to solve the problem, or mystery, of diagnosis in each patient you see. In the diagnosis of musculoskeletal disorders and injuries you should conduct the investigation in the following order: (1) history taking (symptoms); (2) physical examination (signs); (3) radiographic examination (x-ray signs); (4) laboratory examinations (including examinations of various body fluids as well as examination of a specimen, or biopsy, of diseased tissue). Symptoms provide *subjective data*, whereas physical signs, radiographic signs and the results of laboratory tests provide *objective data*.

The Patient's Story (History)

As a medical student of the present you will have many opportunities to obtain the clinical history from patients assigned to you in the wards and outpatient clinics of your teaching hospitals. You will be wise to develop good habits of history taking during these formative years of your clinical training; they will serve you well as a medical doctor of the future.

In order to obtain a complete and accurate history, you must be a discerning listener and an intelligent questioner. Furthermore, you must have certain attitudes of mind toward your patient, and these include a sincere and kindly interest in him as a fellow human being, compassion, understanding, patience and tact. Remember that for many persons, consulting a doctor may be an anxious experience; regardless of their age or level of intelligence, your patients will be quick to sense *your attitude toward them* and they will either be put at ease or be made to feel ill at ease by it.

Under certain circumstances (infancy, mental retardation, language barrier, loss of consciousness), your patient will be unable to tell you his story himself, in which case you must rely on the "hearsay" history given by a relative or friend. In present times, when so much medical information (and misinformation) is reported in newspapers, lay magazines, radio and television programs, you must be discerning about your patient's interpretation of his symptoms or his attempts at self-diagnosis; not that they should be automatically discounted (they may even be correct) but they may have misled your patient and you must not allow them to mislead *you*.

IMPORTANT DATA IN THE PATIENT'S HISTORY

Preliminary Data

Your patient's name, sex, date of birth and present age, occupation and family responsibilities.

The Presenting Problem or Chief Complaint

The chief complaint is the main symptom, or group of symptoms, that have prompted your patient to seek your help and advice. Your opening inquiry about this should not be "What is wrong with *you*?" since such a question invites the obvious reaction, either silent or expressed: "But that is just what I have come to find out from *you!*" A preferable beginning would be, "What have you *noticed* or *felt* that does not seem right to you?" Having listened to your patient describe his chief complaints in his own words, you will need to obtain more precise information by asking further questions to determine the following: time of onset, type of onset (sudden or gradual), severity, constancy (constant or intermittent), progression, activities that aggravate it and those that relieve it, relation to any injury or other incident, any associated symptoms.

Common Musculoskeletal Symptoms or Complaints

The following are the main reasons why a patient with a musculoskeletal condition will consult you:

1. Pain. By far the most important presenting symptom is pain, and you must inquire about it in great detail, with respect to its onset, precise location, character (dull, sharp, burning), severity, duration, factors that relieve the pain as well as those that aggravate it and its variation with day and night. There is a very wide variation from person to person in relation to pain threshold and pain tolerance; the patient who "feels" more pain, or who tolerates it less well than average, may not be exaggerating at all, and requires kindly consideration. Most musculoskeletal pain is aggravated by local movement and relieved by local rest; this will suggest to you that during movement, such pain is caused by a sudden increase in either tension or pressure in sensitive soft tissues such as periosteum (movement in a fracture site) or joint capsule and ligaments (movement in a joint). Any such painful movement initiates muscle spasm, which in itself is painful, and this pain is superimposed upon the initial pain. Pain that persists in spite of local rest will suggest progressively increasing pressure in a closed space, such as occurs with an increasing amount of purulent exudate within the confines of a bone (osteomyelitis) or within a joint cavity (septic arthritis) and as occurs also with a progressively expanding bone neoplasm. Pressure on a nerve, or nerve root, produces *radiating pain* in the sensory area of that nerve or nerve root; the commonest example is "sciatica," pain radiating down the leg in the distribution of the sciatic nerve from pressure of a protruded intervertebral disc on a nerve root. Remember also, the phenomenon of *referred pain*, the most important example of which is pain felt in the knee (referred to the knee) but arising from a painful lesion in the hip due to the obturator nerve pattern of hip pain. Neurological lesions may produce alterations in skin sensation including increased or painful feeling (*hyperesthesia*) or peculiar feeling (*paresthesia*).

2. Decrease in Function. Decreased ability to use a part is also a very common presenting complaint (chief complaint) of patients with musculoskeletal conditions. Your patient may be concerned about decreased ability (disability) due to muscle weakness or fatigue, giving way (instability) of a joint, or stiffness of a joint.

3. Physical Appearance. Your patient's chief complaint may be the physical appearance of a *deformity* such as a crooked limb or limbs (angulatory deformity), twisted limb (torsional or rotational deformity), a wasted limb (atrophy), a short leg (leg length discrepancy), or a crooked back (scoliosis). He may be concerned about the physical appearance of an abnormal way of walking (limp, or abnormal gait). Deformities and abnormal gaits are physical signs rather than symptoms but they may still be the patient's chief complaint or presenting problem. You must determine when the problem was first noticed, its character, clinical course (getting better, getting worse or remaining unchanged) and the extent of any associated disability. As with tolerance to pain, patients vary widely in their tolerance, or acceptance, of deformities and abnormal gaits. A given deformity or a given limp may be quite acceptable to one patient and yet be a source of great concern (and therefore a problem) to another.

Relevant Past History

It is important to obtain a history of previous illnesses, previous injuries and previous related treatment, including operations. Your patient may have a tendency to ascribe his present symptoms or signs to a specific incident such as previous illness, an injury or treatment, whereas you may discern that, in fact, the incident merely served to draw the patient's attention to a pre-existing and previously unrecognized condition.

Functional Inquiry

Patients with disorders of the musculoskeletal system may have coexistent disorders of some other body system, or systems, and hence the reason for inquiring into the function of all systems (*functional inquiry*). Some of the more important conditions to include are: heart disease, diabetes, kidney disease, respiratory conditions and psychic disturbances with either exaggeration or falsification of symptoms. It is important to ascertain not only what kind of disease the person has, but also what kind of person has the disease. Nevertheless, you should diligently search for an organic explanation of your patient's symptoms, even though he may appear to be "neurotic," lest you do him the injustice of jumping to the wrong conclusion.

Social, Economic and Work History

Since orthopaedic problems and their treatment frequently extend over long periods of time, you must obtain the relevant details of your patient's social, economic and work history in order that your proposed plan of treatment may be feasible for your particular patient.

Family History

Since some musculoskeletal conditions, both congenital and acquired, show a distinct tendency to appear in members of the same family, either in the same or in different generations, it is important to obtain such data concerning relatives by means of a *family history*.

Physical Examination

In a sense, the physical examination begins the moment the patient comes into your sight. Certain striking features about your patient, his body build (habitus), his facial appearance (facies), his way of walking (gait) as he approaches you, or his sitting or lying position if you are approaching him, may have already provided you with useful clues almost before you have had time to say "How do you do?" Your eager eyes (like those of Sherlock Holmes) will pick out every clue and by the time you have completed taking your patient's history you will have detected many things about him (and he will have detected certain things about *you* also). Your attitude of mind toward your patient will be reflected by your methods of examination. A compassionate attitude of mind will result in an awareness of your patient's feelings, as well as a respect for them. You will, therefore, respect your patient's modesty in his or her necessary degree of undress and you will endeavor to be as gentle as possible in your examination so as not to produce unnecessary pain—not any more than is necessary to detect that a certain pressure or movement is, in fact, painful.

Apart from your own common sense and your keen senses of sight, touch and hearing, the equipment you require for the musculoskeletal examination of your patient is simple (Fig. 5.2). The examination is conducted in systematic order: (1) *looking (inspection)*, (2) *feeling (palpation)*, (3) *moving (assessment of joint motion)*, both active and passive, (4) *listening (auscultation)* over joints and vessels, (5) *special physical tests* to elicit or exclude specific physical signs and (6) *neurological examination*.

LOOKING (INSPECTION)

Your patient must be sufficiently exposed that you will not overlook some important sign. Confirm your earlier observations of the patient's habitus and facies; observe the skin (redness, cyanosis, pigmentation) (Fig. 5.3), atrophy, hypertrophy, scars of previous injury or operation; look for any deformity (Fig. 5.4), swelling (Fig. 5.5), lump (Fig. 5.6), measure any limb shortening (Fig. 5.7) or atrophy (Fig. 5.8), always comparing the abnormal limb with the opposite limb. If your patient is able to walk, you should request him to do so, back and forth in an unobstructed area, at least 20 feet long, since careful observation of the patient's gait may provide many important clues. Many of the abnormal physical signs apparent on inspection will be described and shown in subsequent chapters.

FEELING (PALPATION)

All patients appreciate a doctor who has a "warm heart"; they also appreciate one

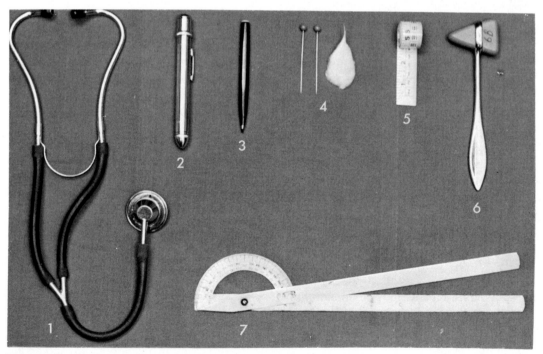

Figure 5.2.   Equipment for musculoskeletal examination. *1*, stethoscope; *2*, pocket flashlight; *3*, skin marker; *4*, pins and cotton wool; *5*, tape measure; *6*, reflex hammer; *7*, goniometer (to measure angles).

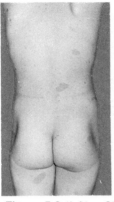 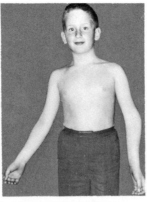

Figure 5.3 (*left*).   Skin pigmentation. The areas of light brown skin pigmentation (café au lait spots) in this boy are a clue to the diagnosis of neurofibromatosis (Von Recklinghausen's disease).
Figure 5.4 (*right*).   Deformity. The cubitus varus deformity of this boy's left arm is the result of an old supracondylar fracture of the humerus that had been allowed to heal with varus angulation.

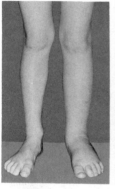 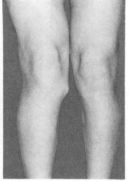

Figure 5.5 (*left*).   Swelling. The diffuse swelling of this boy's left leg is due to chronic edema secondary to lymphatic vessel obstruction.
Figure 5.6 (*right*).   The lump on the medial side of this woman's knee is a bony prominence due to a type of benign bone lesion, an osteochondroma (osteocartilaginous exostosis) arising from the upper end of the tibia.

who has *warm hands* and furthermore, warms hands elicit less muscle spasm than those that are cold and clammy. By palpation you will obtain data concerning skin temperature; pulse; tenderness; nature of swelling (indurated or edematous "pitting"); characteristics of a lump or a mass (consistency, fluctuation, size, relationship to adja-

cent structures); muscle bulk; abnormal relationships of bones at their joints (dislocations). With the combination of joint movement and palpation you will also detect joint crepitus as well as muscle tone.

MOVING (ASSESSMENT OF JOINT MOTION)

Active movement of a joint by your patient should be assessed first; it may be *limited* by pain and associated muscle spasm, muscle weakness, ruptured muscle or tendon, joint stiffness or joint contracture or a bony block. *Passive movement* of a joint by *you*, the examiner, should be assessed gently; it may be *decreased* for any of the reasons mentioned above (except muscle weakness and ruptured muscle or tendon) (Fig. 5.9) or it may be *increased* as in joint instability due to a lax capsule or torn ligaments (Fig. 5.10). Abnormal ranges of joint motion, both active and passive, should be *recorded*. In patients with healing fractures, the clinical state of the union can be assessed by the presence or absence of passive motion at the fracture site.

LISTENING (AUSCULTATION)

Sounds arising from bones (fracture crepitus), joints (joint crepitus) or muscle action (snapping tendons) are sometimes sufficiently loud that they can be heard by both your patient and yourself without any effort. However, it is often informative to listen to a joint during movement, either through direct contact of your ear on the skin or through a stethoscope for more accurate assessment of the quality and localization of the sound (Fig. 5.11). The stethoscope is also of value in detecting the murmur of a peripheral arteriovenous fistula.

SPECIAL PHYSICAL TESTS

Certain important physical signs will escape your detection during physical examination unless you perform special tests that have been developed for their detection. The hip joint, being deeply situated and of complex structure and function, is more difficult to examine accurately than other joints and therefore, it is not surprising that three of

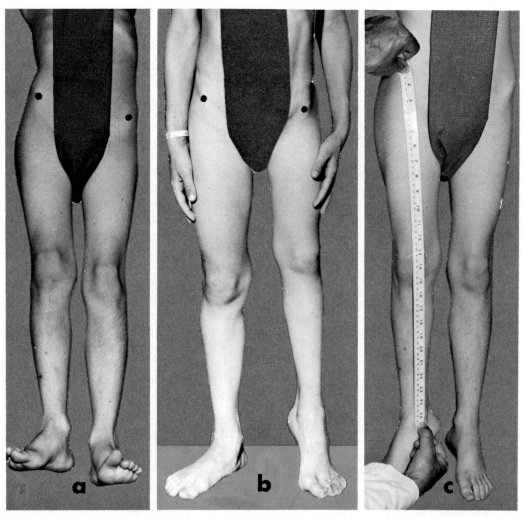

Figure 5.7. Limb shortening. *A*, apparent shortening. This boy's right lower limb appears to be shorter than his left; however, they are actually the same length. The apparent shortening is due to an adduction contracture of the right hip and resultant obliquity of the pelvis (the black dots are on the anterior superior spine). *B*, true shortening. This boy's left lower limb is truly shorter than his right. He is almost able to compensate for this by standing on tip toe on the shorter side. *C*, method of measuring true limb length from the anterior superior spine to the medical malleolus. Apparent limb length is measured from the umbilicus to the medial malleolus with the lower limbs in line with the trunk.

these special tests have been developed to demonstrate specific signs in the hip. Two of these signs are present (the test is positive) in a variety of clinical conditions and accordingly they will be considered now:

Hip flexion deformity—Thomas test (Fig. 5.12).

Ineffectual hip abduction mechanism—Trendelenburg test (Fig. 5.13).

Other specific signs are present in one condition only and are therefore more appropriately considered along with a discussion of that condition; they will be merely listed at present:

Instability (dislocatability) of the newborn hip—Barlow and Ortolani test (Chapter 8).

Sciatic nerve irritation—Lasègue test (Chapter 11).

Torn tag of medial meniscus of the knee—McMurray test (Chapter 17).

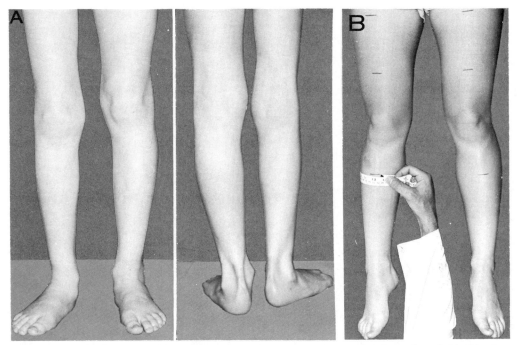

Figure 5.8. Atrophy. *A*, the decrease in circumference of this boy's right calf and thigh is due to muscle atrophy secondary to paralytic poliomyelitis. *B*, method of measuring limb circumference. The levels for comparable circumferential measurements should first be measured from comparable bony landmarks and marked.

NEUROLOGICAL EXAMINATION

Since many musculoskeletal disorders and injuries are associated with neurological deficits, you will appreciate that neurological examination is an important part of the musculoskeletal examination. It is of particular importance when there is evidence of either muscle weakness or muscle spasticity, involuntary movements of muscle, symptoms of altered skin sensation, incoordination of movement and loss of balance. The neurological examination will include assessment of the motor system (muscle tone, power, coordination), sensory system (touch, pain, temperature, position sense, vibration), reflexes (tendon reflexes and plantar reflex) and rectal sphincter tone.

Radiographic Examination

Prior to Roentgen's serendipitous discovery of "X-rays" in 1895, physicians and surgeons relied on clinical evidence to make a musculoskeletal diagnosis and to follow the results of treatment. This important dis-

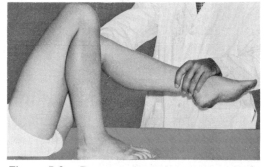

Figure 5.9. Decreased passive movement of a joint. Passive flexion of this girl's left knee was limited to 90° as a result of dense adhesions between the quadriceps muscle and the distal end of the femur following a severely displaced fracture at this site.

covery revolutionized medical and surgical diagnosis and treatment in general, but especially in the musculoskeletal system. It is remarkable that the X-ray filament tube designed by Coolidge in 1913 has been changed very little during the ensuing decades.

Examination of the musculoskeletal system by means of X-rays (radiographic examination) is, in a sense, an extension of physical examination. You might consider it a form of "*internal inspection*" and, as such, it is of extreme value, not only in the accurate diagnosis of musculoskeletal disorders and injuries but also in following the subse-

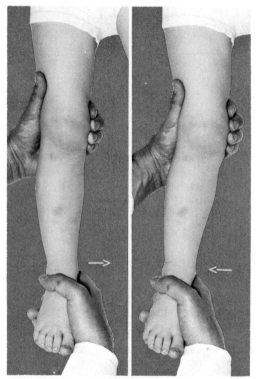

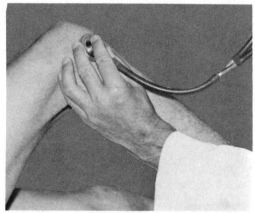

Figure 5.10.   Increased passive movement of a joint. Passive adduction followed by passive abduction of this boy's right knee joint reveals an increased range of passive movement indicating instability of the joint due to joint laxity.

Figure 5.11.   Auscultation of a joint. By means of a stethoscope the source of joint crepitus, such as the "clunk" from an internal derangement of the joint, can usually be accurately localized during passive movement of the joint.

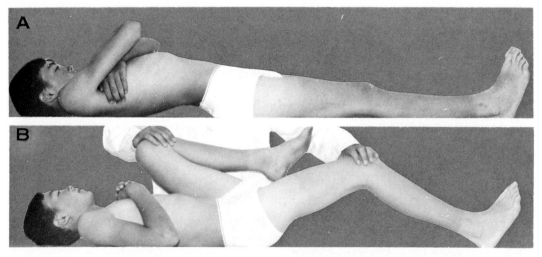

Figure 5.12.   Thomas test for hip flexion deformity. *A*, when the patient is lying supine, a hip flexion deformity can be masked by an increase in the lumbar lordosis. *B*, passive complete flexion of the opposite hip straightens out the lumbar spine and reveals the true extent of the hip flexion deformity. This boy's hip flexion deformity was due to the residual effects of a septic arthritis.

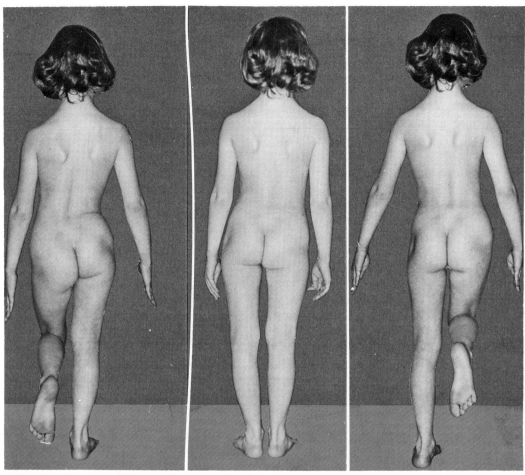

Figure 5.13.   Trendelenburg test for ineffectual hip abduction mechanism in a 4-year old girl with congenital dislocation of the right hip. *Left*, when the child stands on her right foot (the side of the dislocated hip), the hip abductor muscles, having no fulcrum, cannot hold the pelvis level and it drops on the opposite side; the child, in an effort to maintain balance, shifts her trunk toward the involved side. The Trendelenburg sign is also seen in the presence of coxa vara, paralysed hip abductor muscles and painful conditions about the hip. *Center*, the dislocation is not apparent when the child is standing with both feet on the floor (apart from the slight shortening of the right lower limb). *Right*, when the child stands on her left foot (the side of the normal hip) the hip abductor muscles, having a normal function, hold the pelvis level.

quent course of these conditions. A brief explanation of "X-ray shadows" will make your interpretation of X-ray films more interesting and more meaningful. An X-ray film (radiograph) is studied against a bright light because it is a photographic "negative" rather than a "print." You will observe in radiographs that bone appears relatively white (radio-opaque) while the soft tissues appear relatively dark (radiolucent). The ra-

diographic density of a tissue depends upon its thickness as well as its atomic weight. The thicker the tissue and the higher its atomic weight, the more radiation is absorbed and therefore the less radiation "penetrates" the tissue to expose the film, and the whiter it will appear. Conversely, the thinner the tissue and the lower its atomic weight, the less radiation is absorbed and therefore the more radiation "penetrates" the tissue to expose the film, and the darker it will appear. Fat has the lowest atomic weight of all the solid tissues and therefore appears darkest (most radiolucent) in the radiographic negative. Muscle, cartilage and osteoid (not yet calcified) have approximately the same atomic weight, which is higher than that of fat, and consequently they are more radio-opaque than fat. Bone, however, because of its mineral content of calcium, phosphorus, magnesium and other minerals, has a much higher atomic weight and is therefore much more radio-opaque than the various soft tissues (Fig. 5.14). Furthermore, bone as a structure varies in its radiographic density depending on its thickness or structural density and on its calcification. Radiographically, an abnormally increased density in bone is called *sclerosis*, whereas an abnormally decreased density is called *rarefaction* (Fig. 5.15). You will recall from Chapter 3 that the radiographic density of bone clearly demonstrates the altered deposition and altered resorption of the bone as it reacts to abnormal conditions.

A gas, of course, is the most radiolucent substance seen in a radiograph. Air is expected in the lungs as is gas in the gastrointestinal tract. Air in the soft tissues at the base of the neck, however, signifies surgical emphysema while widespread gas within the soft tissues of a limb is an ominous sign of gas gangrene (Fig. 5.16).

A radiograph, like a photograph, is only two dimensional and a single radiograph represents but one view—which could mislead you. Therefore, a second view (at right angles to the first) is essential so that you can study the structures at least from the front (*anteroposterior projection*) and from the side (*lateral projection*) (Fig. 5.17). Sometimes, additional views are required such as *oblique projections*. The third dimension can be best appreciated by studying two *stereoscopic projections*. By means of a special technique called *tomography* or *laminography*, many films are taken, each of which shows a different layer, or slice, of the tissue in focus.

INSPECTION OF A RADIOGRAPH

Just as in the inspection of your patient, so also in the inspection of his radiographs, you must know what to look for. The following are some of the important features to look for in a radiograph:

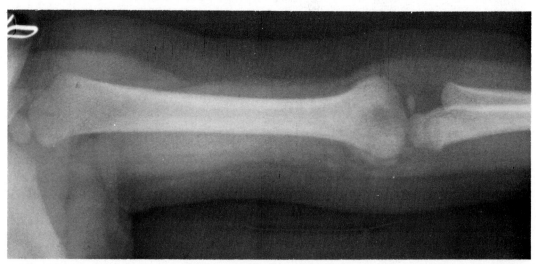

Figure 5.14. Radiographic density of various tissues. In this radiograph the bones, muscles and subcutaneous fat are clearly differentiated from one another by their specific radiographic density. Note the extreme radiographic density of the metal object.

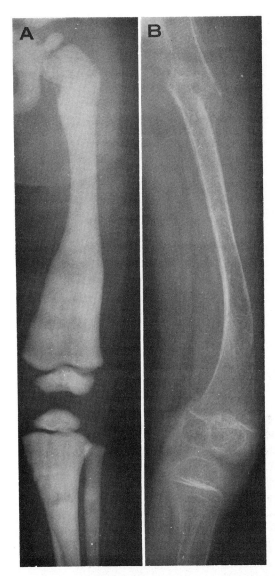

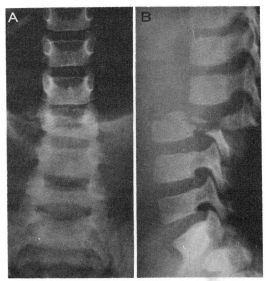

Figure 5.17. The importance of at least two projections. *A*, the anteroposterior projection of the lumbar spine of this severely injured boy reveals relatively little distortion of the spine. *B*, the lateral projection of the lumbar spine of the same boy reveals a severe fracture-dislocation of the spine. Two projections at right angles to each other are essential.

Figure 5.15. General density of bone. *A*, increased density of bone (sclerosis) due to osteopetrosis ("marble bones"). Note also the deficit in the femoral neck. *B*, decreased density of bone (rarefaction) due to osteogenesis imperfecta ("fragile bones"). Note also the healed fracture in the upper third of the femur.

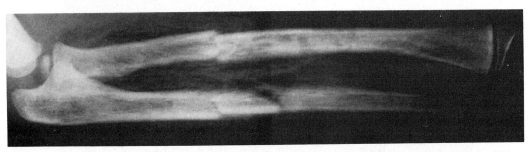

Figure 5.16. Radiograph of the forearm of a 10-year-old boy who had sustained an open ("compound") fracture of the radius and ulna three days previously. Note the widespread gas within the soft tissues of the forearm which is a sign of gas gangrene. So fulminating was the gas gangrene that amputation was required to save the boy's life.

General density of bone—increased or decreased (Fig. 5.15).

Local density of bone—increased or decreased (Fig. 5.18).

Relationship between bones—dislocation or subluxation (Fig. 5.19).

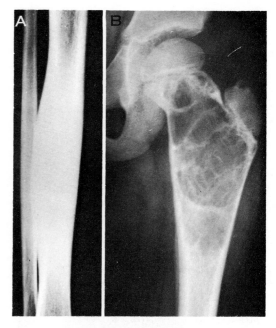

Figure 5.18.   Local density of bone. *A*, increased local density of bone (sclerosis). The localized area of sclerosis in this boy's tibia is due to new bone formation as a reaction to an osteosclerotic lesion (an osteoid osteoma) within the bone. In this radiograph the osteoid osteoma itself (which is only 1 cm in diameter and is actually osteolytic) is obscured by the extensive reaction of osteosclerosis in the surrounding bone of the lateral cortex of the tibia. *B*, decreased local density of bone (rarefaction). The localized area of rarefaction in the upper end of this girl's femur is due to an osteolytic lesion (a simple bone cyst) within the bone.

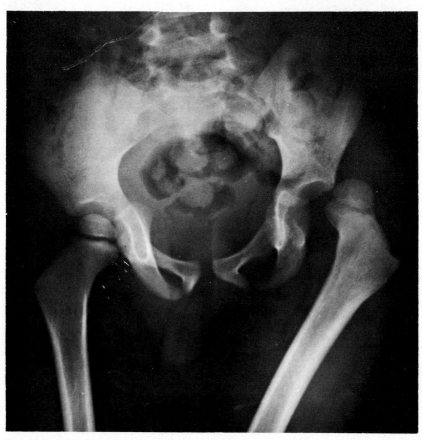

Figure 5.19.   Relationship between bones. This child's left hip joint is completely dislocated as the result of a severe injury (traumatic dislocation).

Break in bone continuity—fracture (Fig. 5.20).

General contour of a bone—deformity (Fig. 5.21).

Local contour of a bone—internal or external irregularity (Fig. 5.22).

Thickness of articular cartilage—the cartilage space (Fig. 5.23).

Changes in soft tissues—swelling, atrophy (Fig. 5.24).

You will be wise to inspect, or study, a radiograph as you would inspect, or study, a patient, initially from a distance and then from close range. In this way your eyes move from the general to the particular and you are less likely to miss an important radiographic clue. Remember also that there may be more than one clue or sign in a given radiograph (Fig. 5.20). Comparison of a limb with the opposite limb, which has already been stressed in clinical examination, is equally important in radiographic examination, particularly in children, because of the varying appearance of epiphyses and epiphyseal plates during the period of growth.

Special types of radiographic examination demonstrate certain soft tissue outlines not clearly depicted in an ordinary radiograph. These examinations involve the injection of a contrast medium (either a fluid that is radio-opaque, or air, which is radiolucent) into a body space. The following are three examples of contrast radiographs:

Arthrogram

Injection of a radio-opaque dye or air (or a combination of the two for a "double contrast" examination) into the synovial cavity

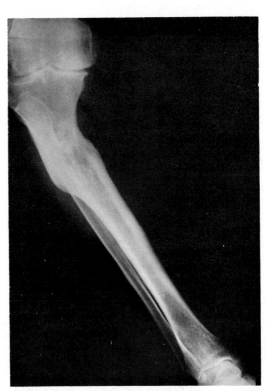

Figure 5.21. General contour of a bone. The varus deformity in this 60-year-old man's right tibia is the result of an old fracture that had been allowed to heal with deformity (malunion).

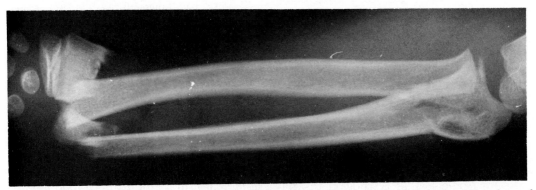

Figure 5.20. Break in bone continuity. The displaced fractures of the distal metaphyseal regions of the radius and ulna are obvious. However, there may be more than one clue in a given radiograph. Can you also detect the less obvious fracture of the proximal end of the ulna?

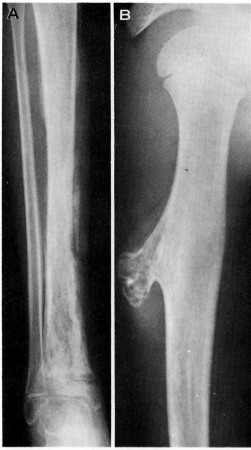

Figure 5.22. Local contour of a bone. *A*, internal irregularity of the distal half of the tibia of a child due to chronic osteomyelitis. *B*, external irregularity of the humerus of a child due to an osteochondroma (osteocartilaginous exostosis).

to detect injuries or other abnormalities of the articular cartilage, fibrocartilaginous menisci, capsule and ligaments (Fig. 5.25).

Myelogram

Injection of the medium into the subarachnoid space to detect the protrusion of nucleus pulposus or soft tissue neoplasm into the vertebral canal (Fig. 5.26).

Discogram

Injection of a radio-opaque dye into suspected abnormal intervertebral discs under local anesthetic can be of help in localizing the particular disc that is causing the patient's symptoms, not only because the in-

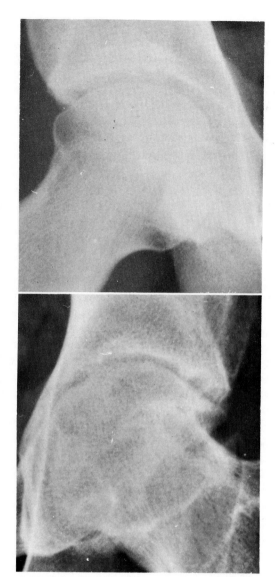

Figure 5.23. Thickness of articular cartilage. The left hip joint of this 14-year-old girl has been the site of pyogenic infection (septic arthritis). Note the decreased thickness of the cartilage space (a more accurate term than ''joint space'') of the left hip, compared to that of the normal opposite hip (*top*) indicating loss of articular cartilage.

jection into the responsible disc reproduces the symptoms but also because the radiographic pattern of the dye in such a disc is abnormal in that it extends beyond the normal confines of the disc.

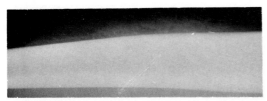

Figure 5.24. Changes in soft tissues. Note the irregular density in the subcutaneous tissues overlying the tibia. This soft tissue shadow is due to a recent hemorrhage and resultant hematoma in the subcutaneous tissues.

Sinogram

Injection of the medium into an external sinus to follow the sinus track to its source in the depths of the tissues (Fig. 5.27).

SCINTIGRAPHY

During the 1970's the specialty of nuclear medicine has made great strides in detection of a wide variety of lesions in bone through the use of bone-seeking radionuclides such as technetium-99m-labeled polyphosphate, its analog, methylene disphosphate, and others. The resultant "bone scans" reflect changes in the local blood flow in bone as well as the degree of local metabolic activity.

Scintigraphy has been useful in detecting and localizing a wide variety of lesions including benign conditions (especially osteoid osteoma), primary malignant tumors, skeletal metastases, early osteomyelitis, infected endoprostheses and even stress fractures, all of which appear on the scan as an area of *increased* radionuclide uptake (a so-called "hot spot") (Fig. 5.28 and 5.29). In addition, bone scans are useful in detecting avascular necrosis of bone in its early stages at which time there is *decreased* radionuclide uptake (a so-called "cold spot").

COMPUTED TOMOGRAPHY

In the entire field of diagnostic radiology, computed tomography has been by far the most important and most exciting advance since 1875 when Roentgen discovered what he called "X-rays". Indeed, radiology has entered what might be called "the era of imaginative imaging" as a result of this marvel of radiation physics, electronics and com-

puter science. Even the word radiology is gradually being replaced by the term "diagnostic imaging."

Computerized tomography, through which accurate images of "slices" of the body are generated, ingeniously overcomes many of the limitations of two-dimensional radiography and provides a degree of diagnostic accuracy not previously attainable. Originally limited to computerized axial (cross-sectional) tomography—and hence the term "CAT" scan—the technology has now made it possible to look also at coronal, sagittal and even oblique slices. Thus the current term, computed tomography (CT), is more appropriate. This sophisticated diagnostic imaging system clearly differentiates between the radiographic densities of various tissues and enables us to see lesions that are not demonstrable by standard radiography—and with less radiation to the patient than with conventional tomograms.

The science and technology of computed tomography is advancing at such a phenomenal rate that each successive generation of CT scanners soon becomes relatively obsolete.

In the musculoskeletal system computed tomography is of tremendous value in the detection of the precise site and extent of such variegated disorders as benign and malignant tumors, pulmonary metastases, osteomyelitis, intervertebral disc herniation (combined with myelography), spinal stenosis, diastematomyelia, meningomyelocele, torsional deformities of the femur, dislocation of the hip and complex fractures of the pelvis. Examples of CT scans of musculoskeletal tissues are shown in Figures 5.30, 5.31 and 5.32.

Ultrasonography

The Doppler phenomenon using ultrasound has been found to be a useful and noninvasive method of assessing arterial blood flow in an extremity; it has an estimated 95% rate of accuracy.

Ultrasound has been used as a safe and non-invasive method of differentiating between solid lesions and fluid-filled cystic le-

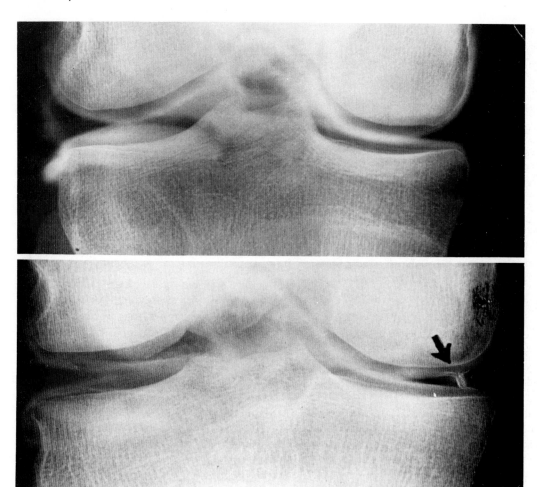

Figure 5.25. Arthrograms of the knee using a radio-opaque dye. *Top*, normal arthrogram of the right knee. Note the smooth wedge-shaped medial and lateral menisci clearly outlined by the dye in the joint. *Bottom*, arthrogram of the right knee revealing penetration of the dye into a vertical tear in the medial meniscus (*arrow*). By means of several oblique projections, the location and extent of the tear can be determined.

sions (such as a popliteal cyst) and may even have a place in the diagnosis of narrowing of the spinal canal (spinal stenosis).

Laboratory Examination

The fourth source of data, or clues, which may be required, at least in some cases, to solve the problem of diagnosis is the laboratory examination of specimens of body fluids and tissues. These examinations, or tests, involve hematology, biochemistry, immunology, bacteriology and pathology. Of the multitude of laboratory examinations available, those of most value in the diag-

nosis of musculoskeletal disorders are the following:

Blood: hemoglobin, red blood cell count, white blood cell count, stained smear or film of blood, sedimentation rate, blood coagulation studies, uric acid, blood culture.

Serum: serum calcium, inorganic phosphate, alkaline phosphatase, acid phosphatase, proteins. Immunological or serological tests include the Wasserman or Kahn reaction for syphilis, the Mantoux test for tuberculosis and the Rose test for rheumatoid disease.

Urine: gross appearance, albumin, sugar,

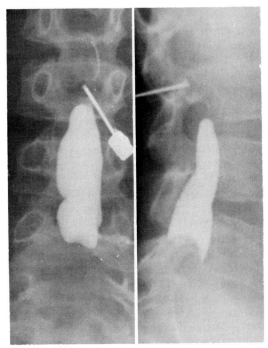

Figure 5.26. Myelogram. The descent of the radio-opaque medium is completely blocked at the level of the fourth lumbar vertebra by a space-occupying lesion, in this patient a neoplasm, within the vertebral canal. Metrizamide is much more satisfactory for this purpose then previously available radio-opaque media.

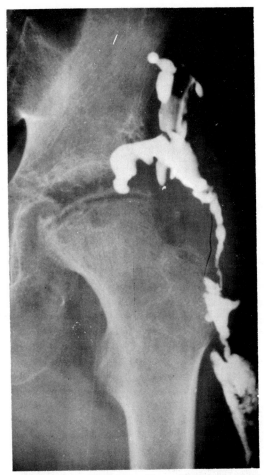

Figure 5.27. Sinogram. The radio-opaque medium has been injected into a sinus on the lateral aspect of this boy's left thigh. The medium outlines the sinus tract and reveals its connection with the hip joint. The medium also outlines a radiolucent foreign body just lateral to the ilium above the hip joint; this was a piece of wood that had been driven into the soft tissues at the time of a penetrating injury and traumatic dislocation of the hip. Note also the evidence of destruction of the femoral head due to the combination of infection and necrosis.

cells, casts, urinary calcium and phosphorus, urine culture.

Cerebrospinal fluid: gross appearance, pressure, protein, cells, culture.

Synovial fluid: gross appearance, protein cells, sugar, culture.

The analysis of synovial fluid obtained by joint aspiration (arthrocentesis) is of considerable value in the laboratory diagnosis of joint disorders. Normal synovial fluid contains a total protein of approximately 1.8 mg/100 ml with relatively more albumin than globulin and is relatively acellular (10 to 200 cells per milliliter, predominantly mononuclear).

Synovial fluid from non-inflammatory joints is usually clear, has few cells (with a normal distribution) and a low protein content whereas the synovial fluid from inflammatory joints is usually turbid (from white blood cells and/or crystals) many more cells

(predominantly polymorphonuclear leucocytes) and a high protein count.

In septic arthritis bacteria may be found as well as a very low level of joint fluid sugar. The presence of crystals in "chemical" arthritis can be diagnostic—monosodium urate crystals for gout and calcium pyrophosphate crystals for pseudogout.

Abnormal fluids (effusions, exudates):

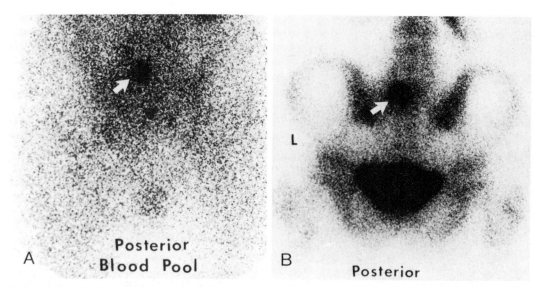

Figure 5.28. *A*, conventional radiograph of the distal end of the left tibia of a 14-year-old boy with a history of sudden onset of severe pain in the region of the ankle three days previously (too early to expect radiographic changes). *B*, scintigram of both ankle regions (viewed from behind) showing a large area of increased radionuclide uptake—a "hot spot"—typical of acute hematogenous osteomyelitis. (Courtesy of Dr. David Gilday)

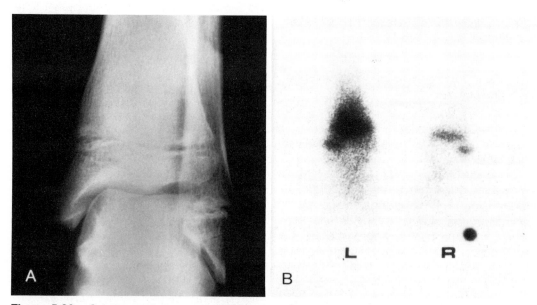

Figure 5.29. Scintigram (bone scan) of the lower lumbar spine and pelvis (viewed from behind) depicting the typical appearance of an osteoid osteoma in the left side of the lamina of the 5th lumbar vertebra in both the blood pool image (*A*) as a vascular localized lesion (*arrow*) and in the delayed image (*B*) as a round localized area of increased radionuclide uptake—a "hot spot" (*arrow*). This is a difficult area in which to make the diagnosis of an osteoid osteoma with conventional radiography. (Courtesy of Dr. David Gilday)

gross appearance, cells, direct smear, culture. When an organism is obtained by culture, further examinations are required to assess its resistance to the various antibiotics.

Body tissues (specimen obtained by biopsy): Bone marrow is usually obtained by

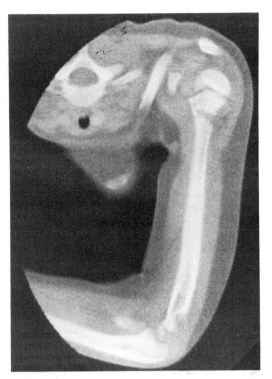

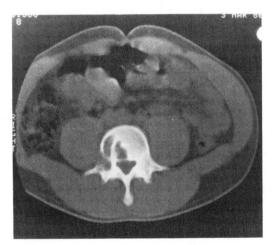

Figure 5.30.   Computed tomogram of the cross-section of the body at the level of the fourth lumbar vertebra. Note the extensive osteolytic lesion of the vertebral body and pedicle. The diagnosis is aneurysmal bone cyst.

Figure 5.32.   Computed tomogram of the sagittal section of the upper limb. Note the destructive lesion in the proximal metaphysis of the humerus. The diagnosis is a leukemic deposit in bone.

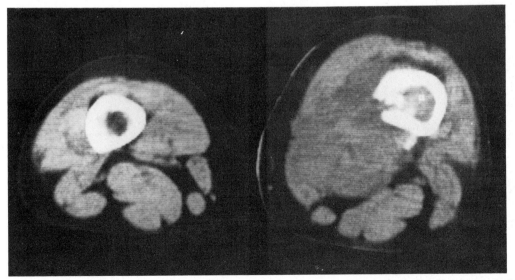

Figure 5.31.   Computed tomogram of the cross-section of both thighs. Note the destructive lesion in the femur on your right and the extensive extension of the lesion into the soft tissues. The diagnosis is a far advanced osteosarcoma.

either sternal or iliac crest puncture (*aspiration biopsy*). Bone and soft tissue specimens are obtained either by open operation (*open biopsy*) or by withdrawing a small piece of tissue through a hollow cannula (*punch biopsy*). The microscopic examination of these tissues is of particular value in the diagnosis of musculoskeletal neoplasms.

Examples of the role of these various laboratory examinations in the diagnosis of specific musculoskeletal disorders are given in subsequent chapters.

Arthroscopy

Despite the efficacy of arthrography, nothing surpasses direct visualization of the interior of a joint. Following the lead of urologists, who for decades have been able to explore the interior of the urinary bladder by means of the cystoscope, orthopaedic surgeons have more recently developed sophisticated fiber optic arthroscopes (especially for the knee) which enable us to increase the accuracy of diagnosis of internal derangements and other disorders to over 95% (Fig. 5.33). Furthermore, it is now feasible even to perform certain surgical procedures using the arthroscope plus specially designed instruments that are inserted either through the scope or into the knee through a separate portal (arthroscopic surgery)—procedures such as removal of a loose body, partial or total menisectomy, drilling defects in the articular surface and shaving or abrading areas of chondromalacia).

Arthroscopy of the knee and even arthroscopic surgery can be performed under either local or general anesthetic and usually on an outpatient or "day-care" basis with considerably less morbidity than is associated with open arthrotomy. Because of the inaccessibility of some areas of the knee joint, arthroscopy may have to be combined with double contrast (air and dye) arthrography in the diagnosis of "problem knees." Arthroscopy has also been developed for other joints including the shoulder, elbow, wrist, ankle and even the hip.

Arthroscopy identifies those patients for whom arthrotomy can be obviated, while for those patients requiring arthrotomy, arthroscopy makes the planning for such open surgery more accurate.

Myeloscopy

Using fiber optics and a very fine needle scope, it is now possible to visualize the extradural and subarachnoid spaces. This

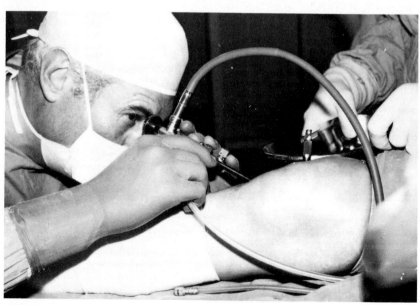

Figure 5.33. Examination of the interior of the knee through an arthroscope. Note the sterile conditions in the operating room. (Courtesy of Dr. R. W. Jackson)

can be very helpful in the precise diagnosis of lesions involving the nerve roots and especially arachonoiditis in patients with recurrent leg pain following spinal surgery.

Antenatal Diagnosis

During the past decade antenatal, or prenatal, diagnosis of certain musculoskeletal disorders, such as meningomyelocele, Down's syndrome, some of the inborn errors of metabolism and others has become possible by means of a study of cells obtained from amniocentesis and even direct visualization of a fetus through an endoscope (fetoscopy). These developments are discussed in Chapter 8.

CORRELATION OF ALL DATA (CLUES)

As you proceed with the investigation of your patient's problem, you are continually thinking of possible diagnoses and are directing the investigation along appropriate lines. Having collected the pertinent data or clues, you, like Sherlock Holmes, will then be ready to review the overall picture and to correlate the data, or relate the clues to each other. By means of logic, deduction and previous experience you will then endeavor to arrive at a probable solution (*provisional diagnosis*) of the problem. When there is insufficient proof, or evidence, for a single solution, you can at least narrow the possibilities down to a few "suspects" (*differential diagnosis*), following which you should continue the investigation by obtaining more data.

From a study of 50 clinicopathological conferences published in the *New England Journal of Medicine* in 1974 and 1979, Eddy and Clanton concluded that the following six steps are taken to arrive at a diagnosis: aggregation of groups of findings into patterns, selection of a "pivot" or key finding, generation of a cause list, pruning of the cause list, selection of a diagnosis, and validation of the diagnosis.

If your personal experience is limited, you would naturally wish, in the interests of your patient, to seek consultation with a more experienced colleague.

COMMUNICATION WITH YOUR PATIENTS

Solving the problem of diagnosis for your patient is but the first of many steps toward the *goal of helping him with his problem*. Having made a diagnosis of the *present situation*, you must then consider the *future outlook (prognosis)* for your patient, and be prepared to *communicate* with him at his level of understanding. He and his close relatives have the right to know (if they wish) just what your diagnosis means *in relation to him and his future*. How often one hears a patient say of his doctor: "He *said* quite a bit, and used some big words which I couldn't understand, but he really didn't *tell* me anything, and I am confused and concerned." No matter how brilliant you have been in the scientific aspect of your investigation, it is of little *comfort* to your patient unless you have developed the *art of communication*. It is, of course, not only necessary, but also unwise, to explain the minutiae of your patient's diagnosis and treatment to him as though he were a medical student, or a medical doctor. Nevertheless, it is *essential* that you give him an *understanding* of his condition and also that you be *aware of his particular needs and fears*. He may either fear *death* from a progressive disease such as cancer, or fear *life* with a painful, crippling or disabling condition. He will *want* and *need* to know the answers to such questions as "What is wrong with me? How serious is it? Can it be treated? How successfully? What is the treatment? How long will I be away from my home, or from my work? What would happen if it is not treated?"

Wilson has written that the medical doctor communicates best when he or she, is honest, compassionate, caring, calm, readily available, sensitive and trustworthy.

The practice of medicine is becoming progressively more *scientific* and this is as it should be, since *science* must always be the *basis of medical knowledge*. At the same time, you must develop the *art of communicating with your patients*, which, in effect, requires that you develop a keen and sympathetic awareness of their needs, for as Sir

William Osler has stated so clearly *"The practice of medicine is an art based on science."*

Suggested Additional Reading

AbuRahma, A. F., Dietrich, E. B. and Reiling, M.: Doppler testing in peripheral vascular disease. Surg. Gyn. Obstet. 150: 26–28, 1980.

Bauer, G.: Progress in the use of radionuclides in orthopaedics. Acta Orthop. Scand. 46: 315–322, 1975.

Chapman, M.: Myeloscopy (personal communication, 1982).

D'Amrosia, R. D. (ed.): *Musculoskeletal Disorders: Regional Examination and Differential diagnosis*. Philadelphia, J. B. Lippincott, 1977.

Dandy, D. J.: Arthroscopic surgery of the knee In *Current Problems in Orthopaedics* Edinburgh, Churchill-Livingstone, 1981.

Eddy, D. M., and Clanton, C. H.: The art of diagnosis. Solving the clinicopathological conference. N. Engl. J. Med. 306: 1263–1268, 1982.

Fan, A. G.: M.S.K. musculoskeletal examination. From *Toronto Physical Examination* series. Collier-Macmillan Canada, 1980.

Genant, H. K., Wilson, J. S., Bovill, E. G., Brunelle, F. O., Murray, W. R., and Rodrigo, J. J.: Computed tomography of the musculoskeletal system. J. Bone Joint Surg. 62A: 1088–1101, 1980.

Haller, O. J. and Shkolnik, A. (eds.): *Ultrasound in Pediatrics*. Edinburgh, Churchill-Livingstone, 1981.

Hoppenfeld, S.: *Physical Examination of the Spine and Extremities*. New York, Appleton-Century-Crofts, 1976.

Hoppenfeld, S.: *Orthopaedic Neurology: A Diagnostic Guide to Neurologic Levels*. Philadelphia, J.B. Lippincott, 1977.

Hughes, S. P. F.: Radionuclides in orthopaedic surgery. J. Bone Joint Surg. 62B: 141–150, 1980.

Ireland, J., Trickey, E. L. and Stoker, D. J.: Arthroscopy and arthrography of the knee: critical review. J. Bone Joint Surg. 62B: 3–6, 1980.

Jackson, R. W. and Danby, D. J.: *Arthroscopy of the Knee*. New York, Grune & Stratton, 1976.

Kirchner, P. T. and Simon, M. A.: Current concepts review: radioisotopic evaluation of skeletal disease. J. Bone Joint Surg. 63A: 673–681, 1981.

Kessel, L.: *Color Atlas of Clinical Orthopaedics*. Chicago, Year Book Medical Publishers, 1980.

McGinty, J. B.: Arthroscopy, a modality of diagnosis or treatment (Abraham Colles Lecture). J. Irish Coll. Phys. Surg. 11: 63–67, 1981.

McLeod, R. A., Stephens, D. H., Beabout, J. W., Sheedy, P. F. and Hattery, R. R.: Computed tomography of the skeletal. Semin. Roentgenol. 13: 1978.

McRae, R.: *Clinical Orthopaedic Examination*. Edinburgh, Churchill-Livingstone, 1976.

Murray, R. O.: Orthopaedic radiology: an expanding discipline. J. R. Soc. Med. 73: 320–323, 1980.

Murray, R. O. and Jacobson, H. G.:O *The Radiology of Skeletal Disorders: Exercises in Diagnosis*, 2nd ed. Edinburgh, Churchill-Livingstone, 1977.

Ozonoff, M. B.: *Pediatric Orthopaedic Radiology*. Philadelphia, W. B. Saunders, 1979.

Paul, D. J. and Gilday, D. L.: Polyphosphate bone scanning of non-malignant bone disease in children. J. Can. Assoc. Radiol. 26: 285–290, 1975.

Paul, D. F., Morrey, B. F. and Helms, C. A.: Computerized tomography in orthopaedic surgery. Clin. Orthop. 139: 142–149, 1979.

Smith, F. W. and Gilday, D. L.: Scintigraphic appearances of osteoid osteoma. Radiology 137: 191–195, 1980.

Sullivan, A. J., Vasileff, T. and Leonard, J. C.: An evaluation of nuclear scanning in orthopaedic infections. J. Pediatr. Orthop. 1: 73–79, 1981.

Wightman, K. J. R.: *Patient Examination and History Taking*. Collier-Macmillan Canada, 1977.

Williams, E. A. and Davies, D. R. A.: Arthroscopy of the knee in general orthopedic practice. J. R. Coll. Surg. Edinb. 25: 91–97, 1980.

Wilson, D.: Communication and the family physician. Can. Fam. Phys. 26: 1710–1716, 1980.

Zohn, D. A. and McMannell, J.: *Musculoskeletal Pain: Diagnosis and Physical Treatment*. Boston, Little, Brown, 1976.

CHAPTER 6

The General Principles and Specific Methods of Musculoskeletal Treatment

The General Principles of Treatment
 1. **Firstly Do No Harm**
 2. **Base Treatment on an Accurate Diagnosis and Prognosis**
 3. **Select Treatment with Specific Aims**
 4. **Cooperate with the "Laws of Nature"**
 5. **Be Realistic and Practical in Your Treatment**
 6. **Select Treatment for Your Patient as an Individual**
A Litany for Medical Doctors
General Forms and Specific Method of Treatment
  Forms of Treatment
  Specific Methods of Treatment
   1. **Psychological Considerations**
   2. **Therapeutic Drugs**
   3. **Orthopaedic Apparatus and Appliances**
   4. **Physical and Occupational Therapy**
   5. **Surgical Manipulation**
   6. **Surgical Operations**
   7. **Electrical Stimulation**
   8. **Continuous Passive Motion (CPM)**
   9. **Radiation Therapy**
Rehabilitation—A Philosophy in Action

You will have come to appreciate from the first five chapters of this textbook, as well as from your own preclinical and clinical experience to date, that man is subject to a large number and wide variety of disorders and injuries of the musculoskeletal system. In addition, a given disorder or injury may present different problems for different kinds of individuals. It will not be surprising to you, therefore, that the specific methods of treatment for patients with musculoskeletal conditions are both numerous and varied. Before discussing the many disorders and injuries of the musculoskeletal system and their treatment in subsequent chapters, it would seem wise at this time to consider the *general principles* as well as the *specific methods* of treatment for musculoskeletal conditions in order that you may become aware of the "therapeutic armamentarium" and that the subsequent discussions may be more meaningful for you.

THE GENERAL PRINCIPLES OF TREATMENT

Principles are those fundamental truths which provide both a basis for reasoning and a guide for conduct. In the practice of medicine, general principles are formulated from natural laws ("laws of nature")—laws of the behavior of body tissues under various conditions, as well as laws of human behavior—laws that you must constantly respect. As Leonardo da Vinci has stated, "Nature never breaks her own laws." Thus, the general principles of treatment must be the *basis for your reasoning* in selecting the specific method of treatment for your patient as well as the *guide for your conduct* during his total care. It is important not only to know *what* you are doing or planning to do, but also to know the reason *why*.

The following general principles are expressed in the form of advice to you as a medical doctor of the future. These principles of treatment—like your own professional conscience—ought always to be obeyed.

1. FIRSTLY DO NO HARM (*PRIMUM NON NOCERE*)

As a result of the many important scientific advances in recent years, you will have powerful and effective methods of treatment to help your patient with his problem. Remember, however, that while these methods have a potential for great benefit, they also have a potential for great harm. Treatment can be a double-edged sword. The expression *"iatrogenic disease"* means a harmful condition produced unwittingly and inadvertently by the physician or surgeon. You must be constantly aware of this danger, and on guard against it. In planning a method of treatment for your patient you must weigh its potential benefit against its potential harm. For your patient, not to be made better by treatment is discouraging—but to be made worse by treatment is devastating!

2. BASE TREATMENT ON AN ACCURATE DIAGNOSIS AND PROGNOSIS

It will be obvious that you will not help your patient with his problem if you treat him on the basis of a wrong diagnosis; for example, if you treat him for rheumatic fever when, in fact, he has acute osteomyelitis; or if you treat him for osteomyelitis when, in fact, he has a sarcoma of bone. Moreover, you will not be helping your patient as much as you should if you treat only a secondary manifestation of his disease (a symptom or a sign) without making an accurate diagnosis of the underlying or primary disease; for example, if you merely treat his pain without diagnosing its cause; or if you treat his paralytic foot deformity without recognizing that the primary cause, or condition, is a spinal cord neoplasm. Furthermore, you will do your patient a disservice if you treat him (other than by reassurance) for a condition with such a good prognosis that it would improve spontaneously without treatment; or if you fail to treat him, thinking his prognosis is good when, in fact, it is not. You may think that all such errors of omission and commission are surely very uncommon, but regrettably, they are not.

3. SELECT TREATMENT WITH SPECIFIC AIMS

While the *general* aim of treatment must always be to help your patient, your treatment must have *specific* aims to deal with his specific problems. You will recall from the preceding chapter that the common presenting problems, or chief complaints, of patients with musculoskeletal conditions are: (1) pain, (2) a decrease in function and (3) the physical appearance of either a deformity or an abnormal gait. Therefore, having made an accurate diagnosis of the underlying, or primary, condition responsible for the presenting problem or complaint and having planned its treatment, you must in addition, select treatment with the specific aim of dealing with the complaint itself. Thus, your treatment will have as its specific aim one or more of the following: (1) the relief of pain, (2) the improvement of function, (3) the prevention or correction of deformity and (4) the improvement of gait.

4. COOPERATE WITH THE "LAWS OF NATURE"

The natural restorative powers in man are truly remarkable and constitute your strongest ally in treating his disorders and injuries. Work *with* these powers and you will accomplish much for your patient; work *against* them and you will accomplish little. You must appreciate the *natural laws of behavior of body tissues* under various circumstances in order to work *with* them through your appropriate choice of the general type of treatment as well as the specific method and particular technique of treatment. Furthermore, with a knowledge of the *natural laws of human behavior*, you will be much more aware of your patient's need for your understanding, kindness and reassurance, as well as his need to have confidence in you—his doctor. As you treat your patient in coöperation with the "Laws of Nature" you will come to realize how much you depend upon these natural powers of restoration, just as Ambroise Paré, a famous 16th century French surgeon, realized when he said, "Je le pansay, Dieu le guarit" ("I dressed his wounds, God healed him").

5. BE REALISTIC AND PRACTICAL IN YOUR TREATMENT

Certain methods of treatment which may seem attractive in theory may be neither realistic nor practical for your particular patient. Common sense and sound judgment will lead you to ask yourself three important questions concerning any proposed treatment:

(i) "Precisely what am I aiming to accomplish by this method of treatment—what is its specific aim or goal?"

(ii) "Am I, in fact, likely to accomplish this aim or goal by this method of treatment?" If the answer to this question is "No," then obviously you must make another choice. If the answer is "Yes," then you must ask yourself a third question.

(iii) "Will the anticipated end result justify the means or method—will it be *worth it for your patient* in terms of what *he* will have to go through—the risks, the discomfort, the period away from his home, work or school?" If the carefully considered answer to this third question is "Yes," then you will have selected a realistic and practical method of treatment for your patient.

6. SELECT TREATMENT FOR YOUR PATIENT AS AN INDIVIDUAL

The treatment of many non-traumatic disorders of the musculoskeletal system is "elective," as opposed to "emergency" in nature. This means that you will have ample time to elect, or select, *the particular method* of treatment most suitable for *your particular patient* with *his particular disorder* in relation to *his particular needs.* In this way you will avoid merely selecting a method of treatment for a "case" or for a diagnosis as though it existed in isolation rather than in a human individual with individual needs. A given disorder may present a very different problem for one individual than it does for

another, not only in relation to age, sex, occupation and any coexistent disease, but also in relation to his personality and his resultant psychological reaction to his problem. Therefore, your choice of treatment will be influenced by all of these factors so that it may be tailored to fit the particular needs of your particular patient. You are, in fact, hoping through your treatment to do something *for* your patient rather than just *to* him.

We must forever remember that our function as medical doctors is "to cure sometimes, to relieve often and to comfort always" (anonymous folksaying of the 15th century).

A LITANY FOR MEDICAL DOCTORS

Some of these important general principles are epitomized by Sir Robert Hutchinson, of The London Hospital, England, in the following litany which he has written for medical doctors (1953):

"From inability to let well alone;

From too much zeal for the new and contempt for what is old;

From putting knowledge before wisdom, science before art, and cleverness before common sense;

From treating patients as cases, and from making the cure of the disease more grievous than the endurance of the same,

Good Lord, deliver us."

GENERAL FORMS AND SPECIFIC METHODS OF TREATMENT

Forms of Treatment

Patients with musculoskeletal conditions are cared for by various *general forms* or *types of treatment* each of which includes a number of *specific methods*; furthermore, each specific method may be achieved by a variety of *specialized techniques*. It will be apparent to you that, at this stage of your training, it is more important for you to learn about the *general principles*, the *general forms* or *types* and the *specific methods* of treatment than it is to learn about the specialized techniques.

The *seven general forms* or *types of treatment* include the following: (1) psychological considerations; (2) therapeutic drugs; (3) orthopaedic apparatus and appliances; (4) physical and occupational therapy; (5) surgical manipulation; (6) surgical repair and reconstruction; (7) electrical stimulation; (8) continuous passive motion; (9) radiation therapy. Treatment is sometimes described as either "conservative" (when no surgical operation is involved) or "radical" (when the treatment consists of operation). However, under many circumstances, these terms lose their significance and meaning and therefore, the terms *non-operative* and *operative* are more appropriate.

The importance of *rehabilitation* is given special emphasis at the end of this chapter.

Specific Methods of Treatment

In subsequent chapters reference will be made to the various forms and specific methods of treatment in relation to specific musculoskeletal disorders and injuries. However, in this chapter, all of the forms and their specific methods are discussed as a group so that you may consider them in perspective and also in order that references to treatment in subsequent chapters may be more meaningful for you.

For each specific method of treatment there are favorable circumstances in which the method *should* be used (*indications*) as well as unfavorable circumstances in which it *should not* be used (*contraindications*). A knowledge of the indications and contraindications is of great importance in selecting a specific method, or methods, of treatment for your particular patient with his particular problem. There is not always unanimity of opinion, even among experts, about indications and contraindications in relation to treatment of many disorders and injuries since these opinions are based, not only on general principles, but also on individual experience and the present state of knowledge. With continuing advances in knowledge and improvements in both methods and techniques, indications and contraindications become modified. You will appreci-ate that there may be more than one therapeutic pathway by which to reach a desired goal, but some pathways are smoother, easier and safer for your patient than others.

1. PSYCHOLOGICAL CONSIDERATIONS

Socrates, circa 400 B.C., admonished that we "ought not treat the body without the mind." Every one of your patients will require—and deserve—some psychological consideration in the form of *sympathetic understanding* as well as the *assurance* that everything possible will be done to help him with his problem. For patients with minor disorders, or with musculoskeletal variations of normal, the only type of treatment needed may be *reassurance.* However, this important form of treatment requires both time and skill; your patient's concern, or anxiety, is usually greater than you realize. He will not be reassured if you merely state that there is nothing seriously wrong with him and that there will be no treatment. Your thoughtful reassurance will do much to allay his fears and restore his peace of mind.

2. THERAPEUTIC DRUGS

Many of the disorders and injuries of the musculoskeletal system are *physical* conditions for which there is no specific drug therapy. For example, there is no specific therapeutic drug available (as yet) that will accelerate the normal healing of injured musculoskeletal tissues, or that will make a weak muscle stronger, a lax ligament tighter, a stiff joint mobile or a deformed bone straight. Nevertheless, certain types of drugs do have an important place in musculoskeletal treatment. Since specific drug preparations are continually changing as a result of pharmaceutical advances, it is preferable in a textbook such as this to discuss types of drugs rather than specific preparations.

Analgesics

The relief of pain, which is of such immediate importance to your patient, can and should be provided by appropriate analgesics. However, the underlying *cause* of the pain must be determined lest you make the error of treating only a symptom of an underlying condition which, in itself, requires specific treatment. Salicylates and other mild analgesics are effective in relief of mild musculoskeletal pain; narcotics must be used with great caution, particularly for chronic pain because of the danger of *iatrogenic* drug addiction.

Chemotherapeutic Agents

Antibiotics and other chemotherapeutic agents can be of great value in the treatment of specific musculoskeletal infections, particularly osteomyelitis and septic arthritis. However, they must be administered intelligently by determining, insofar as is possible, the specific causative organism as well as its sensitivity, or its resistance, to the various agents. Antibiotic therapy is discussed in Chapter 10.

During the past two decades, the use of powerful cytotoxic agents in the chemotherapy of cancer has done much to increase the survival rate and to prolong life, although not necessarily to improve its quality. These anticancerous agents are discussed in Chapter 14.

Another form of chemotherapy developing during the past two decades is "chemonucleolysis," i.e. the intradiscal injection of the enzyme chymopapain to degrade, and hence shrink, the nucleus pulposus for the purpose of alleviating the distressful symptoms of intervertebral disc protrusion. This form of chemotherapy is discussed further in Chapter 11.

Corticosteroids

The anti-inflammatory action of corticosteroids has been of some value in decreasing certain of the manifestations of non-specific inflammations associated with conditions such as bursitis and rheumatoid arthritis, but these drugs do not cure the underlying disease. Furthermore, the prolonged systemic administration of corticosteroids can produce many harmful effects. Therefore these drugs should be used with caution in the treatment of chronic musculoskeletal conditions.

Vitamins

Vitamin C is the specific therapeutic agent for scurvy and vitamin D is specific for the classical type of vitamin D deficiency rickets.

Other types of rickets are refractory to ordinary doses of vitamin D; the treatment of the various generalized disorders of bone is presented in Chapter 9.

Specific Drugs

Colchicine is one of the few examples of a specific therapeutic drug that provides dramatic relief for one specific condition—acute gouty arthritis.

3. ORTHOPAEDIC APPARATUS AND APPLIANCES

Prior to the advent of anesthesia in the 19th century, much of the treatment of musculoskeletal disorders and injuries involved the use of various types of orthopaedic apparatus and appliances designed to provide local rest, support and corrective forces. These methods, which are still important—and will continue to be important in the future—are best considered in relation to their specific aims in musculoskeletal treatment.

Rest

For centuries it was thought—on the basis of empiricism—that total body rest (bed rest) was necessary for certain severe disorders and injuries of the musculoskeletal system. However, prolonged and continuous bed rest is associated with many harmful effects including (1) disuse atrophy of muscles with resultant generalized weakness; (2) disuse atrophy of bone (generalized osteoporosis); (3) increased calcium excretion; (4) deep vein thrombosis with the threat of pulmonary embolism; (5) pressure sores (decubitus ulcers) which can be prevented only by excellent nursing care. Therefore, bed-ridden patients should be encouraged to exercise uninvolved limbs, and whenever feasible, should be helped from their bed to a chair, or wheel chair, for at least a part of each day.

For centuries it has also been thought—on the basis of the same empiricism—that *local rest* of varying degree aids the healing of inflamed and injured musculoskeletal tissues, and also helps to relieve pain that is related to movement. *Relative rest* for a limb may be provided by simply preventing its usual function, with a sling for an upper limb, or with crutches for the relief of weight bearing in a lower limb. For relief of weight bearing, a sling for the lower limb may be used with crutches (Fig. 6.1). Another form of relative rest for a limb is provided by *continuous traction* which can be achieved by many techniques. Continuous traction is used for the following purposes: (1) to maintain length of the limb and alignment of fracture fragments in unstable fractures of the shafts of long bones (Fig. 6.2); (2) to relieve painful muscle spasm associated with joint inflammation or injury; (3) to gradually stretch soft tissues that have become shortened secondary to a long standing joint deformity or dislocation (for example, continuous traction prior to reduction of a congenital dislocation of the hip).

Fairly rigid and continuous local rest (*immobilization*) is used to maintain or stabilize the position of a fracture or a dislocation following its reduction and also to maintain the desired position of a part following injury, surgical manipulation or surgical operation. This type of immobilization is most commonly obtained by the application of plaster of Paris casts of varying design (Fig. 6.3).

You must realize, however, that prolonged immobilization of a limb, including its synovial joints, is associated with many harmful effects including (1) disuse atrophy of local muscles and resultant muscle weakness; (2) disuse atrophy of local bone (localized osteoporosis); (3) local venous thrombosis with resultant edema; (4) the complication of pressure sores (cast sores); and, most importantly, muscle contractures, joint capsule contractures and intra-articular adhesions, all of which lead to persistent joint stiffness. These iatrogenic effects may take many months to be reversed—with or without physiotherapy. If the involved limb has been immobilized for a very long time (more than one or two months), especially after an intra-articular injury or operation, the joint may never recover and consequently may develop secondary post-traumatic arthritis.

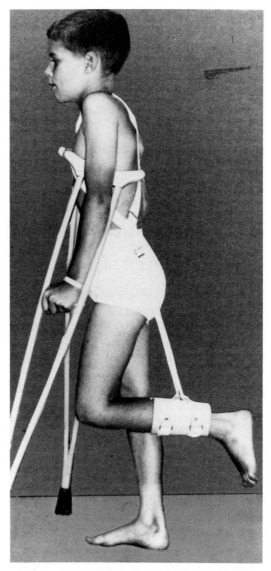

Figure 6.1. A Snyder sling for the relief of weight bearing in a lower limb. This form of management is acceptable for short term treatment but for long term treatment the problem, understandably, is lack of patient compliance.

Support for Muscle Weakness and Joint Instability

A patient with extensive muscle weakness in the upper limb can be helped by the use of *functional braces* which are designed to transmit movement to the weak part of the limb from some other muscle group (Fig.

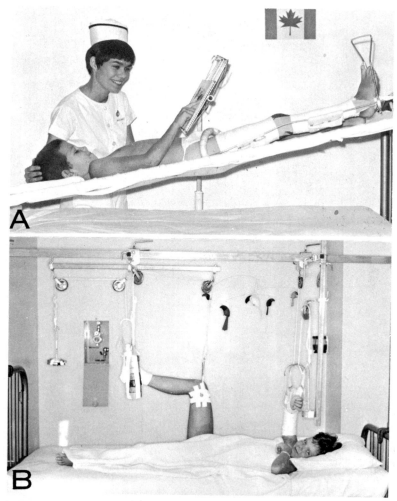

Figure 6.2. Continuous traction. *A*, skin traction through special adhesive tape. The child's body tends to move away from the elevated end of the frame and provides the counteraction. This boy is being treated for an unstable fracture of the shaft of right femur. *B*, skin traction through special adhesive tape for an unstable fracture of the humerus and skeletal traction through a metal pin in the distal end of the femur for an unstable fracture of the upper third of the femoral shaft.

6.4). A weak or unstable and painful spine can be given some degree of support by a *spinal brace* (Fig. 6.5). In the lower limb, when either muscle weakness or joint instability interfere with weight bearing and walking, the involved limb can be supported by means of an appropriate *brace* which prevents unwanted motion while permitting desired motion (Fig. 6.6*A*). Hypermobile joints in the feet occasionally require temporary support by appropriate *shoe corrections* such as arch supports and sole wedges. Mild soft tissue injuries of joints may be given temporary support by means of carefully applied *adhesive tape strapping*.

In recent years the time honored terms "braces" and "splints" have been replaced by the sophisticated collective term "orthoses" and those individuals who produce such devices are no longer "brace makers" or "splint makers" but rather "orthotists." By the same token, artificial limbs have become "prostheses" and are produced not by "limb makers" but by "prosthetists."

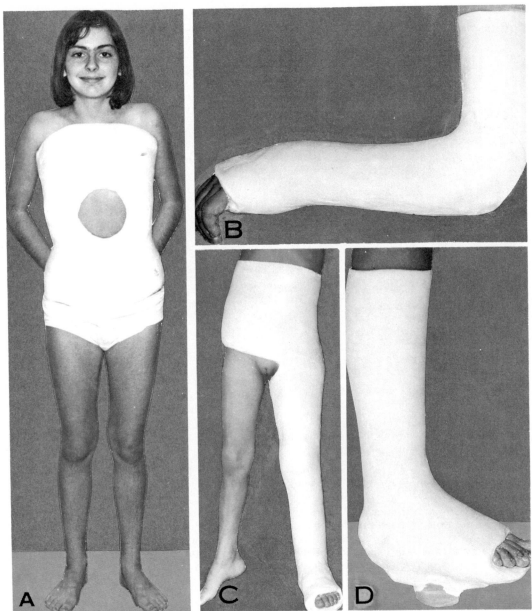

Figure 6.3.   Plaster of Paris casts of varying design to provide immobilization. *A*, body cast; *B*, above elbow cast. *C*, hip spica cast. *D*, below knee walking cast.

Light plastic materials such as polypropylene have made present-day orthoses not only lighter but cosmetically more acceptable (Fig. 6.6*B*)

Prevention and Correction of Deformity.

When the development of a joint deformity is anticipated, as with muscle imbalance in either spastic or flaccid paralysis, or with muscle spasm in chronic arthritis, it is frequently possible to *prevent* the deformity by means of *intermittent immobilization* in a removable splint (Fig. 6.7*A*). Following correction of a joint deformity and the subsequent period of continuous immobilization, it is sometimes necessary to use a removable

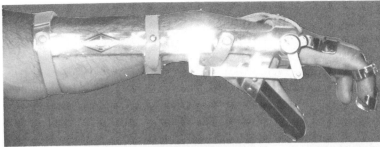
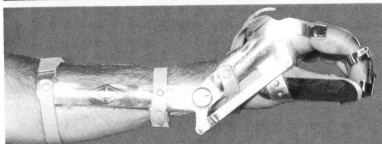
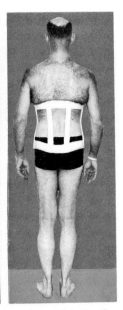

Figure 6.4 (*left*).   Functional brace. This brace is used to compensate for loss of power in the finger flexors. It is so designed that active dorsiflexion of the wrist causes the paralyzed fingers to flex and the thumb to oppose them.
Figure 6.5 (*right*).   Spinal brace. This type of lumbosacral brace is designed to limit the extremes of motion of the spine and is used to relieve certain types of low back pain. It is not possible to immobilize the spine completely by any type of brace.

splint for intermittent immobilization in order to *prevent recurrence* of the deformity. The gradual *correction* of certain torsional deformities in growing long bones is possible over a period of months by means of removable night splints specially designed to transmit corrective forces to the epiphyseal plates (Fig. 6.7*B*).

4. PHYSICAL AND OCCUPATIONAL THERAPY (Fig. 6.8)

The *aims* of these closely related forms of treatment are *to regain and maintain joint motion*, *to increase muscle strength* and *to improve musculoskeletal function.* Although there is considerable overlap, physical therapy (physiotherapy) has more application for problems of the lower limbs and trunk, whereas occupational therapy is more applicable for those of the upper limbs. The specific methods of physical and occupational therapy are carried out by trained *therapists* at the request, and on the prescription

of, the patient's own physician or surgeon who, of course, is the coordinator of all the forms of treatment required for his patient. The following are some of the specific methods of such therapy in relation to their specific aims.

Joint Motion

The safest method of *regaining motion in a painful stiff joint* is *active movement* (by the patient's own muscle action) which is encouraged and directed by the therapist; the pain which arises at each end of the range of motion produces a reflex inhibition of muscle action which "protects" the joint from being forced. *Intermittent passive movement* (by the therapist) of such a joint is potentially dangerous, especially if it is forceful, because it may produce further irritation and injury to the abnormal synovial membrane and joint capsule and thereby result in more stiffness. Intermittent passive movement is of greatest value in *maintaining joint motion* and thereby *preventing deform-*

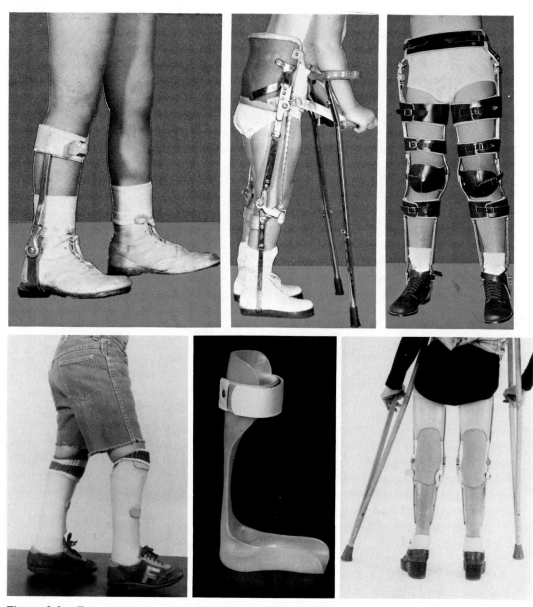

Figure 6.6. *Top*, standard metallic lower limb braces which prevent unwanted motion while permitting desired motion in weak or unstable limbs. *Bottom*, present day orthoses constructed of light plastic materials.

ity in a joint which the patient cannot move actively because of paralysis. Passive movement is also of some help in the gradual stretching of existing muscle contractures.

Muscle Strength

A muscle is strengthened only by *active exercise.* Even when a limb is immobilized, as in a cast, muscles can be strengthened by *static* exercises (muscle action without joint motion). *Dynamic* exercises (producing joint motion) serve the dual purpose of increasing muscle strength and helping to regain motion. Muscle exercises performed against progressively increasing resistance are particularly effective for increasing

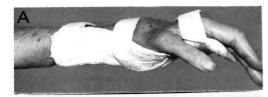

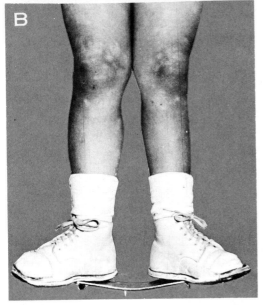

strength. When a muscle has an intact nerve supply but is "inhibited" following injury or operation, it can be electrically stimulated to contract by means of a *faradic* current applied to its motor nerve. A muscle that has lost its nerve supply gradually atrophies and becomes fibrosed; but if there is hope of nerve recovery, these changes can be minimized pending nerve recovery by means of a *galvanic* current which stimulates muscle fibres directly.

Improvement of Musculoskeletal Function

Functional training involves more than joint motion and muscle strength; it involves coordination of muscles in skilful and purposeful activity by the patient. The therapist

Figure 6.7. Removable splints. *A*, this splint is being worn at night and during part of the day to help prevent deformity in the patient's hand, which is affected by rheumatoid arthritis. *B*, this Denis-Browne night splint is being worn at night by a child with internal tibial torsion. It is designed to exert a torsional force on the epiphyseal plates of the tibiae.

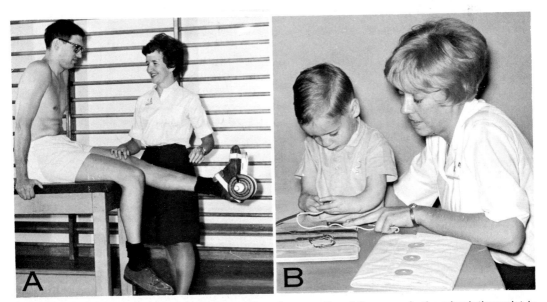

Figure 6.8. Physical therapy (physiotherapy) and occupational therapy. *A*, the physiotherapist is instructing this man to actively extend his left knee against the resistance of weights attached to his foot. The purpose of this dynamic exercise is to strengthen the quadriceps muscle. *B*, the occupational therapist is training the child to develop skill in his weak and deformed hands.

helps the patient to help himself by training him in musculoskeletal activities required for daily life, such as walking, going up and down stairs, dressing and eating. The occupational therapist encourages purposeful manual activities (including handicrafts) which are designed to improve coordinated hand function, and at the same time to provide interesting and absorbing mental diversion.

5. SURGICAL MANIPULATION

The *aims* of surgical manipulation are to *correct deformity* either in a bone that is fractured or in a joint that is dislocated and to a lesser extent, to *regain motion* in a stiff joint. Such manipulations, which are usually performed under anesthesia, involve passive movement of the parts by a surgeon. The great majority of fractures and dislocations can be treated by manipulation of the parts into satisfactory position (*closed reduction*). Likewise, many congenital dislocations can be treated by closed reduction—at least in very young children. The *gradual correction of joint deformities* due to contracture of muscle and capsule can often be obtained by *repeated gentle stretching* of the tight structures at intervals; immobilization of the joint in a position of correction not only helps to maintain correction, but also allows the contractures to soften somewhat so that further correction may be obtained at the time of the next stretching. This gentle type of manipulative treatment can be performed without anesthesia and is of particular value in the gradual correction of such congenital deformities as clubfeet. *Forceful manipulation* of stiff joints under anesthesia carries the risk of either producing further joint damage, or causing a fracture through osteoporotic bone. Nevertheless, manipulation of a large joint, under anesthesia, and without undue force, is of value in regaining motion when the stiffness is due to simple joint adhesions rather than to severe contractures of muscle or joint capsule. Such manipulation, of course, must be followed by active exercises in order to maintain the increased motion that has been gained. The

anatomical effects of manipulation of the cervical or lumbar spine are not well understood as yet but some surgeons believe that such manipulations frequently relieve pain arising from the musculoskeletal tissues in these areas. Manual fracture of a bone (*"osteoclasis"*) under anesthesia was commonly used in the past to correct deformities but is seldom used now except with abnormally weakened bone.

6. SURGICAL OPERATIONS

As a result of advancing clinical and experimental knowledge, improved surgical techniques and improved anesthesia, open surgical operations have come to play an increasingly important role in the treatment of musculoskeletal disorders and injuries. Nevertheless, you will appreciate that the operative form of treatment is *indicated* only for certain specific musculoskeletal problems. *Many patients can be treated successfully without an operation and therefore do not need one, while others cannot be helped by an operation and therefore should not be subjected to one.* Surgical operations have a potential for providing great benefit *to* the patient, but they also have a potential for producing great harm *to* him. Thus, the *general principles of treatment* discussed at the beginning of this chapter, as well as the *indications* and *contraindications* of the various surgical operations, must be thoughtfully considered by the orthopaedic surgeon—primarily a *physician* who has also been trained and taught *how* to operate, *when* to operate, and most important, *when not* to operate. Indeed, the *decision* is more important than the *incision*.

The *aims* of surgical operations for musculoskeletal conditions include *relief of pain*, *improvement of function and ability*, and *the prevention or correction of deformity*. The *general methods* of operative treatment by which these aims are achieved involve various combinations of *repair, release, resection, reconstruction* and *replacement* of involved tissues. For each general method there are several *specific methods* and for each specific method there are a variety of *surgical techniques.* As a medical student of the present, and as a practising physician of future, you should know about the available surgical methods, but you do *not* need to know the details of surgical techniques. The numerous surgical methods will be discussed briefly in relation to the *tissue* involved and the *aim* of the operation.

Operations on Muscles, Tendons and Ligaments

Increased pressure from bleeding or edema within a closed muscle compartment ("compartment syndrome") can be relieved by surgical division of the fascia (*fasciotomy*). A cut tendon is repaired by suture (*tenorrhaphy*) (Fig. 6.9). If a segment of the tendon has been irreparably damaged, that segment may be replaced by a *free tendon graft* using an autogenous, but unimportant tendon (such as the tendon of the plantaris muscle) (Fig. 6.10). When a tendon is tethered by adhesions, it may be freed (*tenolysis*) or if its range of excursion is limited by a constricting fibrous tunnel, the tendon may be *released* by either *incision* or *excision* of the tunnel. A shortened muscle may be dealt with by simple division of its tendon (*tenotomy*), subcutaneously or at open operation, or by formal *tendon lengthening* (Fig.

6.11). The action of a paralyzed or damaged muscle may be replaced by transferring the tendinous insertion (or origin) of a nearby normal muscle to improve muscle balance (*muscle transfer*) or (*tendon transfer*) (Fig. 6.12). In order to check, or limit, an undesired joint motion the tendon of a muscle (usually a paralyzed muscle) may be separated from its muscle and implanted into bone to serve as a check rein, or ligament (*tenodesis*) (Fig. 6.13). A major ligament that has been completely torn may be sutured (*ligamentous repair*), but if it is irreparably damaged, it may have to be replaced by a tendon, or by a free graft of fascia lata (*ligamentous reconstruction*).

Operations on Nerves

A cut nerve is repaired by *nerve suture*, but if the gap is too large a *nerve graft* may be required. Abnormally thickened perineural sheath, or other constricting soft tissues, may compress the nerve which then

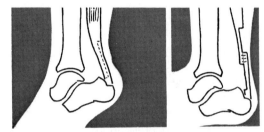

Figure 6.11. Tendon lengthening. Following the long step-cut in this Achilles' tendon, the ends are allowed to shift in relation to each other and are then sutured in the elongated position.

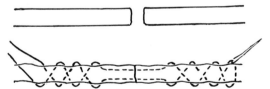

Figure 6.9. Tenorrhaphy (tendon suture). The external surface of the repaired tendon must be smooth in order that it may glide within its sheath.

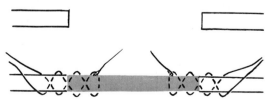

Figure 6.10. Free tendon graft. The autogenous graft replaces an irreparably damaged segment of tendon.

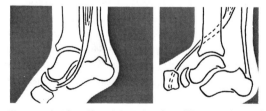

Figure 6.12. Tendon transfer. The tendon of the tibialis posterior muscle has been rerouted through the interosseous membrane and transferred to the lateral cuneiform bone on the dorsum of the foot. In its new position, it will serve as a dorsiflexor of the ankle and an evertor of the foot.

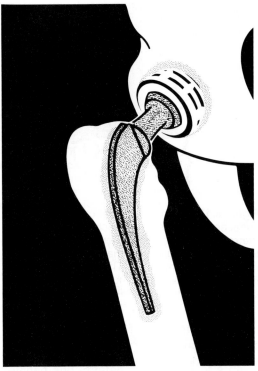

Figure 6.18. One type of prosthetic hip joint replacement. Note the metallic femoral component (head, neck and intramedullary stem) and the plastic acetabular component, both of which are held firmly in place by bone cement.

designed "clean-air surgical enclosures" to minimize this risk. More recently, porous coated prostheses have been developed to allow living bone to grow into the interstices and thereby to eliminate the need for bone cement.

The early clinical results of prosthetic hip joint replacements or "total hips" are dramatic and even published results after 10 years reveal a high rate of success in older patients.

A more recent modification of prosthetic hip replacement is a "surface replacement" in which the reshaped head and neck of the femur is covered by a metallic cup that articulates with a plastic cup in the acetabulum ("double cups") (Fig. 6.19). Initially thought to be an answer for arthritis of the hip in younger adults, the surface replacement type of prosthetic hip replacement has much the same types of complications as the con-

ventional type and hence has much the same limitations.

Although the concept of prosthetic joint replacement began with the hip, it has now been applied to virtually every joint in the upper and lower extremities—finger, thumb, wrist, elbow, shoulder, ankle and knee. A multiplicity of prosthetic knee joint replacements have been developed, including the hemi-arthroplasty of MacIntosh in 1957 and the hinged prosthesis of Waldius; the first non-hinged prosthetic knee joint replacement was designed by Gunston in 1968 while working with Charnley. The relatively high failure rate with the fully constrained, or hinged, prostheses has been reduced by the use of semi-constrained prostheses (Fig. 6.20). Nevertheless, the arthritic knee has been found to be a more challenging problem to solve through prosthetic joint replacement than the hip and the early good results of "total knees" do not seem to stand up as long as those of "total hips."

Prosthetic finger joint replacements, especially of the Swanson type, have proven to be very successful. Early designs of prosthetic elbow replacements were rather unsatisfactory but newer designs are more promising as are those for the shoulder joint.

After an external amputation of an extremity the external prosthesis, or artificial limb, can be revised or replaced without re-operation. By contrast, however, total joint excision is an "internal amputation" with an "internal prothesis" or artificial joint—a prosthesis that cannot be revised or replaced without re-operation. Furthermore, the results of such revision operations are rather discouraging.

In the current phase of phenomenal and widespread enthusiasm for total joint excision and prosthetic joint replacements it is important to appreciate that they are neither biological nor physiological and hence they may not be the final answer to the problem of arthritis. In the meantime, however, prosthetic joint replacements represent a tremendous advance in surgical technology. Nevertheless, it is essential to adhere strictly to their indications and contraindications lest

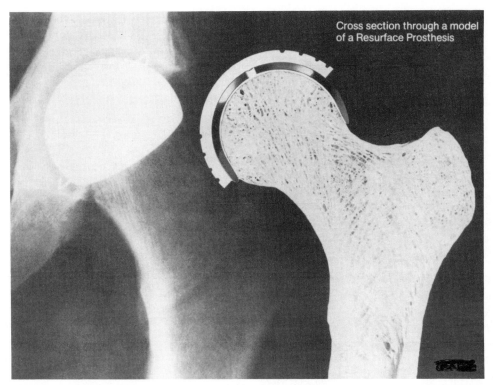

Cross section through a model of a Resurface Prosthesis

Figure 6.19. One type of "surface replacement" prosthetic hip joint in coronal section accompanied by the radiograph of such a hip. Note the metallic cup on the femoral head and neck and the plastic cup in the acetabulum ("double cups"), both of which are cemented to the underlying bone.

surgical technology be allowed to triumph over surgical judgment.

Osteocartilaginous Allografts

As an alternative to prosthetic knee joint replacement in young and middle aged adults with only one side of the joint being arthritic (unicompartmental arthritis), Gross and Langer have used small osteocartilaginous allografts (from fresh cadavers) with encouraging results since 1971 without clinical or radiographic evidence of graft rejection despite the fact that no immunosuppressive therapy has been given. In addition, they, and also Mankin, have also used massive osteocartilaginous allografts or transplants to replace defects from extensive local resection of malignant bone tumors.

Arthroscopic Surgery

As mentioned in Chapter 5, certain surgical procedures on the knee joint can now be performed—without an open arthrotomy—using an arthroscope and specially designed surgical instruments that are inserted either through the scope or into the knee joint through a separate portal. The current scope of arthroscopic surgery includes removal of a loose body, partial or total meniscectomy, drilling defects in the articular surface and shaving or abrading areas of chondromalacia. Understandably, the post-operative morbidity is less than with open arthrotomy.

Operations on Bones

Drainage of pus from within the metaphysis of a bone may become necessary in acute hematogenous osteomyelitis and is accomplished by *bone drilling*. In chronic osteomyelitis, a sequestrum, which is a separated piece of infected dead bone, is removed (*sequestrectomy*). Occasionally, in severe and extensive chronic osteomyelitis,

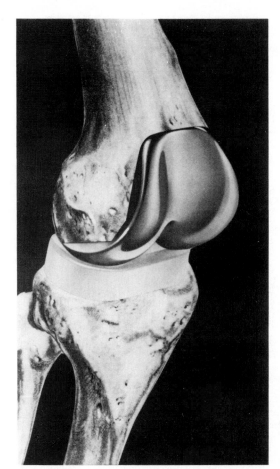

Figure 6.20. One type of prosthetic knee joint replacement. Note the metallic femoral component and the plastic tibial component, both of which are fixed to the underlying cancellous bone with bone cement.

it is necessary to lay a bone open for drainage by removing the cortex on one side (*saucerization*). Removal of a part or all of a bone (*bone resection*) is frequently necessary in the treatment of certain localized neoplasms.

Division of a bone with a sharp instrument (*osteotomy*) is a particularly effective type of reconstructive operation. Osteotomy is used to correct either an angulatory or rotational deformity in a bone (Fig. 6.21); to deal with a joint deformity by producing a compensatory bony deformity near the joint (Fig. 6.22); to redirect a joint surface and thereby improve the line of weight bearing forces or

decrease pressure between the joint surfaces (Fig. 6.23); to permit either surgical shortening of a bone (by resection of a segment or overlapping the fragments) or sur-

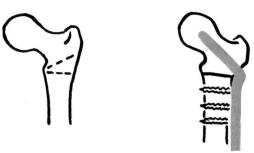

Figure 6.21. Osteotomy to correct angulatory deformity in a long bone. Following removal of a suitably shaped wedge of bone, the fragments are placed in the desired position, held by internal fixation and allowed to unit like a fracture (closed wedge osteotomy).

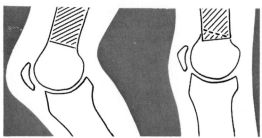

Figure 6.22. Osteotomy to deal with a joint deformity by producing a compensatory bony deformity near the joint. The knee flexion deformity persists, but the limb is made straight by the compensatory osteotomy in the supracondylar region of the femur.

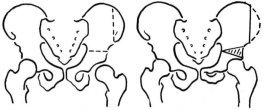

Figure 6.23. Osteotomy to redirect a joint surface. The innominate bone is divided, the distal fragment redirected and a bone graft placed in the opening to maintain the position (open wedge osteotomy). The redirected acetabulum provides better coverage of the femoral head and a larger weight bearing surface of articular cartilage.

gical lengthening of a bone in children (by gradual distraction of the osteotomy site in the presence of an intact periosteum) (Fig. 6.24). In the treatment of certain difficult and unstable fractures, it is sometimes necessary to expose the fracture site in order to replace the fragments under direct vision (*open reduction of a fracture*) and also to fix

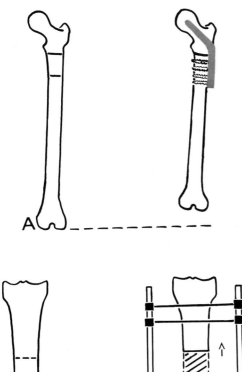

Figure 6.24. *A*, osteotomy to shorten a bone. Following resection of a segment of bone the fragments are brought together, held by internal fixation and allowed to unite like a fracture. *B*, osteotomy to lengthen a bone. Following simple division of the bone (usually by drilling and osteoclasis) the fragments are very slowly distracted over a period of weeks to gain length. New bone from the surrounding periosteum eventually fills the gap.

the fragments rigidly together by means of metallic devices such as screws, staples, plates or intramedullary nails (*internal skeletal fixation*). The various methods of internal fixation of fractures, including the AO/ASIF method, are discussed in Chapter 15.

Removal of the contents of a bone cyst or a benign intramedullary neoplasm is achieved by *curettement* and is usually followed by *intracavity bone grafting* to strengthen the residual defect (Fig. 6.27). In leg length discrepancy, an epiphyseal plate in the shorter limb can be stimulated to grow a little faster by increasing its circulation (*epiphyseal plate stimulation*), or an epiphyseal plate in the longer limb can be prevented from further growth (*epiphyseal plate arrest*) either by bone grafts (*epiphyseodesis*) or by metal staples (*epiphyseal plate stapling*).

Transplantation of bone from one location (donor site) to another site (host site), or *bone grafting*, may involve the use of multiple small fragments, or strips, of cancellous bone, or solid pieces of dense cortical bone. The transplanted (donor) bone graft (the cells of which are, for the most part, dead) is slowly united or fused to the host bone by inducing deposition of new bone at the host site; eventually, the dead graft, which acts as a skeletal framework, is gradually replaced by new living bone through the simultaneous process of donor bone resorption and host bone deposition. The ideal bone graft is from the patient himself (*autograft*) because there is no immunological graft rejection phenomenon. Less satisfactory, but sometimes practical, is stored or "banked" bone from another individual (*homograft, allograft*); least satisfactory and seldom indicated is bone from another species (*heterograft, xenograft*). Bone grafting is used to promote bony union in a fracture that has failed to unite (nonunion) or that is unduly slow in uniting (delayed union) (Fig. 6.25); to promote fusion of a joint (arthrodesis) (Fig. 6.26) or of an epiphyseal plate (epiphyseodesis); to maintain the angulation of an "open wedge" osteotomy (Fig. 6.23); and to fill a bony defect following local bone

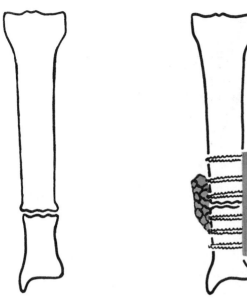

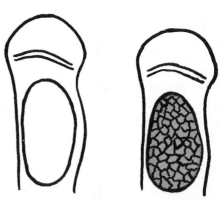

Figure 6.27. Transplantation of bone (bone grafting) to fill a bony defect following curettement of the lining of a cystic lesion in bone.

Figure 6.25. Transplantation of bone (bone grafting) to promote bony union for non-union or delayed union of a fracture. The bone graft may be cortical and held with screws, or it may consist of multiple small chips of cancellous bone.

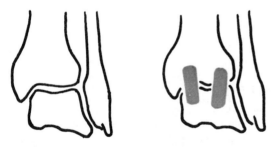

Figure 6.26. Transplantation of bone (bone grafting) to promote fusion of a joint (arthrodesis). In this example, two bone grafts are shown crossing the ankle joint.

resection or curettement of a cystic lesion (Fig. 6.27).

For certain serious conditions of a limb, such as a radio-resistant malignant neoplasm, irreparable injury, gangrene, or a severe congenital deformity that cannot be corrected by reconstructive operations, it may be necessary to remove part (or all) of the limb through bone (*amputation*), or through a joint (*disarticulation*) and to provide the patient with an artificial limb (*prothesis*).

Microsurgery

Surgery performed under the magnification of an operating microscope using microinstruments and microsutures (*microsurgery*) has developed extremely rapidly since 1960 (Fig. 6.28). This exciting advance in surgical technology has had a significant impact on surgical disorders and injuries of the musculoskeletal system in that it is now possible to replant completely severed digits and limbs, to repair with great accuracy divided peripheral nerves, to transfer free vascularized autogenous bone grafts with or without skin and other soft tissues, to transfer a toe to replace a lost thumb, and even to transfer vascularized and re-innervated autogenous muscle grafts that will function as soon as the motor nerve regenerates down the transplanted motor nerve.

7. ELECTRICAL STIMULATION OF FRACTURE HEALING

During the last two decades electricity has been used both in experimental animals and in humans as an alternative to bone grafting to stimulate osteogenesis in the treatment of established non-union of fractures. To date, the following three electrical systems have been developed: constant direct current through percutaneous wire cathodes (semi-invasive) (Brighton); constant direct current through implanted electrodes and power pack (invasive) (Dwyer and also Paterson); and inductive coupling through electromagnetic coils (non-invasive) (Bassett

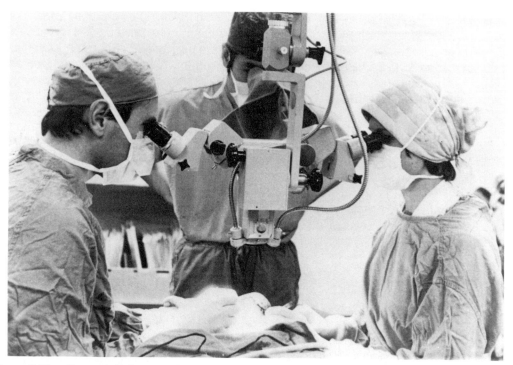

Figure 6.28.   Surgeon (*left*) and assistant performing microsurgery through an operating microscope. A third surgeon is observing the operation through a "teaching arm" of the microscope.

and also de Haas). Each method has its advantages as well as its disadvantages but all three provide the same over-all success rate of approximately 80%. Continuing investigations, both experimental and clinical, will provide more data on this important development.

8. CONTINUOUS PASSIVE MOTION

You will recall from Chapter 3 that since 1970 the concept of continuous passive motion (CPM) has been studied—and continues to be studied—in our laboratory in the Research Institute of The Hospital for Sick Children, Toronto, using experimental models of a wide variety of joint disorders and injuries in rabbits. Encouraged by the results of the first eight years of these scientific investigations and convinced of the comfort and efficacy of CPM, we have now applied the concept to the post-operative management of carefully selected patients.

The *indications* for post-operative CPM in our preliminary clinical trials have been ad-

olescent and adult patients who have had the following types of surgical procedures: (1) arthrotomy, capsulotomy and debridement of joints with painful restriction of motion secondary to post-traumatic arthritis; (2) open reduction of intra-articular fractures; (3) patellectomy; (4) repair of ligamentous injuries; (5) synovectomy for rheumatoid arthritis and hemophilic arthropathy; (6) arthrotomy for acute septic arthritis.

A carefully monitored prospective clinical investigation of CPM is currently under way in our Teaching Hospitals of the University of Toronto; in the meantime, the results of the preliminary clinical trials have been gratifying. As with the rabbits, the CPM devices have been applied to the involved limb of the patients at the completion of the operation while they are still under general anesthesia. The device moves the joint continuously day and night at a rate of approximately one cycle per minute for at least one week during which the patients are remarkably comfortable and after which they can usually maintain an excellent range of motion by their own active exercises.

We have collaborated with Professor David James and John Saringer, mechanical engineers at the University of Toronto, in the design of these electric motor-driven devices to provide continuous passive motion for the ankle-knee-hip, the elbow and the finger— devices that have been designated "CPM Mobilimbs (Figs. 6.29, 6.30 and 6.31).

9. RADIATION THERAPY

The value of ionizing radiation as a form of treatment lies in its relatively selective destruction of rapidly multiplying cells in ma-lignant neoplasms and certain other condi-tions. Immature cells and undifferentiated cells are particularly vulnerable, or sensitive, to the effects of ionizing radiation (*radiosen-sitive*). Thus, it is possible by means of highly developed techniques to deliver a *lethal tu-mor dose* of radiation to a malignant lesion and yet produce relatively little radiation ef-fect in the surrounding normal tissues. Ra-diation at therapeutic levels produces pro-found chromosomal changes in cells but the effects of these changes are not apparent until the time of the next cell division (*mito-sis*), when the cell will either fail to divide or will do so in an abnormal way. Thus, the

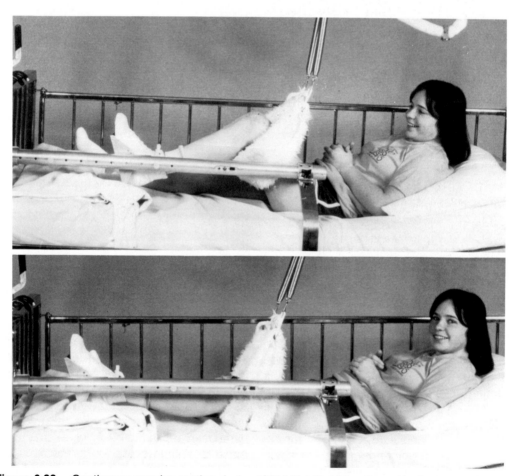

Figure 6.29. Continuous passive motion device (CPM Mobilimb) for the ankle, knee and hip. Note the range of flexion and extension in this girl's knee a few days after extensive intra-articular surgery. The electric motor is incorporated in the hollow tube; during the day the motor is battery powered and the device can be removed from the bed and attached to a crutch so that the patient may be ambulatory. At night the electrical system is plugged into a wall socket to recharge the batteries.

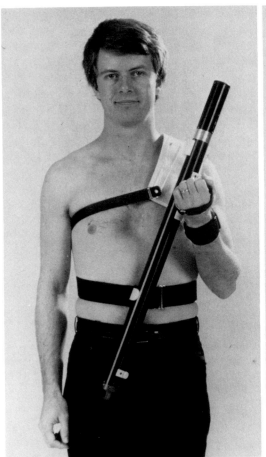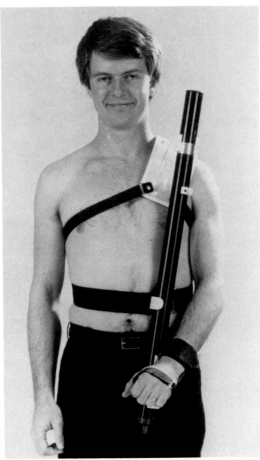

Figure 6.30. Continuous passive motion device (CPM Mobilimb) for the elbow. Note that as the elbow is flexed the forearm is supinated and as the elbow is extended the forearm is pronated, thereby providing an excellent range of both types of elbow motion.

radiation effect is related to the turnover rate of the cell population of the various types of irradiated tissue cells. The cells of the neoplasm, having a very rapid turnover rate, show the radiation effect early, while those in the bed of the neoplasm (fibrous tissue and blood vessels), having a slow turnover rate, show the radiation effect later. The most significant changes in the bed of the neoplasm are slowly progressive fibrosis and ischemia. The *total* effect of radiation therapy, therefore, is delayed rather than immediate.

The source of therapeutic ionizing radiation is usually either a high-voltage X--ray machine or a radioactive isotope such as cobalt ("the cobalt bomb"). Of the three types of energy released during the disintegration of radium (alpha rays, beta rays and gamma rays), the gamma rays have by far the greatest ability to penetrate tissues and are therefore the most effective in radiation therapy. The quantitative physical unit of *emitted* radiation is *a roentgen* (r) but the unit of *absorbed* radiation is a *rad*. Compared to neoplasms arising in other tissues, those arising in bone are relatively *radioresistant* and require high dosages of radiation (7,000 r or more over a period of several weeks). However, certain skeletal neoplasms, such as Ewing's sarcoma and reticulum cell sarcoma, may be at least locally

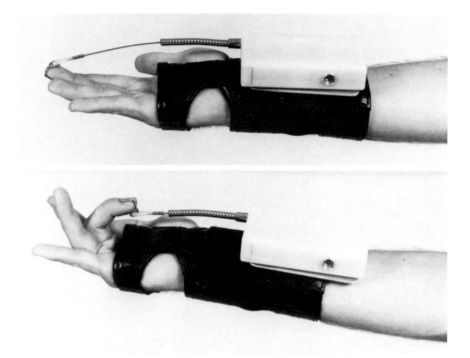

Figure 6.31.   Continuous passive motion device (CPM Mobilimb) for a finger. The flexible cable (which is glued to the fingernail through a small metal plate) pushes the finger into extension and pulls it into flexion. As with the other CPM Mobilimbs the range of motion is adjustable.

destroyed by appropriate radiation techniques even though they may recur subsequently, either locally or elsewhere. For such neoplasms, radiation therapy may be the treatment of choice, whereas neoplasms which are more radio-resistant, such as osteogenic sarcoma and chondrosarcoma, usually require radical surgical resection or amputation either with or without radiation.

Radiation therapy has been used empirically in the treatment of such poorly understood conditions as histiocytosis X and ankylosing spondylitis but is employed with great caution. In general, any nonmalignant condition that can be treated satisfactorily by some other form of treatment should not be treated by radiation. The most serious radiation effects on normal skeletal tissues are the following: epiphyseal plate damage with resultant growth disturbance; radiation necrosis of bone with subsequent pathological fracture; and rarely, radiation-induced malignancy.

REHABILITATION—A PHILOSOPHY IN ACTION

As a medical doctor of the future, regardless of whether you are a family physician or a specialist, you will be involved in the *rehabilitation* of those of your patients who suffer from either chronic or permanent disabling problems. Rehabilitation is not a specialized technique of treatment, not a method of treatment, not even a principle of treatment; rehabilitation is a *philosophy in action*—the philosophy of total care *of* your patient as well as continuing care *for* him. The broad *aim*, or *goal*, of rehabilitation is to correct, insofar as is possible, your patient's problem (whether it be physical, mental or social) and *in addition* to continue to help him by treatment, training, education and encouragement to cope with the residual uncorrectable portion of his problem and his attitude toward it, in order that his life may be changed from one of dependency to one of independence, from one that is empty to one that is full. In a sense, rehabilitation is *"going the second mile"*—and often farther—with your patient, and it is applicable to the disabling problems of all fields of medicine and surgery.

Those of your patients with disabling disorders and injuries of the musculoskeletal system will require, and deserve, rehabilitation in its broad sense. Some examples of such disabling musculoskeletal conditions are extensive *paralysis* from spina bifida with meningomyelocele, poliomyelitis, spinal cord injury (paraplegia), head injury, cerebral palsy, and cerebral vascular accidents ("strokes"); extensive congenital *deformities* and deficiencies of limbs and acquired *amputations*; severe and multiple musculoskeletal *injuries*; generalized *muscle diseases* such as muscular dystrophy; and chronic generalized *rheumatoid arthritis*. The rehabilitation of such patients, the total care *of* them as well as a continuing care *for* them, cannot be accomplished by one person; indeed the philosophy of rehabilitation requires the coordinated efforts of a large group, or *team of professional persons* including the physician or surgeon (who is the captain and coordinator), the nurse, the physical therapist and occupational therapist, the brace maker (orthotist), the limb maker (prosthetist), the psychologist, the medical social worker, the teacher and the vocational adviser. Through continuing advances in all these fields, rehabilitation is becoming progressively more realistic and effective, and it will be of even greater importance in the future than it has been in the past.

Suggested Additional Reading

Amstutz, H. C., Graff-Radford, A., Mai, L. L. and Thomas, B. J.: Surface replacement of the hip with the Thaires system. J. Bone Joint Surg. 63A: 1069–1077, 1981.

Bassett, C. A. L., Mitchell, S. N. and Gaston, S. R.: Treatment of ununited tibial diaphyseal fractures with pulsing electromagnetic fields. J. Bone Joint Surg. 63A: 511–523, 1981.

Becker, R. O.: The significance of electrically stimulated osteogenesis: more questions than answers. Clin. Orthop. 141: 266–274, 1979.

Brighton, C. T.: The treatment of non-unions with elec-

tricity. Current concepts review. J. Bone Joint Surg. 63A: 847–851, 1981.

Brighton, C. T.: Present and future of electrically induced osteogenesis. In *Clinical Trends in Orthopaedics*, edited by Straub, L. R. and Wilson, P. D., Jr. New York, Thieme-Stratton, 1982.

Brown, K. L. B. and Cruess, R. L.: Bone and cartilage transplantation in orthopaedic surgery. A review. J. Bone Joint Surg. 64A: 270–280, 1982.

Charnley, J.: *Low Friction Arthroplasty of the Hip—Theory and Practice.* Berlin, Springer-Verlag, 1979.

Charnley, J.: Trends in arthroplasty of the hip. In *Clinical Trends in Orthopaedics*, edited by Straub, L. R. and Wilson, P. D., Jr. New York, Thieme-Stratton, 1982.

Chung-Wei, C., Yun-Aing, Q. and Zhong-Jia, Y.: Extremity replantation. World J. Surg. 2: 513–523, 1978.

Dandy, D. J.: Arthroscopic surgery of the knee. In *Current Problems in Orthopaedics* Series. Edinburgh, Churchill-Livingstone, 1981.

Daniel, R. K.: Microsurgery: through the looking glass. medical progress. N. Engl. J. Med. 300: 1251–1257, 1979.

Daniel, R. K. and Terzis, J. K. (eds.): *Reconstructive Microsurgery.* Boston, Little, Brown, 1977.

deHaas, W. G., Watson, J. and Morrison, D. M.: Noninvasive treatment of united fractures of the tibia using electrical stimulation. J. Bone Joint Surg. 62B: 465–470, 1980.

Dwyer, A. F. and Wickham, G. G.: Direct current stimulation in spine fusion. Med. J. Aust. 1: 73, 1974.

Edmonson, A. .S. and Crenshaw, A. H. (eds.): *Campbell's Operative Orthopaedics*, 6th ed. St. Louis, C.V. Mosby, 1980.

Freeman, M. A. R.: Trends in arthroplasty of the knee. In *Clinical Trends in Orthopaedics*, edited by Straub, L. R. and Wilson, P. D., Jr. New York, Thieme-Stratton, 1982.

Freeman, M. A. R., Swanson, S. A. V., Day, W. W. and Thomas, R. J.: Conservative total replacement of the hip. J. Bone Joint Surg. 57B: 114, 1975.

Friedenberg, Z. B. and Brighton, C. T.: Bioelectricity and fracture healing. Plast. Reconstr. Surg. 68: 435–443, 1981.

Gross, A. E., Silverstein, E. A., Falk, J., Falk, R. and Langer, F.: The allotransplantation of partial joints in the treatment of osteoarthritis of the knee. Clin. Orthop. 108: 7–14, 1975.

Gunston, F. and McKenzie, R. I.: Complications of polycentric arthroplasty. Clin. Orthop. 120: 11, 1976.

Harris, W. H.: Total joint replacement. N. Engl. J. Med. 297: 650, 1977.

Hunter, G. A., Welsh, R. P., Cameron, H. U. and Bailey, W. H.: The results of revision of total hip arthroplasty. J. Bone Joint Surg. 61B: 419–421, 1979.

Judet, H., Judet, J. and Gilbert, A.: Vascular microsurgery in orthopaedics. Int. Orthop. 5: 61–68, 1981.

Kleinert, H. E.: Microsurgery in trauma: its evolution and future. (Scudder Oration on Trauma). Bull. Am. Coll. Surgeons 67: 10–19, 1982.

Lord, G. A., Hardy, J. R. and Kummer, F. J.: An uncemented total hip replacement. Clin. Orthop. 141: 2–16, 1979.

Lovell, W. W. and Winter, R. B. (eds.): *Paediatric Orthopaedics.* Philadelphia, J. B. Lippincott, 1978.

MacIntosh, D. L.: Arthroplasty of the knee. J. Bone Joint Surg. 48B: 179, 1966.

Mankin, H. J., Fogelson, F. S., Thrasher, A. Z. and Jaffer, F.: Massive resection and allograft transplantation in the treatment of malignant bone tumours. N. Engl. J. Med. 294: 1247–1255, 1976.

Manktelow, R. T. and McKee, N. H.: Digital replantation: a functional assessment. Can. J. Surg. 22: 47–53, 1979.

Murray, D. G.: In defense of becoming unhinged (editorial). J. Bone Joint Surg. 62A: 495–496, 1980.

O'Brien, B. McC.: *Microvascular Reconstructive Surgery*. Edinburgh, Churchill-Livingstone, 1977.

Paterson, D. C., Lewis, G. N. and Cass, C. A.: Treatment of delayed union and nonunion with an implanted direct current stimulator. Clin. Orthop. 148: 117–128, 1980.

Price, C. T. and Lovell, W. W.: Thompson arthrodesis of the hip in children. J. Bone Joint Surg. 62A: 1118–1123, 1980.

Redford, J. B.: *Orthotics Etcetera*. Baltimore, Williams & Wilkins, 1980.

Samson-Fisher, R. W., and Poole, A. D.: Training medical students to empathize—an experimental study. Med. J. Aust. 1: 473–476, 1978.

Serafin, D., and Buncke, H. J., Jr.: *Microsurgical Composite Tissue Transplantation*. St. Louis, C. V. Mosby, 1979.

Swanson, A. B.: Flexible implant arthroplasty for arthritic finger joints: rationale, technique and results of treatment. J. Bone Joint Surg. 54A: 435–455, 1972.

Swanson, S. A. V. and Freeman, M. A. R.: *The Scientific Basis of Joint Replacement*. Tunbridge Wells, Putnam Medical, 1977.

Tachdjian, M. O.: *Pediatric Orthopaedics*. Philadelphia, W. B. Saunders, 1972.

Wadsworth, T. G.: *The Elbow*. Edinburgh, Churchill-Livingstone, 1982.

Wagner, H.: Surface replacement arthroplasty of the hip. Clin. Orthop. 134: 102–130, 1978.

Walldius, P.: Arthroplasty of the knee joint using endoprosthesis. Acta Orthop. Scand. (Suppl.) 24: 19, 1957.

Weiland, A. J.: Vascularized free bone transplants. Current concepts review. J. Bone Joint Surg. 63A: 166–169, 1981.

Zenni, E. J., Jr. and Carothers, T. A.: Total knee arthroplasty: current state of the art. Orthop. Rev. 19: 51–60, 1980.

PART 2

Musculoskeletal Disorders—General and Specific

CHAPTER 7

Common Normal Variations

When you consider the astronomical number of permutations and combinations of genes and chromosomes that determine the form and function of each human being—as well as the influence of innumerable environmental factors—it is not surprising that, apart from uniovular twins, each person in this world is different from every other person. While one speaks of an *average* infant, an *average* child and an *average* adult, it is important to appreciate that there exists *an extremely wide range of normal* in body form and function. However, the normal variations change with age so that a normal variation which is present at birth, and which normally changes spontaneously with age, may no longer be considered normal if it persists into adult life.

It will be obvious to you that you must come to know the wide range of normal variations in man so that when you see patients, you will be able to distinguish the normal (physiological) from the abnormal (pathological) and will not make the error of treating a condition that neither requires nor merits treatment. Nevertheless, the borderline between the extremes of normal variation and the beginning of abnormal variation is not always clearly defined, particularly in the musculoskeletal system; therefore, if the normal variation is extreme and is a source of reasonable concern to your patient, or to his relatives, simple methods of treatment are justifiable provided they are both effective and safe.

For each of these very common normal variations, you should come to understand its underlying *causes*, its *natural course*, or *prognosis*, and whether or not any *treatment* is indicated.

COMMON NORMAL VARIATIONS IN CHILDREN

As a practising doctor you will see many children with normal variations of musculoskeletal form and function, particularly in the lower limbs. The commonest group of such conditions in childhood are (in lay terms) flat feet, knock knees, bow legs, toeing out and toeing in. These conditions are extremely common in young children but become progressively less common toward adoles-

cence, indicating that they tend to improve spontaneously. Nevertheless, these normal variations in perfectly healthy children are the cause of much concern in the minds of the child's parents, grandparents, neigh-

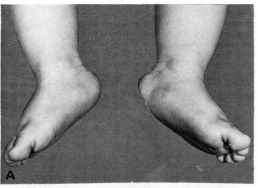

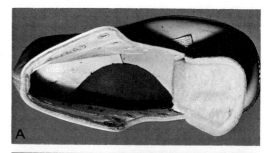

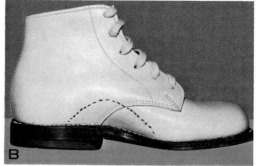

Figure 7.1. Flexible flat feet (hypermobile pes planus) in a 1½-year-old child. *A*, the feet look normal when the child is not standing. *B*, they look flat only when weight bearing.

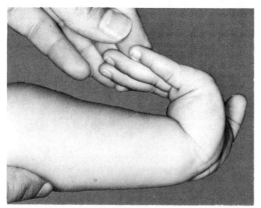

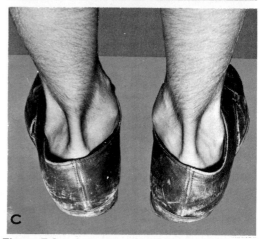

Figure 7.2. Hypermobility of the joints in the upper limb of the child in Figure 7.1 indicating generalized joint laxity. If this child walked on his hands he would have "flat hands."

Figure 7.3. *A* and *B*, sturdy boot for pre-school children with flexible flat feet. A sponge rubber arch support ("scaphoid pad") and a 3/16" inside heel wedge have been added simply to prevent further stretching of the lax joints of the feet. *C*, excessive correction in the shoes of a 6-year-old boy with flexible flat feet. The feet slide to the lateral side of the shoe; the shoes are pushed out of shape and cause the boy discomfort.

bours and well-meaning friends to say nothing of shoe salesmen. An appreciation of the underlying *cause* and the *natural course* (*prognosis*) of these variations will enable you to deal with them intelligently. They are best considered in two main groups based on their underlying cause—those due to looseness, or hypermobility, of joints (joint laxity) and those due to twisting, or torsional, deformities of the growing long bones of the lower limbs.

Variations Due to Hypermobility of Joints (Joint Laxity)

The degree of mobility of joints varies widely in normal children. Hypermobile joints throughout the body are due to lax ligaments and are extremely common in infancy, less common in childhood and relatively uncommon in adult life. The lax ligaments, which are probably an inherited variation, seem to become less lax as the child gets older with the result that the hypermobility of the joints tends to improve spontaneously; only the most severe degrees of the condition persist into adult life. Two very common clinical variations that are secondary to hypermobility or joint laxity are *flexible flat feet* (hypermobile pes planus) and *knock knees* (genu valgum).

FLEXIBLE FLAT FEET (HYPERMOBILE PES PLANUS)

At the age of one year, when most children have begun to stand, all their joints are normally hypermobile and as a result, their feet, being very flexible, look flat—but only with weight bearing (Fig. 7.1). Indeed, if these children walked on their hands they would have flat hands since the hypermobility of the joints is generalized rather than localized (Fig. 7.2). As the ligamentous laxity and associated hypermobility of the joints improve spontaneously, the flat appearance of the child's feet becomes less marked, which explains why flexible flat feet are so common in young children and yet relatively uncommon in adults. The term *"flexible flat feet"* avoids the stigma of the term *"congenital flat feet,"* while the frequently used expression of "fallen arches" and "weak arches" are not only inaccurate, but also sound unnecessarily ominous to the already anxious parents.

Once you appreciate the underlying *cause* as well as the *natural course* of flexible flat

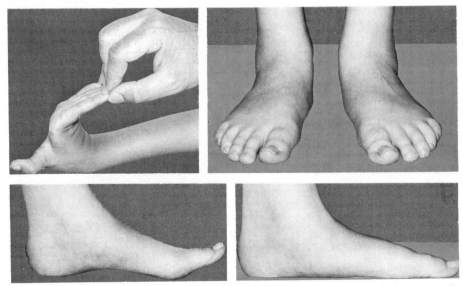

Figure 7.4.   Flexible flat feet and flexible hands in a 10-year-old boy with persistent generalized joint laxity. The feet appear flat only when bearing weight (*upper right* and *lower right*). This boy was very active and did not have any pain in his feet.

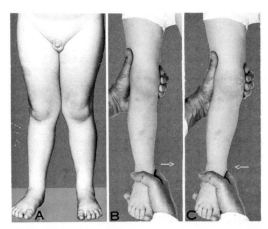

Figure 7.5. Knock knees (genu valgum) in a 4-year-old boy with generalized joint laxity. *A,* the deformity is most noticeable on weight bearing since it occurs through the lax knee joints. *B* and *C,* the hypermobility of the knee is demonstrated by passive adduction, which corrects the deformity, and passive abduction, which aggravates it.

In adolescence only those individuals with the more severe degree of joint laxity still exhibit flexible flat feet (Fig. 7.4). Of these, the majority are completely comfortable, even with ordinary footwear, in spite of being active. A very small percentage of adolescents and adults with flexible flat feet complain of either discomfort or tiredness in their feet and limit their activities as a result. Carefully molded arch supports usually relieve these symptoms, but under the very rare circumstances when they do not—and only under these circumstances—some form of operative treatment such as fusion (arthrodesis) of the subtalar joint is justifiable.

Flexible flat feet associated with a tight tendoachillis should make you think of the possibility of either mild cerebral palsy or early muscular dystrophy. Flexible flat feet must also be differentiated from the less

feet, it becomes obvious that the milder degrees of this condition require no treatment whatsoever—apart from reassurance of the parents. For more severe degrees of flexible flat feet, the *aim* of treatment is simply to prevent further stretching of the already lax ligaments of the feet until such time as the generalized ligamentous laxity has improved spontaneously. This is readily accomplished in pre-school children by means of sturdy boots to which have been added a sponge rubber arch support ("scaphoid pad") and a 3/16″ inside heel wedge (Fig. 7.3*A* and *B*). However, the child need not be denied the joy of running barefoot, or in soft shoes, at least part of the time. For the school age child the same type of corrections added to low shoes have relatively less effect on the natural course of the flexible feet, but do serve to make the shoes last longer. Excessive corrections in low shoes, however, force the child's foot to slide to the lateral side of the shoe and cause unnecessary discomfort (Fig. 7.3*C*). Exercises designed to strengthen supposedly weak muscles are, quite understandably, of no value in the management of flexible flat feet.

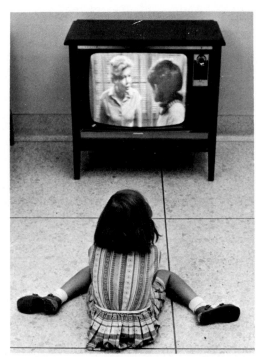

Figure 7.6. The "television position" of sitting. This habitual position of sitting should be avoided, for it not only applies a torsional force to the femora but also stretches the medial collateral ligaments of the knees.

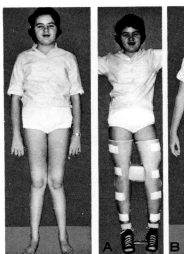

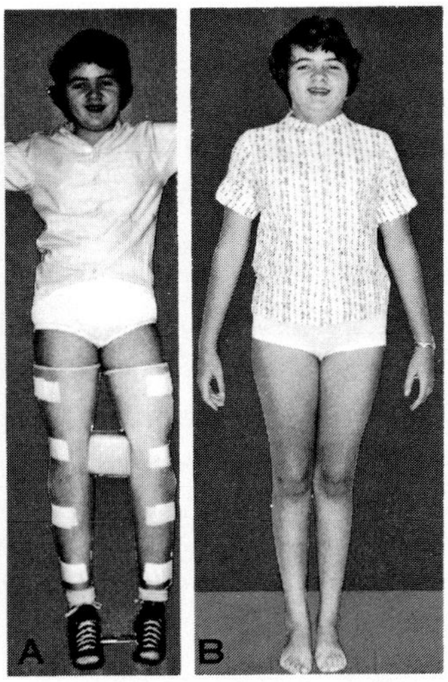

frequently prescribed with the idea of altering the line of weight bearing and thereby decreasing the strain on the medial collateral ligaments of the knees, but their efficacy is difficult to assess.

In those few older children with persistent joint laxity and associated marked knock knees, secondary bony deformity may gradually develop because of uneven epiphyseal plate growth in the region of the knee (Fig. 7.7). Under these circumstances a specially designed night splint may be used to overcome the bony component of the deformity by influencing subsequent growth (Fig. 7.8). Day braces are both cumbersome and ineffectual, and operative treatment is almost never necessary.

Figure 7.7 (*left*). Knock knees (genu valgum) in a 12-year-old girl with persistent generalized joint laxity. A secondary bony deformity has developed.
Figure 7.8 (*right*). *A*, this specially designed corrective splint was worn at night for nine months to influence epiphyseal plate growth at the knees. *B*, the bony deformity was gradually corrected by the use of the night splint.

The common type of knock knees, or genu valgum, must be differentiated from the much less common, but more serious type of genu valgum that occurs through bone secondary to epiphyseal plate disturbance from congenital abnormalities (Chapter

common, but more serious conditions of rigid valgus feet and accessory tarsal scaphoid (Chapter 8).

KNOCK KNEES (GENU VALGUM)

By far the commonest cause of knock knees in young children is hypermobility of the knee joint which, in turn, is simply another manifestation of generalized joint laxity. Thus, knock knees, like flexible flat feet, are much more common in young children than in adolescents, and for the same reason. Since the valgus deformity is secondary to the lax medial collateral ligaments of the knee, it is most noticeable when the child is standing (Fig. 7.5). The *aim* of treatment should be simply to prevent further stretching of the already lax medial collateral ligaments. The habitual position of sitting on the floor with the knees in front and the feet out to the side (which has become known as the "television position") should be avoided because it further stretches these ligaments (Fig. 7.6). Boots with inside heel wedges are

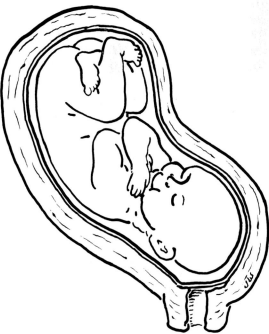

Figure 7.9. Intrauterine position. The hips are always flexed and externally rotated, while the knees are usually flexed and the feet turned inward.

8), metabolic conditions (Chapter 9), or injury (Chapters 15 and 16).

Variations Due to Torsional Deformities in the Lower Limbs

The growing long bones of children respond to repeated twisting, or torsional, forces by an alteration of the normal growth pattern in their epiphyseal plates. The affected long bone becomes twisted in its long axis; that is, it develops either an internal, or an external, torsional deformity. Prenatal intrauterine positions and certain postnatal habitual sleeping and sitting positions place torsional forces on the growing long bones and are responsible for the torsional deformities that cause either toeing out or toeing in.

Before birth the hips are always flexed (there being no "standing room" *in utero*) and externally rotated, while the knees are usually flexed and the feet turned inward (Fig. 7.9). As a result of the torsional forces associated with this position, all newborn infants exhibit some degree of external femoral torsion and internal tibial torsion, both of which normally correct spontaneously with subsequent growth. However, certain common habitual positions of sleeping and sitting during childhood exert torsional forces on the growing lower limbs and either

prevent the spontaneous correction of those deformities present at birth, or even create new torsional deformities. An appreciation of this basic concept is pivotal in an understanding of the *causes* and the *natural course* (*prognosis*) of the common clinical variations of toeing out and toeing in.

TOEING OUT DUE TO EXTERNAL TORSIONAL DEFORMITIES

External Femoral Torsion

Toeing out, which is very common in young children, is nearly always due to external femoral torsion (Fig. 7.10). Examination reveals that when the extended lower limbs are rotated outward (externally), the knees turn out to about 90°; whereas when they are rotated inward (internally), the knees can be brought only to the neutral position (Fig. 7.11). If the child habitually sleeps face down with the femora externally rotated (Fig. 12), the external femoral torsion persists and, in addition, external tibial torsion may develop as a result of the associated outward torsional force on the tibia. This sleeping position, however, is seldom assumed after the age of two years. Thus, the prognosis for external femoral torsion is good. Rarely, in the older child, it may be necessary to use a simple night splint in which the feet are turned inward to correct the residual external femoral torsion.

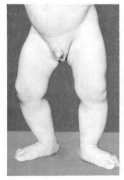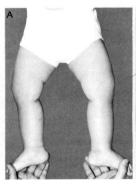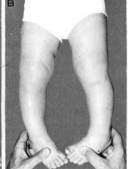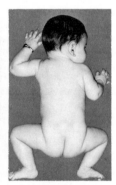

Figure 7.10 (*left*).   External femoral torsion with resultant toeing out in a 1-year-old boy.
Figure 7.11, *A* and *B*.   External femoral torsion. When the extended lower limbs are rotated outward, the knees turn out to 90°, whereas when they are rotated inward, the knees can be brought only to the neutral position indicating that the torsional deformity is in the femora.
Figure 7.12 (*right*).   This sleeping position with the femora and tibiae externally rotated prevents spontaneous correction of the external femoral torsion and may even produce external tibial torsion.

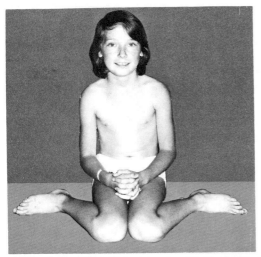

Figure 7.13. The "television position" of sitting has gradually produced an acquired internal femoral torsion and external tibial torsion in this 9-year-old girl.

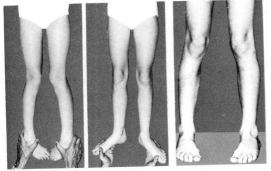

Figure 7.14 (*left*). Internal femoral torsion. When the extended lower limbs are rotated inward the knees turn in to about 90°. When they are rotated outward the knees can be brought only slightly beyond the neutral position indicating that the torsional deformity is in the femora.

Figure 7.15 (*right*). Internal femoral torsion in a 9-year-old girl. Note that both the knees and the feet are turned inward.

External Tibial Torsion

Toeing out due to external tibial torsion alone is rare, although external tibial torsion may aggravate the toeing out due to external femoral torsion as already mentioned; it may also compensate to some extent for internal femoral torsion, as will be mentioned later. In addition, external tibial torsion may develop secondary to the muscle imbalance

of such paralytic conditions as spina bifida, cerebral palsy and poliomyelitis (Chapter 12).

External rotation of the entire lower limb at the hip, without any torsional deformity, can be due to congenital dislocation of the hip in the younger child (Chapter 8), and to slipped upper femoral epiphysis in the older child (Chapter 13).

TOEING IN DUE TO INTERNAL TORSIONAL DEFORMITIES

Internal Femoral Torsion

Since the femora are never internally rotated *in utero*, internal femoral torsion is never seen in the newborn, nor even during infancy. However, if the child subsequently develops the habit of sitting on the floor with the knees in front, the femora internally rotated and the feet out to the side (the "television position") (Fig. 7.13), the associated torsional force on the growing femur gradually produces an internal femoral torsion by the time the child is about five years of age. Examination reveals that when the extended lower limbs are rotated inward (internally), the knees turn in to about 90°; whereas when they are rotated outward (externally), the knees can be brought only slightly beyond the neutral position (Fig. 7.14). As a

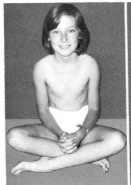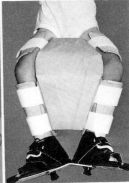

Figure 7.16 (*left*). The "tailor" or cross-legged position, in which an external torsional force is applied to the femur, helps to correct the internal femoral torsion.

Figure 7.17 (*right*). This specially designed corrective splint is used at night to apply a mild external torsional force to the growing femur and thereby to correct internal femoral torsion.

result, the child walks with both the feet and the knees turned inward (Fig. 7.15). If the child continues to assume this sitting position, the associated external force on the tibia gradually produces an external tibial torsion in which case the child comes to walk with the knees turned in but the feet pointing straight ahead. Internal femoral torsion, being a gradually acquired torsional deformity in older children, exhibits much less tendency to correct spontaneously than do the other torsional variations.

The *aim* of treatment is simply to prevent

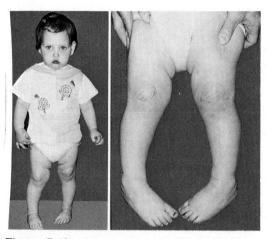

Figure 7.18. Internal tibial torsion. When the knee is facing forward, the foot is turned inward.

further internal torsional forces from being exerted on the femora by training the child to stop sitting in the position that has caused the deformity; in addition, corrective external torsional forces can be applied to the femora by training the child to sit in the "tailor" or cross-legged position (Fig. 7.16). For more severe and persistent internal femoral torsion, in children over the age of eight years, it may be necessary to use a specially designed night splint in which the lower limbs are kept externally rotated (Fig. 7.17). Straight last shoes may minimize the appearance of the toeing in but wedges in the soles are of no value. Rotation osteotomy of the femur is not necessary for simple internal femoral torsion in the growing child.

In-toeing due to internal rotation contracture of the hip joint secondary to the muscle imbalance of paralytic conditions such as spina bifida, cerebral palsy and poliomyelitis should present little difficulty in differential diagnosis (Chapter 12).

Internal Tibial Torsion

In young children the commonest cause of toeing in is internal tibial torsion. Examination reveals that when the knee is facing forward, the foot is turned inward (Fig. 7.18). Some degree of this deformity is present in almost all infants due to the common intra-

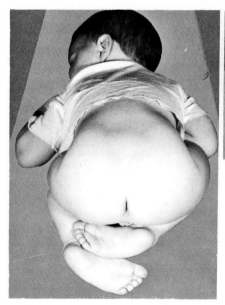

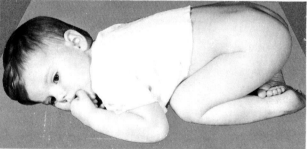

Figure 7.19. This sleeping position with the feet turned in and underneath the infant applies further torsional force to the tibiae and not only prevents spontaneous correction of the internal tibial torsion but actually aggravates it.

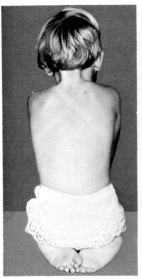
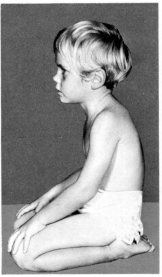
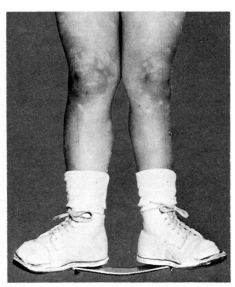

Figure 7.20. This sitting position with the feet turned in and underneath the girl applies further torsional force to the tibiae and not only prevents spontaneous correction of the internal tibial torsion, but may actually aggravate it.

Figure 7.21 (*right*). A Denis-Browne night splint with the feet externally rotated applies a mild external torsional force to the growing tibiae and gradually corrects internal tibial torsion over a period of several months.

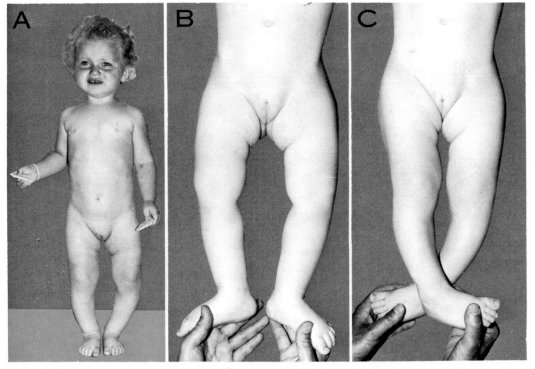

Figure 7.22. *A*, bow legs (genu varum) due to a combination of internal torsion and varus of the tibia along with external torsion of the femur in a 2-year-old girl. *B* and *C*, passive rotation of the extended limbs outward and inward reveals the combination of torsional deformities responsible for the appearance of bow legs.

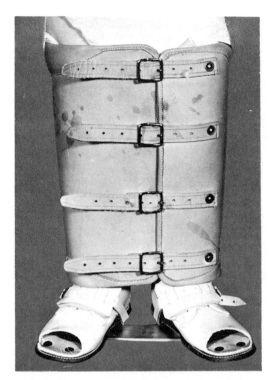

Figure 7.23. This specially designed corrective splint for children over the age of 2 years is used at night to influence epiphyseal plate growth and thereby to correct the genu varum.

uterine position (Fig. 7.9). Normally, the internal tibial torsion corrects spontaneously with subsequent growth. However, if the infant adopts the habitual position of sleeping on the knees with the feet turned in (Fig. 7.19), or of sitting on top of inturned feet (Fig. 7.20), the internal tibial torsion not only fails to correct spontaneously, but may even increase over the years.

The *aim* of treatment is to prevent internal torsional forces from being applied to the tibiae by training the child to avoid the aforementioned harmful positions of sleeping and sitting. When this is accomplished, the internal tibial torsion gradually corrects spontaneously over a period of several years. If, however, in a child over the age of two years, the internal tibial torsion is sufficiently severe that the child is repeatedly tripping over his own feet, treatment is justifiable since it consists of simply holding the feet in

external rotation in a night splint (Fig. 7.21). The mild external torsional force exerted by this splint each night gradually corrects the internal tibial torsion by influencing epiphyseal plate growth over a period of from four to eight months, depending upon how rapidly the child is growing at the time. Straight last shoes may minimize the appearance of the toeing in, but wedges in the soles of the shoes are of no value. Rotation osteotomy of the tibia for simple internal tibial torsion in young children is not necessary and could even be considered meddlesome.

Toeing in due to foot deformities such as metatarsus varus (forefoot adduction) and clubfeet should be obvious, although it should be remembered that in both of these conditions there is usually an element of internal tibial torsion as well (Chapter 8).

BOW LEGS (GENU VARUM)

The commonest cause of bow legs in children is a combination of internal torsion and varus of the tibia along with external torsion of the femur (Fig. 7.22). Thus, the common type of bow leg deformity is not simply the opposite deformity to knock knees. These combined deformities are frequently present at birth due to intrauterine position, but usually improve spontaneously.

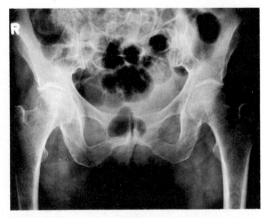

Figure 7.24. Generalized osteoporosis seen in the pelvis and femora of a 76-year-old lady. In this condition the femoral necks are weak and are particularly susceptible to fracture with minimal trauma.

However, they may even be increased by the aforementioned habitual positions of sleeping and sitting (Figs. 7.19 and 7.20).

In more severe degrees of persistent genu varum in children over the age of two years, it may be necessary to use a specially designed night splint to correct the varus element in the tibia while the opposing torsional deformities in the femora are allowed to correct spontaneously (Fig. 7.23). Day braces for bow legs are ineffectual and osteotomy of the tibia is not necessary for this physiological type of bow legs in young children.

The marked bow leg deformities associated with the various types of rickets (Chapter 9), tibia vara (Chapter 13), and epiphyseal plate injuries (Chapter 16) are readily differentiated from the common type of bow legs by radiographic examination.

NORMAL VARIATIONS IN ADULTS

The normal variations of joint laxity and torsional deformities just described in children may, if severe and untreated, persist into adult life in which case they can no longer be considered to be within the normal range *for adults*. Indeed, the more severe degrees of residual flat feet, knock knees and bow legs, though relatively rare in adults, may produce symptoms because of premature degenerative changes in the associated joints.

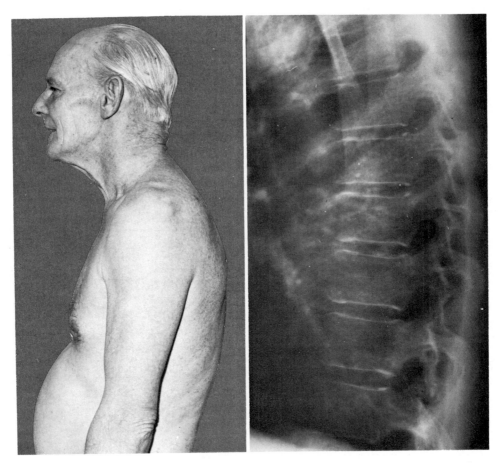

Figure 7.25.   Dorsal kyphosis (round back) associated with osteoporosis of the spine in a 61-year-old man. Note the generalized rarefaction of the vertebral bodies.

The Normal Aging Process in the Musculoskeletal System

As man grows older many changes gradually take place in his tissues as part of the aging process, changes that are as normal as greying of the hair and wrinkling of the skin. Changes of normal aging in the musculoskeletal system include a gradual decrease in muscle strength and a very gradual decrease in joint motion. Synovial joints normally "last a lifetime" in spite of gradual thinning of articular cartilage. Chondromalacia (softening of cartilage), however, is seen to some extent in the patella of almost all adults over the age of thirty years. In addition, there is a gradual decrease in the water content of the intervertebral discs with resultant narrowing of the disc spaces and, in turn, a gradual decrease in body height during the later decades of adult life.

In the senior years, particularly in women, there is always some degree of generalized osteoporosis with resultant weakening of bone (Fig. 7.24). This type of "senile" osteoporosis renders certain areas of the skeleton, such as the femoral neck, especially susceptible to fracture from minor injury. Other sites of osteoporotic cancellous bone, such as in the vertebral bodies, may gradually become deformed over the years thereby producing the familiar "round back" or dorsal kyphosis of the elderly (Fig. 7.25).

It is important that you learn to distinguish the normal (physiological) from the abnormal (pathological) for each of the ages of man, in order that you may deal with them intelligently.

Suggested Additional Reading

Dyment, P. G. and Bogan, P. M.: Pediatricians' attitudes concerning infants' shoes. Pediatrics 50: 655–657, 1972.

Lloyd-Roberts, G. C.: Children's feet (editorial). Proc. Roy. Soc. Med. 70: 375–377, 1977.

Rang, M.: The Easter Seal Guide to Children's Orthopaedics: Prevention, Screening and Problem Solving. Toronto, The Easter Seal Society of Ontario, 1982.

Sharrard, W. J. W.: Knock knees and bow legs. Br. Med. J. 1: 827, 1976.

Sharrard, W. J. W.: In-toeing and flat feet. Br. Med. J. 1: 888–889, 1976.

Staheli, L. T., Giffin, L.: Corrective shoes for children: a survey of current pediatric practice. Pediatrics 65: 13–17, 1980.

"When I look upon a child I am filled with admiration—not so much for what that child is today as for what it may become."

—LOUIS PASTEUR

CHAPTER 8

Congenital Abnormalities

GENERAL FEATURES

Definition and Variety

Congenital abnormalities may be defined as those defects in development of body form or function that are present *at the time of birth*. When you consider the remarkable speed and complexity of the embryonic development of the human, discussed in Chapter 2, it is hardly surprising that some children are born with a congenital abnormality; indeed, what is surprising is that the vast majority of children are perfectly normal at birth.

The congenital musculoskeletal abnormalities vary greatly, both in extent and severity. They may be *localized*, as in a single clubfoot, or *generalized*, as in osteogenesis imperfecta (fragile bones). Furthermore, a clubfoot, for example, may be a mild and readily correctable deformity, or it may be a very severe deformity that is resistant to simple methods of treatment; in either case, the deformity is easily detected at birth. Osteogenesis imperfecta may be mild and not clinically detectable at birth—indeed not until several years after birth when the affected child sustains the first pathological fracture—or it may be so severe that pathological fractures have occurred even before birth.

Incidence

The exact incidence of congenital abnormalities is understandably difficult to determine, not only because some of the abnormalities are not detectable at birth and therefore not reported at that time, but also because of the indefinite borderline between minor abnormalities and normal variations. Even large surveys differ, but the incidence of abnormalities detectable at birth (including stillbirths) is approximately 3%, while the incidence of abnormalities detectable at one year of age is approximately 6%. Significant congenital abnormalities of the musculoskeletal system are quite common, being exceeded in frequency only by those of the central nervous system and cardiovascular system. Furthermore, the presence of one congenital abnormality should always make you search diligently for others since it is not unusual for two, or even more, abnormalities to coexist in a given child.

Etiological Factors

Congenital abnormalities may be caused by a variety of factors including genetic defects (autosomal dominant or recessive, X-linked dominant or recessive, and mutations) and environmental, or teratogenic factors (for example, rubella and thalidomide). They may also be multifactorial in origin due to the combination of genetic predisposition and environmental factors.

Types of Congenital Musculoskeletal Abnormalities

LOCALIZED ABNORMALITIES

All localized congenital abnormalities of the skeleton are manifestations of one or more of the various types of disturbances in its normal growth and development. Thus, a bone may fail to form entirely (*aplasia*); it may fail to grow to a normal size (*hypoplasia*); its growth may be abnormal (*dysplasia*); or it may overgrow (*Hypertrophy* or *local gigantism*). Extra, or supernumerary parts of the skeleton, may form (*duplication*), as in extra digits (*polydactyly*). Skeletal development may be *arrested* at any stage during intrauterine life; for example, when the normal descent of the scapula is arrested (Sprengel's deformity), or when the normal bony closure of the posterior part of the spinal canal is arrested, as in the various degrees of spina bifida.

Localized congenital abnormalities of joints include those in which a joint is either merely *unstable*, or actually *dislocated*, as in congenital dislocation of the hip; those in which a joint has failed to form (*failure of segmentation*), as in congenital radioulnar synostosis; and those in which a severe and resistant contracture of one or more joints is present at birth, as in a congenital clubfoot.

GENERALIZED ABNORMALITIES

The generalized congenital abnormalities involving many parts of the musculoskeletal system include developmental defects of epiphyseal plate growth, as in achondroplasia; congenital imbalance between bone deposition and bone resorption, as in osteogenesis imperfecta; and inborn errors of metabolism, as in certain types of refractory rickets. In addition, all joints of the body may be unduly *hypermobile* (congenital generalized joint laxity), or they may be unduly *rigid*, as in arthrogryposis.

Diagnosis of Congenital Abnormalities

ANTENATAL DIAGNOSIS

The rapidly developing field of antenatal, or prenatal, medicine (also called "fetology") is primarily concerned with the diagnosis of certain abnormalities in the fetus around the 16th week of intrauterine life in "high risk" pregnancies. Its greatest impetus has come from the development of the safe and reliable technique of *amniocentesis* whereby the aspirated amniotic fluid is studied biochemically and cytogenetically. Thus, it is now possible to diagnose chromosomal abnormalities (such as Down's syndrome), open neural tube defects (i.e. spina bifida with either meningomyelocele or myelocele) and certain inborn errors of metabolism (such as the mucopolysaccharidoses). Consequently, a completely new dimension has been added to genetic counseling.

Of prime importance concerning antenatal diagnosis in the musculoskeletal system are open neural tube defects, i.e. open spina bifida with either a meningomyelocele or a myelocele. When the fetus does have an open spina bifida the level of α-fetoprotein (AFP) in the mother's serum is elevated and indeed can be used as a screening test. A raised serum AFP, in turn, is an indication for amniocentesis, which usually demonstrates an elevated level of both AFP and one form of acetylcholinesterase in the amniotic fluid. In this condition a "high risk" pregnancy would be one in which the expectant mother has an affected close relative—a parent, a sibling or a previous child—in which case the risk of her unborn child being affected is about 3%, and this justifies amniocentesis. Additional techniques available for antenatal diagnosis of open spina bifida are ultrasound (ultrasonography) and direct inspection of the fetus by means of a fetoscope (fetoscopy).

Once the antenatal diagnosis of open spina bifida has been established, the parents must make what can be an agonizing decision concerning whether or not the life of their afflicted unborn child should be terminated. Although the antenatal diagnosis of open spina bifida has raised the possibility of eliminating at least some of the children with this abnormality through abortion, it has also, quite understandably, raised a number of controversial moral and ethical issues.

POSTNATAL DIAGNOSIS

The responsibility for the early diagnosis of congenital abnormalities is shared by the family physician, obstetrician and pediatrician who first see the child. Some abnormalities, such as clubfeet, are so obvious at birth that their recognition presents no difficulty. However, others, such as congenital dislocation of the hip, are not at all obvious at birth and will be detected only by very careful and specific methods of examination; you may be surprised to learn that this serious and potentially crippling condition is one of the most frequently undetected congenital abnormalities in the newborn period simply because of the failure on the part of the attending physician to search for it. Still other congenital abnormalities are not detectable at birth, but can and should be diagnosed at the time of their first clinical manifestation. Failure to recognize a congenital abnormality at the earliest possible time is an injustice, not only to the unfortunate child, but also to his devoted parents.

Principles and Methods of Treatment

Most of the localized congenital musculoskeletal abnormalities are compatible with longevity and therefore, their total care demands farsighted planning, skilful orthopaedic treatment and prolonged supervision since the results must last a lifetime. At this time you may wish to review the general principles and specific methods of musculoskeletal treatment discussed in Chapter 6, because they are as applicable to congenital abnormalities as they are to acquired disorders and injuries.

A knowledge of the *significance* and *prognosis* of a given congenital musculoskeletal abnormality is essential in relation to its treatment. Many localized abnormalities involving joints, such as congenital clubfoot and congenital dislocation of the hip, become progressively more difficult to treat as time goes on because of progressive secondary changes in the involved joints and surrounding muscles. For these conditions, early recognition and early treatment are mandatory in order to obtain the most satisfactory result. Other abnormalities, such as a single hemivertebra, have a reasonably good prognosis in that significant curvature of the spine (scoliosis) is unlikely to develop with subsequent spinal growth. By contrast, asymmetrical fusion (failure of segmentation) of the spine always leads to a progressive scoliosis with growth and therefore requires early treatment.

The parents of a child who is afflicted with a congenital abnormality need kindly and considerate counseling so that needless and harmful feelings of *guilt* and *negative self-pity* may be replaced by the more *positive* and helpful attitudes of *acceptance* of the problem and *cooperation* with its treatment. These parents are anxious and entitled to know something of the prognosis, particularly with respect to anticipated future appearance and function of the involved part as their child grows and reaches adult life. In addition, a geneticist can be of considerable help to such parents who are concerned about the likelihood of a similar abnormality occurring in their subsequent children as well as in their children's children.

LOCALIZED CONGENITAL ABNORMALITIES OF THE LOWER LIMB
The Foot
METATARSUS PRIMUS VARUS

A varus, or adduction, deformity of the first (prime) metatarsal in relation to the other four metatarsals is designated *metatarsus primus varus*. The medial border of the forefoot is curved inward and there is a wide space between the first and second toes (Fig. 8.1). If treated early by the application of a series of corrective plaster casts, the deformity is readily overcome. Unfortunately, this relatively mild deformity is frequently overlooked for several years during which time the pressure of shoes gradually pushes the first toe (hallux) laterally, thereby producing the secondary deformity of *adolescent hallux valgus* (Fig. 8.2). When hallux valgus occurs during adolescence, it is usually progressive; and, since the prognosis is bad, the deformity should be corrected by a soft tissue procedure around the metatarsophalangeal joint combined with corrective osteotomy at the base of the medially deviated first metatarsal.

METATARSUS VARUS (METATARSUS ADDUCTUS)

A varus, or adduction, deformity of all five metatarsals in relation to the rest of the foot is referred to as *metatarsus varus* or *metatarsus adductus* (Fig. 8.3). Although these two terms are often used interchangeably, the term metatarsus adductus is actually more correct. The whole forefoot is not only adducted, but also supinated, and there is usually an associated internal tibial torsion. The normal appearance of the heel and ankle readily distinguish this condition from a congenital clubfoot (talipes equinovarus). Metatarsus varus is quite common (incidence of 2 per 1,000 live births) and is frequently bilateral; occasionally, it occurs in the opposite foot of a child with a unilateral clubfoot.

In many children the forefoot deformity is both mild and flexible, in which case the prognosis is good with simple stretching by the parent and the avoidance of sleeping face down with the feet curled in (Fig. 8.4). When the deformity is more marked and more rigid, or resistant, the prognosis is not good and treatment should be started at least within the first few weeks of life. It is regrettable that metatarsus varus of the resistant type frequently escapes detection for several months, or even longer, because the deformity becomes progressively resistant with each passing month. *Treatment* involves the careful application of a series of plaster casts in which the heel is maintained in neutral position and the forefoot is molded

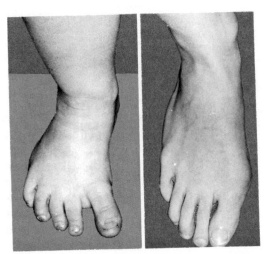

Figure 8.1. (*left*).   Congenital metatarsus primus varus in a 3-year-old girl. Note the inward curve of the medial border of the foot and the increased space between the first and second toes due to medial deviation of the first metatarsal. This deformity should be corrected early in life to prevent the development of adolescent hallux valgus.

Figure 8.2. (*right*).   Adolescent hallux valgus in a 13-year-old girl. In the presence of an underlying metatarsus primus varus, pressure from footwear has gradually produced a valgus deformity at the metatarsophalangeal joint (hallux valgus). When this deformity develops during adolescence, it tends to be progressive and should be corrected surgically.

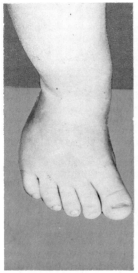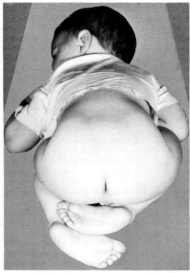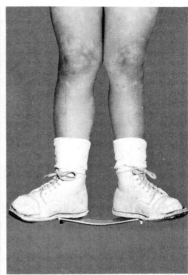

Figure 8.3. Congenital matatarsus varus (metatarsus adductus) in a 3-month-old child. The whole forefoot is deviated medially (adducted) and supinated, but the hindfoot is normal. There is frequently an associated internal tibial torsion. This child's deformity was corrected by a series of plaster casts over a period of 3 months and the correction was maintained by the use of a Denis Browne night splint.

Figure 8.4. Habitual sleeping position with the feet curled in. This position tends to aggravate metatarsus varus and the associated internal tibial torsion.

Figure 8.5. Denis Browne night splint. This is used following plaster cast correction of metatarsus varus to maintain the correction and also to overcome the internal tibial torsion.

into abduction and pronation. The casts are changed every two weeks and the duration of cast treatment varies from six to twelve weeks depending on the resistance to correction. A Denis Browne type of boot splint is then applied nightly for a few months, not only to maintain correction but also to overcome the associated internal tibial torsion (Fig. 8.5). Outflare boots (in which the front of the boot is deviated laterally) help to maintain correction during the day for the ensuing year.

Untreated congenital metatarsus varus in a child over the age of two years may require a soft tissue releasing operation and, if the child has reached the age of four years without correction, it may be necessary to perform an osteotomy at the base of each metatarsal.

CLUBFOOT (TALIPES EQUINOVARUS)

The most important congenital abnormality of the foot is *clubfoot* or *talipes equino-varus*, a deformity easy to diagnose but difficult to correct completely, even in the hands of an experienced orthopaedic surgeon. A congenital clubfoot consists of a combination of deformities including forefoot adduction and supination through the mid-tarsal joint, heel varus through the subtalar joint, equinus through the ankle joint and medial deviation of the whole foot in relation to the knee (Fig. 8.6). The medial deviation of the foot is due partly to an angulation in the neck of the talus and partly to internal tibial torsion. The degree of severity of the deformity, which may be mild, moderate or severe, is better assessed by its feel of rigidity, or resistance, than by its appearance.

Incidence

Congenital clubfoot is quite common (incidence of 2 per 1,000 live births), is bilateral in half of the afflicted children and affects boys twice as often as girls. A genetic factor

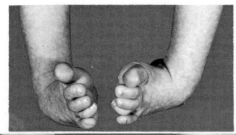
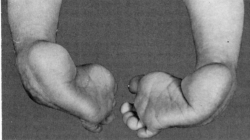

Figure 8.6. Congenital clubfeet (talipes equino-varus) in a newborn infant. Note the forefoot adduction and supination, the heel varus, the ankle equinus and the internal tibial torsion. The deformities of this infant's feet were assessed as moderately severe on the basis of the feel of resistance to passive correction.

would seem to be responsible in about 10% of the children, but in the remainder the abnormality appears inexplicably for the first time in the family tree.

Etiology and Pathology

The etiology of congenital clubfoot remains one of the many unsolved puzzles of the musculoskeletal system although the recent ultrastructural and histochemical studies of Handelsman suggest a neuromuscular cause. The deformity is known to exist from the very early stages of embryonic development when the foot first begins to form. The muscles on the posterior and medial aspect of the leg (particularly the calf muscle and the tibialis posterior) are unduly short and, in addition, the fibrous capsules of all the deformed joints are thick and contracted on the concave side of the deformity. These soft tissue contractures become progressively resistant to correction as the weeks go by—both before and after birth—and lead to *secondary* changes, not only in the shape of the actively growing bones, but

also in the involved joints. The pathological anatomy of clubfoot (as well as its surgical correction) is well described by Carroll. An appreciation of this observation should serve to emphasize the tremendous importance of very early treatment.

Diagnosis

While the typical clubfoot of moderate severity is easily diagnosed, the *mild* clubfoot must be distinguished from the condition of "*positional equinovarus*," which is simply due to intrauterine position and can therefore be readily placed in a normal position. The *severe* clubfoot must be differentiated from the less common, but more troublesome type of clubfoot deformity associated with either *spina bifida* or *arthrogryposis*.

Treatment

One of your responsibilities is to reassure the anxious parents at the outset that with early and expert treatment, their child will not be "crippled"—rather that he will be able to enjoy a reasonably normal life, both as a child and as an adult. The general principles of treatment, which should be applied very early—at least within the first few days of life—include gentle passive correction of the deformities (proceeding from the forefoot adduction to the heel varus to the ankle equinus), maintenance of correction for a very long period and supervision of the child until the end of growth. Even after full correction of a clubfoot, the apparent failure of the contracted soft tissues to grow adequately in length tends to produce a *recurrence* of deformity in about half of the children, particularly during periods of rapid skeletal growth.

The specific methods of treatment of clubfoot vary considerably but the following general plan of treatment, which has proven to be very satisfactory, is suggested for the average clubfoot seen within the first month of life. Nevertheless, it must be remembered that the treatment of an individual clubfoot must be tailored to fit the needs of that particular foot.

1. Weekly application of plaster casts (following gentle and progressive correction of

the deformities in the aforementioned order) which requires about six weeks (Fig. 8.7).

2. Denis Browne type of clubfoot splint to which the feet are strapped by adhesive tape and in which the affected foot is progressively turned outward and into valgus (Fig. 8.8). The adhesive is changed weekly for about twelve weeks and, during this phase of treatment, correction of the deformity is maintained while some movement is allowed in the involved joints.

3. Denis Browne type of boot splint which is to be worn day and night (and removed only for bathing) during the ensuing three months, following which it is left off for longer and longer periods until the child is walking (Fig. 8.9). It is most important that the splint be used at night for at least another year or longer in order to decrease the chances of recurrence.

4. Straight last or outflare boots for day wear until age three years, and occasionally the addition of an outside sole wedge.

Approximately 60% of congenital clubfeet treated early by these non-operative methods will have responded satisfactorily within the first three months of treatment. The remaining 40% are *resistant* to these methods and consequently, under these circumstances, continuation of non-operative treatment leads to eventual failure, due either to incomplete correction, or recurrence of the deformity. In such resistant clubfeet it is better judgment to perform a meticulous soft tissue correction of all tendon and joint contractures at this time for *resistance* rather than to delay surgical treatment and be forced to perform a major operation at a later date for *recurrence*, at which time the results are less satisfactory. Following this type of early surgery, the aforementioned non-operative plan is resumed to maintain

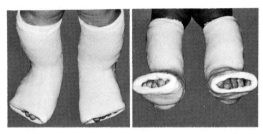

Figure 8.7. Carefully molded plaster casts for the initial correction of clubfeet. The skin has been painted with tincture of benzoin (Friar's balsam) and covered by a bandage before the cast is applied in order to prevent the child from kicking the cast off. These casts are changed at weekly intervals and at the time of each change, further correction is obtained.

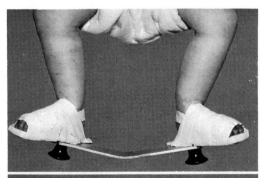

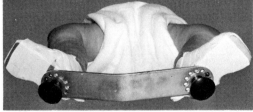

Figure 8.8. Denis Browne clubfoot adhesive splint. This exercise splint maintains correction of the deformity while allowing movement in the involved joints.

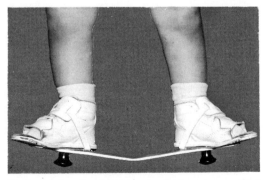

Figure 8.9. Denis Browne clubfoot boot splint. This removable splint is worn at night for at least one year and usually longer, following correction of the clubfoot, and is the best type of prevention of recurrence of the deformity.

the correction. Neglected clubfeet and re-current clubfeet always require operative treatment, the extent of which depends on the severity of the various components of the residual deformity. In general, soft tissue operations (such as capsulotomies, tendon lengthenings, tendon transfers) are effective in the first five years of life, but become less effective in older children because of the increasingly abnormal shape of the bones. Thus, in the older child, bony operations (such as arthrodesis of the subtalar and midtarsal joints) are usually necessary to correct any residual deformity but are best deferred until the age of about ten years.

The relatively recent emphasis on early minor operation for *resistant* clubfeet at three months of age has greatly decreased the number of recurrences and has been an important factor in improving the overall re-sults of treatment for this important congen-ital abnormality.

TALIPES CALCANEOVALGUS

Some children at the time of birth are found to have one or both feet maintained in a dorsiflexed and everted position, a con-dition commonly referred to as *congenital talipes calcaneovalgus*. (Fig. 8.10). This mild and transient deformity of an otherwise nor-mal foot is probably the result of intrauterine position rather than a true congenital abnor-

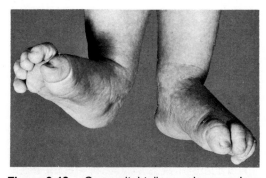

Figure 8.10. Congenital talipes calcaneovalgus in a newborn infant. Note the everted and dorsi-flexed position of the foot, which is probably related to intrauterine position. This infant's foot was normal 3 months later, the only treatment having been daily stretching of the foot by the mother.

mality of development; thus it is comparable to a "positional equinovarus" rather than to a talipes equinovarus. Daily passive stretch-ing of the soft tissues by the mother usually produces excellent and permanent correc-tion of the deformity; indeed, many of these feet improve spontaneously. Only the more resistant deformities require the application of one or two plaster casts.

TARSAL COALITION (RIGID VALGUS FOOT)

Any two of the tarsal bones in the hindfoot may be congenitally joined together by a bridge or bar (*coalition*), which at birth and in early childhood is still cartilaginous (a syn-chondrosis) but which in adolescence be-comes ossified (a synostosis). As a result of such coalitions as *talocalcaneal bridge* and *calcaneonavicular bar*, movement in the in-volved tarsal joints is restricted (Fig. 8.11). The foot, which almost always goes into a position of valgus, looks flat, but unlike the hypermobile, or flexible type of flatfoot, this type of flatfoot gradually becomes both rigid and painful and is associated with secondary spasm and contracture of the peroneal mus-cles (it is also called "peroneal spastic flat-foot") (Fig. 8.11). These congenital abnor-malities usually pass undetected during the first ten years of life, after which time sec-ondary degenerative arthritis in the talonav-icular joint produces a painful foot which causes the child to walk with a shuffling type of gait. Non-operative measures of treat-ment are of only temporary value; excision of the area of coalition is often inadequate (especially if secondary degenerative changes are present in the talonavicular joint). The most certain form of treatment is combined subtalar and mid tarsal (triple) ar-throdesis.

ACCESSORY TARSAL NAVICULAR

The tarsal navicular, which is cartilaginous at birth, is sometimes congenitally larger than normal and over the years a separate center of ossification appears within it on the medial side. This accessory bone (some-times referred to as an "os tibiale exter-num"), into which part of the tibialis posterior

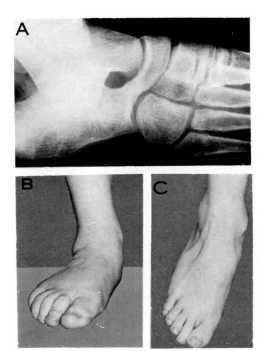

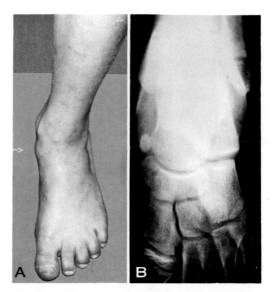

Figure 8.12. *A*, congenital accessory tarsal navicular in a 13-year-old girl's left foot. Note the bony prominence on the medial side of the foot in the region of the navicular which was associated with local tenderness (*arrow*). *B*, a congenital accessory tarsal navicular demonstrating the separate center of ossification in the abnormally large navicular to which is attached one portion of the tibialis posterior muscle. A false joint develops between the two bony parts of the navicular and is the site of pain. Relief of symptoms followed surgical excision of the separate center (accessory bone) along with the prominent medial portion of the navicular.

Figure 8.11. Oblique radiograph of a congenital calcaneonavicular bar (coalition) in the right foot of a 15-year-old boy. The abnormal bony bar joining the calcaneus to the navicular is cartilaginous in early childhood, but ossifies during adolescence and blocks normal midtarsal movement. Rigid valgus foot (peroneal spastic flat foot) due to congenital calcaneonavicular bar in the 15-year-old boy whose radiograph is shown above. Note that the foot is flat and in valgus even when not bearing weight. This boy's foot was very painful and required surgical treatment consisting of arthrodesis of the subtalar, talonavicular and calcaneocuboid joints ("triple arthrodesis").

tendon is inserted, is not rigidly joined to the body of the navicular and produces on the medial side of the foot a bony prominence which may become painful and tender in early adolescence (Fig. 8.12). If symptoms persist, it is necessary to excise the accessory bone along with the prominent portion of the navicular preserving the deep insertion of the tibialis posterior tendon.

The Long Bones

PSEUDARTHROSIS OF THE TIBIA

In this rare but serious abnormality, the tibia, which has failed to grow normally in width, becomes angulated in its lower third resulting in an anterior bowing of the leg before birth. The abnormality may be related to neurofibromatosis but the exact etiology is not clear. The thin, sclerotic bone at the site of angulation is brittle and consequently a pathological fracture occurs, either at birth or in early childhood. Since the abnormal bone is avascular at this site, the fracture fails to unite and a *pseudarthrosis* (false joint) develops with a resultant increase in the angulatory deformity (Fig. 8.13). Congenital pseudarthrosis of the tibia is the most difficult type of non-union confronting the orthopaedic surgeon and requires special techniques of bone grafting for its correction. In recent years encouraging results have been obtained from free vascularized autogenous bone grafts (performed by mi-

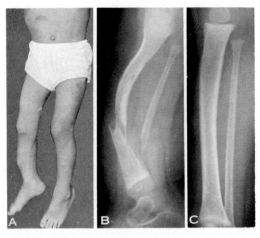

Figure 8.13. *A*, congenital pseudarthrosis of the tibia in a 2-year-old child. Note the anterior angulation of the right tibia and also the area of pigmentation—a café au lait spot—on the child's abdomen and left thigh suggestive of a relationship with neurofibromatosis. *B* and *C*, congenital pseudarthrosis of the tibia in the same child demonstrating the pathological fracture which has failed to unite and has produced a pseudarthrosis (false joint). Note also the thin diameter of the tibia in this area compared to the normal tibia.

crosurgery) as well as from electrical stimulation.

The Knee

DISCOID LATERAL MENISCUS

In this isolated abnormality the lateral meniscus (semilunar cartilage) is thicker than normal, somewhat disc-shaped and lacks adequate attachment posteriorly. As the child's knee extends, the thick meniscus is suddenly pushed forward and the femoral condyle rides over it, pushing it suddenly backward and accounting for the loud "clunk" that occurs during movement of the knee. The discoid meniscus usually produces pain in early childhood, in which case it should be excised.

The Hip

(DEVELOPMENTAL) COXA VARA

In this condition a localized congenital defect of ossification in the femoral neck results in the gradual development of a progressive varus deformity of the upper end of the femur (*coxa vara*) over the years (Fig. 8.14). For this reason the coxa vara is sometimes referred to as *developmental* rather than congenital. The clinical examination reveals mild shortening of the lower limb and limitation of passive abduction of the hip. The child develops a positive Trendelenburg sign, since the distance from the greater trochanter to the iliac crest is less than normal, and the efficiency of the hip abductor muscles is decreased. Accordingly, the child walks with a painless Trendelenburg, or lurching, type of limp. There would seem to be some relationship between congenital coxa vara and hypoplasia of the femur since in the former, the femoral shaft is frequently short, and in the latter, there is always a coexistent and severe coxa vara. The most effective treatment for congenital coxa vara is abduction subtrochanteric osteotomy of the femur, which not only corrects the adduction, or varus deformity, but also encourages ossification of the defect in the femoral neck. The operation is most effective if performed before a marked deformity has developed.

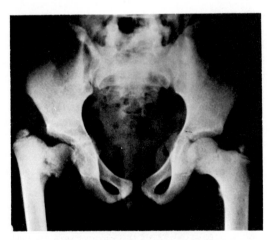

Figure 8.14. Congenital (developmental) coxa vara of the right hip in a 10-year-old boy. Note the defect of ossification in the right femoral neck which has allowed a progressive varus deformity. The boy walked with a Trendelenburg type of limp on the right side. Following abduction subtrochanteric osteotomy of the right femur, the femoral neck defect ossified and the boy's gait became normal.

DISLOCATION AND SUBLUXATION OF THE HIP

One of the most challenging and most important congenital abnormalities of the musculoskeletal system is *congenital dislocation of the hip*—an abnormality that is almost as common as clubfoot and yet not so obvious at birth; an abnormality that demands a specific method of examination for its detection in the newborn and yet one that, regrettably, is still not being recognized sufficiently early (and may even escape detection until after the child has started to walk); and finally, an abnormality that, unless treated early and well, leads inevitably to painful crippling degenerative arthritis of the hip in adult life. Indeed, at least one third of all degenerative joint disease of the hip in adults is caused by the sequelae of congenital dislocation of the hip (Fig. 8.15). In no other congenital abnormality of the musculoskeletal system is the effort to make an early diagnosis so rewarding—and the failure to make this effort so tragic! You can meet this challenge by *resolving* that throughout your professional lifetime you will *always* examine the hip joints of *every* infant entrusted to your care.

The condition of congenital dislocation of the hip is best considered in a temporal sense as a process, or chain of events which, in the beginning at least, can be arrested and even reversed. A description of certain terms will be helpful at this time. *Dislocation (luxation)* of the hip refers to the femoral head being completely outside the socket, or acetabulum, but still within the stretched and elongated capsule (intracapsular). *Subluxation* of the hip refers to the femoral head riding on the edge of the acetabulum; such a hip is usually reduced and stable when the hip is flexed and abducted, but is subluxated when the hip is extended and adducted. When the hip is either dislocated or subluxated, the bony development of the acetabulum becomes progressively abnormal (*acetabular dysplasia*). The present discussion concerns only the common and typical type of congenital dislocation in

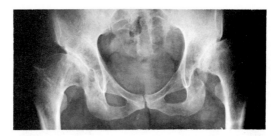

Figure 8.15. Degenerative joint disease of both hips in a 38-year-old woman secondary to residual subluxation following inadequate treatment of congenital dislocation of the hips in childhood. The patient walked with a marked limp and suffered pain in both hips. This serious and disabling condition could have been prevented by diagnosis and adequate treatment at birth.

otherwise normal children, as opposed to the less common prenatal (teratologic) type of congenital dislocation associated with spina bifida and arthrogryposis.

Incidence

Congenital dislocation and subluxation of the hip are quite common (incidence of 1.5 per 1,000 live births). The abnormality is bilateral in more than half of the afflicted children (dislocation of both hips, subluxation of both hips, or one of each) and affects girls eight times as often as boys. A study of the geographic incidence, which varies tremendously throughout the world, suggests that the higher incidence is related, in part, to the custom of maintaining the hips of newborn infants in extension and adduction by various means, including tightly wrapped blankets (Fig. 8.16). Infants with either congenital muscular torticollis or metatarsus varus have a much higher incidence of congenital dislocation than do otherwise normal infants.

Etiology and Pathology

Unlike most of the congenital musculoskeletal abnormalities, congenital dislocation and subluxation of the hip are the end results of combined genetic and environmental factors. Although this complex subject is still controversial due to lack of adequate data, the following explanation seems most rea-

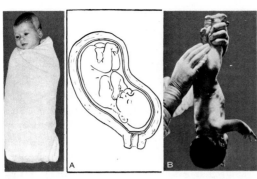

Figure 8.16. (*left*). Newborn infant tightly wrapped in a blanket which maintains the newborn hips in the harmful position of extension and adduction. This custom is one factor in the cause of the initial dislocation of a congenitally unstable hip and therefore should be avoided.

Figure 8.17. *A*, fetal position *in utero*. The hip joints are always constantly maintained in complete flexion. *B*, sudden, passive extension of the previously flexed hips immediately after birth should be avoided because it is one factor in the initial dislocation of a congenitally unstable hip.

sonable and is presented briefly at this time without discussing the available evidence. The hip joint develops well *in utero* and is constantly held in acute *flexion* (Fig. 8.17*A*). At birth, one child in 80 exhibits an undue degree of congenital hip joint laxity and this is probably genetically determined. If at the moment of birth, or even within the first few weeks, the previously flexed hips are passively *extended* in the presence of such marked hip joint laxity, the femoral head may dislocate, and then either reduce (relocate) or remain dislocated (Fig. 8.17*B*). Thus, at birth, the abnormal hip is *dislocatable* but not permanently dislocated. Indeed, the majority of such hips become stable spontaneously within the first two months. However, if a vulnerable hip is *maintained* in extension, it tends to *remain* either dislocated or subluxated (Fig. 8.16). Persistent dislocation and subluxation cause progressive *secondary* changes in all the structures in and around the hip joint. These important secondary changes include abnormal development (*dysplasia*) of the acetabulum which becomes *maldirected*; increase in the normal *femoral neck anteversion*; hypertrophy

of the elongated capsule; and contracture and shortening of the muscles that cross the hip joint, especially the adductor and the iliopsoas.

It will be obvious to you, even from this very brief description, that each and every one of the progressive secondary changes increases the difficulty, not only of reducing the hip, but also of maintaining its reduction. Furthermore, as time goes on, these changes not only become progressively more marked—they also become progressively *less reversible*. All of these facts should serve to emphasize the extreme importance of *early diagnosis*, the responsibility for which rests with the family physician, obstetrician and pediatrician who are the first to see and examine infants. Indeed, it is quite possible that if a newborn infant's hips were *never* passively extended and *never* maintained in extension during the first few months of life, the great majority of genetically vulnerable hips could be *prevented* from dislocating or subluxating and would therefore go on to develop *normally*. Thus, the possible *prevention* of at least *most* congenital dislocations and subluxations of the hip and all their tragic sequelae becomes an exciting challenge.

Diagnosis and Treatment

The clinical and radiographic diagnosis, as well as the orthopaedic treatment, of congenital dislocation and subluxation of the hip vary so greatly with the child's age that they are best considered in relation to several specific age groups. Nevertheless, the importance of *very early diagnosis* and *very early treatment* merits repeated emphasis. The general principles of treatment include gentle reduction of the hip followed by maintenance of the reduction with the hip in a stable position until the various components of the hip have developed well and the hip has become stable even in the position of weight bearing.

Birth to Three Months

During this most important period of greatest opportunity, the abnormality is *never obvious*, which means that *you must seek it out* by careful examination of *every* infant you see. The instability of the *dislocatable* hip can be detected at birth by the Barlow "provocation" *test*, in which the flexed hips are alternately adducted while pressing the femur downward, and abducted while lifting the femur upward (Fig. 8.18). In the presence of instability you will feel—and see —the hip dislocate as it is adducted and reduce as it is abducted.

If the hip is already *dislocated*, the femoral head lies posterior to the acetabulum when the hip is in the flexed position and it can be reduced by abduction while lifting the femur forward (i.e. it is reducible); this is the Ortolani sign. Limitation of passive abduction of the flexed hip (due to contracture of the adductor muscles) is a very important sign, particularly after the first month (Fig. 8.19). Limitation of abduction does not necessarily indicate a complete dislocation, but does indicate an abnormal hip and should always be investigated further by radiographic examination (Fig. 8.20). Because there is a wide range of normal at this age, the radiographs should be interpreted by an expe-

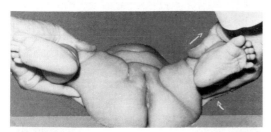

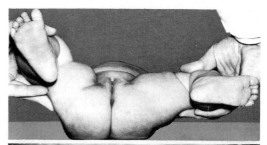

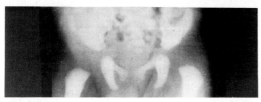

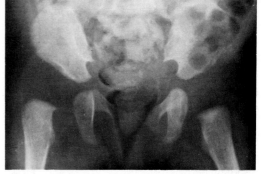

Figure 8.18. *Top*, Barlow test to demonstrate instability of the hip in the newborn period. When the flexed hip is adducted slightly while pressing downward along the long axis of the femur, the femoral head slides posteriorly out of the acetabulum. When the flexed hip is then abducted slightly while lifting the femur upward and pressing forward on the greater trochanter, the femoral head is suddenly reduced into the acetabulum with a "jerk." The instability can be both felt and seen. You must perform this test in every newborn infant you see in order to avoid the serious error of overlooking the diagnosis of congenital dislocation of the hip in the newborn period. *Bottom*, radiograph of infant shown at top. The left hip is dislocated in the extended position as evidenced by the slight upward and lateral displacement of the adducted femur. Note that the acetabulum in this newborn infant has not yet become dysplastic.

Figure 8.19 (*top*). Limitation of passive abduction of the right hip in a 2-month-old infant with congenital dislocation of the right hip. This sign is more apparent after the first month of life. Note also the asymmetry of the skin folds on the medial aspect of the thighs.

Figure 8.20 (*bottom*). Congenital dislocation of the right hip in the 2-month-old infant shown in Fig. 8.19. Note the upward and lateral displacement of the right femur and the delayed development (dysplasia) of the bony part of the right acetabulum.

rienced individual. Extra skin creases on the inner side of the thigh and external rotation of the lower limb should make you at least suspicious of congenital dislocation of the hip even though both of these signs may also be seen in normal infants.

Treatment during this most favorable period involves gentle *reduction* of the hip, which is usually not difficult at this stage, followed by the *maintenance* of the hip in the stable position of flexion and abduction in some type of device such as the Frejka pillow splint (Fig. 8.21). An alternate form of management during the first three to six months is the Pavlik harness which maintains the hips in flexion while permitting motion in other directions; when properly used this harness produces excellent results with few complications (Fig. 8.22). Occasionally, even at this age, the hip is too unstable to be kept reduced by any type of splint, in which case a plaster hip spica cast is indi-

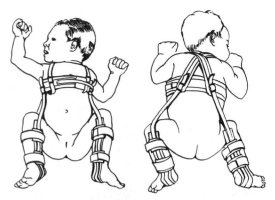

Figure 8.22. The Pavlik harness which prevents both active and passive extension of the hips but permits all other movements and thereby helps to stimulate the development of the reduced hip.

cated. A period of about four months protection is usually necessary for the capsule to become tighter and for the reduced femoral head to stimulate development of the hip and thereby reverse the secondary changes. The effects of treatment must be assessed both clinically and radiographically.

Three Months to Eighteen Months

In this period the adduction contracture is more marked, and physical signs resulting from this contracture, such as limitation of passive abduction, apparent and real shortening of the involved lower limb and prominence of the hip, become progressively more obvious (Fig. 8.23). With unilateral dislocation, shortening of the thigh is most apparent when the hips are flexed and the level of the knees is compared (*Galeazzi's sign*) (Fig. 8.24). The presence of a dislocation is confirmed by feeling the hip go in and out of the joint during the previously mentioned Ortolani test, but this phenomenon becomes progressively more difficult to elicit the longer the hip has remained out of joint—and it cannot be elicited with a subluxation. In the presence of a complete dislocation, a push-pull maneuver on the femur will demonstrate the phenomenon of *telescoping* as the femur moves to and fro within the thigh (Fig. 8.25). Radiographs reveal an excessive slope of the *ossified* portion of the acetabulum (an indication of acetabular

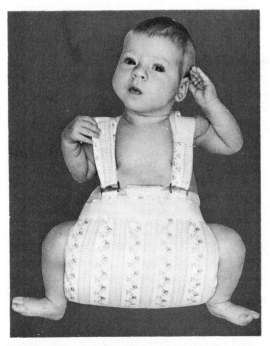

Figure 8.21. Frejka pillow splint. This 2-month-old girl had a congenitally unstable left hip joint with a positive Ortolani test. The pillow splint keeps the hips in the stable position of flexion and abduction while still allowing some active movement of the hips.

dysplasia and maldirection), delayed ossification of the femoral head and varying degrees of upward and lateral displacement of the head of the femur (Fig. 8.26).

Treatment in this age group involves preliminary lengthening of the tight adductor muscles by continuous traction for a few weeks (Fig. 8.27) (and always a subcutaneous adductor tenotomy) followed by very gentle *closed reduction* of the hip under anesthesia and *maintenance* of the reduced hip in a hip spica cast in a stable position of marked flexion and only moderate abduction (that we have called the "human" position—as opposed to the traditional "frog" position) (Fig. 8.28). Retention of the hip in an

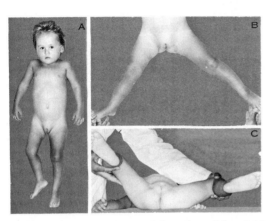

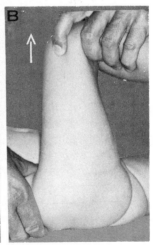

Figure 8.23. Congenital dislocation of the right hip in a 14-month-old girl. Note the adduction contracture of the right hip resulting in apparent shortening of the right lower limb (added to the true shortening from the dislocation), the prominence of the right hip and the external rotation of the lower limb. Note also the limitation of passive abduction of the right hip.

Figure 8.26. Congenital dislocation of the right hip in a 14-month-old girl. Note upward and lateral displacement of the right femur, delayed ossification of the right femoral head and delayed ossification of the right acetabulum (acetabular dysplasia).

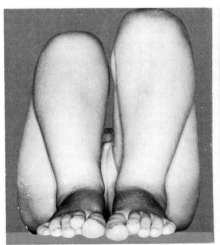
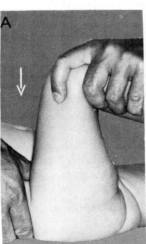
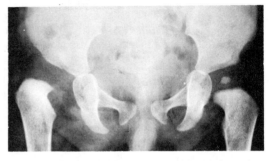

Figure 8.24 (*left*). Galeazzi's sign (also called Allis' sign) of congenital dislocation of the right hip in a 14-month-old girl. This sign, which is of value only with a unilateral dislocation, demonstrates that when the hips are flexed to 90°, the femoral head lies posterior to the acetabulum and as a result the thigh on the dislocated side is shortened as evidenced by the lower level of the knee.

Figure 8.25 (*middle* and *right*). Telescoping of the thigh in congenital dislocation of the hip in a 14-month-old girl. With the involved hip flexed, a push-pull maneuver demonstrates that the femur, being dislocated at the hip, moves to and fro within the thigh.

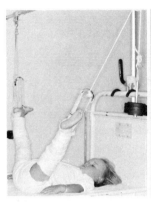
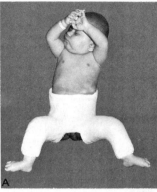
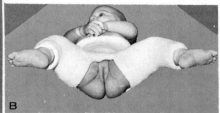

Figure 8.27 (*left*).   Continuous skin traction via adhesive tape on the lower limb for congenital dislocation of the hip in a 1-year-old girl. The traction, which is maintained for a few weeks, gradually stretches the shortened muscles about the hip in preparation for a safe and gentle closed reduction.
Figure 8.28 (*right*).   Bilateral hip spica plaster cast for congenital dislocation of the hip in a 1-year-old girl. This type of cast is applied following adductor tenotomy and gentle closed reduction and maintains the reduced hip in the stable position of marked flexion and moderate abduction (the "human" position). This child required a total period of 12 months in a cast, during which time the hip responded well. Earlier diagnosis and treatment would have shortened the period of immobilization.

extreme or forced position of abduction or internal rotation must be avoided since it is probably the most important cause of *avascular necrosis* of the femoral head, which is a serious complication of treatment. The hip spica cast is changed every two months until radiographs reveal satisfactory development of both the acetabulum and femoral head. The period of immobilization of the reduced hip required to bring about reversal of the secondary changes varies directly with the number of months the hip had been dislocated before treatment, but is usually between 6 and 18 months. During the last part of this period of retention, adequate *protection* of the reduction can usually be obtained by the use of two long leg casts separated by an abduction bar; this type of cast allows some movement of the hip within a safe range and thereby provides further stimulation for development of the acetabulum and femoral head.

The results of gentle and careful closed treatment instituted between 3 and 18 months of age are good in approximately 80% of patients. However, it must be remembered that the percentage of good re-sults is much higher when treatment is started at 3 months than at 18 months.

Eighteen Months to Five Years

In this age group the secondary changes are not only more severe but also less reversible. By this time the child is walking and a typical limp is added to the aforementioned clinical signs, all of which are more marked. When the child is asked to stand on one foot (on the side of the dislocated hip), the hip abductor muscles, having no fulcrum, cannot hold the pelvis level and it drops on the opposite side; the child, in an effort to maintain balance shifts her trunk toward the involved side. These observations indicate a positive *Trendelenburg sign* (Fig. 8.29). The limp is another manifestation of this phenomenon. When the dislocation is unilateral, the child walks as though the lower limb on that side were too short and shifts the trunk toward the involved side when weight is borne on that hip. When the dislocation is bilateral, the child shifts the trunk from one side to the other while walking and gives the impression of *waddling* like a duck. In a subluxation the Trendelenburg sign and the

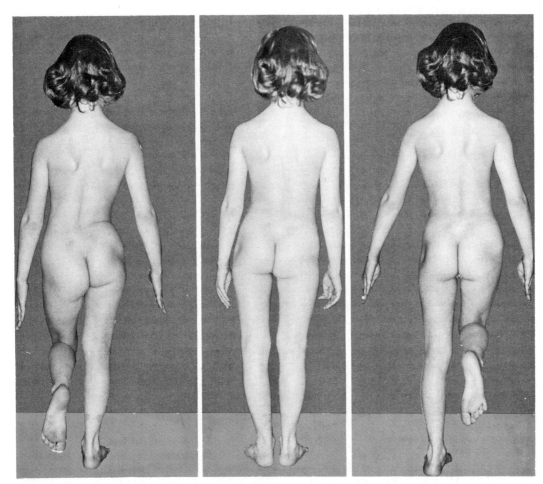

Figure 8.29. Trendelenburg sign in a congenital dislocation of the hip in a 4-year-old girl. *Left*, when the child stands on the right foot (the side of the dislocated hip), the hip abductor muscles, having no fulcrum, cannot hold the pelvis level and it drops on the opposite side; the child, in an effort to maintain balance, shifts her trunk toward the involved side. *Middle*, the dislocation is not apparent when the child is standing with both feet on the floor (apart from the slight shortening of the lower limb). *Right*, when the child stands on left foot (the side of the normal hip) the hip abductors, having a normal fulcrum, hold the pelvis level. The Trendelenburg sign is also seen in the presence of coxa vara, paralyzed hip abductors and painful conditions about the hip.

limp are not nearly so apparent as in a dislocation, but they are more readily detected when the muscles are fatigued, for example, after a long period of walking.

Treatment in this age group is fraught with difficulties, dangers and disappointments even in the most experienced hands. The muscle contractures, which by this time have become very resistant, must be overcome by a longer period of traction as well as by subcutaneous adductor tenotomy.

The likelihood of obtaining a satisfactory closed reduction becomes progressively less and if closed reduction fails to produce a perfect repositioning of the femoral head in the acetabulum, *operative reduction* is indicated. At the time of open reduction the secondary soft tissue abnormalities, particularly those related to the joint capsule, must be dealt with. The *main* problem in this age group is not so much the reduction, but rather *maintaining the reduction*; this is a manifestation of the marked instability of the reduced, but poorly developed, hip joint. Many bony operations involving either the femur or the acetabulum have been designed to overcome this problem of instability but the most reliable in our experience has been innominate osteotomy, which is designed to provide stability of the reduced hip by redirecting the entire acetabulum (Fig. 8.30).

The long term results of closed reduction in this age group are depressing since only 30% are good. Following careful open reduction and the improvement of stability by bony operations, the results are much better but still cannot compare with the results of closed treatment instituted in the first three months of life—all of which provides mute testimony to the extreme importance of early diagnosis and treatment.

Over the Age of Five Years

Fortunately, few children now reach the age of five years with previously untreated congenital dislocation of the hip—though the same cannot be said for congenital subluxation. By this time the secondary changes in a complete dislocation are so marked and their reversibility so limited that even extensive operative procedures (including femoral shortening) cannot be expected to meet with success, particularly in children over six or seven years of age; beyond this age, it is unwise even to attempt reduction (Fig. 8.31). Residual subluxation is less difficult to treat in this age group than dislocation and can be improved considerably by innominate osteotomy up to the end of the growing period and beyond. For those unfortunate older children with irreducible congenital dislocation of the hip, palliative and salvage types of operative procedures are frequently required for the relief of pain in early adult life.

Neonatal screening for congenital dislocation of the hip in *all* infants during the first few days of life has been effective in reducing the incidence of "missed" dislocations—and hence in reducing the number of children

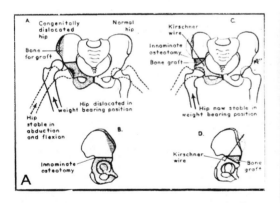
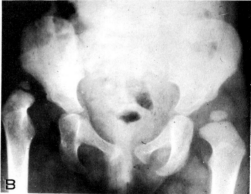
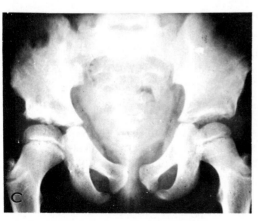

Figure 8.30. *A*, the principle of innominate osteotomy is redirection of the entire acetabulum in such a way that the reduced hip, which previously was stable only in a position of flexion and abduction, is rendered stable with the limb in the normal position of weight bearing. *B*, congenital dislocation of the right hip and congenital subluxation of the left hip in a 3-year-old girl. Note the severity of the secondary dysplastic head. *C*, the same girl 4 years after open reduction and innominate osteotomy of the right hip, and innominate osteotomy of the left hip. The girl walked normally. Early diagnosis and treatment would have rendered such surgical treatment unnecessary.

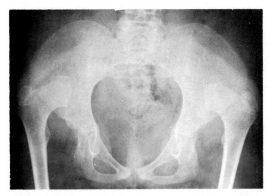

Figure 8.31. Bilateral congenital dislocation of the hip in a 9-year-old girl. The secondary changes in the acetabulum and femur, as well as in the soft tissues, are so severe and so irreversible at this age that it is not possible to obtain a good result by *any* form of treatment. Therefore, this girl is doomed to a disability for the rest of her life, a disability that could have been prevented by early diagnosis and early treatment.

requiring extensive surgical treatment. Subluxations are more difficult to detect at birth but routine physical and radiographic examination at three months would be useful in their detection as well.

It is to be hoped that you and your contemporaries during your professional lifetime will *never* allow a newborn infant with congenital dislocation of the hip to go unrecognized!

LOCALIZED CONGENITAL ABNORMALITIES OF THE UPPER LIMB

The Hand

TRIGGER THUMB

A constantly flexed interphalangeal joint of the thumb in children is usually due to a congenital constriction (*stenosis*) of the fibrous sheath of the flexor pollicis longus tendon and a *secondary* enlargement in the tendon at the proximal edge of the constriction. This combination always prevents active extension of the interphalangeal joint, and frequently prevents even passive extension so that the "trigger phenomenon" of sudden, snapping flexion is seldom seen in the congenital type, even though the abnormality is commonly referred to as trigger thumb. Under the proximal skin crease the

enlargement in the tendon is readily felt as a nodule which moves with the tendon during passive movement of the interphalangeal joint (Fig. 8.32). Surgical treatment, which consists of longitudinal division of the constricted fibrous sheath through a transverse skin incision, allows free gliding of the tendon following which the secondary enlargement in the tendon gradually disappears.

The Forearm

HYPOPLASIA OF THE RADIUS (*CLUBHAND*)

This relatively uncommon, but serious, abnormality consists of varying degrees of hypoplasia, or even aplasia, of the radial ray of the upper limb including the radius, scaphoid, trapezium, first metacarpal and thumb as well as the associated muscles, nerves and blood vessels. When the abnormality is severe, radial deviation of the hand is invariably present, the ulna is short as well as curved and even the proximal part of the upper limb may be hypoplastic (Fig. 8.33).

The principles of treatment of this difficult problem include very early correction of the radial deviation of the hand, maintenance of this correction during growth and finally, improvement of hand function. Passive stretching of the contracted soft tissues on

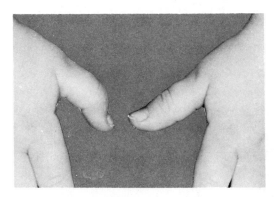

Figure 8.32. Congenital right trigger thumb due to a congenital constriction (stenosis) of the fibrous sheath of the flexor pollicis longus tendon. This 1-year-old child could not actively extend the interphalangeal joint of the right thumb; a nodule was palpable on the flexor tendon just proximal to the fibrous sheath (under the proximal skin crease). This anomaly responded well to simple division of the fibrous sheath.

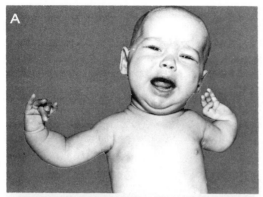

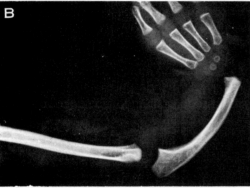

Figure 8.33. Congenital hypoplasia of the radius (clubhand). *A*, in this little girl the anomaly is bilateral but much more severe in the left upper limb than in the right. Note the absence of a thumb, the radial deviation of the hand and the short, curved forearm. This child also had congenital heart disease requiring operative correction. *B*, radiograph of the left arm of the same patient reveals absence of the radius, curvature of the hypoplastic ulna, radial deviation of the hand and absence of the thumb and first metacarpal.

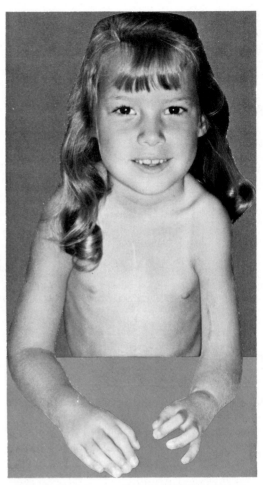

Figure 8.34. Congenital hypoplasia of the radius (clubhand). The same patient in Figure 8.33 shown 6 years after surgical correction of the radial deviation of each hand and pollicization of the left index finger.

the concave side of the deformity is of limited and temporary value. Much more effective is early soft tissue operation consisting of Z-plasty of the skin, division of the fibrous band (anlage) in the location of the defective radius, maintenance of correction for several months in casts followed by appropriate removable splints. Permanent correction of the radial deviation may necessitate bony operations, such as implantation of the distal end of the ulna into a slot fashioned in the carpus (Fig. 8.34). If the condition is bilateral and both thumbs are absent, the index finger of the dominant hand can be surgically repositioned to function as a thumb (*pollicization*) in order to improve pinch and grasp. It should be remembered, however, that resourceful individuals with congenital absence even of both thumbs may develop surprisingly good function of the hands without operation.

LOCALIZED CONGENITAL ABNORMALITIES OF THE SPINE

SPINA BIFIDA

The commonest congenital abnormality of the spine, by far, is *spina bifida*, which includes varying degrees of incomplete bony closure of one or more neural arches. The defect may occur at any level, but the most frequent site is the lumbosacral region, which is normally the last part of the vertebral column to close. Although minor defects are very common indeed, spina bifida of sufficient degree to be obvious at birth has an incidence of 2 per 1,000 births.

At the beginning of this chapter, reference is made to the antenatal diagnosis of the open types of spina bifida through the detection of elevated levels of AFP in the expectant mother's serum as well as in the amniotic fluid, and also through ultrasonography and fetoscopy. These measures have markedly reduced the incidence of open spina bifida in those countries (such as Great Britain) in which programs of antenatal diagnosis have been well established for a number of years. The most significant aspect of this abnormality is not the bony defect itself but rather the frequently associated neurological deficit which is due to defective development of the spinal cord (*myelodysplasia*). When present, the neurological deficit may vary from mild muscle imbalance and sensory loss in the lower limbs to complete paraplegia. Thus, spina bifida must always be considered as a possible cause of neurogenic deformities and trophic ulcers in the lower limbs as well as of bladder and bowel incontinence. Some severe teratologic types of congenital clubfeet and congenital dislocation of the hip are secondary to the prenatal paralysis and failure of muscle development associated with spina bifida. Furthermore, during childhood, various neurogenic deformities of the lower limbs may appear and increase in severity with growth as a result of residual muscle imbalance secondary to spina bifida.

The varying degrees of spina bifida are best classified morphologically and discussed on this basis.

Spina Bifida Occulta

The mildest degree of spina bifida occurs without any external manifestation and is truly hidden (occult) being detectable only

by radiographic examination (Fig. 8.35). This extremely common form of spina bifida occurs in about 10% of the population and is least serious since it is rarely associated with a neurological deficit. When there is some external manifestation of the abnormality, such as a dimple, hairy patch, pigmented area or hemangioma (Fig. 8.36), the underlying spina bifida is more likely to be complicated by a midline spur that splits the spinal cord (*diastematomyelia*) or by a *congenital neoplasm* such as a lipoma, hemangioma or

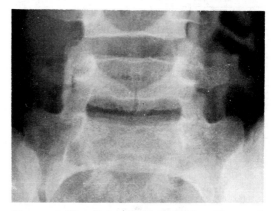

Figure 8.35. Spina bifida occulta. The radiograph reveals incomplete closure of the neural arch of the fifth lumbar vertebra in the midline, the commonest site of spina bifida occulta. The defect was an incidental finding in this 12-year-old boy and was not associated with any symptoms or any neurological deficit.

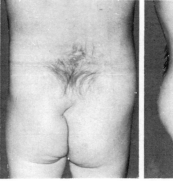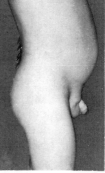

Figure 8.36. Spina bifida of the fifth lumbar neural arch associated with an overlying hairy patch. This 2-year-old child had a neurogenic deformity in one foot due to muscle imbalance.

dermoid cyst, either inside or outside the spinal canal. Under these circumstances a neurological deficit may be present at birth, or it may develop gradually during the subsequent years of spinal growth.

Spina Bifida with Meningocele

The meninges may extrude through a larger defect in the neural arches thereby forming a *meningocele* covered by normal skin and containing cerebrospinal fluid and some nerve roots (Fig. 8.37). The spinal cord remains confined to the spinal canal and there is usually little or no neurological deficit clinically detectable at birth. However, as in the type of spina bifida occulta with some

external skin manifestation, a neurological deficit may develop gradually during the subsequent years of spinal growth.

Spina Bifida with Meningomyelocele

When the abnormality is more severe, the spinal cord as well as the nerve roots are involved and may either lie free within the sac or constitute part of its wall. The overlying muscles and subcutaneous fat are usually deficient and under these circumstances the covering skin is thin and translucent. In severe meningomyeloceles the skin may be absent, in which case the cord is covered by the arachnoid and dura, and sometimes by the arachnoid alone (Fig. 8.38). As might

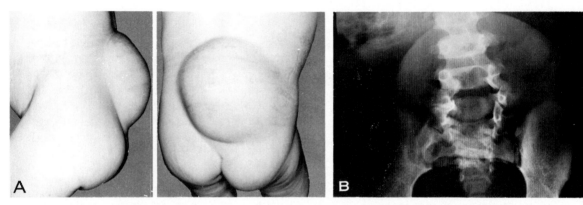

Figure 8.37. *A*, spina bifida with meningocele. The prominent meningocele is well covered by normal skin and subcutaneous tissue. *B*, the same patient. Note the wide defect in the neural arch of the fourth and fifth lumbar vertebrae. The curved line of density proximal to the bony defect represents the outline of the proximal edge of the meningocele.

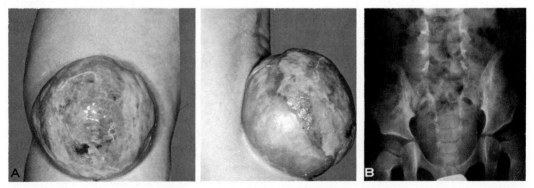

Figure 8.38. *A*, spina bifida with meningomyelocele. The meningomyelocele is partly covered by thin skin but in the central area the dura is exposed. This infant had extensive paralysis in the lower limbs. *B*, a child with a meningomyelocele. Note the very large defect in the neural arch of the last three lumbar vertebrae and of the sacrum. Note also the paralytic subluxation of this child's left hip joint and secondary dysplasia of the acetabulum.

be expected, a meningomyelocele is always associated with a serious neurological deficit which often includes bladder and bowel incontinence as well as sensory and motor loss in the lower limbs with typical deformities. When nerve roots only are involved in the meningomyelocele, the resultant paralysis is flaccid, whereas spinal cord involvement results in a spastic type of paralysis; thus, in a given child there may be a *mixed* flaccid and spastic paralysis. In almost half of these children hydrocephalus coexists as either a potential or an actual complication. The hydrocephalus is secondary to either downward prolongation of the brain stem and part of the cerebellum through the foramen magnum (*Arnold-Chiari malformation*) or other developmental defects of the brain, such as *aqueduct stenosis.*

Spina Bifida with Myelocele (Rachischisis)

In this, the most severe degree of spina bifida, even the skin and dura have failed to close over the neural tube so that the spinal cord and nerve roots lie completely exposed (Fig. 8.39). Inevitable infection usually results in death during early infancy.

Clinical Course of the Neurological Deficit

Although the neurological deficit is usually present from the beginning and tends to remain static, it may actually increase during the first few days or weeks as a result of increasing nerve root tension and infection. Even when the deficit remains static, the resultant muscle imbalance in the lower limbs produces deformities that are accentuated by longitudinal growth of the limbs (Fig. 8.40). Furthermore, abnormal fixation of the neural elements to the defective area of the spine may interfere with the normal ascent of the distal end of the spinal cord by a tethering effect and thereby produce an increasing traction lesion of the cord and a resultant increasing neurological deficit, particularly during periods of rapid vertebral growth.

Treatment of Spina Bifida with Neurological Deficit

In no other congenital abnormality of the musculoskeletal system is the *team* approach of greater importance than in the management of children afflicted by spina bifida with neurological involvement. *Neurosurgical treatment* includes careful removal of the sac whenever feasible and as early as possible, followed by the provision of good skin coverage; in addition, any associated

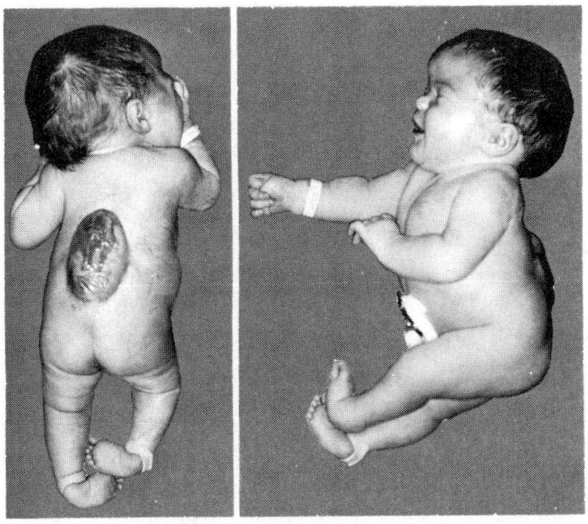

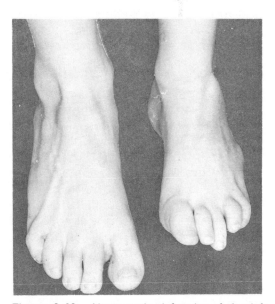

Figure 8.39.   Spina bifida with myelocele (rachischisis). In this newborn infant the spinal cord and nerve roots lie completely exposed on the surface. Note also the poorly developed lower limbs and the neurogenic clubfeet.

Figure 8.40.   Neurogenic deformity of the left foot (cavus and varus) due to muscle imbalance that was secondary to spina bifida with a meningocele.

hydrocephalus is decompressed by appropriate shunting operations with plastic tubes (ventriculoperitoneal shunt, ventriculocardiac shunt) in order to prevent irreversible brain damage.

During the past two decades the indications for immediate surgical "closure" of the open type of spina bifida in newborn infants have been controversial.

In the 1960's surgeons in some major centers recommended "emergency operations" to excise the sac and provide skin coverage for *all* newborn infants with the open type of spina bifida within the first few hours of life. It was hoped that such operations might prevent the otherwise inevitable progression of the neurological deficit and thereby decrease the residual paralysis and sensory loss. The early enthusiasm for such "routine" surgery has waned as it became apparent that those infants with extremely *severe* forms of spina bifida (thoracolumbar lesions with complete paralysis of the lower limbs, severe spinal deformities and hydrocephalus) were not really helped by such an approach. Such infants (who without surgical treatment are destined to die from the complications of their abnormality within the first six months) could be kept alive but the end results of multiple operations—neurosurgical, urological, orthopaedic and plastic—were so dismal that most neurosurgeons feel that for these extremely affected infants, surgical treatment on the first day of life is not justifiable. Nevertheless excision of the sac and provision of skin coverage in the first few weeks may be justified even in this severely involved group of infants to facilitate their nursing care. For newborn infants with all lesser degrees of involvement most neurosurgeons would recommend surgical "closure" in the first hours of life. Thus the initial decision to operate or not at birth is made on the basis of sound surgical judgement tempered by the wishes of the distressed parents; understandably, such a decision, which raises philosophical and ethical issues, can be exceedingly difficult for everyone concerned.

The principles of *orthopaedic treatment* for flaccid paralysis are similar to those to be discussed for poliomyelitis; and when the paralysis is of the spastic type, the principles are comparable to those to be discussed for cerebral palsy (Chapter 12). Particular care is required, however, to prevent pressure sores in areas of skin deprived of normal sensation. *Urological treatment* is of great importance, not only in overcoming the distressing problem of urinary incontinence, but also in preserving renal function by preventing or controlling recurrent urinary infection. Thus, the neurosurgeon, the orthopaedic surgeon and the urological surgeon each have a significant contribution to make and all three must be cognizant of the importance of the overall *rehabilitation* of the afflicted child in relation to his social development, special education and vocational guidance in order that he may reach his full potential in life, limited though it may be.

SCOLIOSIS

Lateral curvature of the spine (*scoliosis*) due to congenital abnormalities of the vertebral column and associated tissues varies widely both in severity and prognosis. Failure of one half of a vertebral body to form (*hemivertebra*) results in a short, relatively mild curvature which is usually well compensated above and below by the normal spine (Fig. 8.41). The clinical deformity is usually inconspicuous and the diagnosis is frequently made when a radiograph is taken for some other purpose. Progression of such a curvature is unlikely, but the child should be seen at least at yearly intervals for clinical and radiographic reassessment.

Multiple congenital abnormalities of the spinal column and ribs, including multiple hemivertebrae, asymmetrical fusion of vertebral bodies and absent ribs or fused ribs, are seldom balanced in their distribution and result in a severe congenital scoliosis that is unrelentingly progressive with subsequent growth (Fig. 8.42). Severe and progressive congenital scoliosis necessitates early operative treatment, including spinal fusion, even in growing children, in order to prevent extreme deformity. The prognosis of con-

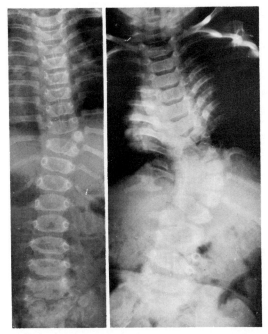

Figure 8.41 (*left*).   Congenital scoliosis due to a hemivertebra at the level of the ninth thoracic vertebra in a 1-year-old child. The scoliosis involves a short segment of the thoracic spine, is well compensated above and below and is clinically inconspicuous. The prognosis for this type of congenital scoliosis is good.

Figure 8.42 (*right*).   Congenital scoliosis due to multiple congenital anomalies of the spine including multiple hemivertebrae, fused ribs and a congenital synostosis of pedicles on the concave side of the curve. The prognosis for this 2-year-old child's scoliosis is bad in that the curvature will definitely increase with growth. Early correction and spinal fusion are indicated.

genital scoliosis in any given child, however, may be difficult to predict and therefore, repeated clinical and radiographic examinations at regular intervals are required to choose the most appropriate form of treatment.

MUSCULAR TORTICOLLIS (*WRY NECK*)

The exact etiology of this congenital muscular abnormality remains a mystery although at least 40% of the infants have experienced a difficult delivery. The deformity is minimal at birth but within the first few weeks of life a large, firm swelling develops in one sternocleidomastoid muscle. This swelling, called a "sternocleidomastoid tumor," which is probably the result of hypertrophy of the fibrous tissue elements within the muscle, gradually disappears but leaves a *contracture* (shortening) of the involved muscle. As a result the head becomes tilted, or laterally flexed, toward the affected side and rotated toward the opposite side (Fig. 8.43). The contracture of the muscle prevents its normal growth in length and therefore, as the cervical spine grows, the muscle fails to keep pace and becomes relatively shorter. This relative shortness of the muscle on one side not only causes an increase in the tilting and rotation of the head, but also results in progressive facial asymmetry during the growing years (Fig. 8.44). Radiographic examination is helpful in differentiating congenital muscular torticollis from the uncorrectable bony type of torticollis seen in cervical synostosis (Klippel-Feil syndrome).

It is important to remember that 20% of all infants with congenital muscular torticollis also have congenital dislocation of one or both hips.

Early recognition and treatment are important since, during the first few months of

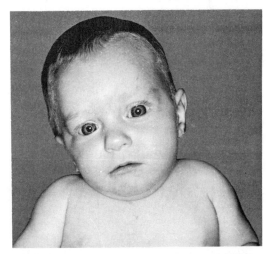

Figure 8.43.   Congenital muscular torticollis in a 1-year-old girl. The girl's head is tilted to the right and slightly turned to the left, indicating that the involved sternocleidomastoid muscle is on the right side (as it is in 85% of afflicted children).

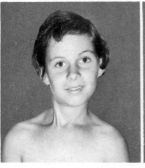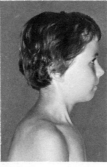

Figure 8.44. Congenital muscular torticollis in a 10-year-old girl. Note the prominent, shortened right sternocleidomastoid muscle and also the facial asymmetry which is due to delayed development of the right side of the face. This girl's face became more symmetrical over a 5-year period of growth following surgical division of the tight sternocleidomastoid muscle.

life at least, the shortened muscle seems to respond well to daily stretching. Initially, the *treatment* is best carried out by an experienced physiotherapist who subsequently trains the parents in the exact method of stretching required. Such treatment, if instituted within the first month and continued for at least a year, results in complete and permanent correction of the torticollis in 90% of the children. In children untreated during the early months, the torticollis becomes progressively resistant to stretching. Resistant and recurrent muscular torticollis require operative division of the contracted sternomastoid muscle and, in older children, secondary contractures of surrounding soft tissue must also be released.

GENERALIZED CONGENITAL ABNORMALITIES
Generalized Abnormalities of Bone

Of the multitude of generalized congenital abnormalities of bone formation and growth, only the six most significant will be discussed. Lest you be confused by their terminology, the various synonyms for these abnormalities are included in brackets. Some of the bone disorders that reflect inborn errors of metabolism are dealt with in Chapter 9.

OSTEOGENESIS IMPERFECTA (*FRAGILITAS OSSIUM*) (*BRITTLE BONES*)

The salient feature of this relatively common and very serious abnormality is the weakness and fragility of all bones of the body. It is transmitted by an autosomal dominant gene. The underlying defect is a failure of periosteal and endosteal intramembranous ossification and probably excessive osteoclasis as well. As a result of imbalance between bone deposition and bone resorption, the cortical bone and the trabeculae of cancellous bone are extremely thin—a congenital type of *osteoporosis*. The delicate bones are not only susceptible to gross pathological fractures with minor trauma, but also prone to bend, probably as a consequence of repeated microscopic fractures. Although these pathological fractures unite, the healed bone is still fragile.

The severity of the defect, which varies considerably, is indicated by the age at which the first fractures occur. In the most severe form (*fetal type*), multiple fractures have already occurred *in utero*, and more occur during the birth process. In this type the mortality during early infancy is high. In the moderately severe form (*infantile type*) the afflicted infant suffers many gross fractures during early childhood (usually several each year), develops severe limb deformities from bending of the bones, and is always stunted in growth. The child's head seems large in relation to his body but not in relation to his age. (Fig. 8.45). The radiographic appearance of the very slender, deformed and relatively radiolucent bones is characteristic (Fig. 8.46). In the least severe form (*juvenile type*) the first pathological fracture occurs in later childhood.

The bones in osteogenesis imperfecta seem to become stronger after puberty and hence fractures occur less frequently in afflicted adults (although it is possible that the adults have learned to be more cautious). In later years the complication of otosclerosis with resultant deafness may arise. In addition to weak and fragile bones, some affected individuals exhibit thin skin and marked joint laxity; some, but by no means all, have blue sclerae. (The underlying cho-

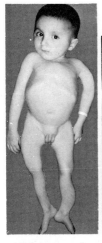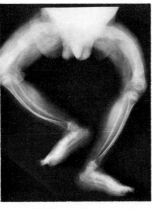

Figure 8.45 (*left*). Osteogenesis imperfecta (fragile bones) in a 4-year-old boy. Note the multiple deformities in the poorly developed limbs from a long series of pathological fractures, and the short trunk relative to the head size. This boy's sclerae are blue.

Figure 8.46 (*right*). Osteogenesis imperfecta (fragile bones) in the same boy as shown at left. Note the multiple healed fractures of both femora. Note also the slender, bent tibiae with very thin cortices, and the generalized osteoporosis.

roid plexus of vessels appears blue through the abnormally translucent sclera just as a bruise or subcutaneous hematoma appears blue through thin, translucent skin).

No effective *treatment* is as yet available for the underlying defect of osteogenesis imperfecta. The prevention of fractures is virtually impossible, but reasonable precautions should be taken by the child and by his parents; frequently, protective long leg braces and crutches are necessary. The pathological fractures are usually treated by ordinary means but prolonged immobilization must be avoided since it adds the problem of disuse atrophy (disuse osteoporosis) to the already weak bones. In the moderately severe infantile type, the operative procedure of multiple segmental osteotomies of long bones and intramedullary metal rod fixation, developed by Sofield, serves the dual purpose of correcting severe bony deformities and providing internal support to prevent further fractures and recurrence of deformity. This method of treatment has

certainly saved many severely afflicted children from a wheelchair existence.

Bailey has designed an extensible intramedullary rod, or nail, like a telescope that elongates as the child's bone grows in length and offers an advantage over the conventional type.

ACHONDROPLASIA (CHONDRODYSTROPHIA FETALIS)

The most striking feature of *achondroplasia*, and one that can be detected even in infancy, is dwarfism of the short limb type, the limbs being disproportionately shorter than the trunk (Fig. 8.47). It is transmitted by an autosomal dominant gene. The underlying defect is a failure of longitudinal growth in the cartilage of the epiphyseal plate (achondroplasia). Thus, all bones that form by endochrondral ossification, including the long bones and facial bones, are affected, while the membrane bones, as in the cranium, grow normally. This accounts for the very short limbs (about half normal length) and the typical facial appearance due to the disproportion between the size of the face and that of the head (Fig. 8.48). The total height seldom exceeds four feet. Radi-

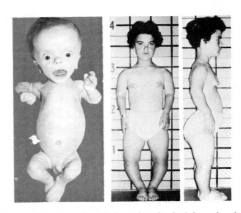

Figure 8.47 (*left*). Achondroplasia (chondrodystrophia fetalis) in a 3-month-old infant. Note the short limbs relative to the trunk and the small face relative to the large head.

Figure 8.48 (*right*). Achondroplasia (chondrodystrophia fetalis) in a 15-year-old girl. Note the dwarfism of the short limb type, the limbs being disproportionately shorter than the trunk. The limbs are bowed and there is an increase in the lumbar lordosis. The face is small relative to the head.

ographically, the bones are thick (because the periosteal intramembranous ossification is normal) but are frequently deformed as indicated by cubitus varus, genu varum, coxa vara and lumbar lordosis. Operative correction of bony deformities in the lower limbs is sometimes indicated to improve both function and appearance.

The achondroplastic dwarf has a normal mentality and a normal life expectancy. Therefore an important aspect of his total care concerns helping him to accept and to adjust to his obvious dwarfism and also helping to provide him with adequate education and vocational guidance in order that he may pursue a meaningful and satisfying occupation rather than merely exist as a circus midget. The dignity of the deformed should always be respected.

ARACHNODACTYLY (HYPERCHONDROPLASIA) (MARFAN'S SYNDROME)

The most characteristic feature of *arachnodactyly* (which means "spider fingers") is the excessive length of the limbs, and to a lesser extent of the trunk (Fig. 8.49). The etiology of this condition is unknown but it tends to have a familial incidence. The underlying abnormality is excessive longitudinal growth in the cartilage of the epiphyseal plate (*hyperchondroplasia*), and in this sense, it is the antithesis of achondroplasia. The child is always considerably taller and thinner than average, is generally weak and exhibits marked joint laxity. Associated skeletal deformities may include a resistant and progressive type of scoliosis, depressed sternum (pectus excavatum) and very long, extremely flexible flat feet. In addition there is a high incidence of associated heart disease and dislocation of the lens. The orthopaedic *treatment* of arachnodactyly involves operative correction of the associated skeletal deformities, if and when they begin to interfere with the child's function.

MULTIPLE HEREDITARY EXOSTOSES (DIAPHYSEAL ACLASIS)

The characteristic feature of this relatively common and deforming abnormality is the gradual development of multiple outgrowths

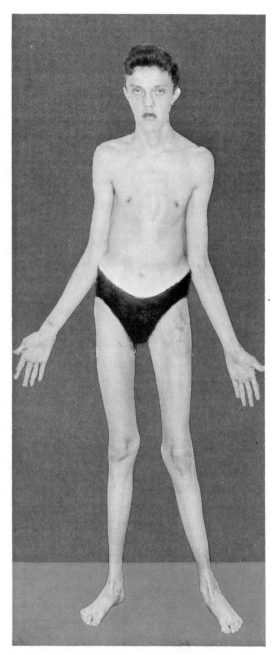

Figure 8.49. Arachnodactyly (hyperchondroplasia, Marfan's syndrome) in a 13-year-old boy. Note the excessively long and slender limbs relative to the length of the trunk. This boy also demonstrates poor chest development, genu valgum and hypermobile feet.

of bone and cartilage (*osteocartilaginous exostoses*) from the abnormally broad metaphyseal region of long bones (Fig. 8.50). The abnormality is transmitted by an autosomal

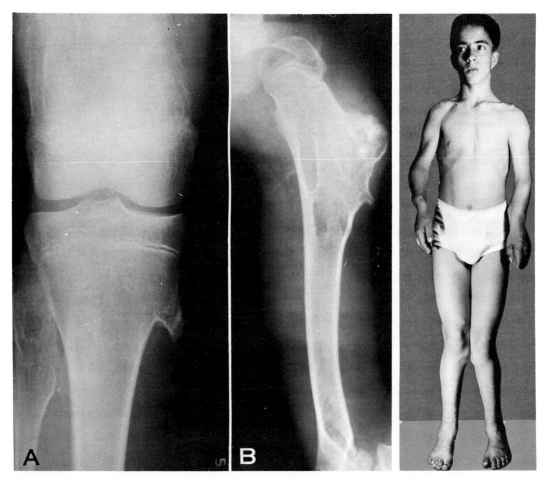

Figure 8.50 (*left*).   Multiple hereditary exostoses (diaphyseal aclasis). *A*, multiple osteocartilaginous exostoses arising from the abnormally broad metaphyseal regions of the long bones in the area of the knee. The exostoses always point away from the neighboring epiphysis. *B*, large osteocartilaginous exostosis arising from the upper end of the humerus.

Figure 8.51 (*right*).   Multiple hereditary exostoses (diaphyseal aclasis) in a 14-year-old boy. Some of the exostoses are sufficiently large that they produce obvious local deformities, particularly in the region of the wrists and knees. Each exostosis, being covered by a cap of cartilage, is always larger clinically than it appears radiographically.

dominant gene. The underlying defect is a lack of the normal osteoclastic activity (*aclasis*) in the process of remodeling of the metaphysis during longitudinal growth. As a result, the metaphysis, rather than becoming trumpet shaped, persists as a broad cylinder. Bony outgrowths, each capped by cartilage and a type of growth plate, develop during early childhood and always point away from the neighboring epiphysis. It is not unusual for a given patient to have 20 or more such osteocartilaginous exostoses.

A rare complication in adult life is the malignant change of one of the osteocartilaginous exostoses to a chondrosarcoma which is always associated with a rapid increase in its size. The longitudinal growth in the long bones is somewhat decreased but never strikingly so. However, bony deformities sometimes develop as a result of uneven epiphyseal plate growth.

The exostoses may become sufficiently large in superficial locations that their mere presence causes deformity (Fig. 8.51). They may cause symptoms, either from pressure on soft tissues, or by interference with the gliding of tendons, particularly in the region of the knee. Operative *treatment* is indicated only for those exostoses that are causing symptoms, producing deformity, or enlarging rapidly, and involves excision of the exostosis along with its periosteal covering and its cartilaginous cap.

Generalized Abnormalities of Nerve and Muscle

AMYOTONIA CONGENITA (INFANTILE SPINAL MUSCULAR ATROPHY)

This generalized congenital abnormality of muscle is characterized at birth by an extreme lack of muscle tone (*amyotonia*) which gives the infant the appearance and feel of a floppy rag doll (Fig. 8.52). Associated with the decreased muscle tone are decreased tendon reflexes and generalized muscle weakness. The child has difficulty in learning to hold his head up, to sit up and to stand up and therefore these milestones of musculoskeletal development are delayed. There is usually a marked degree of coexistent joint laxity and when the child does manage to stand up, he exhibits flexible flat

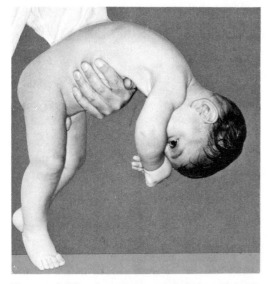

Figure 8.52. Amyotonia congenita (infantile spinal muscular atrophy) in a 1-year-old boy. The extreme lack of muscle tone prevented this child from sitting up or even holding his head up. The child looks and feels like a floppy rag doll.

feet and knock knees. The prognosis in the more severe forms of amyotonia congenita is poor. *Treatment* is limited to the support of weak and floppy limbs and trunk by appropriate braces.

AMYOPLASIA CONGENITA (ARTHROGRYPOSIS MULTIPLEX CONGENITA) (MYODYSTROPHIA FETALIS)

This crippling congenital abnormality of muscle development is characterized by marked stiffness and severe deformity in many joints of the limbs (hence the term *arthrogryposis*, which means "bent joints"). The abnormality, which is immediately apparent at birth, gives the infant the appearance and feel of a wooden doll (Fig. 8.53). It is not genetically determined. The underlying defect is aplasia and hypoplasia of many muscle groups during embryonic development (*amyoplasia*) and is sometimes secondary to a defect in the anterior horn cells of the spinal cord. Thus, there is a marked decrease in the amount of muscle in the spindly limbs. Microscopically, fatty and fibrous infiltration is seen between the scant muscle fibers. As a result the joints controlled by involved muscles have never moved normally *in utero* and consequently, they likewise fail to develop normally, not only before birth but also after. Excessive fibrous tissue infiltration is found in the periarticular soft tissues as well as in the subcutaneous fat and even the skin is tight and inelastic. The muscle abnormality is static rather than progressive, but the secondary changes in and around the joints tend to become more severe during the growing years.

The more common clinical deformities that result from amyoplasia congenita include severe and extremely resistant clubfeet, knee flexion or knee extension deformity (sometimes with resultant dislocation of the knee), a severe and irreducible prenatal (teratologic) type of congenital dislocation of the hip, flexion deformity of the fingers and wrists, extension deformities of the elbows and adduction deformity of the shoulders. The trunk is usually spared, but when it is

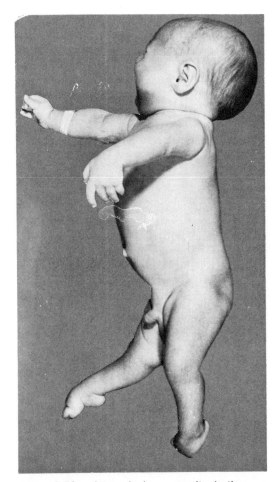

ents may improve the passive joint motion somewhat, but any gain is seldom maintained because of lack of muscle power. In this abnormality there is a vicious tendency to form excessive amounts of dense fibrous scar tissue about the joints following soft tissue operations such as capsulotomy and tendon lengthening and, as might be expected, the results of such procedures are disappointing. Bony operations such as osteotomy and arthrodesis are more effective and the results more permanent. Sound orthopaedic judgment is required in the planning of operative treatment for these severely handicapped children in order that following a given operation the child may be better—and not just different.

Perhaps one of *you* will accept the challenge of working—through clinical and experimental investigation—to solve the perplexing problems posed by these generalized congenital abnormalities of the musculoskeletal system.

Figure 8.53. Amyoplasia congenita (arthrogryposis multiplex congenita, myodystrophia fetalis) in a newborn infant. The limbs are deformed and rigid giving the child the appearance and the feel of a wooden doll. Note the associated clubfeet and the congenital hyperextension of the right knee.

involved, scoliosis may be present. Occasionally, the deformities are limited to the hands and feet. The child's mentality is within normal limits.

Treatment of the joint deformities associated with amyoplasia congenita represents one of the most difficult problems in the musculoskeletal system and demands all the patience, ingenuity and skill of the most experienced orthopaedic surgeon. Daily passive stretching of the stiff and deformed joints by a physiotherapist and by the par-

Suggested Additional Reading

Albright, J. A.: Systemic treatment of osteogenesis imperfecta. Clin. Orthop. 159: 88–95, 1981.

Bailey, R. W.: Further experience with the extensible nail (for osteogenesis imperfecta). Clin. Orthop. 159: 171–176, 1981.

Barlow, T. G.: Early diagnosis and treatment of congenital dislocation of the hip. J. Bone Joint Surg. 44B: 292, 1962.

Benzie, R. J.: Antenatal genetic diagnosis: current status and future prospects. Can. Med. Assoc. J. 120: 685–692, 1979.

Brown, L. M., Robson, M. J. and Sharrard, W. J. W.: The pathophysiology of arthrogryposis multiplex congenita neurologica. J. Bone Joint Surg. 62B: 291–296, 1980.

Carroll, H. C., McMurtry, R. and Leete, S. F.: The pathoanatomy of congenital club foot. Orthop. Clin. North Am. 9: 225–232, 1978.

Coleman, S. S.: *Congenital Dysplasia and Dislocation of the Hip.* St. Louis, C. V. Mosby, 1978.

Duthie, R. B. and Townes, P. L.: The genetics of orthopaedic conditions. J. Bone Joint Surg. 49B: 229–248, 1967.

Gibson, D. A. and Urs, N. D. K.: Arthrogryposis multiplex congenita. J. Bone Joint Surg. 52B: 483–493, 1970.

Golbus, N. S., Loughman, W. D., Epstein, C. J., Halbasch, G., Stephens, J. D. and Hall, B. D.: Prenatal genetic diagnosis in 3000 amniocenteses. N. Engl. J. Med. 300: 157–163, 1979.

Gray, C.: Prenatal diagnosis: the demand is increasing. Can. Med. Assoc. J. 126: 64–71, 1982.

Gray, D. H., and Katz, J. M.: A histochemical study of

muscle in club foot. J. Bone Joint Surg. 63B: 417–423, 1981.

Hagan, K. F. and Buncke, H. J.: Treatment of congenital pseudarthrosis of the tibia with free vascularized bone graft. Clin. Orthop. 166: 34–44, 1982.

Handelsman, J. E. and Badalamente, M. A.: Neuromuscular studies in club foot. J. Pediatr. Orthop. 1: 23–32, 1981.

Johnson, A. H., Aadelen, R. J., Eilers, V. E. and Winter, R. B.: Treatment of congenital hip dislocation with the Pavlik harness. Clin. Orthop. 155: 25–29, 1981.

Jones, D.: Assessment of value of examination of the hip in the newborn. J. Bone Joint Surg. 59B: 318–322, 1981.

Kalamchi, A., and MacFarlane, R. VI: The Pavlik harness: results in patients over three months of age. J. Pediatr. Orthop. 2: 3–8, 1982.

King, J. D. and Bobechko, W. P.: Osteogenesis imperfecta—an orthopaedic description and surgical review. J. Bone Joint Surg. 53B: 72–89, 1971.

Klenerman, L.: Problems of club feet (editorial). Br. Med. J. 284: 1427–1428, 1982.

Kort, J. S., Schink, M. M., Mitchell, S. N. and Bassett, C. A. L.: Congenital pseudarthrosis of the tibia: treatment with pulsing magnetic fields—the international experience. Clin. Orthop. 165: 124–137, 1982.

Kupka, J., Geddes, N. and Carroll, N. C.: Comprehensive management in the child with spina bifida. Orthop. Clin. North Am. 9: 97–113, 1978.

Lorber, J.: Some pediatric aspects of myelomingocele. Acta Orthop. Scand.: 46: 350–355, 1975.

Lorber, J. and Salfield, S. A. W.: Results of selective treatment of spina bifida cystica. Arch. Dis. Child. 56: 822–830, 1981.

Lovell, W. W. and Winter, R. B.: *Paediatric Orthopaedics*. Philadelphia, J. B. Lippincott, 1978.

McAndrew, I.: Adolescents and young people with spina bifida. Dev. Med. Child Neurol. 21: 619–629, 1979.

McKusick, V. A.: The growth and development of human genetics as a clinical discipline. Am. J. Hum. Genet. 27: 261–273, 1975.

McVay, V.: Parental reactions to birth-defective children. Postgrad. Med. 65: 183–189, 1979.

Paterson, D. C., Lewis, G. N. and Cass, C. A.: Treatment of congenital pseudarthrosis of the tibia with direct current stimulation. Clin. Orthop. 148: 129–135, 1980.

Ramsay, P. L., Lasser, S. and MacEwen, G. D.: Congenital dislocation of the hip. J. Bone Joint Surg. 58A: 1000, 1976.

Rang, M.: *The Easter Seal Guide to Children's Orthopaedics: Prevention, Screening and Problem Solving.* Toronto, The Easter Seal Society of Ontario, 1982.

Rodeck, C. H.: Value of fetoscopy in prenatal diagnosis. J. Roy. Soc. Med. 73: 29–33, 1980.

Salter, R. B.: Etiology, pathogenesis and possible prevention of congenital dislocation of the hip. Can. Med. Assoc. J. 98: 933–945, 1968.

Salter, R. B.: Osteotomy of the pelvis (editorial comment). Clinical Orthop. 9B: 2–4, 1974.

Salter, R. B.: Modern medicine, genetics and the future of mankind (Hugh Smith Oration on Moral and Ethical Issues). Ann. R. Coll. Phys. Surg. Can. 3: 209–217, 1978.

Salter, R. B. and Dubos, J. P.: The first 15 years' personal experience with innominate osteotomy in the treatment of congenital dislocation and subluxation of the hip. Clin. Orthop. 98: 72–103, 1974.

Salter, R. B., Kostuik, J., Dallas, S.: Avascular necrosis of the femoral head as a complication of treatment for congenital dislocation of the hip in young children: a clinical and experimental investigation. Can. J. Surg. 12: 44–60, 1969.

Sharrard, W. J. W.: *Pediatric Orthopaedics and Fractures.* Oxford and Edinburgh, Blackwell Scientific Publications, 1971.

Simpson, N. E., Dallaire, L., Miller, J. R., Siminovitch, L., Miller, J. and Hammerton, J. L.: Antenatal diagnosis of neural tube defects in Canada: Extension of a collaborative study. Can. Med. Assoc. J. 120: 653–657, 1979.

Sofield, H. A. and Millar, E. A.: Fragmentation, realignment and intramedullary rod fixation of deformities of long bones in children. J. Bone Joint Surg. 41A: 1371–1392, 1959.

Tachdjian, M. O.: *Pediatric Orthopaedics*. Philadelphia, W. B. Saunders, 1972.

Tredwell, S. J. and Bell, H. M.: Efficacy of neonatal hip examination. J. Pediatr. Orthop. 1: 61–65, 1981.

Turco, V. J.: *Club Foot*. Edinburgh, Churchill-Livingstone, 1981.

CHAPTER 9

Generalized and Disseminated Disorders of Bone

Generalized Bone Disorders Due to Metabolic Disturbance (Metabolic Bone Disease)
   Rickets
   Osteomalacia
   Scurvy
   Osteoporosis
   Hyperparathyroidism
   Hyperpituitarism
   Hypopituitarism
   Hypothyroidism in Childhood (Cretinism)
Disseminated Bone Disorders of Unknown Etiology
   Polyostotic Fibrous Dysplasia
   Osteitis Deformans (Paget's Disease)
   Skeletal Reticuloses

You will recall from the discussions in Chapter 2, that whereas each *individual bone* of the skeleton may be considered as a *structure*, *bone* of the entire skeleton may be considered as an *organ*. Bone, as an organ, is the major storehouse for calcium and phosphorus and is normally the site of very active *turnover* at a cellular level in relation to its physiology. You may find it helpful at this stage to review the brief description of *biochemistry and physiology of bone* in Chapter 2, as well as the *reactions of bone to disorders and injuries* in Chapter 3.

Bone reacts to a wide variety of diseases, many of which have their origin outside the skeletal system. These reactions of bone serve as a *mirror of disease* in that they *reflect* the nature of the underlying abnormality. These bony reflections, or *manifestations*, of disease are of practical importance since they can be detected by clinical and radiographic methods; furthermore, they are often serious in themselves since they may cause pain, deformity and disability in patients. Therefore, the reactions of bone

as an organ and as a structure are equally important to you in the diagnosis and treatment of patients. Without an understanding of bone, both as an organ and as a structure, you run the risk, as a surgeon, of becoming a mere carpenter of cortical bone and as a physician, of becoming a mere purveyor of pills. Indeed, as you will see, the problems presented by many bone diseases require the combined efforts of physician and surgeon.

It will be apparent to you that any abnormal metabolic disturbance affecting bone as an organ will be reflected by a *generalized* reaction in *all* bones of the skeleton and that the result will be a *generalized disease of bone*. Other, and less clearly understood, disturbances are reflected by a *localized* reaction in parts of a number of bones. Since the unaffected bones, as well as the uninvolved parts of the affected bones, are completely normal, the widely scattered lesions constitute a *disseminated disease of bone*.

GENERALIZED BONE DISORDERS DUE TO METABOLIC DISTURBANCES (METABOLIC BONE DISEASE)

The generalized reactions of bone include alterations (an increase or decrease) in either bone deposition or bone resorption, or both. Bone deposition, however, involves the two major processes of osteoblastic formation of organic matrix (osteoid) and calcification of the matrix to form bone. Bone resorption involves osteoclastic removal of formed bone and the release of bone minerals. In some metabolic disturbances, such as *rickets* and *osteomalacia*, the generalized reaction of bone is inadequate calcification of matrix (hypocalcification). In others, such as *scurvy* and *osteoporosis*, the generalized reaction is either a decreased osteoblastic formation of matrix or an increased osteoclastic bone resorption (or both) with a resultant decrease in the total amount of bone. In addition, combinations of these reactions may coexist as seen in the osteoporosis that coexists with hypocalcification in certain types of refractory rickets. It is important to appreciate that one-third of the total amount of bone mineral may be lost before the resultant decrease in radiographic density of the bones is readily detectable by ordinary radiographic techniques.

In some of these generalized disorders the causative factor is either nutritional or hormonal and the disorder is said to be metabolic, whereas in other disorders, a combination of factors, including physical stresses and strains, are responsible. Nevertheless, in all of these disorders there is a disturbance of the *metabolism of bone* and accordingly, they are best considered together in the broad category of *"metabolic bone disease."*

Rickets

Rickets may be defined as a generalized disease of *growing* bone characterized by a failure of calcium salts to be deposited promptly in organic bone matrix (osteoid) as well as in the pre-osseous cartilage of the epiphyseal plate at the zone of calcifying cartilage. The normal deposition of calcium in osteoid and pre-osseous cartilage is largely dependent upon the maintenance of physiological levels of calcium and phosphorus in the serum which, in turn, is dependent upon a balance between the three factors of *absorption* of each element from the intestine, their *excretion* by the kidneys and intestine, and their *rates of movement* into and out of bone. Important factors in maintaining this balance are vitamin D, parathyroid hormone and calcitonin. Thus, several types of disturbance are capable of causing the one generalized bone reaction of rickets. The various clinical forms of rickets are best classified on the basis of their cause; the three main causes of rickets are vitamin D deficiency, chronic renal insufficiency and renal tubular insufficiency. The latter two forms of rickets do not respond to *normal* amounts of vitamin D and are therefore *"vitamin D-refractory"*.

PATHOLOGY

The pathological changes in rickets include a *generalized decrease in calcified matrix (bone)* and an *increase in uncalcified matrix (osteoid)*, with a resultant generalized decrease in radiographic density (*rarefaction*) in all bones. In addition, a wide zone of *uncalcified pre-osseous cartilage* forms at the usual site of calcifying cartilage in the epiphyseal plate (Fig. 9.1). Since calcium provides the "hardness" of bone, the uncalcified areas are "soft" and consequently, progressive deformities occur not only in the substance of bones but also through their epiphyseal plates (Fig. 9.2).

DIAGNOSIS

In infants the possibility of rickets must be considered in the presence of convulsions, tetany, irritability, delayed physical develop-

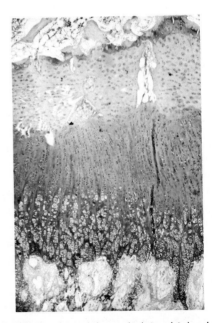

Figure 9.1. An epiphyseal plate obtained postmortem from a 1-year-old child with rickets. (He had died of an unrelated condition.) Note the wide zone of uncalcified pre-osseous cartilage and the disorganized columns of hypertrophic cartilage cells in the epiphyseal plate, as well as the uncalcified bone matrix (osteoid) in the metaphyseal region.

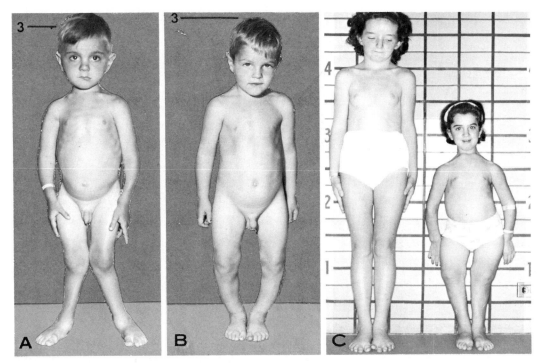

Figure 9.2. Clinical deformities due to rickets. *A*, genu valgum in a 5-year-old boy with vitamin D-refractory rickets. Note also the enlargement of the sites of epiphyseal plates, particularly at the ankles, knees, wrists and costochondral junctions. *B*, genu varum with internal tibial torsion and external femoral torsion in 4-year-old boy with vitamin D-refractory rickets. *C*, small stature, genu varum of the right lower limb and genu valgum of the left in an 11-year-old girl with vitamin D-refractory rickets. The 11-year-old girl on the left is normal.

ment, weakness and failure to thrive. In children who have started to walk, the possibility of rickets must also be considered in the presence of deformities of the lower limbs (particularly severe genu valgum, genu varum, and torsional deformities) and a small stature (Fig. 9.2).

The diagnosis of rickets, whatever the cause, is *suggested* by clinical enlargement at the sites of epiphyseal plates, particularly at the distal end of each radius and at the costochondral junctions, the latter being known as a "rachitic rosary" (Fig. 9.3). However, the diagnosis is *established* by the typical radiographic changes in the growing ends of long bones which demonstrate a widened radiolucent zone in the epiphyseal plate (due to uncalcified preosseous cartilage) and also by the generalized rarefaction of all bones (Fig. 9.4). The serum alkaline phosphatase is elevated in all types of rickets. However, the differentiation between the various etiological types of rickets necessitates the use of a number of standard diagnostic methods. For example, an elevated blood urea and serum inorganic phosphorus indicate a renal *glomerular* lesion, whereas a normal blood urea and lowered serum inorganic phosphorus (hypophosphatemia), in the absence of vitamin D deficiency, indicate a renal *tubular* defect.

Clinical Aspects of the Three Main Forms of Rickets

Vitamin D Deficiency Rickets (Simple Rickets). Although the incidence of this nutritional type of rickets has diminished greatly since the recognition of the importance of sunlight and vitamin D, it is still seen in clinical practice. The child is usually

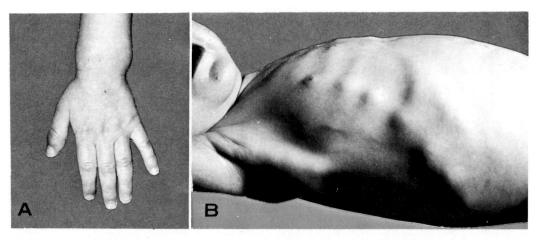

Figure 9.3. Clinical enlargement at the sites of epiphyseal plates. *A*, enlargement at the sites of the distal radial and distal ulnar epiphyseal plates in a 1-year-old boy with vitamin D-refractory rickets. *B*, enlargement at the sites of the epiphyseal plates at the costochondral junctions in the same child. Because of the beaded appearance, this is known as a "rachitic rosary."

around the age of one year, is rather sickly and is retarded in growth. The aforementioned clinical and radiographic signs are readily detected. This type of rickets responds well to *treatment*, which includes normal doses of vitamin D and improvement in diet. In the early stages of vitamin D deficiency, the child may develop severe hypocalcemia with resultant tetany, or even convulsions, but with minimal radiographic changes. Vitamin D deficiency can also be caused by its defective absorption from the intestinal tract due to steatorrhea caused by chronic intestinal or hepatic disorders.

Renal Osteodystrophy (Azotemic Osteodystrophy). This relatively uncommon type of rickets (formerly called "renal rickets") is complex in that chronic renal disease produces not only the bony lesion of rickets already described, but in addition it produces a secondary hyperparathyroidism which results in the superimposition of hyperparathyroid bone lesions (irregular disintegration of metaphyses, erosion of cortical bone and generalized osteoporosis) (Fig. 9.5). This type of rickets is understandably refractory to ordinary doses of vitamin D. *Treatment* is directed toward the renal insufficiency, the rickets and the secondary hyperparathyroidism. Previously the associated rickets was treated by large doses of vitamin D but in recent years, an active metabolite of vitamin D, namely 1,25-dihydroxy vitamin D_3 is preferred.

Rickets Due to Renal Tubular Defect. The

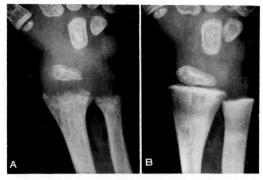

Figure 9.4. *A*, the wrist of a 3-year-old child with rickets. Note the widened radiolucent zone in the epiphyseal plate (due to uncalcified preosseous cartilage and osteoid), the generalized rarefaction of the bones and the coarse trabecular pattern of cancellous bone. This radiograph can be correlated with the histological changes in Figure 9.1. *B*, the same patient following treatment with vitamin D. Note the normal ossification in the metaphyseal regions and the normal generalized density of the bones.

mechanism by which the various renal tubular dysfunctions cause the bony reaction of rickets is defective tubular reabsorption of phosphate and consequent excess loss of phosphate in the urine with resultant hypophosphatemia. The commonest type of such rickets is designated "*hypophosphatemic vitamin D-refractory (resistant) rickets*" (also known as familial hypophosphatemic rickets or X-linked hypophosphatemia). This form of rickets is usually inherited as an X-linked dominant trait but occasionally autosomal dominant inheritance is observed. The child exhibits the clinical and radiographic signs already described but is otherwise healthy and has a normal life expectancy.

The medical treatment of the various types of vitamin D-refractory rickets includes the oral administration of phosphates and either massive doses of vitamin D or smaller doses of its active metabolite, 1,25-dihydroxy vitamin D_3. Careful monitoring of the patient's progress is required to achieve an optimal therapeutic response as well as to avoid the harmful effects of vitamin D intoxication.

Other less common types of rickets due to renal tubular insufficiency include the following: hypophosphatemic vitamin D-refractory rickets with aminoaciduria, (vitamin D dependency rickets, Type I and Type II), Fanconi Syndrome, cystinosis and oculocerebral-renal syndrome of Lowe. In addition, renal tubular acidosis may result in rickets.

The Orthopaedic Management of Deformities in Rickets

The recognition of rickets as the underlying cause of the deformity is essential since correction of such a deformity, without controlling the rickets, invariably leads to its recurrence. Furthermore, once the rickets has been controlled, bony deformities tend to regress somewhat. This improvement can often be enhanced by the use of appropriate night splints of the type described for torsional deformities genu varum and genu valgum in Chapter 7. If, despite adequate medical therapy and non-operative orthopaedic measures, severe rachitic deformities persist, operative correction by osteotomy is indicated. Under these circumstances, vitamin D therapy should be discontinued one month prior to operation in order to avoid the risk of severe hypercalcemia which would otherwise occur during the postoperative period of immobilization.

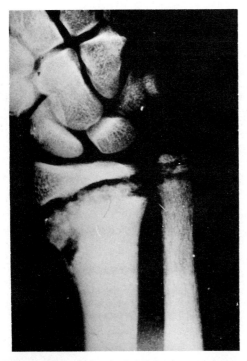

Figure 9.5. Osteodystrophy due to chronic renal insufficiency in a 14-year-old boy. Note the widened radiolucent zone in the epiphyseal plates (due to rickets) and in addition, the irregular disintegration of metaphyses, and the erosion of cortical bone (due to secondary hyperparathyroidism).

Osteomalacia

Osteomalacia, which means "soft bones," is a generalized disease of *adult* bone characterized by a failure of calcium salts to be deposited promptly in organic bone matrix (osteoid). It is, in effect, "adult rickets," but the absence of epiphyseal plates in adults, of course, precludes the epiphyseal plate changes seen in rickets. The causes and types of osteomalacia are comparable to those already described for rickets.

PATHOLOGY

The pathological changes in osteomalacia, like those in rickets, include a generalized *decrease in calcified matrix (bone)* and an *increase in uncalcified matrix (osteoid)* with resultant radiographic rarefaction in all bones. The bone changes may become very severe with the result that the markedly weak and "soft" bones gradually bend and become progressively deformed. Microscopically, wide *osteoid seams* are seen adjacent to the relatively sparse areas of calcified bone (Fig. 9.6). In addition, *pseudofractures*, known as Looser's zones, may develop in the moderately severe form of osteomalacia known as *Milkman's syndrome* (an eponym rather than an occupational hazard in milkmen).

DIAGNOSIS

The *possibility* of osteomalacia should be considered in the presence of anorexia, weight loss, muscle weakness, widespread bone pain as well as bone tenderness and progressive bony deformity of the spine and limbs (Fig. 9.7). The diagnosis is *established* by the typical radiographic changes of gross skeletal deformity (compression of vertebral bodies, distortion of the pelvis and bending of the long bones) and a generalized rarefaction of all bones. In Milkman's syndrome, pseudofractures may be seen in the ribs, pelvis, upper ends of the femora and elsewhere (Fig. 9.8). The serum alkaline phosphatase is usually elevated and the serum phosphate is lowered.

TREATMENT

As with rickets the underlying cause of the osteomalacia must be corrected insofar

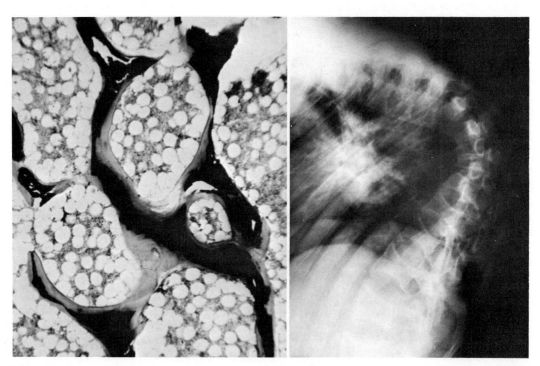

Figure 9.6 (*left*).   Osteomalacia. Undecalcified cancellous bone reveals a decrease in the amount of calcified matrix, or bone, (dark areas) and an increase in the amount of uncalcified matrix, or osteoid (light areas), the latter forming wide "osteoid seams" on sparse areas of bone.
Figure 9.7 (*right*).   Osteomalacia. Shown is a progressive kyphosis of the thoracic spine due to compression of vertebral bodies in a 23-year-old woman with osteomalacia. Note also the generalized rarefaction of all the bones.

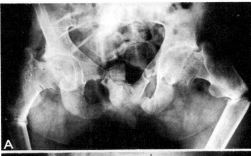

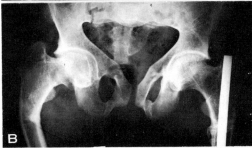

Figure 9.8. Milkman's syndrome in a 25-year-old woman. *A*, a deformity of the pelvis and femora with multiple pseudofractures, as well as a displaced pathological fracture in the subtrochanteric region of the left femur. *B*, the same patient after treatment with vitamin D and a high-calcium diet. The pathological fracture has been treated by means of a large intramedullary nail. Note the healing of the fracture and of the pseudofractures as well as the improvement in the generalized density of all the bones.

as is possible. The administration of vitamin D and a high calcium diet usually improve the calcification of the organic matrix and thereby result in healing of the pseudofractures, as well as in a general strengthening of the bones. Following adequate medical treatment of the osteomalacia, residual bony deformities may require correction by appropriate osteotomies.

Scurvy (Avitaminosis C)

Scurvy is a generalized disease characterized by a failure of osteoblastic formation of bone matrix with a resultant decrease in the total amount of bone (osteoporosis) and accompanied by subperiosteal and submucous hemorrhages. This disease, which is caused by a lack of vitamin C (ascorbic acid), occurs in children between the ages of six months and a year. Severe scurvy is now

relatively uncommon; nevertheless mild scurvy can occur, not only in children, but also in the elderly who tend to eat too little food containing vitamin C.

PATHOLOGY

The decreased osteoblastic formation of bone matrix in the presence of normal osteoclastic resorption of bone accounts for the generalized osteoporosis. Since bone matrix is not being formed on the calcified cores of cartilage in the epiphyseal plate, the zone of calcifying cartilage persists and becomes thicker. Avitaminosis C, however, also increases capillary fragility and consequently, spontaneous hemorrhages occur, not only under the loosely attached periosteum, but also under the mucous membrane of the gums and intestine. When the subperiosteal hemorrhage is massive, the normal attachment of the epiphysis and its epiphyseal plate to the metaphysis is disrupted and an epiphyseal separation ensues.

CLINICAL FEATURES

The scorbutic child experiences the fairly rapid onset of irritability, swelling of the limbs (particularly the thighs), and pain that may be so severe that he refuses to move the limbs (pseudoparalysis). Examination reveals marked swelling, warmth and exquisite tenderness over the affected bones as well as evidence of hemorrhage elsewhere, especially in the gums.

RADIOGRAPHIC FEATURES

The typical radiographic signs of severe scurvy include a generalized rarefaction of all bones (osteoporosis), a dense white line on the metaphyseal side of the epiphyseal plates and a similar line ringing the epiphyses (both of which represent thick zones of calcifying cartilage), and evidence of epiphyseal separations (Fig. 9.9). A soft tissue shadow surrounding the long bones represents the subperiosteal hematomata, which become ossified with remarkable rapidity following treatment (Fig. 9.10).

DIFFERENTIAL DIAGNOSIS

While severe scurvy is not readily confused with other conditions, less severe degrees of the condition must be differentiated from paralysis, osteomyelitis, congenital syphilis, and "child abuse" with multiple epiphyseal separations. In untreated scurvy the blood ascorbic acid is always markedly decreased.

TREATMENT

The administration of vitamin C (ascorbic acid) leads to rapid and complete correction of all aspects of the disease. Ossification of the subperiosteal hematomata secures the epiphyseal separations and the prognosis for subsequent epiphyseal plate growth is excellent.

Osteoporosis (Osteopenia)

Osteoporosis, which means "porous bones" is a generalized disease of bone characterized by decreased osteoblastic formation of matrix combined with increased osteoclastic resorption of bone and a resultant marked decrease in the total amount of bone in the skeleton (*osteopenia*, which

means "too little bone"). While decreased bone deposition has long been considered to be the major factor in the imbalance that leads to osteoporosis, recent data suggest that increased bone resorption may be the more important—if not the only—factor. Although the bones are thin and porous and there is too little bone, the bone that is present is well calcified and its microscopic appearance is normal (in contradistinction to osteomalacia).

ETIOLOGICAL FACTORS

Since generalized osteoporosis represents a disturbance not only in bone deposition but also in bone resorption, there are several types of osteoporosis based on the most prominent factor in their etiology, even though the resultant skeletal lesion is the same. Osteogenesis imperfecta, a congenital type of osteoporosis, has been described in Chapter 8. The many etiological factors in the production of osteoporosis include hormonal disturbances, disuse and senility,

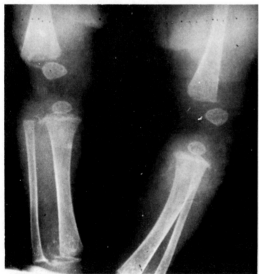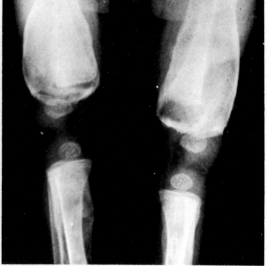

Figure 9.9 (*left*).   Scurvy in a 1-year-old girl. The lower limbs reveal generalized rarefaction of all bones (indicating osteoporosis), a dense white line on the metaphyseal side of the epiphyseal plates and a similar line ringing the epiphyses (both of which represent thick zones of calcified cartilage), as well as separation of both lower femoral epiphyses and both lower tibial epiphyses.

Figure 9.10. (*right*).   Treated scurvy in the same 1-year-old girl (Fig. 9.9) after 10 days of therapy with vitamin C (ascorbic acid). Note the ossification of the massive subperiosteal hematomata and the increased generalized density of the bones. The epiphyseal separations are now securely healed and the prognosis for subsequent epiphyseal plate growth is excellent.

though in any given patient, two or more factors may be combined.

HORMONAL OSTEOPOROSIS

In some patients with osteoporosis, the underlying cause is hormonal imbalance in that there is an increased secretion of anti-anabolic hormones relative to the secretion of anabolic hormones. Thus, osteoporosis is a feature of hyperparathyroidism, hyperpituitarism, hyperthyroidism and hyperadrenocorticism (either from adrenal cortical hyperactivity or from prolonged cortisone therapy). Disorders due to various types of hormonal disturbances are discussed in a subsequent section.

DISUSE OSTEOPOROSIS

All tissues of the body atrophy when they are not used and bone is no exception. The intermittent pressures of weight bearing and the tensions of muscle pull transmitted to the skeleton exert stresses and strains which seem to stimulate bone deposition by osteoblastic activity. In a person who, for any reason, is either confined to bed or grossly restricted in his activities, bone deposition is soon overbalanced by bone resorption and the result is disuse atrophy of bone (disuse osteoporosis). This type of osteoporosis, of course, is most marked in those parts of the skeleton that are being used the least, namely, the lower limbs and spine. Indeed, in a single limb, prolonged immobilization, relief of weight bearing and paralysis can all produce a *localized* disuse osteoporosis limited to the bones that are not being used.

POSTMENOPAUSAL AND SENILE OSTEOPOROSIS

These two types of generalized osteoporosis are considered together because they have so much in common. The distinction is somewhat arbitrary in that when women develop osteoporosis between the menopause and the age of 65 years, the osteoporosis is termed *postmenopausal*, whereas when either men or women develop the condition after the age of 65 years, it is termed *senile*. Postmenopausal and senile osteoporosis represent by far the commonest generalized bone disease that you will see in patients. It has been estimated to be radiographically detectable in 50% of all persons over 65 years and when you realize that the total amount of bone must be decreased by one third before the decrease can be readily detected radiographically, you will appreciate that less severe degrees of postmenopausal and senile osteoporosis are very common indeed. Hypogonadism in the elderly, as well as an inadequate dietary intake of calcium would seem to be factors in the etiology of this type of osteoporosis and furthermore, the condition may well be aggravated by a superimposed "disuse osteoporosis" associated with the usual decline in physical activity of the elderly.

PATHOLOGY

In all types of osteoporosis, the earliest and most striking change is in *cancellous* bone where the normally calcified trabeculae become thin and sparse. (Fig. 9.11). Thus, the osteoporosis is most marked in the vertebral bodies and the metaphyses of long bones, both of which normally consist largely of cancellous bone. The cortical bone eventually becomes thin and porous. As a result, the individual bones, rather than becoming "soft" as in osteomalacia, become fragile, or brittle, and are very susceptible to pathological fractures of either the gross or microscopic type as a result of even the most trivial trauma. Gross pathological fractures are very common, particularly in the predominantly cancellous metaphyses of long bones (neck of femur, neck of humerus, distal end of radius) and in the predominantly cancellous vertebral bodies. In addition, repeated microscopic fractures in the spine produce a gradual wedge-shaped deformity of the vertebral bodies with a resultant slowly progressive dorsal kyphosis and loss of total height. The pressure of the resilient intervertebral discs gradually deforms the less resilient bone of the subjacent surface of each vertebral body and as a result, the vertebral bodies become biconcave as the intervertebral discs become biconvex or balloon-shaped.

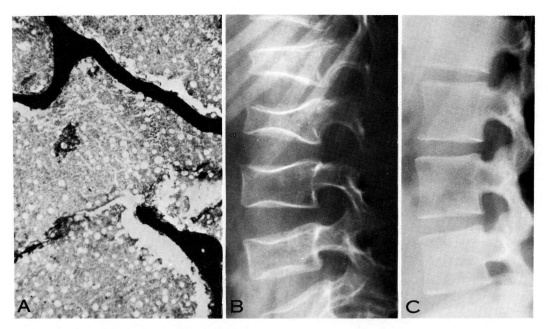

Figure 9.11. Osteoporosis. *A*, undecalcified cancellous bone from a 70-year-old woman with senile osteoporosis. Note the sparse and thin trabeculae of bone which are normally calcified. *B*, lateral radiograph of the lumbar spine of an adult with osteoporosis. Note the compressed, biconcave vertebral bodies with "ballooning" of the intervertebral discs, as well as the generalized rarefaction of all the bones. *C*, normal lumbar spine of an adult for comparison.

CLINICAL AND RADIOGRAPHIC FEATURES

The symptoms of generalized osteoporosis include chronic and intermittent back pain (which is probably related to repeated microscopic fractures) as well as bone pain at other sites. The patient usually exhibits an abnormal degree of dorsal kyphosis (Fig. 9.12). Gross pathological fractures in the aforementioned sites are a very common clinical complication. The radiographic features include a generalized rarefaction of all bones (but most marked in cancellous bone), thin cortices and evidence of deformity, particularly in the vertebral bodies (Fig. 9.13). The serum calcium, phosphorus and alkaline phosphatase are all normal but metabolic studies may reveal a negative calcium balance.

TREATMENT

Because of the magnitude of the morbidity related to postmenopausal and senile osteoporosis (especially gross and microscopic pathological fractures) it is not surprising that metabolic bone physicians have striven for many years to prevent, arrest, or even reverse such osteoporosis by medical treatment, i.e. therapeutic agents. The many agents investigated to date (either alone or in various combinations) include estrogens (for women only) anabolic hormones, calcitonin, diphosponates, vitamin D (or its active metabolites), calcium and sodium fluoride. Each of these agents in high doses may produce undesirable side effects in some patients and hence must be administered with caution and only with regular supervision. It has been shown that sodium fluoride in "toxic" doses stimulates formation of bone, the matrix of which, however, may be slow to become mineralized; calcium supplements would seem to correct this deficit (although time may be a factor). In many patients with osteoporosis, some degree of true osteomalacia coexists and this component of the problem is correctable by adequate doses of vitamin D. Although much scientific investigation remains to be done in both animals and in humans before widespread medical treatment of all osteoporotic patients is justifiable, the currently reco-

mended combination of sodium fluoride and calcium seems to be very promising even though, for reasons that are not yet understood, not all patients respond to fluoride. A

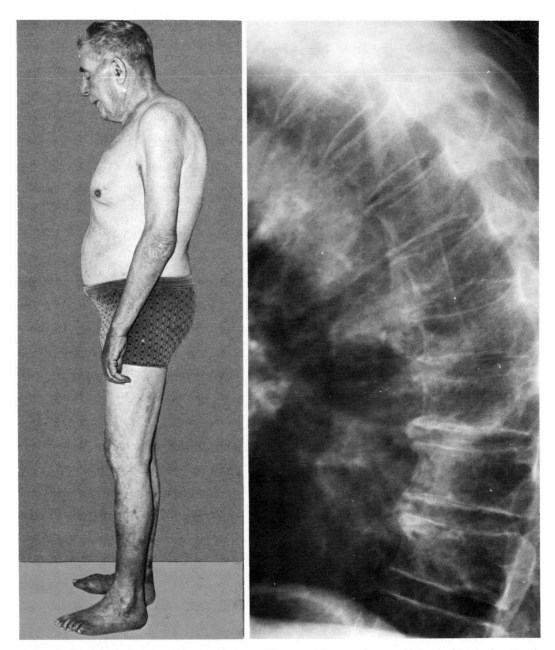

Figure 9.12. (*left*).   Senile osteoporosis in an 82-year-old man who complained of intermittent pain in his back. Note the increased dorsal (thoracic) kyphosis.
Figure 9.13 (*right***).**   The thoracic spine of the patient shown at left. Note the compression of the vertebral bodies with resultant kyphosis. The osteophyte formation at the edges of the vertebral bodies indicates secondary degenerative joint disease of the spine. Note also the generalized rarefaction of all the bones.

program of regular and vigorous physical exercises has been shown to help overcome at least the disease atrophy component of the osteoporosis that is secondary to the sedentary life of postmenopausal women as well as of the elderly, both men and women. The back pain caused by microfractures in osteoporotic vertebrae can be diminished by the use of a light, close fitting spinal brace.

Hyperparathyroidism (Parathyroid Osteodystrophy) (Osteitis Fibrosa Cystica)

Parathyroid osteodystrophy is a rare generalized bone disease resulting from hyperparathyroidism and characterized by a combination of generalized and localized excessive osteoclastic resorption of bone with marrow fibrosis. The resultant bone disease, therefore, consists not only of a generalized form of osteoporosis but also of disseminated osteolytic lesions.

ETIOLOGY AND PATHOLOGY

Primary hyperparathyroidism is the result of a parathyroid adenoma in one or more glands; occasionally, the involved gland is abnormally situated (aberrant). Rarely, the hyperparathyroidism is due to primary hyperplasia of all four glands. The associated excessive bone resorption liberates both calcium and phosphorus into the blood stream but the phosphorus is more readily excreted in the urine; the calcium-phosphorus product remains constant and therefore, there is hypercalcemia and hypophosphatemia. *Secondary hyperparathyroidism*, however, is secondary to the hypocalcemia associated with chronic renal insufficiency, in which case neither calcium nor phosphorus is readily excreted by the kidneys. The generalized bone lesion, which is a form of osteoporosis, is exemplified by thin trabeculae and cortices.

The disseminated osteolytic lesions vary greatly in that they may be *solid* and filled with vascular fibrous tissue, hemosiderin and giant cells ("brown tumors"), or they may be truly *cystic* and filled with old blood. In either case, the bone is greatly weakened by the disseminated lesions through which

pathological fractures may occur. The hypercalcemia associated with hyperparathyroidism leads to the complication of renal calculi of the calcium type.

DIAGNOSIS

The patient with hyperparathyroidism experiences two types of clinical manifestations: those due to the hypercalcemia (anorexia, lethargy, weakness and symptoms of renal calculi) and those due to the associated bone disease (bone pain, progressive bony deformity, pathological fractures and loosening of the teeth). The radiographic changes include generalized rarefaction of all bones and disseminated osteolytic lesions of multiple bones (Fig. 9.14). The earliest radiographic change is resorption of the lamina dura of the tooth sockets and of the cortical bone in the phalanges. The serum calcium is always elevated and usually the urinary calcium is also elevated. The serum phosphorus is lowered, but the urinary phosphorus is elevated (except in secondary hyperparathyroidism in which the reverse is true). The serum alkaline phosphatase is elevated. An important advance in the diagnosis of hyperparathyroidism has been the determination of the serum level of parathyroid hormone by means of radioimmunoassay.

TREATMENT

In primary hyperparathyroidism the causative parathyroid adenoma must be sought and surgically excised, after which a considerable improvement may be expected in the bone disease. Residual deformity may require operative correction by osteotomy. In secondary hyperparathyroidism, treatment is directed toward the underlying chronic renal insufficiency; the associated bone disease may be improved by high doses of vitamin D and, in carefully selected cases, by parathyroidectomy.

Hyperpituitarism

Excessive hormone secretion by the anterior lobe of the pituitary gland exerts a variety of profound generalized effects on bone depending upon the state of skeletal growth at the time, as well as upon the type

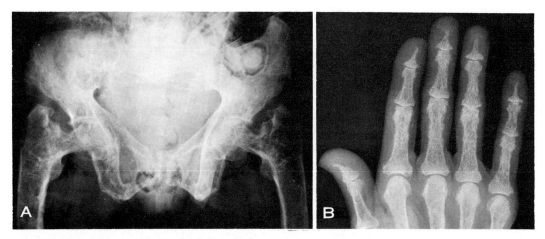

Figure 9.14. Hyperparathyroidism due to a parathyroid adenoma in a 60-year-old woman. *A*, revealed are generalized rarefaction of the bones, coarse trabeculae of cancellous bone (due to loss of minor trabeculae and preservation of major trabeculae), cystic lesions of the pelvis and femora, deformity of the pelvis, bilateral coxa vara and subperiosteal absorption of bone in the femoral necks. *B*, note the generalized rarefaction of all the bones; also coarse trabeculae of cancellous bone and subperiosteal absorption of cortical bone in the phalanges.

of abnormal cell in the gland. Thus, an eosinophil (chromophil) adenoma during the growth period produces *gigantism*, whereas the same neoplasm after growth, produces *acromegaly*. By contrast, a basophil adenoma at any age produces *Cushing's syndrome* (which can also be caused by hyperadrenocorticism).

GIGANTISM

During *childhood*, excessive hormone secretion from an eosinophil adenoma stimulates epiphyseal plate growth to a remarkable degree with the result that the affected child reaches an unusual height, sometimes over seven feet (Fig. 9.15). The condition is usually associated with subnormal sexual development and is occasionally complicated by slipping of the upper femoral epiphysis (adolescent coxa vara). If the hyperpituitarism persists, the adult counterpart, acromegaly, is superimposed upon the gigantism in adult life.

ACROMEGALY

During *adulthood*, excessive hormone secretion from an eosinophil adenoma cannot affect longitudinal growth but it does stimu-

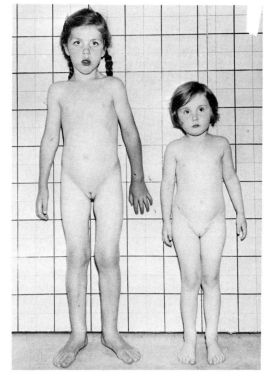

Figure 9.15. Gigantism due to hyperpituitarism in a 5-year-old girl. Note the long limbs and somewhat coarse features compared to those of the normal 5-year-old girl on the right.

late circumferential growth from periosteal intramembranous ossification so that the bones become progressively thicker. The clinical disorder is easily recognized by the coarse facial features (due to enlargement of the jaw, nose and supraorbital ridges) and the thick extremities (Fig. 9.16). The patient may be unusually strong in the early stages, but general weakness frequently supervenes.

CUSHING'S SYNDROME

The generalized bone disease that is associated with Cushing's syndrome is a severe and progressive *osteoporosis* with all the previously described features of that disorder. The neurosurgical removal of pituitary adenomas has been made possible by the development of the operating microscope and the use of the transphenoidal approach to the pituitary gland. In addition, the patient exhibits obesity, particularly of the face ("moon face"), increased body hair and hypertension (Fig. 9.17). This syndrome is the result of *hyperadrenocorticism*, which

in turn may be *primary* due to either hyperplasia or neoplasm of the adrenal cortex, or *secondary*, due either to a basophil adenoma of the anterior lobe of the pituitary gland, or to prolonged cortisone therapy. Indeed, cortisone therapy is presently the commonest cause of Cushing's syndrome and is a disturbing example of "iatrogenic disease." In Cushing's syndrome the urinary

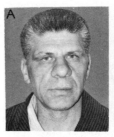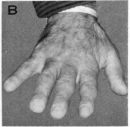

Figure 9.16. Acromegaly due to hyperpituitarism in a 40-year-old man. *A*, the facial features are coarse due to enlargement of the jaw, nose and supraorbital ridges as a result of excessive periosteal intramembranous ossification. *B*, the fingers are coarse and unduly thick.

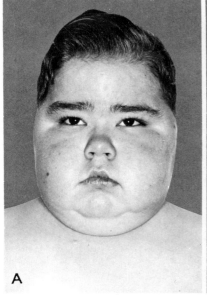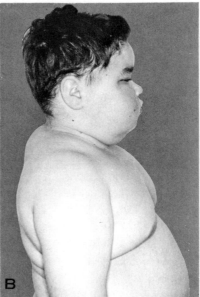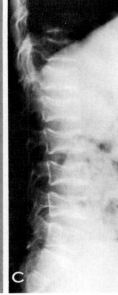

Figure 9.17. Cushing's syndrome, due to hyperadrenocorticism from prolonged cortisone therapy in a 10-year-old boy. *A* and *B*, note the obesity, particularly of the face ("moon face"). *C*, the spine reveals compressed, biconcave vertebral bodies, "ballooning" of the intervertebral discs and generalized rarefaction of all the bones due to osteoporosis.

excretion of 17-hydroxycorticoids is increased. The complications of gross and microscopic pathological fractures with progressive bone deformity are common because of the severe degree of generalized osteoporosis.

Hypopituitarism

A deficient amount of anterior pituitary hormone during *childhood* retards epiphyseal growth and thereby results in a perfectly proportioned *Lorain type of dwarfism* (Fig. 9.18). Hypopituitarism may also produce various degrees of *dystrophia-adiposo-genitalis (Fröhlich's syndrome)* characterized by prominent obesity, subnormal sexual development, relatively normal growth and a predisposition to slipping of the upper femoral epiphysis (adolescent coxa vara) (Fig. 9.19).

Hypothyroidism in Childhood (Cretinism)

Congenital deficiency of thyroid function is manifest in children by delayed epiphyseal plate growth as well as by delayed, irregular ossification of epiphyses (which may mimic the appearance of avascular necrosis). Mental impairment is usual and the child exhibits a large tongue, dry skin and dull facial expression. The significance of cretinism lies in the fact that if it is recognized early and treated by thyroid extract for life, marked improvement in all aspects of the disorder can be achieved. Fortunately, because of widespread neonatal screening programs to determine the level of thyroid stimulating hormone (TSH), even mild forms of hypothyroidism can be diagnosed—and hence treated—very early so that the full-blown clinical picture of cretinism is becoming progressively less common.

DISSEMINATED BONE DISORDERS OF UNKNOWN ETIOLOGY

The heterogenous group of disorders included in this section are manifest in the skeleton by widely disseminated, but discrete, lesions in bone. They are not associated with generalized bone disease in that the uninvolved bone is completely normal. These disorders include *polyostotic fibrous dysplasia*, *osteitis deformans (Paget's disease)* and the various *skeletal reticuloses*.

Polyostotic Fibrous Dysplasia

This curious disseminated disorder of bone is probably a developmental fault of bony development, but its cause remains a mystery. It is characterized by multiple areas of fibrous tissue replacement within multiple bones without any evidence of generalized osteoporosis.

PATHOLOGY

The slowly progressive lesions appear in early childhood and consist of fibrous tissue accumulations within the marrow spaces. The lesions gradually expand the host bone

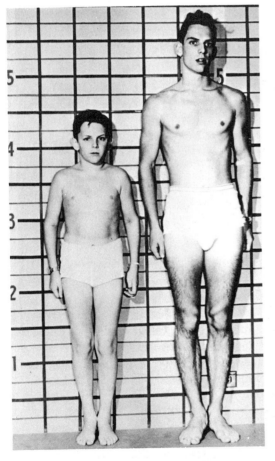

Figure 9.18. Lorain type of dwarfism due to hypopituitarism. These 15-year-old boys are identical twins. Note that the hypopituitary twin, though very short, is normally proportioned.

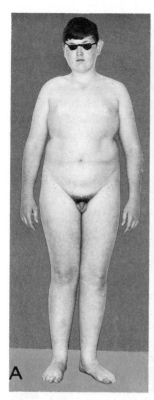
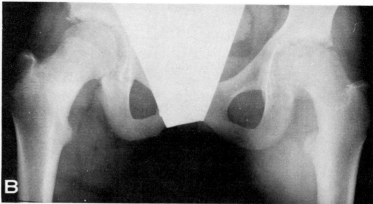
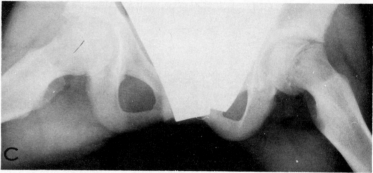

Figure 9.19. Dystrophia-adiposo-genitalis (Fröhlich's syndrome). *A,* this 14-year-old boy demonstrates prominent obesity. His stature is normal for his age, but his sexual development is subnormal. Note that his left lower limb is externally rotated. He complained of pain in his left knee (referred from the hip) due to a slipped left upper femoral epiphysis. *B,* the anteroposterior radiograph reveals a posteromedial slip of the left upper femoral epiphysis. *C,* the lateral radiograph (frog position) reveals the slip of the left upper femoral epiphysis more clearly.

from within as they erode and replace bone, but they are always confined by at least a thin layer of cortical bone since the periosteal intramembranous ossification is uninvolved. The locally destructive lesions weaken the bone considerably, resulting in pathological fractures, but these usually unite well. Microscopically, there is dense fibrous tissue in which spicules of bone are embedded. Rarely, the condition may be limited to one bone (*monostotic* fibrous dysplasia). An unusual variant is *Albright's syndrome,* which occurs in girls and in which there is a combination of sexual precocity, skin pigmentation and polyostotic fibrous dysplasia.

DIAGNOSIS

Polyostotic fibrous dysplasia is usually detected in early childhood because of a deformity or a pathological fracture. The progressive radiographic changes include expanded osteolytic lesions enclosed by a thin shell of cortical bone and frequently severe bony deformities, particularly in the upper end of the femur (Fig. 9.20). The blood chemistry is normal, which helps to differentiate this condition from the generalized disease of hyperparathyroidism.

TREATMENT

There is, as yet, no specific treatment for polyostotic fibrous dysplasia. The complications of pathological fracture and severe bony deformities may necessitate operative procedures such as currettement of a fibrous tissue lesion followed by packing of the defect with bone grafts; osteotomy may be indicated to correct residual deformity.

Osteitis Deformans (Paget's Disease)

The disseminated bone disorder of *osteitis deformans* is characterized by slowly progressive enlargement and deformity of multiple bones associated with unexplained acceleration of both deposition and resorption of bone. This condition, particularly in its milder forms, is very common, affecting approximately 3% of all persons over the age of 40 years.

ETIOLOGY

Although the precise etiology of Paget's disease is not proven, it is now thought that a "slow virus" affecting primarily osteoclasts may be involved.

PATHOLOGY

The pathological process of osteitis deformans (which was originally thought to be inflammatory) involves a markedly accelerated bone turnover with excessive osteoclastic resorption and excessive osteoblas-

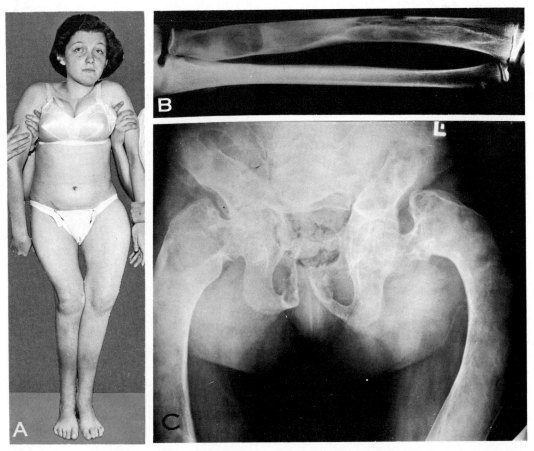

Figure 9.20. Polyostotic fibrous dysplasia. *A,* this 14-year-old girl exhibits severe deformities, particularly of her lower limbs and is unable to stand without support. *B,* the forearm reveals expanded osteolytic lesions in the radius enclosed by a thin shell of cortical bone. *C,* the hips reveals severe deformities of the pelvis and femora with multiple expanded osteolytic lesions enclosed by a thin shell of cortical bone. Note the evidence of previous pathological fractures.

tic deposition taking place simultaneously. The involved areas of bone are extremely vascular and may even exhibit arteriovenous shunts. During the early and more active phase, resorption exceeds deposition and the bone, although enlarged, becomes sponge-like, weakened and deformed. This *osteolytic phase* is followed by an *osteosclerotic phase* in which the balance swings in favor of deposition, with the result that the enlarged bones become thick and dense. The bones most commonly involved are the tibia, femur, pelvis, vertebral bodies and skull. Although the disease is usually polyostotic, it is occasionally limited to one bone (*monostotic* osteitis deformans). Microscopically, the normal lamellar pattern of bone is lost and is replaced by an irregular mosaic pattern of alternating mature and immature bone. Complications of this bizarre process include progressive deformities due to the enlargement and bending of bones in the osteolytic phase, pathological fractures (which are usually transverse and somewhat slow to unite) and occasionally malignant change in the hyperactive osteoblasts resulting in an exceedingly malignant and invariably fatal type of osteogenic sarcoma.

DIAGNOSIS

While osteitis deformans is common, the milder forms are subclinical in that they do not cause symptoms and are discovered only incidentally. The more severe forms cause bone pain which may be very severe indeed. The patient observes that his lower limbs are becoming progressively bowed, his head is becoming gradually larger (his hats seem too small) and he is becoming shorter (Fig. 9.21). The radiographic changes include enlargement, deformity and porosity of involved bones during the osteolytic phase and increased, but irregular density of the bones, in the osteosclerotic phase (Fig. 9.22). The serum alkaline phosphatase and urinary hydroxyproline are always markedly elevated when the disease is disseminated but they are not always elevated when the disease is localized.

TREATMENT

As yet there exists no medical treatment that is specific for Paget's disease. Nevertheless, at least three therapeutic agents (calcitonin, diphosphonates and mithramycin) have been shown to reduce both bone resorption and bone formation in this disorder of rapid bone turnover and thereby to relieve the associated bone pain. Of the available calcitonins (porcine, salmon and synthetic human) the most potent and the one with fewest side effects is salmon calcitonin—even though neutralizing antibodies may be produced eventually. Diphosphonates also inhibit bone resorption and secondarily, osteoblastic matrix synthesis; in addition, they inhibit mineralization of newly formed matrix by physiochemical

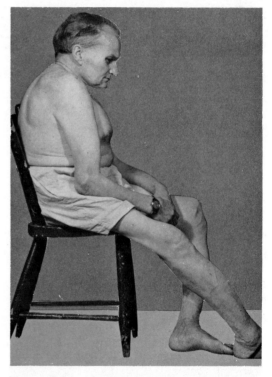

Figure 9.21. Osteitis deformans (Paget's disease). This 60-year-old man complained of severe pain in his lower limbs which were becoming progressively bowed. He also has deformities in his upper limbs. He noticed that he was becoming shorter but that his head was becoming larger.

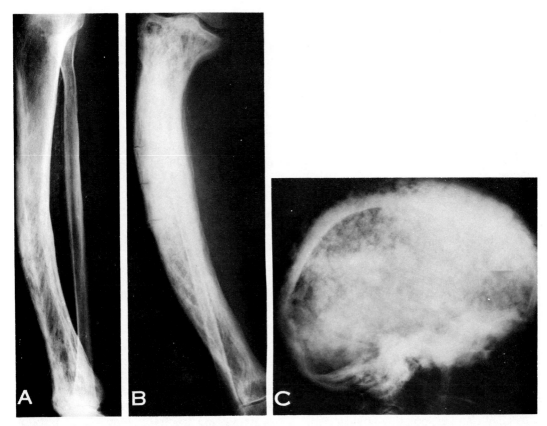

Figure 9.22. Osteitis deformans (Paget's disease). *A*, the tibia in the early osteolytic stage. The lesion, which is most marked in the distal half of the tibia, is advancing proximally. *B*, the tibia in the late osteosclerotic phase. The tibia is thickened and bowed. Horizontal pseudofractures can be seen on the convex side of the deformed tibia. *C*, the skull reveals irregular sclerosis of bone. The new bone formation on the outer surface of the skull accounts for the increasing size of the head.

means, i.e., adsorption of calcium to bone. These two agents, which are administered in intermittent courses of therapy, seem to potentiate each other's effects.

More recently, mithramycin, a cytotoxic agent, has also been found to be effective in reducing the pain of widely disseminated, painful Paget's disease.

Skeletal Reticuloses

Proliferation of the cells of the reticuloendothelial system within bone occurs in a number of poorly understood granulomatous conditions. Although these conditions differ considerably, they are all capable of producing disseminated lesions in bone and are referred to collectively as "*the skeletal reticuloses.*" The non-lipid reticuloses include *Letterer-Siwe's disease, Hand-Schüller-Christian disease* and *eosinophilic granuloma.* Since the predominant cell is the histiocyte, these three conditions are designated "*histiocytosis X.*" The lipid reticulosis known as *Gaucher's disease* is a manifestation of abnormal lipid metabolism and is, in fact, a lipid storage disease.

NON-LIPID RETICULOSES (HISTIOCYTOSIS X)

Letterer-Siwe's Disease

In this rare but very serious type of histiocytosis X, the onset is in infancy and the progress is extremely rapid. The clinical manifestations involve mainly soft tissues

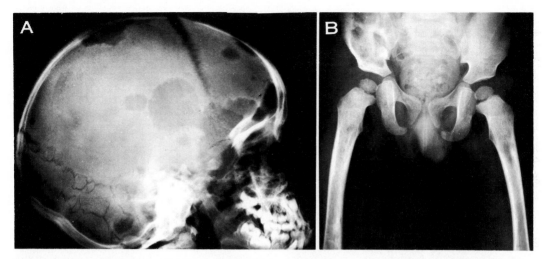

Figure 9.23. Hand-Schüller-Christian disease. *A*, the skull in a 4-year-old boy showing numerous round, clearly demarcated osteolytic defects. Note also the spreading of the suture lines. *B*, the hips of the same boy showing numerous osteolytic lesions of the right innominate bone and the right femur.

(enlarged spleen, liver and lymph nodes) and are accompanied by thrombocytopenic purpura with petechial hemorrhages. The condition usually results in early death before significant bone lesions have developed.

Hand-Schüller-Christian Disease

In this variety of histiocytosis X, proliferation of histiocytes within the bone causes disseminated, but discrete, destructive lesions, particularly in the skull, but also in other bones. Deposits of similar cells around the pituitary gland result in diabetes insipidus. The onset is in early childhood and the progress of the condition is moderately rapid. Microscopically, the lesions in bone contain histiocytes (which become secondarily laden with lipids eventually), eosinophils and giant cells. Radiographically, the lesions in the skull are seen as clearly demarcated osteolytic defects, whereas the lesions elsewhere are osteolytic but less clearly defined (Fig. 9.23). Radiotherapy causes the skeletal lesions to heal, at least temporarily, but when the involvement is extensive the prognosis is unfavorable.

Eosinophilic Granuloma

A less serious and more localized variety of histiocytosis X is *eosinophilic granuloma*, which is encountered in children and young adults. The osteolytic lesion, which is usually single, is composed of histiocytes as well as an impressive accumulation of eosinophils. Pathological fractures may occur through the osteolytic lesions but they always heal. When a vertebral body is involved, the primary center of ossification becomes dense and thin, but subsequently is reconstituted to a large extent. (This type of vertebral lesion, originally described by Calvé, was formerly thought to represent avascular necrosis.) The osteolytic lesions develop rapidly and are accompanied by periosteal new bone formation.

Clinically and radiographically, eosinophilic granuloma is an imitator of several bone diseases including osteomyelitis, tuberculosis, simple bone cyst, fibrous dysplasia and various malignant bone neoplasms (Fig. 9.24). Although the discrete lesions are similar to those of the other varieties of histiocytosis X, the prognosis of eosinophilic granuloma is extremely good in that it seems to be a self-limiting condition in which the bony lesions gradually heal spontaneously. However, the ominous clinical and radiographic features usually merit biopsy to exclude a more serious lesion. Curettement of the lesion at the time of biopsy seems to accelerate healing.

LIPID RETICULOSIS-GAUCHER'S DISEASE

Gaucher's disease is an uncommon inborn error of lipid metabolism in which proliferating reticuloendothelial cells in the bone marrow, spleen and liver are filled with the lipid, *kerasin*. The kerasin filled cells, called Gaucher's cells, infiltrate the bone marrow and cause localized osteolytic lesions of bone. Such lesions may be complicated by avascular necrosis of bone, particularly when they occur in the femoral head (Fig. 9.25). The more severe forms of Gaucher's

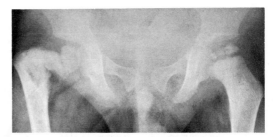

Figure 9.25. Gaucher's disease. This 3-year-old boy's hips reveal a pathological fracture at the base of the neck of the right femur (through a localized osteolytic lesion) and avascular necrosis of the left femoral head.

disease, which become manifest in early childhood, have a bad prognosis; but the milder forms, which are encountered later, do not seem to shorten the patient's life expectancy. The diagnosis is established by the demonstration of Gaucher's cells in the bone marrow (obtained by either sternal or iliac crest puncture). Radiotherapy usually results in regression of the bony lesions and splenectomy may be indicated solely to relieve local discomfort from the gross splenomegaly.

Suggested Additional Reading

Aloia, J. F., Cohn, S. H., Ostani, J. A., Cane, R. and Ellis, K.: Prevention of involutional bone loss by exercise. Ann. Intern. Med. 89: 356–358, 1978.

Avioli, L. V.: Osteoporosis: diagnosis and treatment. Myology Monogr. Contin. Ed. 4: 3–10, 1979.

Copp, D. H. Calcitonin—recent advances and clinical implications. Mod. Med. Can. 28: 41–45, 1973.

Evans, I., Hughes, S., and Taylor, S.: Metabolic bone disorders. In *The Basis and Practice of Orthopaedics*, edited by Hughes, S. and Sweetnam, R. London, William Heinemann Medical Books, 1980.

Fraser, D., Kind, H. P., and Kooh, S. W.: Disturbances of parathyroid hormone and calcitonin. In *Textbook of Pediatrics*, 2nd ed., edited by G. C. Arneil and J. D. Forfar. Edinburgh, Churchill Livingstone, 1978, pp. 1001–1004.

Fraser, D., Kooh, S. W., and Scriver, C. R.: Rickets with high hereditability relatively refractory to vitamin D: challenges and prospects. Part 1. Mod. Med. Can. 37: 199–209, 1982.

Fraser, D. and Salter, R. B.: The diagnosis and management of the various types of rickets. Pediatr. Clin. North Am. Vol. 5, 417–444, 1958.

Harrison, J. E., McNeill, K. G., Sturtridge, W. C., Bayley, T. M., Williams, M. C., Tam, C., and Fornasier, V.: Three-year changes in bone mineral mass of postmenopausal osteoporotic patients based on neutron activation analysis of the central third of the skeleton. J. Clin. Endocrinol. Metab. 52: 751–758, 1981.

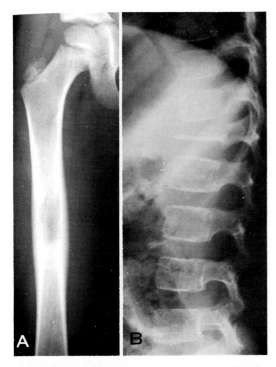

Figure 9.24. Eosinophilic granuloma. *A,* the femur of a 10-year-old boy who complained of pain in his thigh. The osteolytic defect is associated with subperiosteal new bone formation (reactive bone) and is frequently difficult to differentiate from other bone lesions radiographically. *B,* the spine of a 7-year boy who complained of back pain. The first lumbar vertebra has collapsed. Formerly this radiographic appearance was invariably thought to represent avascular necrosis of the primary center of ossification (Calvé's disease).

Harrison, J. E., Murray, T. M., and Bright-See, E. (co-ordinating editors): Recent advances in osteoporosis. Clin. Invest. Med. 5: 137–201, 1982.

Hosling, D. J.: Paget's disease of bone. Br. Med. J. 283: 686–683, 1981.

Jowsey, J.: *Metabolic Diseases of Bone.* Philadelphia, W. B. Saunders, 1977.

Milgram, J. W.: Orthopaedic management of Paget's disease of bone. Clin. Orthop. 127: 63–69, 1977.

Nordin, B. E. C., Peacock, M., Aaron, J., Crilly, R. G., Heyburn, P. J., Horsman, A., and Marshall, D.: Osteoporosis and osteomalacia. Clin. Endocrinol. Metab. 9: 177–203, 1980.

Riggs, B. L., Hodgson, S. F., and Hoffmann, D. L.: Treatment of primary osteoporosis with fluoride and calcium. J.A.M.A. 243: 446–449, 1980.

Riggs, B. L., Seeman, E., Hodgson, S. F., Taves, D. R., O'Fallon, W. M.: Effect of the fluoride/calcium regimen on vertebral fracture occurrence in postmenopausal osteoporosis. Comparison with conventional therapy. N. Engl. J. Med. 306(8): 446–50, 1982.

Schatzker, J., Chapman, M., Ha'eri, G. B., Fournasier, V. L., Sumner-Smith, G., and Williams, C.: The effect of calcitonin in fracture healing. Clin. Orthop. 141: 103, 1979.

Singer, F. P.: Human calcitonin treatment of Paget's disease of bone. Clin. Orthop. 127: 86–93, 1977.

Solomon, L.: Bone loss in aging individuals. Orthopaedic Proceedings of the Orthopaedic Department, University of Witwatersrand, Johannesburg, South Africa. 6 (No. 2): 1–21, 1978.

Sturtridge, W. C.: Osteoporosis and Paget's disease. Medicine, North America, Vol. 1, pp. 1171–1180, May 11, 1981.

Turek, S. L.: *Orthopaedics, Principles and Their Application*, 3rd ed. Philadelphia, J. B. Lippincott, 1977.

CHAPTER 10

Inflammatory Disorders of Bones and Joints

A wide variety of disorders of the musculoskeletal system are manifest clinically by the phenomenon of *inflammation* and are therefore best considered as a broad group in relation to this basic pathological process. For some of these clinical disorders, such as osteomyelitis and septic arthritis, a specific causative microorganism can be incriminated; however, for others, such as ankylosing spondylitis and rheumatoid arthritis, the exact etiology remains an unsolved and challenging mystery.

Before learning about the various disorders as clinical entities, you will find it helpful to review some of the general features of the inflammatory process as well as the reactions of the musculoskeletal tissues to this process.

THE INFLAMMATORY PROCESS: GENERAL FEATURES

Inflammation, a process of biological events, is best defined as "the local reaction of living tissues to an irritant" (Boyd). In this reactive process, cells and exudates accumulate in the irritated tissues and usually (but not invariably) tend to protect them from further injury. Once considered a disease entity in itself, inflammation is now known to be a tissue response, or reaction, to any one of many types of irritants. The four clinical manifestations of inflammation originally described by Celsus are: *rubor*, *tumor*, *calor* et *dolor* (redness, swelling, heat and pain). To these Galen later added a fifth— *functio laesa* (loss of function). These five clinical manifestations are readily explained by the nature of the inflammatory process.

The *redness* and the *heat* are due to the vascular response, namely a dilatation of local blood vessels combined with an increased rate of flow. The *swelling* represents the formation of an exudate which results from the combination of increased hydrostatic pressure within the capillaries and increased capillary permeability. To this inflammatory exudate is added the emigration of various types of leukocytes from the capillaries. The *pain*, which is most severe in the acute type of inflammatory process, is related to the marked increase in local pressure within the tissues. When the inflammatory process develops in a closed space, such as a bone or a synovial joint, it is easy to understand why the pain may be severe. The initial *loss of function* of the involved part is due to pain and swelling; however, subsequent loss of function may result from a combination of actual destruction of tissue, such as articular cartilage, and dense scar formation in soft tissues.

In the central zone of the inflammatory process, local tissue necrosis and liquefaction are frequently seen. By contrast, the reaction in the peripheral zone is hyperplasia of connective tissue cells, a reaction that initially serves to localize the process and subsequently aids in the repair of the inflammatory lesion.

REACTIONS OF THE MUSCULOSKELETAL TISSUES TO INFLAMMATION

Each specialized type of tissue in the body reacts in a characteristic way to the general process of inflammation. Thus, a knowledge of the characteristic reactions of the various musculoskeletal tissues will enhance your *understanding*, not only of the clinical, radiographic and laboratory *manifestations* of inflammatory musculoskeletal disorders in your patients, but also of the underlying *reason* for the principles and methods of their treatment. The characteristic reactions to infection and other types of inflammation in bone, epiphyseal plate, articular cartilage, synovial membrane, capsule and ligaments are discussed and illustrated in Chapter 3. They are of sufficient importance that you may wish to review them in Chapter 3 before proceeding to a discussion of the various

clinical disease entities that result from inflammation of musculoskeletal tissues.

TYPES OF INFLAMMATORY DISORDERS OF BONES AND JOINTS

The various musculoskeletal disorders discussed in this chapter have in common, as their most prominent feature, the phenomenon of inflammation. They are best considered in four broad groups.

First is the broad group of *specific infections* for which causative organisms can be detected. Of these, many are *pyogenic* (pus producing) infections, such as osteomyelitis, septic arthritis and tenosynovitis. Others are *granulomatous* (granuloma producing) infections, such as tuberculous osteomyelitis and tuberculous arthritis.

A second broad group of inflammatory disorders includes the nonspecific and idiopathic *inflammatory types of rheumatic diseases* which include such entities as rheumatic fever, transient synovitis, rheumatoid arthritis and spondylitis.

A third group includes inflammation of musculoskeletal tissue secondary to a chemical irritant, as seen in the form of *metabolic arthritis* known as gout.

A fourth group is characterized by chronic inflammation due to *repeated physical injury*—usually minor injury (microtrauma) or mechanical irritation. Bursitis and tenovaginitis stenosans are examples of this type of inflammation.

PYOGENIC BACTERIAL INFECTIONS

Pyogenic bacterial infections in bones and joints continue to represent a serious threat to both life and limb. Although chemotherapeutic and antibiotic drugs have dramatically reduced the *mortality* of the various pyogenic infections involving the musculoskeletal system, the *incidence* of these infections and their *morbidity* have been less dramatically reduced. Indeed, drug therapy may mask the clinical manifestations of infection without completely controlling the local lesion and thereby create an altered clinical picture.

Principles of Antibacterial Therapy

Acute pyogenic infection is an exceedingly rapid process measured in hours and days. Thus, even a short delay in treatment may lead to serious consequences for the patient. Antibiotics (at least in low doses, such as tetracycline, chloramphenicol and erythromycin) exert their effect on the metabolism of bacteria and thereby markedly decrease their rate of multiplication; their action, therefore, is *bacteriostatic.* Other antibacterial drugs, such as the penicillins and cephalosporins, actually kill bacteria and hence are *bacteriocidal.*

To control an infection the concentration of the appropriate antibiotic in the blood and at the site of infection must exceed the level necessary to kill the infecting organism. The ideal antibiotic is *bacteriocidal* (as opposed to *bacteriostatic*), should be known to be effective against the most likely infecting bacteria, must reach the infected tissues in high concentrations (which can be difficult in bone) should be non-toxic and should have little effect on the normal flora.

The parenteral (intravenous or intramuscular) route of administration is more effective than the oral route in achieving adequate serum and tissue levels of the antibiotic and is therefore preferable in the initial treatment.

Since patients vary in their response to antibiotics and since the infecting organisms vary in their resistance, both clinical and laboratory monitoring of the patient are essential. An effective laboratory method of such monitoring is the weekly determination of the serum bacterial titer as recommended by Prober.

Antibacterial therapy must be continued for a longer perior to control infection in bone than in soft tissues in order to achieve a permanent cure and thereby prevent either chronic, or recurrent infection. Empirically, this period is from four to six weeks.

The relatively slow diffusion of antibacterial agents into the area of bacterial inflammation is dependent upon an intact local blood supply. When the local pressure within the inflamed tissues becomes excessive with resultant ischemia, the circulating antibacterial agents are no longer able to reach the causative organism to exert their effect. Likewise, accumulation of a purulent exudate (*pus*) in an abscess prevents the agents from reaching bacteria. These facts emphasize the very real value of surgical decompression of the increased pressure within a closed space—such as a bone or a joint—and surgical evacuation of accumulated pus.

Acute Hematogenous Osteomyelitis

One of the most serious inflammatory disorders of the musculoskeletal system is *acute hematogenous osteomyelitis*, a rapidly developing blood-borne bacterial infection of bone and its marrow in children.

INCIDENCE

At the beginning of the era of specific antibacterial drugs there was a sharp fall in the incidence of acute hematogenous osteomyelitis; indeed, some clinicians optimistically predicted the eradication of this disease. Subsequently, however, the incidence has returned almost to its former level. This phenomenon—which has been paralleled by bacterial infections involving other tissues—is explained by a combination of the emergence of resistant strains of bacteria (especially staphylococci) and the failure of too many clinicians to understand and apply the principles of antibacterial and surgical therapy in relation to bone and joint infections.

Hematogenous osteomyelitis is primarily a disease of growing bones and therefore, of children; boys are afflicted three times as often as girls. The long bones most frequently involved (in order of decreasing frequency) are the femur, tibia, humerus, radius, ulna and fibula, the characteristic site in any given bone being the metaphyseal region—possibly because of the unique blood supply to this part of the bone during childhood.

ETIOLOGY

Staphylococcus aureus is by far the commonest causative organism being responsible for at least 90% of acute hematogenous osteomyelitis. The *portal of entry* is usually through the skin secondary to infected scratches, abrasions, pimples or boils; sometimes it is through the mucous membranes of the upper respiratory tract as a complication of a nose or throat infection. In the presence of a bacteremia, local trauma seems to play a significant role in determining the particular bone in which osteomyelitis develops (perhaps because of local thrombosis and hence decreased resistance to infection); this may account, in part, for the higher incidence, not only in boys but also in the lower extremities. Streptococcus, *Hemophilus influenzae* or pneumococcus may, on occasion, be the offending bacteria, particularly in infants.

PATHOGENESIS AND PATHOLOGY

The early and rapid development of untreated hematogenous osteomyelitis is characterized by an initially small focus of bacterial inflammation with early *hyperemia* and *edema* in the cancellous bone and marrow of the metaphyseal region of a long bone (Fig. 10.1). Unlike soft tissues, which are capable of expanding to accommodate swelling, the bone represents a rigid closed space; therefore, the early edema of the inflammatory process produces a sharp rise in the intraosseous pressure which explains the symptom of severe and constant local pain. Pus forms, thereby increasing the local pressure even further with resultant compromise of the local circulation which, in turn, leads to vascular thrombosis and consequent *necrosis of bone.*

The untreated infection rapidly spreads by several routes, destroying bone by *osteolysis* in its path (Fig. 10.2). Through damaged vessels in the local lesion, large numbers of bacteria re-invade the bloodstream; the clinically undetectable bacteremia become a *septicemia* which is manifest by the onset of malaise, anorexia and fever. Local spread of the infection by direct extension, aided by increased local pressure, penetrates the relatively thin cortex of the metaphyseal region and involves the highly sensitive periosteum, which accounts for the exquisite local tenderness. The periosteum, being loosely attached to bone during child-

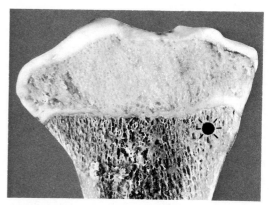

Figure 10.1.   Site of the initial focus of hematogenous osteomyelitis in the metaphyseal region of the upper end of the tibia showing the cut surface of the tibia; note the architectural arrangement of the cancellous bone in the metaphysis which is different from that in the epiphysis.

hood, is readily stripped up and the result is a *subperiosteal abscess* which may either remain localized or spread along and around the entire shaft of the bone; such elevation of the periosteum disrupts the blood supply to the underlying cortex thereby increasing the extent of bone necrosis.

After the first few days the infection penetrates the periosteum to produce a *cellulitis* and eventually a *soft tissue abscess.* In those sites where the metaphyseal region is within the synovial joint, as in the upper end of the femur and the upper end of the radius, penetration of the periosteum carries the infection directly into the joint with a resultant *septic arthritis* (Fig. 10.3). In other sites, where the metaphyseal region is outside, but close to the joint, a sterile synovial effusion frequently develops.

Meanwhile, local spread of the infection within the medullary cavity further compromises the internal circulation. The resultant area of bone necrosis, which may vary in extent from a small spicule to the entire shaft, eventually becomes separated, or sequestrated, from the living bone thereby forming a separated fragment of infected dead bone, a *sequestrum.* Extensive new bone formation from the deep layer of the elevated periosteum produces an envelop-

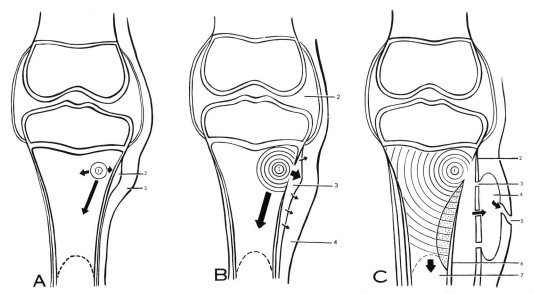

Figure 10.2.   Routes of spread of untreated acute hematogenous osteomyelitis in the upper end of the tibia. *A*, (1) initially the infection spreads in three directions as shown by the *arrows*; (2) periosteal edema; (3) edema in the soft tissues. *B*, (1) original focus of infection has increased in size; (2) there may be an inflammatory exudate in the knee joint but no direct extension of the infection; (3) subperiosteal abscess; (4) cellulitis in the overlying soft tissues. *C*, (1) the area of osteomyelitis has become extensive; (2) the periosteum has been elevated from the underlying bone over a large area; (3) infection has penetrated the periosteum to produce (4) a soft tissue abscess. (5) The abscess has drained onto the skin surface through a sinus; (6) an area of bone necrosis which will subsequently sequestrate; (7) continuing spread of the infection in the medullary cavity.

ing bony tube, or *involucrum*, which maintains continuity of the involved bone, even when large segments of the shaft have died and sequestrated (Fig. 10.2). The epiphyseal plate usually acts as a barrier to direct spread of infection, but if it is damaged in the process, a serious growth disturbance will become apparent at a later date.

At any time the septicemia, if uncontrolled, may produce metastatic foci of infection in other bones, or more important in other organs, particularly the lungs and the brain. Indeed, in the days before antibacterial drugs 25% of all children with acute hematogenous osteomyelitis died from the associated septicemia. If the child survives the septicemia, the local bone lesion—unless adequately treated—gradually passes into a chronic state. Chronic osteomyelitis, which is perpetuated by the presence of infected dead bone, is discussed in a subsequent section of this chapter.

CLINICAL FEATURES AND DIAGNOSIS

The clinical features of acute hematogenous osteomyelitis are readily correlated with the foregoing description of its pathogenesis. The onset is acute and the infection progresses with remarkable rapidity. There is a history of recent local injury in 50% of the children; frequently you will find evidence of a pre-existing bacterial infection either in the skin or in the upper respiratory tract.

The first and most significant symptom the afflicted child experiences is severe and constant pain near the end of the involved long bone; this is accompanied by exquisite local tenderness and the child's unwillingness to use the limb (Fig. 10.4). Within 24 hours the associated septicemia is evidenced by malaise, anorexia and fever; the child appears acutely ill. Increasing pain and local tenderness near the end of a long bone combined with systemic manifestations of

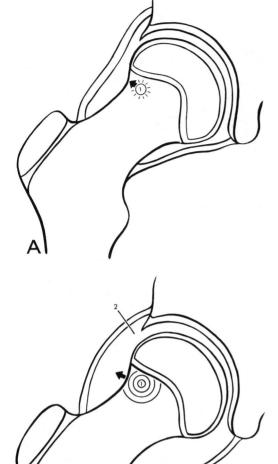

has already spread beyond the confines of the bone (Fig. 10.5).

It is extremely important for you to appreciate that the early diagnosis of acute hematogenous osteomyelitis must be made on *clinical* grounds alone. During at least the first week of illness, despite severe local involvement of bone, there is absolutely no concrete radiographic evidence of bone infection. There may be radiographic evidence of soft tissue swelling after the first few days (Fig. 10.6). However, only after the first week does the radiograph reveal the first evidence of destruction of bone in the metaphysis and the first signs of reactive new bone from the periosteum (Fig. 10.7). During this first week before radiographic changes

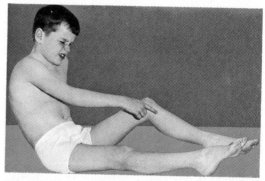

Figure 10.4. This boy, who has early acute hematogenous osteomyelitis of the upper end of the left tibia, is unable to bear weight on his left foot and is unwilling to move his knee. He is able to localize the point of pain and tenderness very accurately.

Figure 10.3. Acute hematogenous osteomyelitis of the upper end of the femur in a child. *A,* (1) initial focus of infection in the metaphyseal region. *B,* (1) the focus of infection has spread through the metaphyseal cortex directly into (2) the synovial cavity of the hip joint.

infection in a child always justify the *clinical* diagnosis of acute hematogenous osteomyelitis—at least until there is definite evidence to the contrary. Soft tissue swelling is a relatively late sign appearing only after a few days and indicating that the infection

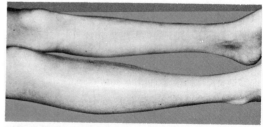

Figure 10.5. Soft tissue swelling secondary to osteomyelitis of the right tibia in a child. This child had severe pain in the right leg for seven days prior to this photograph. The infection has already spread from the bone into the soft tissues to produce an extensive cellulitis.

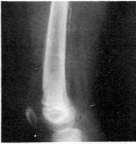

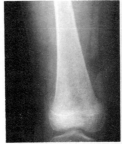

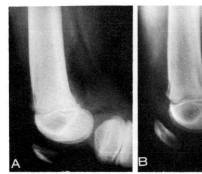

Figure 10.6. Radiographic evidence of soft tissue swelling secondary to acute hematogenous osteomyelitis. *A*, normal lower end of soft tissue swelling posterior to the lower end of the femur in a child with acute hematogenous osteomyelitis 3 days after the onset of symptoms. At this stage there is no evidence of bone destruction.

Figure 10.7. Radiographic evidence of bone destruction in the metaphyseal region of the lower end of the femur of a child with acute hematogenous osteomyelitis of 10 days' duration. Note also the evidence of subperiosteal new bone formation along the shaft of the femur.

become apparent, scintigraphy, i.e. a bone scan, may be of value in establishing the diagnosis (as discussed in Chapter 5).

In infants the systemic manifestations of infection are often less apparent than they are in children. Furthermore, the localization of the osteomyelitis is obviously more difficult, due to lack of communication, and requires careful examination of all the major long bones and joints.

The white blood cell count and the sedimentation rate are usually elevated, but despite the underlying bacteremia, and later the septicemia, a single blood culture is positive in only about half of the patients.

The clinical manifestations of acute hematogenous osteomyelitis—particularly the systemic manifestations—may be masked during the first few days of the illness by the casual and speculative use of inadequate antibacterial therapy for what is loosely considered "a little infection." This deplorable type of management obscures the true diagnosis until irreparable changes in the bone have developed and the local infection has progressed relentlessly to chronic osteomyelitis (Fig. 10.8).

In its early stages, acute hematogenous osteomyelitis must be differentiated from rheumatic fever, cellulitis of soft tissues and local trauma to soft tissues or bone. After the first week or more, particularly if the systemic manifestations have been masked by antibacterial drugs, the radiographic changes of irregular metaphyseal rarefaction and subperiosteal new bone formation can mimic such bone lesions as eosinophilic granuloma, Ewing's sarcoma and osteosarcoma.

TREATMENT

Acute hematogenous osteomyelitis represents an extremely serious infection which demands urgent and vigorous treatment. As soon as the *clinical* diagnosis is strongly suspected on the basis of the above mentioned symptoms and signs, the child should be admitted to hospital for intensive treatment. As soon as one blood sample has been taken for culture to seek the causative bacteria as well as their sensitivity to the various antibacterial drugs, antibacterial therapy is instituted. Since the bacterial environment varies not only from one locality to another but also from year to year, the choice of the specific drug to be used initially will depend upon existing conditions in your locality at the time. Nevertheless, general guidelines can be stated.

Currently, penicillin is still the safest antibiotic drug but in many communities over 70% of the Staphylococci are penicillin-resistant. Therefore, at least initially, one of the newer antibiotics such as methicillin or cloxacillin should be given or, alternatively,

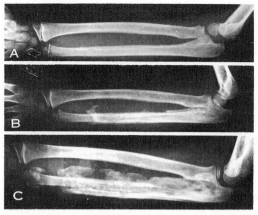
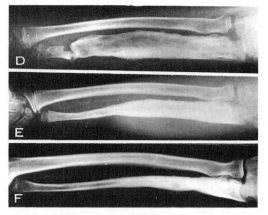

Figure 10.8.   The relentless progression from acute hematogenous osteomyelitis to chronic osteomyelitis. This series of radiographs of a girl's forearm extends over a period of 10 years and demonstrates many of the radiographic changes of acute and chronic osteomyelitis of the ulna.

A, one week after the onset of symptoms. There is soft tissue swelling, a small area of destruction in the metaphyseal region of the distal end of the ulna and beginning new bone formation along the shaft of the ulna. This child had been thought to have a "a little infection" and had received a small amount of antibacterial therapy for a few days. At the end of one week her arm was markedly swollen and tender. The infection had already spread throughout the length of the ulna and at this stage even extensive therapy could not eradicate all the infection.

B, ten days later there is evidence of further destruction in the ulna and more subperiosteal new bone formation.

C, one month later there is involucrum formation and sequestration of the distal third of the ulna. At this stage a large sequestrum was removed.

D, eight months later there is still chronic osteomyelitis; there is a pathological fracture in that portion of the lower end of the ulna that has reformed from the deep surface of periosteum.

E, three years later there is evidence of premature cessation of growth at the distal ulnar epiphyseal plate secondary to the infection. There is still marked thickening of the proximal two-thirds of the ulna because of residual chronic osteomyelitis.

F, ten years after the onset of the osteomyelitis there is a small abscess in the upper end of the ulna and additional evidence of chronic osteomyelitis in the entire upper third of the ulna.

This relentless progression from acute hematogenous osteomyelitis to chronic osteomyelitis could have been prevented by early adequate treatment.

one of the cephalosporins such as cephalothin (all of which are effective in the presence of penicillinase). As soon as the culture and sensitivity results are known, antibiotic therapy can be modified appropriately if necessary. A consultant in the rapidly changing field of infectious diseases can be of much help in advising about the antibacterial therapy for these patients.

The following general plan of treatment has been found to be most effective:

1. Bed rest and analgesics for the child.

2. Supportive measures including intravenous fluids and, when necessary, blood transfusion.

3. Local rest for the involved extremity with either a removable splint or traction—to reduce pain, retard the spread of infection and prevent soft tissue contractures.

4. Immediate parenteral administration of appropriate antibacterial therapy (as soon as a blood sample has been taken for culture), not only to control the bacteremia and septicemia, but also to reach the area of osteomyelitis before it has become ischemic and therefore inaccessible to the circulating drug. After the first two weeks—provided there has been a good clinical response—the antibiotic may be given orally (which has been proven to be effective and is certainly more comfortable for the child).

5. If local and systemic manifestations

have not improved dramatically after 24 hours of intensive treatment, surgical decompression of the involved area of bone (evacuation of subperiosteal pus, drilling of bone) to reduce the intraosseous pressure and to obtain pus for culture. Postoperatively, continuous local infusion of saline with an antibiotic, combined with drainage for at least a few days (Fig. 10.9).

6. Continuation of antibacterial therapy for a minimum period of four weeks, even if clinical improvement during the first few days has been satisfactory. (After four weeks, treatment is discontinued only when the sedimentation rate begins to approach a normal level.)

PROGNOSIS

Four important factors determine the effectiveness of antibacterial treatment for acute hematogenous osteomyelitis and consequently its prognosis:

1. *The time interval between onset of the infection and the institution of treatment.* Treatment begun during the first three days of illness is ideal because at this stage the local area of osteomyelitis has not yet become ischemic. Such early treatment, provided the causative organism is sensitive to the drug chosen, usually controls the infection completely so that osteolysis, bone necrosis and reactive new bone formation are prevented; under these circumstances radiographic changes in the bone may not appear later (Fig. 10.10).

Treatment begun between three and seven days usually attenuates the infection both systemically and locally, but is too late to prevent bone destruction (Fig. 10.11).

Treatment instituted after the first week of illness may control the septicemia and therefore still be life-saving, but it has little effect on the relentless progression of the local pathological process within the bone (Fig. 10.8).

2. *The effectiveness of the antibacterial drug against the specific causative bacteria.* This depends on whether the bacteria is

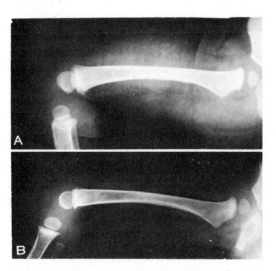

Figure 10.10. Complete resolution of acute hematogenous osteomyelitis of the femur following early adequate treatment. *A,* two days after the onset of pain in the lower end of the thigh of a young child. There is soft tissue swelling but no evidence of bone destruction. At this time the child was acutely ill and exhibited the classical signs of acute hematogenous osteomyelitis. *B,* one month later there is no evidence of bony changes, because the osteomyelitis had been completely controlled by effective antibacterial therapy that had been instituted within the first three days of its onset.

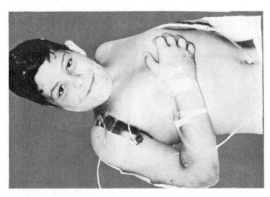

Figure 10.9. Ten-year-old boy two days after surgical decompression of an area of osteomyelitis of the upper end of the right humerus. You will observe from the boy's facial expression that he is completely comfortable. Note the continuous intravenous infusion in the right forearm, the plastic tube for infusion in the region of the shoulder and the second plastic tube at the lower end of the wound for continuous drainage. The incision, which has been closed, is under the blood stained dressing.

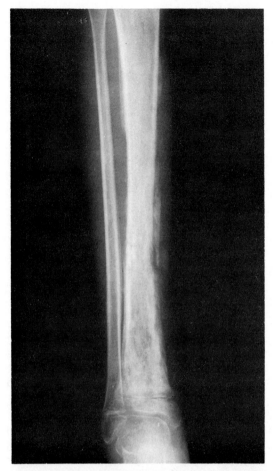

Figure 10.11. Right tibia of a child with acute hematogenous osteomyelitis 5 weeks after the onset of infection. Treatment had been started 5 days after the onset of symptoms and although the infection had been controlled systemically, the treatment was started too late to prevent bone destruction. Note evidence of destruction in the distal two-thirds of the tibia and also the subperiosteal new bone formation.

sensitive to the drug or resistant to it, and emphasizes the importance of culture and sensitivity studies.

3. *The dosage of the antibacterial drug.* The local factor of compromised circulation within the area of bone infection necessitates much larger doses of antibacterial drugs for osteomyelitis than for soft tissue infections.

4. *The duration of antibacterial therapy.* Premature cessation of therapy, especially

under four weeks, frequently results in either chronic or recurrent osteomyelitis.

COMPLICATIONS OF ACUTE HEMATOGENOUS OSTEOMYELITIS

The early *complications* include: (1) *death* from the associated septicemia; (2) *abscess formation*, (3) *septic arthritis*, especially in the hip joint.

The *late complications* include: (1) *chronic osteomyelitis* either persistent or recurrent; (2) *pathological fracture* through a weakened area of bone; (3) *joint contracture*; (4) *local growth disturbance* of the involved bone, either overgrowth from the stimulation of prolonged hyperemia, or premature cessation of growth from epiphyseal plate damage. (Fig. 10.12)

Chronic Hematogenous Osteomyelitis

Inadequate treatment of the acute phase of hematogenous osteomyelitis allows the

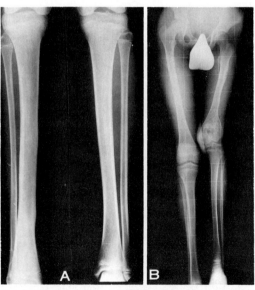

Figure 10.12. Local growth disturbance in the involved bone complicating osteomyelitis. *A*, overgrowth of the right tibia in a 14-year-old girl with chronic osteomyelitis involving the distal end of the tibia. The infection has been chronic for 5 years. *B*, premature cessation of growth in the left lower femoral epiphysis complicating osteomyelitis in early childhood. In this full length radiograph (orthroentogenogram) a severe leg length discrepancy is apparent.

local pathological process either to persist and become chronic or to become relatively quiescent for a time, only to recur, or flare up at a later date. Both the persistent chronic form and the recurrent chronic form of osteomyelitis are exceedingly difficult to eradicate.

INCIDENCE

The continuing prevalence of chronic hematogenous osteomyelitis testifies to the frequent failure to diagnose acute osteomyelitis within the first few days of onset as well as the failure to provide effective antibacterial therapy and the failure to intervene surgically, when indicated, in the acute phase.

PATHOGENESIS AND PATHOLOGY

The most significant pathological lesion in the chronic phase of hematogenous osteomyelitis, and the one which prevents its spontaneous resolution, is *infected dead bone.* Unlike a segment of sterile dead bone, which is gradually revascularized, resorbed and replaced by living bone, infected dead bone always separates, or sequestrates from the remaining living bone and thus becomes a *sequestrum.* Bacteria are able to survive and continue to multiply within the tiny Haversian canals and canaliculi of this island of avascular bone; the surrounding lake of pus prevents revascularization of the sequestrum and thereby protects its bacterial inhabitants not only from the living leukocytes of the defensive inflammatory reaction, but also from the action of circulating antibacterial drugs. Furthermore, in the absence of revascularization, the living process of osteoclastic resorption of dead bone cannot reach the sequestrum. As a result, the sequestrum persists as a haven for bacteria and a source of either persistent or recurrent infection. Thus, the infection cannot be permanently eradicated until all sequestra have been eliminated, either by the natural process of spontaneous extrusion through an opening (*cloaca*) in the *involucrum* and thence through a *sinus track* to the exterior, or by surgical removal (*sequestrectomy*). An area of persistent infection within cancellous bone may eventually become walled off from the surrounding bone by fibrous tissue to form a chronic bone abscess (*Brodie's abscess*).

CLINICAL FEATURES AND DIAGNOSIS

The child, having recovered from the septicemia of the acute phase, is no longer acutely ill but has a residual painful lesion in the involved long bone associated with swelling, tenderness and loss of function of the limb; there may be one or more draining sinuses (Fig. 10.13).

The radiographic diagnosis is usually apparent, particularly in the presence of obvious sequestra (Fig. 10.14). Nevertheless, the combination of local rarefaction, sclerosis and periosteal new bone formation

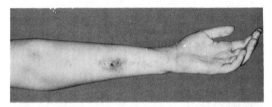

Figure 10.13. Draining sinus in the forearm of a child with chronic osteomyelitis. This type of sinus will not heal until all infected bone (sequestra) have been removed.

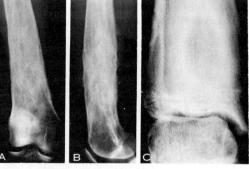

Figure 10.14. *A* and *B*, residual chronic osteomyelitis with several small sequestra in the lower end of the femur of a 40-year-old woman who had acute hematogenous osteomyelitis in this site at age 10 years. *C*, Brodie's abscess in the distal end of the tibia in a young adult. The osteolytic lesion is not unlike that of an osteolytic bone neoplasm.

may mimic other bone lesions such as osteosarcoma, Ewing's sarcoma and eosinophilic granuloma. The radiographic appearance of a Brodie's abscess is not unlike that of an osteolytic bone neoplasm (Fig. 10.14). In the presence of a draining sinus, a sinogram often helps locate the site of underlying infection (Fig. 10.15).

Persistent anemia and elevation of the sedimentation rate reflect the chronic infection.

TREATMENT

Chronic osteomyelitis can seldom be completely eradicated until all the infected dead bone not only has separated, or sequestrated, but also has either been extruded spontaneously through a sinus tract or been removed surgically (*sequestrectomy*). Antibacterial therapy is required both systemically and locally. A residual abscess cavity

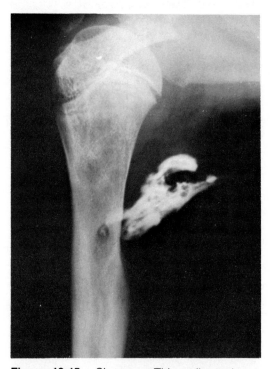

Figure 10.15. Sinogram. This radiograph was taken after radiopaque material had been injected into a draining sinus in the axilla. Note that the contrast medium tracks along the sinus to a small area of osteolysis in the shaft of the humerus. Note also a small sequestrum lying within the osteolytic area.

within the bone usually necessitates an operation in which one surface of the tubular bone is removed to make it open like a saucer (*saucerization*). Following either sequestrectomy or saucerization, antibacterial drugs and a detergent, such as alevaire, are instilled into the area in saline solution by continuous infusion, and pus is removed by drainage. Occasionally, reconstructive operations such as bone grafting and skin grafting are required later to overcome a residual defect in the bone and soft tissues.

COMPLICATIONS

The complications of persistent chronic osteomyelitis include: (1) *joint contracture*; (2) *pathological fracture*; (3) *amyloid disease*; (4) malignant changes in the epidermis (*epidermoid carcinoma*) of a sinus tract in which infection has been allowed to persist for many years.

Acute Septic Arthritis (Pyogenic Arthritis)

When pyogenic bacteria invade a synovial joint, the result is acute septic (pyogenic) arthritis, a rapidly progressive infection which, unless adequately treated, leads to severe destruction of the joint.

INCIDENCE

The incidence of septic arthritis parallels that of hematogenous osteomyelitis with which it is so frequently associated. Septic arthritis, therefore, is primarily a disease of childhood. Newborn infants are particularly susceptible and especially those who have an immunodeficiency, as suggested by Kuo and Lloyd-Roberts. During childhood, the commonest sites are those in which the metaphysis of the bone is entirely intracapsular, namely the hip and the elbow (Fig. 10.3). In adult life, septic arthritis can develop in any joint because it is unrelated to osteomyelitis; the incidence is higher in adults receiving prolonged adrenocorticosteroid therapy.

ETIOLOGY

The spread of pyogenic bacteria from hematogenous osteomyelitis in the metaphysis directly into the joint is the commonest source of septic arthritis in children.

Consequently, as in osteomyelitis, the most frequent causative organism is *Staphylococcus aureus*. However, bacteria, particularly Streptococci and pneumococci and less commonly *Hemophilus influenzae* and Salmonella, may reach the joint by the bloodstream to produce hematogenous septic arthritis. In adults, Staphylococci, pneumococci and gonococci may also invade a synovial joint by the hematogenous route as a complication of systemic infection.

PATHOGENESIS AND PATHOLOGY

Acute septic arthritis is an extremely serious infection because the purulent exudate—particularly that of Staphylococci—rapidly digests articular cartilage. The mechanism of initial cartilage destruction includes enzymatic digestion of the matrix by lysosomal enzymes from both polymorphonuclear leukocytes and bacteria. As a result, the collagen fibers lose their support and the cartilage disintegrates. Granulation tissue may creep over the articular cartilage as a *pannus*, blocking its nutrition from synovial fluid and thereby leading to even further destruction. Since cartilage is virtually incapable of regeneration under ordinary circumstances, its destruction is not only devastating but also permanent. The inflamed synovial membrane becomes grossly swollen. As the joint becomes filled with pus, the fibrous capsule softens and stretches with the result that a pathological dislocation may ensue, particularly in the hip joint of infants and children. Furthermore, in the hip joint, the increased intra-articular fluid pressure of the pus frequently occludes the precarious blood supply to the bone with resultant necrosis of the femoral head. The infantile femoral head, being entirely cartilaginous, may be completely destroyed. Late sequelae of inadequately treated septic arthritis include degenerative joint disease, fibrous ankylosis and occasionally, bony ankylosis.

CLINICAL FEATURES AND DIAGNOSIS

The clinical manifestations of acute septic arthritis in infants are significantly different from those in older children or adults and are best considered separately.

SEPTIC ARTHRITIS IN INFANTS

During infancy, particularly in the newborn period, acute septic arthritis may develop with few clinical manifestations other than irritability of the infant. Local examination reveals tenderness over the joint and obviously painful restriction of joint motion (Fig. 10.16). Fever and elevation of the white blood cell count are misleadingly slight in this age group and unless the major joints of the limbs are examined daily during any febrile illness, the diagnosis of septic arthritis may not be made sufficiently early to prevent necrosis of the femoral head and irreparable damage to the joint. Clinical suspicion of acute septic arthritis is an urgent indication for immediate needle aspiration of the joint, as a valuable diagnostic procedure and as a means of obtaining fluid from the joint for culture.

Radiographic examination during the first week may reveal evidence of soft tissue swelling, but not until the second week is there evidence of a pathological dislocation (Fig. 10.17). Equally delayed are the radiographic changes of osteomyelitis in the intracapsular part of the metaphysis (Fig. 10.18).

SEPTIC ARTHRITIS IN OLDER CHILDREN AND ADULTS

Unlike the uncommunicative infant, the older child or adult with septic arthritis is able to tell you of severe pain in the region of the involved joint and, furthermore, that

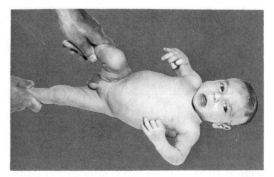

Figure 10.16. Acute septic arthritis of the right hip in an infant. The right hip is held in flexion and abduction and the infant resists passive movement of the hip because of pain.

of the disease are relatively mild and there is little suppuration. Another, and more descriptive term, is *spondylarthritis*, which signifies that the adjacent intervertebral disc is invariably involved and partially destroyed.

The commonest sites are the vertebrae of the lower thoracic and upper lumbar spine, which raises the suspicion that the route of the infection may be via Batson's plexus of paravertebral veins. *Staphylococcus aureus* and *Escherichia coli* are the most frequent causative organisms.

CLINICAL FEATURES AND DIAGNOSIS

In childhood the first symptom is poorly localized back pain, and this is accompanied by the physical signs of protective muscle spasm in the back and local deep tenderness. There may even be signs of meningeal irritation (painful limitation of neck flexion and straight-leg raising). The child is frequently reluctant to sit up or stand and is always reluctant to bend forward (Fig. 10.21).

Systemic manifestations include irritability and loss of appetite but fever is usually mild. The white blood cell count is frequently normal, but the sedimentation rate is always elevated.

Radiographic examination of the spine within the first two weeks of illness fails to reveal any bony abnormality but during this period a bone scan may be helpful (as discussed in Chapter 5). Subsequently, narrowing of the adjacent intervertebral disc space and osteolysis of the involved vertebra become obvious (Fig. 10.22).

The most important differential diagnosis is spinal tuberculosis, which can be excluded if the tuberculin skin test is negative. Vertebral punch biopsy (under anesthesia and with radiographic control) may be necessary to confirm the diagnosis of osteomyelitis, but is safe only in the lumbar region.

In adults afflicted with osteomyelitis of the spine, severe back pain is a prominent feature. The physical signs are similar to those seen in children, but the systemic reaction to the infection is usually more marked. As with children, the radiographic findings of osteolysis of the vertebral body and narrow-

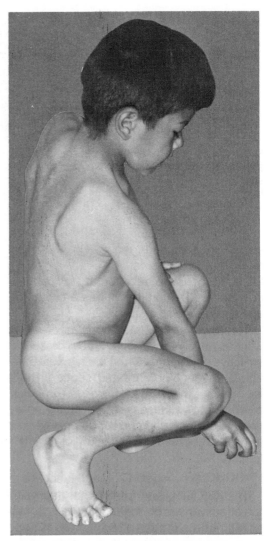

Figure 10.21. Boy with hematogenous osteomyelitis of the spine. On attempting to pick something up from the floor he keeps his spine perfectly straight because of pain and muscle spasm in the lumbar region, the site of osteomyelitis.

ing of the intervertebral disc space become obvious only after the first two weeks of illness (Fig. 10.23).

TREATMENT AND PROGNOSIS

The general plan of treatment for acute hematogenous osteomyelitis of the spine is similar to that described (in a previous section of this chapter) for osteomyelitis of the long bones.

Bed rest for the patient is supplemented

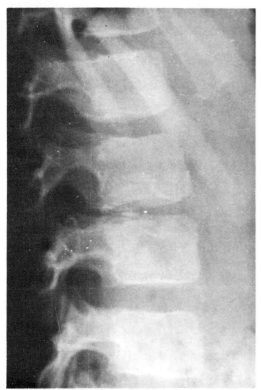

Figure 10.22. Hematogenous osteomyelitis of the lumbar spine in a 7-year-old child. Note the marked narrowing of the involved intervertebral disc space and the osteolytic lesions in the adjacent vertebral bodies.

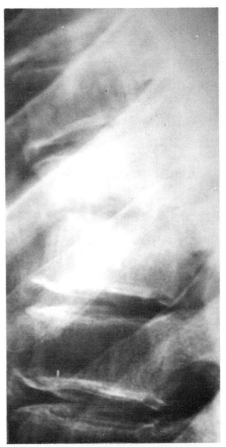

Figure 10.23. Osteomyelitis of the thoracic spine in a 41-year-old adult. Note the marked destruction of the intervertebral disc space and the destruction of the adjacent portions of the involved vertebral bodies.

by local rest for the spine, which is provided by a body cast. Operative drainage of the vertebra and disc space is indicated only if non-operative treatment fails to control the infection; it is seldom necessary.

In children the involved disc space remains permanently narrow but seldom fuses spontaneously, whereas in adults, spontaneous fusion is more frequent. Occasionally, persistent or recurrent back pain arising from the abnormal segment necessitates local spinal fusion.

Osteomyelitis and Septic Arthritis Secondary to Wounds

Bone and joint infection secondary to wounds, whether accidental or surgical, is caused by pathogenic bacteria which have gained access to the skeletal tissues directly from the outside environment. This *exoge-*

nous type of infection, in contradistinction to the hematogenous or endogenous type, can develop in any site and at any age.

Pathogenic bacteria may reach a bone or joint through a variety of wounds, such as a penetrating wound produced by a high velocity missile or even a small puncture wound produced by a sharp object (Fig. 10.24). Furthermore, all open (''compound'') fractures and joint injuries are obviously contaminated by exogenous bacteria and consequently carry the risk of serious infection. Likewise, closed (''simple'') fractures and joint injuries that are treated by operation (*open reduction*) may become infected. Indeed, any operation carries this risk, but it

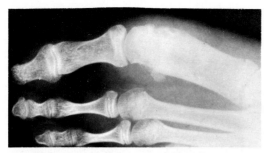

Figure 10.24. Osteomyelitis in the neck of the first metatarsal secondary to a puncture wound in the sole of the foot. This child's puncture wound had occurred 6 months previously and she had experienced recurring pain and swelling in the foot since that time. Note the areas of osteolysis and sclerosis in the neck of the metatarsal. The commonest infecting bacteria in puncture wounds of the foot is Pseudomonas.

is particularly significant in the musculo-skeletal system because the sequelae of bone and joint infection are so serious.

Synovial joints are particularly susceptible to infection and therefore, even simple needle aspiration of a joint demands rigid aseptic precautions. In children with a bacteremia the practice of obtaining a blood sample by femoral artery or vein puncture directly over the hip joint is potentially dangerous because the needle may traverse the vessel, penetrate the joint and thereby inoculate it with bacteria.

The pathological and clinical features of established exogenous infections of bones and joints are comparable to those of the hematogenous, or endogenous variety, and hence need not be repeated here. The preventive aspects of exogenous infection, however, merit emphasis. Since any wound, large or small, that communicates with skeletal tissues is potentially serious, the most important therapeutic aspect of such wounds is careful wound cleansing and, when necessary, debridement of devitalized tissues in an attempt to prevent bone and joint infection (Fig. 10.24).

Should infection develop despite preventive measures, you will be alert to the first manifestations and will be able to institute appropriate therapy at the earliest possible moment. This exogenous type of infection,

once established, does not respond to antibacterial therapy alone and requires exploration of the wound, removal of necrotic tissue, adequate drainage of pus and the local instillation of antibiotic drugs and a detergent.

Pyogenic Infections in the Hand

The soft tissues of the hand are frequently infected by pyogenic bacteria because of the high incidence of minor hand injuries such as lacerations and puncture wounds. Such infections are not only common, but are also potentially serious, since they may spread to the bones, joints or tendon sheaths.

Soft tissue infections in the hand include the following three groups: (1) those involving the nail fold (paronychia) (Fig. 10.25A); (2) those involving potential spaces in the hand—the pulp space (felon) (Fig. 10.25B), the thenar space (Fig. 10.26A) and the mid-palmar space (Fig. 10.26B); (3) those involving a tendon sheath (pyogenic tenosynovitis). Of these, pyogenic tenosynovitis is the most serious and deserves special mention.

PYOGENIC TENOSYNOVITIS

Etiology

Laceration and puncture wounds provide the portal of entry to the tendon sheath for pathogenic bacteria, the most common of which is *Staphylococcus aureus*.

Pathogenesis and Pathology

The synovial lining of a tendon sheath is comparable to the synovial lining of a joint and responds in the same manner to

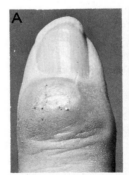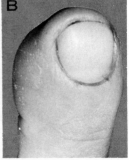

Figure 10.25. *A*, paronychia. *B*, pulp space infection (Felon).

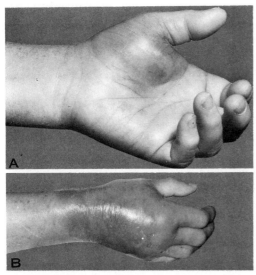

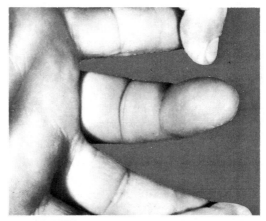

Figure 10.27. Pyogenic tenosynovitis of the finger. Note that the involved finger is swollen and tends to assume a flexed position because of the tension in the inflamed synovial sheath.

Figure 10.26. *A*, thenar space infection. *B*, midpalmar space infection. The swelling rapidly extends to the dorsum of the hand where the areolar planes are loosely arranged.

pyogenic infection, namely by edema, hypertrophy and production of a synovial effusion. The inflamed synovial sheath becomes progressively distended by pus under pressure, which explains the semi-flexed position of the digit, a position in which the synovial sheath can accept the greatest volume of fluid. The blood supply to the tendon may be compromised with resultant tendon necrosis. In the later stages of untreated tenosynovitis, fibrous adhesions between the tendon and its enveloping sheath lead to permanent loss of motion in the involved digit.

Clinical Features and Diagnosis

The symptom of severe local pain and the signs of local swelling, tenderness and severe pain with any passive movement of the digit are readily understood on the basis of the underlying pathological process (Fig. 10.27). Elevation of temperature, white blood cell count and sedimentation rate indicate the systemic reaction to the infection.

Treatment

Pyogenic tenosynovitis requires the same plan of systemic and local treatment as that described (in a previous section of this chap-

ter) for acute hematogenous osteomyelitis. Early operative treatment (through an incision along one side of the digit) is as important for tenosynovitis as for septic (pyogenic) arthritis; pus is evacuated and, in addition, continuous drainage and instillation of antibacterial drugs are instituted in an attempt to preserve the tendon as well as the motion between it and its sheath.

GRANULOMATOUS BACTERIAL INFECTIONS

The terms *granulomatous* or *granuloma-producing* infections refer to a group of chronic inflammatory conditions, some of which are caused by *bacteria*, such as tuberculosis and syphilis and others by *fungi*, such as actinomycosis.

The inflammatory reaction incited by these granulomatous infections is chronic from the beginning, since the *productive* element of inflammation predominates the exudative element. Characteristic of this type of chronic inflammation is the reaction of the local tissue cells (histiocytes including epithelioid cells), which collect to produce small discrete lesions about the size of a *granule* (1 to 2 mm); hence the terms granulomatous or granuloma-producing infections. As the inflammatory reaction progresses, more granules are produced and these subsequently coalesce to form progressively larger lesions.

Of the granulomatous infections involving the musculoskeletal system, the most important is tuberculosis.

Tuberculous Infections: General Features

Improved public health measures concerning prevention and early detection of tuberculosis, as well as the development of effective antituberculous drugs, both have been important factors in the striking reduction of *mortality* and *morbidity* of tuberculous infection. However, the *incidence* of this potentially serious infection has not been reduced so strikingly, even in well developed countries; indeed, in some of the developing countries of the world, tuberculosis continues to be a common and serious problem.

ESTABLISHMENT OF INFECTION

In the past the bovine type of tubercle bacillus, present in the milk of tuberculous cows and ingested by children, was the main cause of tuberculosis involving bowel, lymph nodes, bones and joints. Fortunately, in most areas, this has been well controlled by enforced inspection and tuberculin testing of dairy herds, as well as pasteurization of milk.

At present the human type of tubercle bacillus is responsible for virtually all tuberculous infection in man; the initial, or primary, lesion is in the lung. The mode of infection is inhalation of air and dust particles that contain bacilli from the coughing of a tuberculous patient with a positive sputum. The initial infection usually occurs during childhood in areas where tuberculosis is common; but in areas of low incidence, the initial infection may occur in adult life.

Within the lung the tubercle bacilli incite a granulomatous type of inflammatory reaction. A *miliary tubercle* is formed by histiocytes which, being phagocytic macrophages, engulf the bacilli. Nevertheless, even in this intracellular environment, tubercle bacilli are able to survive and multiply. Groups of macrophages may fuse to form *giant cells*, which are a characteristic part of the histological picture. Since the tubercle is

relatively avascular, its central portion eventually becomes caseous (cheese-like) due to *coagulation necrosis*. Later, the caseous material *liquifies* but all the while the tubercle bacilli continue to multiply.

The child's defense reactions may be sufficiently strong to heal the tubercle by fibrosis with subsequent calcification; indeed, radiographs of the lungs reveal evidence of such healed primary lesions in many apparently healthy individuals (Fig. 10.28). Nevertheless, even in healed tubercles, living tubercle bacilli tend to persist in a dormant state and are capable of *reactivation*, particularly if the defense reaction, or resistance, of the patient is weakened by such factors as poor nutrition and chronic fatigue.

PRINCIPLES OF ANTITUBERCULOUS THERAPY

For many years prior to the development of antituberculous chemotherapy, the traditional treatment of musculoskeletal tuberculosis centered on prolonged immobilization of the involved joint(s) and often total recumbency in a sanitorium. Fortunately, these unphysiological and demoralizing forms of non-specific treatment have been replaced by aggressive chemotherapy. Streptomycin was the first chemotherapeutic agent found to be effective against tu-

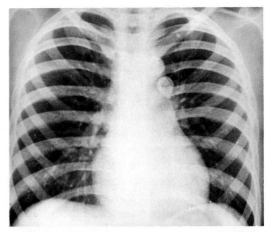

Figure 10.28. Healed primary lesions of tuberculosis in a young adult. Note the two calcified lesions in the left side of the chest along the left side of the heart.

berculosis. Because of the emergence of resistant organisms, however, streptomycin was usually administered in combination with isonicotinic acid hydrazide (INH) and *para*-aminosalicylic acid (PAS). Currently rifampicin is the most effective antituberculous agent and is usually used instead of PAS; indeed, it has almost replaced streptomycin as well. Thus, rifampicin is given in combination with INH, with or without streptomycin. These antituberculous drugs are reasonably effective against early lesions; but once the tubercle bacilli are enclosed within an avascular caseous lesion, they are protected from the action of blood-borne drugs. This fact emphasizes the importance of early diagnosis and the institution of antituberculous drug therapy in the earliest stages of the tuberculous infection. Because of the chronic nature of the infection the combined antituberculous chemotherapy is continued for at least one full year.

The avascularity of well established tuberculous lesions explains the necessity for bold surgical excision of diseased tissues and evacuation of the pus of "cold abscesses."

Tuberculous Osteomyelitis

Tuberculous osteomyelitis, or bone tuberculosis, is always secondary to a tuberculous lesion elsewhere in the body. Like hematogenous pyogenic osteomyelitis, it is a blood-borne infection and usually afflicts children; by contrast, however, tuberculous osteomyelitis, rather than developing in the metaphyseal region of long bones, develops most frequently in vertebral bodies (*tuberculous spondylitis*).

Hematogenous tuberculous osteomyelitis may also develop in the *epiphyses* of long bones and spread into the joint to produce a tuberculous arthritis; sometimes the reverse is true in that the infection in a tuberculous joint spreads into the epiphysis. (Tuberculous arthritis is discussed in a subsequent section of this chapter.) Occasionally, particularly in young children, hematogenous tuberculous osteomyelitis involves the shaft, or diaphysis, of a phalanx (tuberculous dactylitis).

Tuberculosis of the spine merits special attention.

TUBERCULOUS OSTEOMYELITIS OF THE SPINE (TUBERCULOUS SPONDYLITIS) (POTT'S DISEASE)

Tuberculosis of the spine, which accounts for more than half of all bone and joint tuberculosis, usually begins during early childhood. The commonest sites are the lower thoracic and upper lumbar vertebrae and in these sites, as suggested by Hodgson, it is probably secondary to urinary tract tuberculosis, the hematogenous route being Batson's plexus of paravertebral veins.

Pathogenesis and Pathology

The tuberculous infection, a specific type of granulomatous inflammation, is characterized by slowly progressive bone destruction (*local osteolysis*) in the anterior part of a vertebral body and is accompanied by regional osteoporosis. Spreading caseation prevents reactive new bone formation and at the same time renders segments of bone avascular, thereby producing *tuberculous sequestra*, particularly in the thoracic region.

Gradually, *tuberculous granulation tissue* penetrates the thin cortex of the vertebral body to produce a *paravertebral abscess* which spans several vertebrae. In addition, the infection spreads up and down the spine under the anterior and posterior longitudinal ligaments. The intervertebral discs, being avascular, are relatively resistant to tuberculous infection; initially, the adjacent disc becomes narrowed due to dehydration but eventually it may be partially destroyed by tuberculous granulation tissue. Progressive destruction of bone anteriorly and resultant anterior collapse of the involved vertebral bodies lead to progressive *kyphosis* (posterior angulation) of the spine (Fig. 10.29).

Clinical Features and Diagnosis

The patient, usually a child, experiences back pain and is reluctant to sit up, stand up or bend forward, precisely like a child with hematogenous osteomyelitis of the spine (Fig. 10.21). Local deep tenderness is readily elicited and protective muscle spasm is apparent. Systemic manifestations include

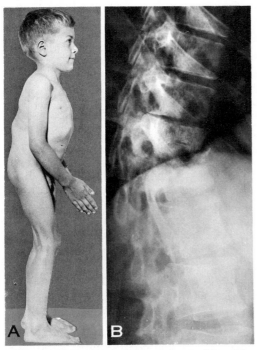

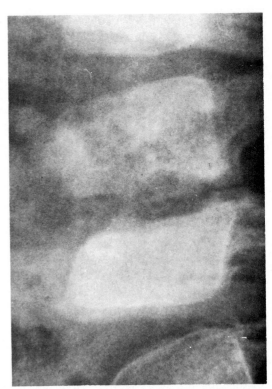

Figure 10.29.   Tuberculous osteomyelitis of the spine. *A*, posterior angulation (kyphosis) due to collapse of the anterior portion of the vertebral bodies in the lumbar region. This type of deformity is sometimes referred to as a "gibbus." *B*, tuberculous osteomyelitis of the spine in the lumbar region. Note the anterior destruction of adjacent vertebral bodies and the resultant anterior collapse with production of a kyphotic deformity. In this lateral radiograph there is also evidence of involvement of the two vertebral bodies above the major area of disease.

Figure 10.30.   Early tuberculous osteomyelitis of the spine in a child. In the lateral radiograph there is obvious narrowing of the intervertebral disc space and osteolytic lesions in the anterior portions of the adjacent vertebral bodies.

chronic ill health and usually evidence of either pulmonary or urinary tract tuberculosis. The sedimentation rate is elevated and the tuberculin skin test is positive.

Radiographic examination of the spine in the early stages reveals an osteolytic lesion in the anterior part of a vertebral body, regional osteoporosis and narrowing of the adjacent intervertebral disc (Fig. 10.30). At a more advanced stage there is evidence of extensive anterior destruction, involvement of other vertebrae and a paravertebral abscess (Fig. 10.31).

The diagnosis can be confirmed by aspiration of paravertebral "pus," which is studied microscopically for tubercle bacilli and

also inoculated into a guinea pig. The sensitivity of the causative tubercle bacillus to various antituberculous drugs should be determined. Tissue obtained either by closed punch biopsy or open surgical biopsy reveals the typical histological picture of tuberculous infection.

Treatment

The care of a patient with tuberculosis of the spine includes the treatment of generalized tuberculosis—antituberculous drugs, general rest, nourishing diet—as well as the treatment of the local disease in the spine by local rest on a turning frame or in a plaster bed. After one month of drug therapy and local rest, the spinal lesion is most effectively treated by bold, direct open operation to evacuate the tuberculous "pus," to remove tuberculous sequestra as well as diseased bone, and to fuse the involved segments of

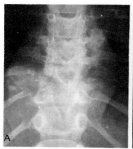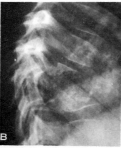

Figure 10.31. Extensive tuberculous osteo-myelitis of the lower thoracic spine with a para-vertebral abscess in a child. *A*, the bulbous soft tissue swelling on each side of the spine represents a paravertebral abscess. Note also the marked destruction of vertebral bodies. *B*, in the lateral radiograph there is evidence of destruction of two vertebral bodies with resultant anterior collapse of the spine and a kyphotic deformity.

the spine, preferably by anterior interbody fusion using autogenous bone grafts.

In countries where adequate surgical facilities are lacking, an acceptable alternative is antituberculous chemotherapy combined with a spinal brace or cast.

Complications of Tuberculous Spondylitis

The most serious complication of spinal tuberculosis is *paraplegia* (Pott's paraplegia) which may occur either early or late in the course of the disease. The *paraplegia of active disease* develops relatively early; it can result either from extradural pressure (tuberculous "pus," sequestra, sequestrated intervertebral disc) or from direct involvement of the spinal cord by tuberculous granulation tissue. Under the latter circumstances, the prognosis for recovery is poor. The *paraplegia of healed disease* always develops late; it can result either from the gradual development of a bony ridge which impinges on the spinal canal or form progressive fibrosis of tuberculous granulation tissue. Myelography is helpful in differentiating between the pressure type of paraplegia (which can be alleviated surgically) and paraplegia due to invasion of the dura and spinal cord.

The development of paraplegia due to pressure during the course of spinal tuberculosis represents a relative emergency which should be treated by surgical decompression of the spinal cord and nerve roots.

A less common complication is rupture of a thoracic paravertebral abscess into the pleura to produce a *tuberculous empyema*. In the lumbar region, tuberculous "pus" may enter the iliopsoas muscle and track distally as a *psoas abscess*, which is an example of a "cold abscess."

Tuberculous Arthritis

Tubercle bacilli may infect a synovial joint by hematogenous spread from a distant tuberculous lesion. More commonly, however, tuberculous arthritis is caused by direct extension of infection into the joint from an area of tuberculous osteomyelitis in the epiphysis; although the underlying epiphyseal lesion may be too small to be detected radiographically, it can usually be seen at operation.

Any synovial joint can be affected but the two most common sites are the hip and the knee. As with tuberculosis in other tissues, the onset is nearly always in childhood.

Pathogenesis and Pathology

The synovial membrane responds to tuberculous infection by villous hypertrophy and an effusion with resultant distension of the joint capsule. Small greyish *tubercles* may be seen on the inflamed synovial surface. Later, tuberculous granulation tissue creeps across the joint surfaces as a *tuberculous pannus* which deprives the articular cartilage of its nutrition from the synovial fluid and thereby causes *cartilage necrosis*. In addition, tuberculous granulation tissue erodes subchondral bone to produce a local area of tuberculous osteomyelitis with subsequent collapse of bone. It also burrows under the articular cartilage causing the cartilage to sequestrate. The combination of cartilage necrosis and destruction of the underlying bone leads to irreparable joint damage.

Clinical Features and Diagnosis

The patient, usually a child, presents with a chronically irritable joint; when the involved joint is in the lower limb, there is an obvious limp. Painful limitation of joint motion, protective muscle spasm and muscle atrophy are apparent. The sedimentation rate is elevated and the tuberculin skin test is positive.

Radiographic examination in the early stages reveals regional osteoporosis as well as evidence of soft tissue swelling around the joint. In the later stages, osteolytic lesions in the epiphysis become apparent (Fig. 10.32). Eventually, loss of the radiographic cartilage space indicates that the articular cartilage has been destroyed (Fig. 10.33).

The diagnosis can be proven by open surgical biopsy of the synovial membrane; the joint fluid obtained at the time of operation is also studied microscopically, as well as inoculated into a guinea pig, in order to

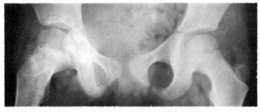

Figure 10.32. Tuberculous arthritis of the right hip in a child. Note the regional osteoporosis as well as small osteolytic lesions in the epiphysis.

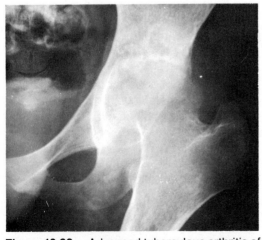

Figure 10.33. Advanced tuberculous arthritis of the left hip in a young adult. There has been considerable destruction of the femoral head. The cartilage space has almost disappeared, indicating destruction of articular cartilage.

isolate the causative tubercle bacillus and subsequently test its sensitivity to the various antituberculous drugs.

Treatment

The care of a patient with tuberculous arthritis involves the treatment of generalized tuberculosis—antituberculous drugs, general rest, nourishing diet—as well as the treatment of the local arthritis. During the early stages of tuberculous arthritis while the infection is predominantly synovial, adequate treatment can prevent damage to joint cartilage and underlying bone and can thereby preserve joint function, particularly in children.

Once the articular cartilage is destroyed, however, the joint is irreparably damaged and, consequently, surgical fusion (*arthrodesis*) of the joint is required, not only to relieve the pain in the arthritic joint but also to bring about permanent healing of the tuberculous infection.

NON-SPECIFIC INFLAMMATORY DISORDERS OF JOINTS

A wide variety of clinical conditions, all of which cause *pain and stiffness in the musculoskeletal system*, are commonly grouped under the broad heading of "*rheumatic diseases*." In the majority of these diseases the predominant lesion is articular (*arthritis, articular rheumatism*), whereas in others it is extra-articular (*nonarticular rheumatism*). Although the venerable term "rheumatism" has no pathological significance, its use is so prevalent that, for want of a better term, it has persisted. (The term "rheumatism" is derived from the Greek word *rheumatismos*, a "flowing of an evil body humor," that was thought to go from the brain to the joints and other parts of the body producing pain). Thus, the clinical study of rheumatic diseases constitutes the medical specialty of *rheumatology* and specialists in internal medicine who devote themselves to the medical care of arthritis and allied conditions are known as *rheumatologists*.

Of course, many others, including family physicians, orthopaedic surgeons, rehabilitation physicians (physiatrists), physiotherapists, occupational therapists and social workers, also share an interest and a responsibility in the over-all management of this unfortunate group of patients.

Classification of Rheumatic Diseases

The large number and variety of clinical diseases that are capable of causing "pain and stiffness in the musculoskeletal system" make their classification difficult and somewhat unsatisfactory. An exhaustive—and exhausting—classification compiled by a committee of the American Rheumatism Association comprises 13 major headings and over 130 sub-headings and individual disorders (See Rodnan, G. P. reference.) The major headings are presented here for the sake of standardized nomenclature.

1. Polyarthritis of unknown etiology
2. "Connective tissue" disorders
3. Rheumatic fever
4. Degenerative joint disease (discussed in Chapter 11)
5. Nonarticular rheumatism (discussed in Chapter 11)
6. Diseases with which arthritis is frequently associated
7. Associated with known infectious agents
8. Traumatic and/or neurogenic disorders (discussed in Chapter 11)
9. Associated with known biochemical or endocrine abnormalities
10. Tumor and tumor-like conditions (discussed in Chapter 14)
11. Allergy and drug reactions
12. Inherited and congenital disorders
13. Miscellaneous disorders

The diseases in which arthritis is the predominant feature can be grouped in the following simple working classification:

1. Inflammatory polyarthritis of unknown etiology, including rheumatoid arthritis, ankylosing spondylitis, rheumatic fever
2. Degenerative joint disease, also called osteoarthritis and osteoarthrosis
3. Infectious arthritis, including septic (pyogenic) arthritis, tuberculous arthritis
4. Traumatic arthritis, secondary to fractures and joint injuries

5. Metabolic arthritis, including gout

From the onset you should appreciate that degenerative joint disease represents a slowly progressive deterioration of a given joint and can be secondary to *any* local disturbance of joint structure and function. Therefore, in a given joint, residual abnormalities from *any other* type of arthritis can initiate the process of degenerative joint disease which is then superimposed upon the original condition.

Prevalence of the Rheumatic Diseases

The rheumatic diseases lead all causes of crippling and economic loss in the general population and therefore represent a major health problem. For example, it has been estimated that over 6% of all persons in North America suffer at some time from arthritis or rheumatism. Since the overall incidence of rheumatic diseases increases with age, increasing longevity will render this particular health problem even more prevalent in the future than it has been in the past.

Rheumatoid Arthritis

Rheumatoid arthritis, which is one type of inflammatory polyarthritis, is characterized by a variable but usually prolonged course with exacerbations and remissions of joint pains and swelling which frequently lead to progressive deformities and may even lead to permanent disability. The arthritis is the dominant clinical manifestation of a more generalized systemic disease of connective tissue (*rheumatoid disease*).

Buchanan has stated that while there is good historical evidence that *degenerative* joint disease (osteoarthritis) has afflicted man for at least 40,000 years, and probably much longer, *rheumatoid* arthritis would seem to have appeared as a relatively new disease in man only 200 years ago.

INCIDENCE

Rheumatoid arthritis is relatively common; indeed, surveys have revealed that approximately 2.5% of the adult population in countries of temperate climate suffer from this disease. Women are afflicted three times more frequently than men and although the disease may begin at almost any age, the peak period of onset is between the ages of 20 and 40 years. The peripheral joints, especially those of the hands, are the most frequent sites of initial involvement by rheumatoid arthritis and the distribution in paired limbs tends to be symmetrical (Fig. 10.34).

ETIOLOGY

Despite intensive clinical and experimental research, the etiology of rheumatoid arthritis has eluded discovery and remains a challenging mystery. However, the observation that this is a relatively new disease has sparked the speculation that the causative agent may be a relatively new microorganism, such as the ubiquitous Epstein-Barr virus or some other virus. Former theories of foci of bacterial infection, vitamin deficiency and hormonal imbalance have been discarded because of lack of scientific proof.

Some of the features of rheumatoid arthritis and the frequent coexistent lesions of rheumatoid disease suggest an exaggeration of normal immune mechanisms, or hypersensitivity—a continuous immunological response to a persistent antigen. In 70% of patients a *rheumatoid factor*, which is a macroglobulin, can be demonstrated by serological means, such as latex and sheep cell agglutin tests. These tests are negative in the early phases of the disease and in most afflicted children, but tend to become positive as the disease progresses. However, the presence of a rheumatoid factor is not only inconsistent in rheumatoid arthritis but also may occur in a variety of unrelated connective tissue diseases. This macroglobulin has been isolated from plasma cells of diseased synovial membrane as well as from regional lymph nodes; this suggests the possibility of an antigenic stimulus which might arise from an altered gamma globulin in the diseased joint, a type of autoimmune mechanism. Nevertheless, these immune responses could be a secondary phenomenon, the result, rather than the cause, of rheumatoid arthritis.

In the past it has been thought that psychological factors may predispose an individual to this disease. The anxiety-ridden and depressed person who tends to suppress feelings of hostility and aggression seemed more prone to develop rheumatoid arthritis than the average, while the psychotic individual seemed less prone. However, the current consensus is that these psychological or personality traits are an understandable reaction to the disease, i.e. an effect, or result rather than a factor in its cause. Nevertheless, in a given patient, emotional stress is often followed by an exacerbation of rheumatoid activity.

Obviously much research remains to be done before the significance and interrelationship of the various etiological factors will be understood.

PATHOGENESIS AND PATHOLOGY

The primary "target" of the disease is the synovial membrane of joints and tendon sheaths. This membrane, normally a thin syncitium of cells, reacts to the inflammation by congestion, edema, fibrin exudation, proliferation and villous formation. Polymorphonuclear leukocytes, though present in large numbers in the synovial fluid, are not found in the membrane; the characteristic inflammatory cells in the synovial membrane in

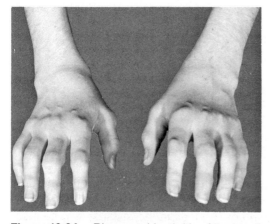

Figure 10.34.   Rheumatoid arthritis of the hands of a 30-year-old woman who has had symptoms for one year. Note the symmetrical involvement in the wrists, metacarpophalangeal joints and proximal interphalangeal joints.

rheumatoid arthritis are monocytes (T and B lymphocytes, plasma cells and macrophages), some of which are grouped in nodular formations with germinal centers.

It is now thought that the T lymphocytes are responsible for cell-mediated immunoregulatory functions while the B lymphocytes become antibody-producing plasma cells. The resultant immune process within the diseased synovium produces immune complexes which, in turn, activate a multitude of chemical mediators of inflammation. In the acute inflammatory exudate in the synovial fluid, polymorphonuclear leukocytes engulf immune complexes but, in so doing, they extrude hydrolytic enzymes (neutral proteases such as cathepsin G, elastase and collagenase) that are capable of degrading the proteoglycans and collagen of cartilage matrix and of thereby inducing an autoimmune response.

Inflammatory granulation tissue infiltrates the subsynovial connective tissue causing it to become swollen and boggy. Even the fibrous capsule and joint ligaments may be involved and, if they become sufficiently softened and stretched, the joint may subluxate or even dislocate. As occurs in other types of inflammation, granulation tissue is eventually replaced by reparative fibrosis or scar formation with resultant *joint contracture* and *deformity*.

The inflammatory granulation tissue also creeps across the joint surface to form a *pannus* which interferes with the normal nutrition of articular cartilage from synovial fluid and causes *cartilage necrosis* (Fig. 10.35). Furthermore, the same tissue erodes subchondral bone at the margins of the joint and burrows beneath the cartilage to produce local areas of *osteolysis* (cysts) in the bone. The remaining bone in the area of the joint exhibits *regional osteoporosis*. If the process continues over a period of months or years, fibrous adhesions eventually form between opposing joint surfaces with a resultant *fibrous ankylosis*. Indeed, the fibrous ankylosis may eventually ossify to become a *bony ankylosis*.

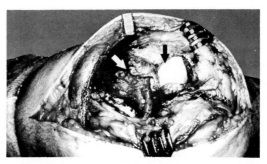

Figure 10.35. The anterior aspect of the left knee at the time of synovectomy. The *black arrow* points to part of the articular surface of the lateral condyle of the femur. The *white arrow* points to the inflammatory granulation tissue that is creeping across the articular cartilage. This pannus had already resulted in some destruction of the underlying cartilage.

The synovial membrane, covering tendons and lining their sheaths, reacts in a similar manner with corresponding disturbance of function. Even the connective tissue elements of the muscles that control the joint become involved by the inflammatory process. Thus, in addition to disuse atrophy of muscle, foci of monocellular infiltrations appear and are subsequently replaced by reparative fibrosis with resultant *contracture* of the muscle, another factor in the pathogenesis of deformity.

Approximately 30% of patients exhibit subcutaneous *rheumatoid nodules* over areas subjected to pressure, particularly in the upper limbs (Fig. 10.36). These extra-articular lesions, which seem to begin as an area of rheumatoid vasculitis with subsequent necrosis, are composed of a central zone of fibrinoid material and cellular debris surrounded by a middle zone of mononuclear cells and an outer zone of granulation tissue.

Other extra-articular lesions of rheumatoid disease may occur in the connective tissue components of the cardiovascular system (pericardial adhesions, myocarditis vasculitis), the reticuloendothelial system and even the respiratory system (pulmonary fibrosis), though they can seldom be detected clinically.

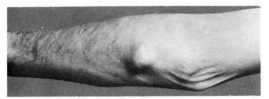

Figure 10.36. Subcutaneous rheumatoid nodule on the extensor aspect of the forearm just below the elbow joint. This is the most common site for such nodules.

CLINICAL FEATURES AND DIAGNOSIS

The clinical manifestations of rheumatoid arthritis are so variable in their mode of onset, distribution, degree of severity and rate of progression that they almost defy brief description.

The onset is usually insidious but can be episodic or even acute. The disease usually begins in several joints (*rheumatoid polyarthritis*), but can begin, and even remain for long periods, in a single joint (*monarticular rheumatoid arthritis*). The commonest joints involved, in order of frequency and progression, are those of the hands, wrists, knees, elbows, feet, shoulders and hips; the distribution of polyarthritis tends to be bilaterally symmetrical (Fig. 10.34).

In the early stages of rheumatoid arthritis the most characteristic distribution of involvement is in certain joints of the hands and feet—the metacarpophalangeal joints of the thumb, index and middle fingers, the proximal interphalangeal joints of the index, middle and ring fingers, and the metatarsophalangeal joints of the four small toes. Occasionally, the larger joints are involved before the small peripheral joints.

In the early phases of the disease, systemic manifestations such as malaise, fatigability and weight loss are common, particularly among young and middle-aged patients. Less common is acute systemic toxicity with high fever, weakness and anemia.

Initially, the most frequent local symptoms are vague pain and stiffness of involved joints; these symptoms are most noticeable as the patient rises each morning and begins to move inflamed joints that have tended to "stiffen up" during sleep. In the early phases, these symptoms tend to abate after the patient has "limbered up," but later they tend to become progressively more severe and more persistent.

In each involved joint the five manifestations of inflammation (redness, swelling, heat, pain and loss of function) become progressively more marked. The joint swelling is due to a combination of synovial thickening plus synovial effusion and its appearance is exaggerated by the rapidly developing atrophy of neighboring muscles (Fig. 10.37). The joints, which have a characteristic boggy feel, are tender to pressure and painful on movement, both active and passive, especially when the involved joint is passively nudged or "stressed" a little beyond the limits of its range of motion. Protective muscle spasm is apparent in the muscles that control the inflamed joints. Subcutaneous rheumatoid nodules become apparent in 30% of patients and are most common in the upper limbs (Fig. 10.36).

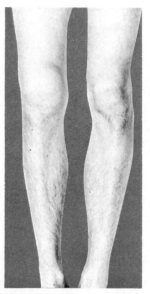

Figure 10.37. Rheumatoid arthritis of the right knee in a young adult. There is thickening of the synovial membrane as well as a massive synovial effusion in the joint. After aspiration of the effusion, atrophy of the quadriceps muscle was obvious in the suprapatellar region.

Deformities develop fairly rapidly with rheumatoid arthritis because of a combination of the following factors: (1) *muscle spasm*, which maintains the joint in the least painful position, usually flexion; (2) *muscle atrophy* with decreasing strength to move the joint; (3) *muscle contracture* due to fibrosis in the inflamed muscles; (4) *subluxation* and *dislocation* due to stretched joint capsule and ligaments; (5) late *capsular and ligamentous contracture* due to fibrosis; (6) *rupture of tendons*, particularly in the hands, due to rheumatoid involvement plus friction against bony spurs. The typical deformities of rheumatoid arthritis are more effectively illustrated than described (Fig. 10.38).

Repeated exacerbations and remissions of the rheumatoid process typify the clinical course for the majority of patients, the remissions being most frequent early in the disease. Nevertheless, 20% of patients have a complete remission following the initial episode with neither recurrent nor residual inflammation. In the remainder of patients the rheumatoid process eventually becomes "burnt out," but the functional state of the joints, as well as of the patient, depends on the amount of structural and irreversible joint damage that has occurred during the active phase of the disease.

Radiographic examination early in the disease reveals evidence of periarticular soft tissue swelling and joint effusion. Subsequently, regional osteoporosis, osteolytic areas in subchondral bone and narrowing of the cartilage space become apparent (Fig. 10.39). Subluxation and dislocation, which are most common in the hands and feet, are late features, whereas bony ankylosis, which is most common in the wrists and

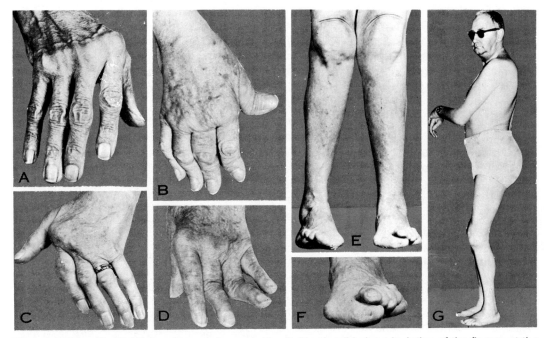

Figure 10.38. Typical deformities of rheumatoid arthritis. *A*, mild ulnar deviation of the fingers at the metacarpophalangeal joints. *B*, Subluxation of the interphalangeal joint of the thumb and the distal interphalangeal joint of the index finger. *C*, marked ulnar deviation of the fingers at the metacarpophalangeal joints. Fusiform swelling of the proximal interphalangeal joints. *D*, subluxation of the proximal interphalangeal joints of the middle and ring fingers. *E*, genu valgum (knock knees) and hallux valgus. *F*, severe hallux valgus and dorsal displacement of the second, third and fourth toes. *G*, flexion deformities of the knees, hips, elbows and wrists.

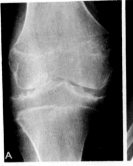
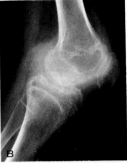

Figure 10.39. Radiographic changes in rheumatoid arthritis of the knee in an adolescent girl. Note the regional osteoporosis, osteolytic areas in the subchondral bone (particularly in the upper end of the tibia) and narrowing of the cartilage space.

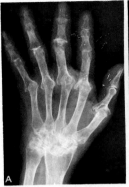
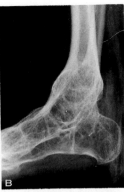

Figure 10.40. Late radiographic changes of rheumatoid arthritis. *A,* note the dislocations of all 5 metacarpophalangeal joints. In addition there is marked narrowing of the proximal interphalangeal joints of the fingers. The wrist joint has been almost completely obliterated. *B,* spontaneous bony ankylosis of the ankle joint and tarsal joints.

ankles, is seen only in advanced rheumatoid arthritis (Fig. 10.40).

Laboratory examinations are useful in the diagnosis and differential diagnosis of rheumatoid disease even though there is, as yet no specific laboratory test. They are also of value in monitoring the activity of the disease in a given patient over a period of time. Anemia, an elevated white blood cell count and an elevated erythrocyte sedimention rate (ESR) are characteristic findings and the elevated ESR usually correlates with acute phase reactants such as fibrinogen and C-reactive protein. Rheumatoid factor, which acts like an autoantibody to γ-globulin, is detectable because of its ability to agglutinate particles of latex coated with the human immunoglubulin IgG. While rheumatoid factor may not be present in the earliest stages, its titer usually reflects the severity of the disease. Examination of the synovial fluid (synovianalysis) reveals it to be turbid because of excessive numbers of leukocytes and it is less viscous than normal. In addition, the synovial fluid exhibits a low glucose concentration and its mucin clots poorly on addition of acetic acid.

PROGNOSIS

It is estimated that in about 30% of patients the disease is so mild that they do not consult a physician for treatment. However, in most patients, rheumatoid arthritis runs either a subacute or a chronic course over a period of many years with multiple exacerbations and remissions. As might be expected, the prognosis is least favorable in those patients in whom the process remains active over several years or longer. Nevertheless, many treated patients recover sufficiently to be able to return to their previous occupation. Indeed, of all treated patients, only 10% are left severely handicapped and largely confined to bed or a wheel chair (Fig. 10.41).

TREATMENT

While there is, as yet, no specific cure for rheumatoid arthritis or the associated rheumatoid disease and while, in a given patient, the rheumatoid process tends to run an almost predetermined course, much can be accomplished for rheumatoid patients therapeutically, provided the treatment, both general and local, is tailored to meet the specific needs of each afflicted individual.

The *aims* of treatment as well as the available *methods* of treatment must all be considered in planning a treatment program for each patient. Ideally, the complex treatment of patients with rheumatoid arthritis should be formulated and at least supervised by a rheumatologist; the initial complete assess-

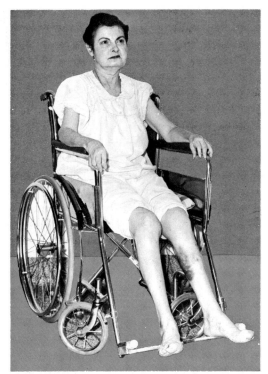

Figure 10.41. A patient with advanced rheumatoid arthritis who is severely handicapped and largely confined to a bed or a wheel chair. Note the multiple deformities of this patient's extremities.

ment of a patient, the institution of treatment for the early phase as well as for exacerbations are most effectively carried out in hospital.

AIMS OF TREATMENT

The overall management of a given patient with rheumatoid arthritis is based on the following aims: (1) to help the patient understand the nature of the disease; (2) to provide psychological support; (3) to alleviate pain; (4) to suppress the inflammatory reaction; (5) to maintain joint function and prevent deformity; (6) to correct existing deformity; (7) to improve function; (8) to rehabilitate the individual patient.

METHODS OF TREATMENT

1. Psychological considerations

In any long term chronic illness such as rheumatoid arthritis, the relationship between physician and patient is particularly important; it must be developed by sympathetic understanding, free discussion of the nature of the disease, the prognosis and the proposed treatment. These patients seldom require psychiatric care but are greatly helped by careful attention to their specific psychological needs, not the least of which is the need to have complete confidence in their physician.

2. Therapeutic Drugs

The multiplicity of drugs prescribed for patients with rheumatoid arthritis can be categorized in the order of frequency of their administration: short- or fast-acting non-steroidal anti-inflammatory drugs (NSAIDs), slow-acting anti-rheumatic drugs (SAARDs), corticosteroids, and immunosuppressive agents.

Of the NSIADs, salicylates such as enteric coated aspirin continue to be the most useful drugs in the "first-line" treatment of rheumatoid arthritis. They not only relieve pain but also have a definite anti-inflammatory effect when administered in sufficiently large doses to provide a blood level of 20 mg/100 ml. The goal is to reach a total dose of 12 to 24 (300 mg) tablets a day within the limits of toxic effects, which include gastrointestinal disturbance, tinnitus and hearing loss.

During the last two decades many new NSAIDs have been developed by medical scientists and the pharmaceutical industry—each drug having its specific beneficial effects as well as its specific undesirable side effects and none having been scientifically proven to be more effective than salicylates. Examples of these newer drugs include: phenylalcanoic or proprionic acids (e.g. naproxen); pyrazolidinediones (e.g. phenylbutazone); indoleacetic acids (e.g. indomethacin). One of the more recently developed drugs, piroxicam, which is chemically unrelated to the NSAIDs, is longer acting and requires administration only once daily. These various newer NSAIDs are particularly useful for patients who, for various reasons, are unable to tolerate salicylates.

When the disease process progresses despite the use of salicylates or other NSAIDs, the "second line" of drugs, namely the SAARDs are indicated. These more powerful, but also more toxic, disease-suppressing agents include gold salts (chrysotherapy), antimalarial agents (e.g. chloroquine) and penicillamine.

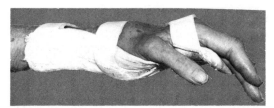

Figure 10.42. Removable splint, designed to relieve pain and prevent deformity.

The "third line" of therapeutic agents, i.e. corticosteroids, which were at one time widely recommended, are now used more sparingly because their non-specific beneficial anti-inflammatory effects must be weighed against their undesirable side effects which include a decreased resistance to infection, generalized osteoporosis, deleterious metabolic effects and steroid dependency. Thus, corticosteroids are usually reserved for extremely severe forms of rheumatoid arthritis and for serious complications of the disease.

For those patients whose disease has been refractory to the above forms of medication and has continued to be progressive there is a place for immunosuppressive drugs and cytotoxic agents, preferably under the direction of a rheumatologist.

Local disease suppressive measures include the intra-articular injection of corticosteroids (which should not be repeated at frequent intervals in a given joint because of the harmful effects on articular cartilage) and "radiation synovectomy" by means of the intra-articular injection of radioactive material such as yttrium-90.

3. Orthopaedic Applicances

In addition to adequate general rest (bed rest), local rest of painfully inflamed joints by *removable splints* is of great value, not only in relieving pain but also in the prevention of deformity (Fig. 10.42). Remedial shoes often make it possible for a patient with painful feet to continue walking. Canes or crutches may become necessary eventually.

4. Physical Therapy

Active movements of involved joints within the limits of pain are important in the attempt to preserve joint motion and maintain muscle strength. A program of physical therapy, though initiated in a hospital setting, must of course be carried out subsequently by the patient at home, and hence, the motivation of the patient is an important factor in the efficacy of physical therapy. When muscles have been involved by the rheumatoid process, the associated atrophy is understandably difficult to overcome by exercises alone.

5. Orthopaedic Surgical Operations

For many years it was thought that surgical operations for rheumatoid arthritis should not be performed during the active stage of the disease for fear of producing an exacerbation of both the local and systemic inflammatory process. Consequently, in the past, operations were performed only as a last resort and in the very late, "burnt out" stage of the disease, by which time the joints had suffered irreparable damage. Such operations included fusion of joints (*arthrodesis*) and reconstruction of joints by various means (*arthroplasty*).

It is now known, however, that surgical operations can be performed with relative safety, even during the active stages of rheumatoid arthritis. Thus, when the rheumatologist and the orthopaedic surgeon work closely together in selecting the patient, as well as the type of operation, much can be accomplished early in the disease to prevent some of the joint and tendon damage as well as the associated deformities (Fig. 10.38).

Excision of the grossly hypertrophied synovial membrane (*synovectomy*) of a severely swollen joint frequently results in an improved range of motion, decreased effusion and less pannus formation; thus, some of the cartilage and subchondral bone destruction may be prevented with resultant preservation of joint function. Although the synovial membrane regenerates following synovectomy, the newly formed membrane seldom becomes severely involved. Synovectomy of tendon sheaths has also proved helpful in preserving the gliding function of the tendons, particularly in the hand. Spontaneous tendon ruptures can be repaired by *tendon grafts*, or their action can be replaced by *tendon transfer*. Subluxations and dislocations of finger joints and displacement of their tendons can be treated surgically before secondary changes occur in articular cartilage.

A nodule within a flexor tendon can produce a "trigger finger" or "trigger thumb" necessitating surgical division of the tendon sheath and, if necessary, excision of the intratendinous nodule. Rheumatoid tenosynovitis of the flexor tendon sheaths at the wrist may cause median nerve compression within the carpal tunnel requiring surgical decompression.

Rheumatoid arthritis involving the synovial joints of the first and second cervical vertebrae may cause a potentially serious degree of spinal instability at this level with the threat of spinal cord compression in which case a C1–C2 arthrodesis (fusion) is indicated.

Prosthetic joint replacement of either the conventional type or the surface replacement type can be very useful in the surgical management of irreparably damaged hip joints. For the knee joint the MacIntosh tibial plateau prosthetic replacement has proven effective unless the damage is severe in which case a semi-constrained prosthetic joint replacement is indicated. In general, prosthetic joint replacements are of most value in the knee, hip, elbow and metacarpophalangeal joints, whereas arthrodesis is most suitable for the ankle, wrist and interphalangeal joints. When walking becomes painful because of depression of the metatarsal heads, excision of the metatarsophalangeal joints corrects the deformity and relieves the pain.

JUVENILE RHEUMATOID ARTHRITIS (JUVENILE CHRONIC ARTHRITIS)

In most children who develop chronic arthritis involving one or more joints, the disease process is quite different—both genetically and immunologically—from that of rheumatoid arthritis in adults. Consequently, the all-inclusive term of *juvenile rheumatoid arthritis*, although hallowed by tradition, is not entirely appropriate and in some European countries has been replaced by the term *juvenile chronic arthritis*. Thus, in 90% of children, this disease is *not* the beginning of the adult type of rheumatoid arthritis and, in general, it carries a better prognosis. Despite the fact that in these children there is a very low incidence of antigen HLA-DW4 and the disease is "sero-negative" (i.e. the rheumatoid factor is absent), the pathogenesis and pathology of the arthritis in a given joint is comparable in the two age groups.

Clinical Varieties

During childhood, at least three varieties of chronic arthritis can be distinguished on the basis of their onset, number of joints involved and clinical features. Consequently, each of these varieties merits separate consideration.

1. Pauci-articular (Oligo-articular) Juvenile Arthritis. In two-thirds of children with chronic arthritis the disease affects only a paucity of joints (less than five) and hence, this is known as the pauci-articular or oligo-articular variety, which includes, of course, single joint involvement, i.e. nonarticular arthritis. The child's general health usually remains good. Most commonly affected joints are the knee, ankle and elbow and less commonly the finger and toe joints. When the knee is involved, the associated hyperemia may cause local overgrowth through the distal femoral and proximal tibial epiphyseal plates. If the disease remains limited to one joint for at least one year, it is unlikely that other joints will become involved but frequently a few joints are involved from the beginning. Although the clinical course is characterized by the ups and downs of exacerbations and remissions over a period of years, the arthritis resolves in over 50% of the patients within five years. Young children with the pauci-articular form of juvenile arthritis are prone to develop the complication of iridocyclitis.

2. Polyarticular Juvenile Arthritis. This variety of chronic arthritis can begin at any age during childhood and affects girls predominantly. Five or more joints are involved, the most frequent sites being knees, ankles, feet, wrists, hands and neck. Usually the disease is limited to the joints. Surprisingly, the prognosis is worse when the onset is insidious than when it is acute; in either case the disease remains active for several years and may be complicated by general retardation of skeletal growth, a phenomenon that is aggravated by the prolonged administration of corticosteroids.

In one sub-variety of polyarticular arthritis which primarily affects girls over the age of ten years, the disease truly resembles the adult type of rheumatoid arthritis in that it runs a similar clinical course and the disease is sero-positive.

3. Systemic Juvenile Arthritis. In this, the least common—but most serious—variety, the disease usually begins in young boys and girls under the age of five years and involves multiple body systems. It is this systemic variety that is known eponymously as *Still's disease*. Typically, the acute onset includes a high fever, an erythematous rash, anemia, generalized lymphadenopathy and, less frequently, hepatosplenomegaly and pericarditis. Indeed, the systemic component of the disease may precede the multiple joint involvement. (Fig. 10.43). Exacerbations and remissions characterize the prolonged clinical course of the disease which in 70% of the children becomes inactive or "burnt out" within ten years.

Laboratory Investigations

The ESR is generally raised while the disease process is active, especially in the systemic variety, and it correlates with an elevated C-reactive protein. The presence of anti-nuclear antibodies is usually associated with the complication of iridocyclitis while the rheumatoid factor is found only in the aforementioned variety that resembles rheumatoid arthritis.

Treatment

The *aims* and *methods* of treatment already outlined in this chapter for rheumatoid

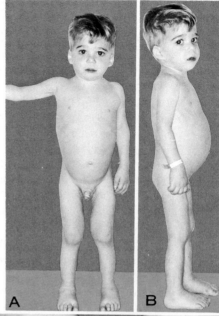

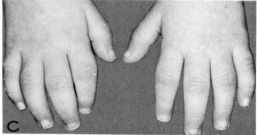

Figure 10.43. Rheumatoid polyarthritis and a visceral involvement (Still's disease) in a 2-year-old boy. *A* and *B*, note the symmetrical swellings of the ankles, knees, fingers and wrists a well as the generalized muscle atrophy. This boy's protruberant abdomen is, in part, due to an enlarged spleen. *C*, the hands of the same boy showing diffuse swelling in the region of the proximal interphalangeal joints.

arthritis in adults are, for the most part, applicable to juvenile chronic (rheumatoid) arthritis. Temporary splints may be necessary to prevent joint deformities but active exercises are essential to help maintain a useful range of joint motion. Salicylates are still the first line form of medical treatment because they relieve pain and decrease inflammation with relatively few side effects. Other non-steroidal, anti-inflammatory drugs are sometimes required, but "slow-acting" drugs such as gold salts, penicillamine or chloroquine are usually reserved for sero-positive disease or for sero-negative poly-articular disease that has not responded to other drugs after one year or more. Corticosteroids have not been proven to improve the ultimate prognosis or to prevent complications of the disease but their cautious use is indicated in the presence of severe systemic disease and in the child with relentless polyarticular arthritis that has not responded to other forms of medical treatment. Excessive corticosteroid therapy, however, decreases the child's resistance to infection, produces generalized osteoporosis and even generalized retardation of skeletal growth.

Orthopaedic surgical operations, as discussed for the adult form of rheumatoid arthritis, may be required, especially synovectomy. However, for children, prosthetic joint replacement is contraindicated except in the case of adolescents with completely disabling involvement of both hip joints.

The poignant pyschological needs of children and adolescents with persistent disability must be met by all those involved with their care as well as by their parents.

Ankylosing Spondylitis

The clinical entity of *ankylosing spondylitis* (Marie-Strumpell disease, Bechterew's disease, pelvospondylitis ossificans, "rheumatoid spondylitis") is a form of chronic seronegative spondyloarthritis characterized by progressive involvement of the sacroiliac and spinal joints with eventual ossification in and around these joints (*bony ankylosis*). The proximal joints of the extremities, particularly the hips may be affected as may the peripheral joints, especially in the lower extremities.

Ankylosing spondylitis differs sufficiently from rheumatoid arthritis in relation to its immunogenetics, age of onset, sex incidence, distribution clinical and radiographic features and response to therapy that it is currently believed to be a separate disease of connective tissue rather than an expression, or variant, of rheumatoid disease.

INCIDENCE

Until the past decade, ankylosing spondylitis was considered to be a relatively un-common rheumatic disease occurring predominantly in young males. It is now known, however, that when less severe forms of the disease are recognized and included, ankylosing spondylitis is almost as common as rheumatoid arthritis and also that young women are affected almost as often as young men. Typically, the onset is in the late teens and seldom after the age of 30. Nevertheless, a juvenile form of ankylosing spondylitis can begin as early as ten years in association with pauci-articular arthritis.

ETIOLOGY

Although the precise cause is unknown, the importance of a genetic predisposing factor has been emphasized by the discovery that 96% of Caucasians suffering from ankylosing spondylitis carry the inherited tissue antigen HLA-B27 which serves as a genetic marker. This particular antigen is found in 5% to 15% of all Caucasians and of those who carry it, only 20% develop ankylosing spondylitis. In certain races in whom HLA-B27 is extremely rare in the general population, ankylosing spondylitis is equally rare.

PATHOGENESIS AND PATHOLOGY

In contrast to rheumatoid arthritis that attacks the synovial membrane, ankylosing spondylitis attacks the site of insertion of tendons, ligaments, fascia and fibrous joint capsules—sites that have been recently named "entheses." The pathological process is one of progressive fibrosis and ossification in these periarticular soft tissues; this process—named "enthesopathy"—eventually leads to bony ankylosis of the entire joint (Fig. 10.44).

Beginning in the sacroiliac joints, the disease slowly spreads upwards along the spine where it affects the capsule of the posterior facet joints (apophyseal joints). The lumbar spine may be spared in the early stages but is eventually involved. Subsequently the periarticular tissues of the intervertebral joints, which are symphyses, are likewise affected. Eventually, the soft tissues of both types of joint ossify thereby producing a bony ankylosis which may come to involve the entire spine converting it into

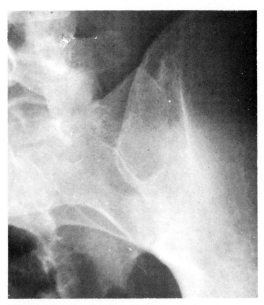

Figure 10.44. Ankylosing spondylitis, involving the left sacroiliac joint. The joint is gradually becoming ankylosed.

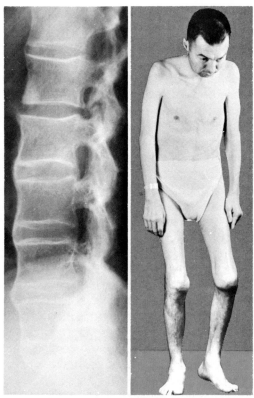

one rigid mass of bone (Fig. 10.45). The extraspinal joints became involved in one-third of patients; the hips are particularly prone to becoming completely ankylosed. A systemic element of ankylosing spondylitis exists as evidenced by lesions that may involve the eyes, lungs, heart or prostate gland.

Figure 10.45. (*left*). Ankylosing spondylitis involving the lumbar spine ("bamboo spine"). Note the ossification across the intervertebral disc spaces and also the ankylosis of the posterior joints.
Figure 10.46 (*right*). Ankylosing spondylitis. This man has ankylosis of most of his spine and also his left hip. He is unable to look up or even to look straight ahead.

CLINICAL FEATURES AND DIAGNOSIS

The patient, usually a young person, first experiences the gradual onset of vague low back pain which is aggravated by sudden movement but is not relieved by rest. Morning stiffness of the spine persists well into the day and, in contrast to "mechanical" low back pain, the pain of ankylosing spondylitis improves with physical exercise. Physical examination reveals local deep tenderness over the sacroiliac joints and spine as well as spinal muscle spasm and a loss of the normal lumbar lordosis. The patient may also complain of pain in the back of the heel at the site of insertion of the Achilles tendon into the os calcis or under the heel at the site of insertion of the plantar fascia. These symptoms are accompanied by local tenderness. Progression of signs and symp-

toms is usually continuous but may be intermittent. After a year or more, by which time the disease has usually spread upwards along the spine, the patient's back becomes progressively stiffer. Involvement of the costovertebral joints causes pain on deep breathing and, as these joints lose motion, there is a measurable decrease in the normal chest expansion.

In the more severe forms of ankylosing spondylitis as the spinal column becomes progressively stiffer ("poker back") it also tends to become progressively flexed ("rocker back"). Furthermore, this progressive flexion deformity of the spine may be dramatically accelerated by a series of vertebral fractures that result from trivial trauma. Eventually, the patient may no longer be able to look straight ahead, a dangerous as well as an embarrassing disability (Fig. 10.46). If, in addition, the hips become ankylosed, the unfortunate victim has extreme difficulty walking. Although the disease process may become arrested spontaneously at any stage, the more common course is one of slow but relentless progression.

Radiographic examination in the early stages reveals narrowing of the sacroiliac cartilage space and subchondral sclerosis (Fig. 10.44); a bone scan, although non-specific, may be positive at an even earlier stage. Eventually these joints may ossify. Subsequently, ossification of the annulus fibrosus of the intervertebral joints produces the classical radiographic picture of the "bamboo spine" (Fig. 10.45).

Clinical manifestations of systemic illness include fatigue, weight loss and a low grade fever.

Laboratory examination may reveal anemia and an elevated ESR. Since only 20% of HLA-B27 positive individuals develop ankylosing spondylitis and since not *all* individuals with the disease carry this antigen, the HLA-B27 antigen is not of absolute diagnostic value. Hence, the diagnosis must be made primarily on clinical and radiographic grounds.

TREATMENT

The *aims* of treatment for ankylosing spondylitis are comparable to those already described for rheumatoid arthritis.

1. Psychological Considerations

These young, previously healthy patients need to be informed that less than one-third of them will develop the full-blown "classical" picture of ankylosing spondylitis. They also need psychological support in accepting the importance of developing good postural habits and of doing daily exercises for the rest of their lives.

2. Therapeutic Drugs

Although salicylates are the safest of the non-steroidal anti-inflammatory drugs, they are not usually very effective in ankylosing spondylitis. Of the many other NSAIDs available, indomethacin is currently the most appropriate, although it, in turn, may be replaced in the future by newer drugs. For those patients in whom indomethacin is not well tolerated, phenylbutazone may be used, but with caution because of its long-term toxicity including bone marrow depression and peptic ulceration. Neither corticosteroids nor gold salts are effective in this disease.

3. Radiation Therapy

Once a common modality of treatment for ankylosing spondylitis because it relieved the pain, radiation therapy is no longer recommended since it has been proven to have the potential for causing either radiation-induced aplastic anemia or leukemia.

4. Orthopaedic Appliances

Spinal braces are ineffectual in preventing the progressive flexion deformity of the spine but a firm flat mattress may be of help during sleep. Sudden increase in the flexion deformity is usually the result of one or more fractures and may necessitate reduction of the fracture(s) and the temporary use of external fixation by means of a halo-pelvic device.

5. Physical Therapy

It is essential for these patients to exercise faithfully several times a day for the rest of their lives. Swimming is especially beneficial.

6. Orthopaedic Surgical Operations

Although one of the basic aims of treatment is the prevention of severe spinal deformity, those patients most severely involved may, nevertheless, develop disabling and permanent deformity (even more severe than that seen in Figure 10.46). For such patients, spinal osteotomy is now feasible in either the lumbar or the cervical region (depending upon the site of the major deformity) and produces dramatic improvement; understandably, this type of major surgery carries a moderate risk, but one that is minimized when the operation is performed under local anaesthesia as recommended by

Simmons. Ankylosis of one or both hips is particularly disabling when combined with ankylosis of the spine, but fortunately this condition can be helped by prosthetic joint replacement of the conventional type ("total hip").

Many of the patients with severe ankylosing spondylitis require vocational rehabilitation.

Chronic Arthritis Associated with Other Conditions

DIFFUSE CONNECTIVE TISSUE DISEASES ("COLLAGEN DISEASE")

Chronic polyarthritis may develop in a variety of other diffuse connective diseases which are frequently referred to as the *collagen diseases*. These include *systemic lupus erythematosus* (formerly disseminated lupus erythematosus), *polyarteritis nodosa* (formerly periarteritis nodosa), *progressive systemic sclerosis* (formerly scleroderma), *polymyositis, dermatomyositis and thrombotic thrombocytopenic purpura.*

REITER'S SYNDROME

This syndrome of urethritis, conjunctivitis and sero-negative asymmetric arthritis is thought to be secondary either to a venereal type of infection or to bacillary dysentery. It afflicts mostly males and the arthritis involves joints of the lower extremities predominantly. As with ankylosing spondylitis, there is a close correlation between Reiter's syndrome and the histocompatibility antigen, HLA-B27.

PSORIASIS

Although the skin disease psoriasis is relatively common, only 2% of patients, both male and female, exhibit an associated polyarthritis. The arthritis characteristically develops in the distal interphalangeal joints of the fingers and toes and seems to be related to psoriatic involvement of the nails.

Rheumatic Fever

Rheumatic fever is an acute inflammatory disease which attacks connective tissues in the heart, blood vessels and joints of children. The cardiac lesions are particularly significant since they may be followed by serious and permanent scarring of the valves (chronic rheumatic heart disease). By contrast, the joint lesions are always transient.

ETIOLOGY

This disease, which usually afflicts children over the age of five years, is a sequel to infection with group A hemolytic streptococci and hence its incidence parallels the incidence of such infections. Consequently, with improved health conditions and the use of effective antibiotics, rheumatic fever occurs less frequently now than in the past. Although the relationship to Group A streptococcal infections has been well established immunologically, by elevated titers of antibodies to streptococcal antigens, the pathogenesis of rheumatic fever is not yet understood.

PATHOLOGY

The acute inflammatory polyarthritis is characterized by an intense synovitis. However, the local inflammatory process is transient, and no pannus forms; hence articular cartilage is spared and the joints always recover completely.

CLINICAL FEATURES AND DIAGNOSIS

Rheumatic fever usually presents as an attack of acute febrile illness accompanied by acute polyarthritis; though more than one joint may be involved at a given time, the transient inflammatory process tends to migrate from joint to joint (Fig. 10.47). The more serious cardiac lesions are manifest by heart murmurs and electrocardiographic changes (prolongation of the P-R interval). The acute phase of rheumatic fever seldom lasts more than two months.

Laboratory examination reveals an elevated erythrocyte sedimentation rate but the diagnosis is strengthened by the demonstration of a changing antistreptolysin-O titer which indicates a recent streptococcal infection. The mucin of the synovial fluid clots well on the addition of acetic acid.

TREATMENT

As with the other rheumatic diseases, there is no specific cure. The joint lesions,

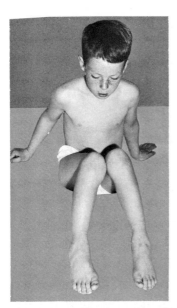

Figure 10.47. Rheumatic fever in a 6-year-old boy. Note the symmetrical swelling of both ankle joints. Two days later the swelling on the left ankle subsided but the right elbow became swollen.

fusion bulges the hip joint capsule and as the intra-articular fluid pressure rises, the child comes to prefer lying down with the hip held in flexion, abduction and external rotation, the position in which the capacity of the hip joint capsule is greatest (Fig. 10.48). Systemic manifestations of inflammation are minimal.

Radiographic examination reveals only evidence of an effusion in the involved hip joint (Fig. 10.49).

The diagnosis of transient synovitis of the hip can be suspected on clinical grounds alone but is established by exclusion of more serious conditions that mimic it—Legg-Perthes' disease, septic arthritis, rheumatic fever, monarticular rheumatoid arthritis and tuberculosis arthritis. Aspiration of the joint is of value when the diagnosis is in doubt.

Treatment consists of bed rest with the hip maintained in the most comfortable position of flexion, abduction and external rota-

however, are so transient that only symptomatic treatment is required. Salicylates in high doses tend to suppress the inflammatory reaction and are much safer than adrenocorticosteroids, though the latter may be required for some patients. Penicillin is administered in large doses during the acute phase and must be continued indefinitely in prophylactic doses in order to prevent recurrent attacks of rheumatic fever by preventing recurrent streptococcal infections.

Transient Synovitis of the Hip Joint in Children

The relative common clinical entity, *transient synovitis of the hip joint* in children (idiopathic monarticular synovitis) ("observation hip"), is a non-bacterial inflammatory disorder of unknown etiology; it develops most frequently in boys between the ages of 3 and 10 years.

Clinically, the synovitis is manifest by pain in the region of the hip, occasionally referred pain in the knee, a painful (antalgic) limp and restriction of hip joint motion with associated muscle spasm. The progressive synovial ef-

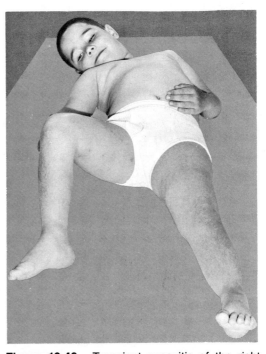

Figure 10.48. Transient synovitis of the right hip joint in a 6-year-old boy. The boy prefers to maintain the inflamed hip in position of flexion, abduction and external rotation. This position, in which the capacity of the hip joint capsule is greatest, is the position of comfort.

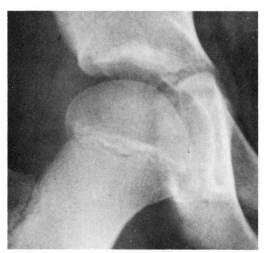

Figure 10.49. Evidence of an effusion in the right hip joint in a child with transient synovitis of the hip. The slightly denser shadow which is lateral to the femoral head and neck indicates a bulging of the hip joint capsule.

tion until a full range of painless motion of the hip has returned, which is usually within one week. Relief of weight bearing on the involved hip by means of crutches is recommended for a further few weeks in an attempt to prevent recurrence.

Approximately 5% of children with transient synovitis of the hip develop radiographic evidence of Legg-Perthes' disease within the ensuing two years. For this reason all children who have synovitis of the hip should be seen, and their hip joints radiographed, at six-monthly intervals in order to detect the earliest evidence of this complication. The possible etiological relationship of transient synovitis of the hip to Legg-Perthes' disease is discussed in Chapter 13.

Gout and Gouty Arthritis

The clinical condition of *gout*, which is the manifestation of a familial *inborn error of purine metabolism*, is characterized by an elevated serum uric acid (*hyperuricemia*), recurrent attacks of *acute gouty arthritis* in peripheral joints and, eventually, *chronic gouty arthritis* associated with periarticular and subcutaneous deposits, or *tophi*, of urate salts; gout may also be associated with renal disease and uric acid nephrolithiasis.

INCIDENCE

Although classical gout is relatively uncommon, milder forms of the disease, which often escape diagnosis, may be more prevalent than previously thought. Gout is predominantly a disease of males, the ratio being 20:1. It may present during adolescence but the peak incidence is after the age of 40, and when females are afflicted, it is seldom before the menopause. Gouty arthritis involves mainly the peripheral joints of the feet and hands, by far the most common site being the metatarsophalangeal joint of the great toe.

ETIOLOGY

In over half the patients there is a definite familial incidence of either clinical gout or hyperuricemia. The etiology of the purine metabolic disorder is unknown, but presumably the hyperuricemia is due to either excessive production or deficient urinary excretion of uric acid. Nevertheless, not all persons with hyperuricemia actually suffer from gout.

Attacks of acute gouty arthritis seem to be precipitated in a given patient by a variety of general factors, including infection, alcoholic or dietary indiscretion, and emotional factors, as well as by local factors including injury and exposure to cold. In certain blood dyscrasias, such as leukemia and polycythemia, *secondary gout* can develop due to overproduction of urates; in patients with chronic renal disease and in patients receiving diuretics, secondary gout can develop due to impaired urinary excretion of urates.

PATHOGENESIS AND PATHOLOGY

Attacks of acute gouty arthritis are caused by the sudden deposition of sodium monourate crystals in the synovial membrane and therefore represent a type of *crystal-induced arthritis*. Leukocytes phagocytose the crystals, then disintegrate, releasing lysosomal enzymes which produce an acute and severe local inflammation. Early in the disease the urate crystals are usually absorbed after each attack and consequently the joint returns to normal.

Several years later in the course of gout,

however, nodular deposits, or *tophi* of urate crystals, eventually develop in one or more sites. In the involved joint, tophi develop in synovial membrane, articular cartilage and even subchondral bone. In addition, they may form in the synovial membrane of bursae and tendon sheaths as well as in the cartilage of the external ear.

Eventually, the chronic inflammatory reaction to urate deposits in and around a given joint plus associated destruction of cartilage and subchondral bone lead to progressive degenerative changes in the joint, a type of degenerative joint disease.

CLINICAL FEATURES

The clinical course of gout varies widely in relation to severity and rate of progression. The commonest pattern is a series of attacks of acute gouty arthritis over a period of years followed by the formation of tophi, both articular and extra-articular, and eventually the development of chronic gouty arthritis.

ACUTE GOUTY ARTHRITIS

During the early stages, attacks of acute gouty arthritis are usually monoarticular, and in at least half the patients the initial attack is in the metatarsophalangeal joint of the great toe ("podagra"); indeed, this particular joint is eventually afflicted in virtually every patient with gout, though other peripheral joints may also become involved.

Each episode may be preceded by forewarning symptoms, such as mood change, constipation and diuresis. The actual attack, which develops with dramatic rapidity, is characterized by intense pain which progresses to the point of being excruciating; even the slightest movement of the joint is intolerable and local tenderness is exquisite. The joint becomes swollen within a few hours and is obviously acutely inflamed. Indeed, the clinical picture, which includes fever and leukocytosis, may simulate cellulitis or even acute septic arthritis (Fig. 10.50). Mild attacks of acute gouty arthritis last for several days, but more severe attacks may persist for as long as several weeks. However, once the attack is over, all signs of

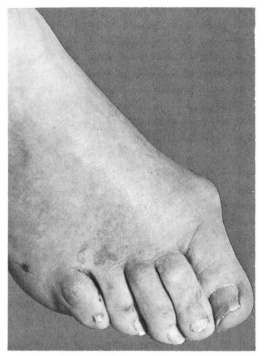

Figure 10.50. Acute gouty arthritis involving the metatarsophalangeal joint of the great toe. The joint is markedly swollen and acutely inflamed.

inflammation subside spontaneously and, at least in the early stages of the disease, the joint returns to normal.

At first the attacks tend to occur at infrequent intervals, even a few years apart, and between attacks the patient is completely free of symptoms. Later, however, the attacks not only occur more frequently but also are more severe and may even involve multiple joints.

CHRONIC TOPHACEOUS GOUT

After several years, half the patients develop tophaceous gout. Tophi, which consist of persistent deposits of urate crystals surrounded by chronic inflammatory tissue, develop in the synovial membrane and may become sufficiently large that they interfere with joint function. Tophi also develop in articular cartilage where they cause local destruction and in the subchondral bone where they incite local osteoclastic resorption with cyst-like lesions (Fig. 10.51). Extra-articular tophi form in bursae (the com-

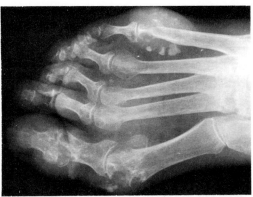

Figure 10.51. Chronic gout in the foot of a 50-year-old man. Note the local osteoclastic resorption with cyst-like lesions in the first metatarsal, the fifth metatarsal and the phalanges of the great toe. Note also the areas of soft-tissue calcification.

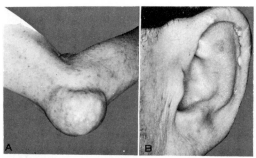

Figure 10.52. Extra-articular gouty tophi. *A*, in the olecranon bursa. *B*, in the cartilage of the external ear.

monest site being the olecranon bursa), in tendon sheaths and in the cartilage of the external ear (Fig. 10.52). Since tophi form slowly, they are usually painless; but those that are subcutaneous may eventually ulcerate through the skin.

CHRONIC GOUTY ARTHRITIS

Articular and subchondral tophi lead to progressive degenerative arthritis with chronic joint pain, swelling and stiffness. Nevertheless, even in this late stage, acute attacks may be superimposed upon the chronic arthritis. Although pure urate deposits are radiolucent, subsequent secondary deposition of calcium renders them radio-opaque.

Laboratory Diagnosis

Hyperuricemia is virtually always demonstrable in patients with gout both during and between attacks. (The normal serum uric acid level by colorimetric methods is 6.0 mg/100 ml for adult males and 5.5 mg/100 ml for adult females.) The demonstration of urate crystals from synovial fluid or from tophi by means of a polarizing microscope is diagnostic; however, tophi develop in only half of all patients with gout.

Treatment

By means of presently available drugs, most patients with gout are able to pursue their normal activities; acute attacks can be reasonably well controlled and tophaceous complications including chronic gouty arthritis can usually be prevented. However, the medical treatment of gout must continue for the rest of the patient's life and is ideally supervised by a rheumatologist.

Treatment of Acute Gouty Arthritis. Colchicine, which is of specific value in the treatment of acute attacks, is taken hourly from the onset until the severe pain is relieved, at least up to 12 hours, or until gastrointestinal symptoms develop; alternatively, it may be given intravenously. *Indomethacin* is equally effective and does not upset the gastrointestinal tract. Subsequent acute attacks can often be prevented, or at least reduced in severity, by moderate dietary restrictions, particularly avoidance of such purine-rich foods as liver, kidney and sweetbreads; prophylactic administration of colchicine in small doses may also be helpful.

Treatment of Chronic Gout and Chronic Gouty Arthritis. In the chronic phase of gout, the hyperuricemia can be reduced by *uricosuric* drugs, which increase the urinary excretion of uric acid presumably by blocking its reabsorption in the renal tubules. The currently limited indications for uricosuric drugs, which must be continued for the rest of the patient's life, are the presence of tophi, a persistent elevation of serum uric acid above 8.0 mg/100 ml and the failure of other drugs to prevent frequent attacks. Two of the more effective uricosurics are *probenecid* and *sulphinpyrazone*. At present, the drug of choice as a uric acid-lowering agent is allopurinal, which helps to inhibit the production of uric acid and is therefore of particular value for patients with uric acid nephrolithiasis. This drug will be required for the rest of the patient's life.

Pseudogout

Like true gout, its imitater *pseudogout* is a form of crystal-induced arthritis but the crystals are composed of calcium pyrophosphate dihydrate rather than uric acid. A relatively common type of metabolic arthritis, it afflicts primarily the elderly and is characterized by recurrent painful attacks of acute arthritis which may be triggered by either trauma or illness. The joints most frequently involved are those of the hand and wrist as well as the knee and hip but there also is a high incidence of pre-existing degenerative arthritis. In the majority of patients, radiographic examination reveals calcium deposits within the hyaline articular cartilage and the fibrocartilage of menisci (*chondrocalcinosis*) and even calcification of periarticular soft tissues such as joint capsules and ligaments. One-third of the patients develop a rapidly progressive and devastatingly destructive degenerative arthritis called *pyrophosphate arthropathy*. While the diagnosis can be suspected on the basis of clinical and radiographic data, it can be confirmed only by the detection of the typical crystals of calcium pyrophosphate dihydrate in the synovial fluid using polarizing microscopy. Phenylbutazone and indomethacin are equally effective in controlling the acute attacks of pseudogout. Although there is no effective prophylactic treatment, joint lavage may provide temporary improvement by reducing the number of crystals in the synovial fluid.

The Rheumatic Disease Unit

The variety and complexity of the rheumatic diseases, which present many problems of diagnosis and treatment, justify the establishment in large general hospitals of special *rheumatic disease units.* In such units the combined team efforts of rheumatologists, family physicians, orthopaedic surgeons, rehabilitation physicians, physical and occupational therapists and medical social workers can most effectively improve the outlook for this unfortunate group of patients. Furthermore, a rheumatic disease unit is a splendid setting for both undergraduate and postgraduate teaching. In addition, such units provide a powerful stimulus for both clinical and experimental investigation which hopefully, will lead to a better understanding of this baffling group of diseases.

Hemophilic Arthritis

Classical *hemophilia and Christmas disease,** which are defects of the first-stage clotting mechanism of blood, are frequently complicated by repeated joint hemorrhages (*hemarthroses*) which, in turn, lead to progressive joint damage (*hemophilic arthritis, hemophilic arthropathy*). Other bleeding disorders are seldom complicated by hemarthrosis.

INCIDENCE

Classical hemophilia (a deficiency of antihemophilic factor, or factor VIII) is relatively uncommon and Christmas disease (a deficiency of plasma thromboplastin, or factor IX) is even less common. Nevertheless, in each of these bleeding disorders, hemarthrosis is the most common hemorrhagic event since it occurs in most of the patients at some time. By far the most frequent site of hemarthrosis is the knee, followed by the ankle and the elbow. The first hemarthrosis usually occurs between the time the child starts to walk and the age of five years. Since hemophilia and Christmas disease are both inherited by boys (by a sex-linked recessive gene carried by the mother), hemophilic arthritis is limited to males.

PATHOGENESIS AND PATHOLOGY

Blood in a synovial joint does not clot even in a normal individual although a clot does form in the torn vessels. In hemophilia, by contrast, a clot fails to form readily in the torn vessels and consequently bleeding into

---

* The term "Christmas" disease comes from the surname of the first boy in whom the disease was discovered.

the joint tends to continue until it is stopped by the raised pressure of the hemarthrosis. In hemophilia, joint hemorrhage is probably always caused by trauma even though the initiating trauma may seem insignificant.

Synovial membrane reacts to the irritation of blood in the joint by an inflammatory proliferation and villous formation. Phagocytes transport the red blood cells from the joint cavity to the synovial membrane where they are broken down with resultant formation of *hemosiderin deposits* which constitute a further source of irritation. Inflammatory granulation tissue creeps across the surface as a *pannus* which interferes with the nutrition of cartilage from the synovial fluid. Furthermore, hemorrhages and inflammatory granulation tissue burrow under the cartilage with subsequent collapse of the joint surface.

After repeated hemarthroses, the grossly thickened synovial membrane tends to become fibrotic with resultant joint adhesions, limitation of motion, contractures and joint deformity. Consequently the stage is set for progressive degenerative changes in the joint which in turn render the joint even more vulnerable to trivial trauma and lead to repeated hemarthroses; thus a vicious repeating cycle is established.

CLINICAL FEATURES AND DIAGNOSIS

The hemophilic patient and his parents are usually aware of the underlying diagnosis due to previous episodes of abnormal bruising or excessive bleeding from minor cuts; in about half the hemophilic children the diagnosis is established following excessive bleeding at the time of circumcision.

Frequently, the patient learns to recognize a vague feeling of joint discomfort which heralds a major hemarthrosis. This is probably due to a minor subsynovial hemorrhage that has not yet penetrated the synovial membrane to enter the joint. Once a progressive hemarthrosis begins, the joint becomes swollen, warm, painful and limited in motion. After repeated hemarthroses in a given joint, the clinical picture is that of superimposed chronic arthritis with persistent swelling of the joint and atrophy of the surrounding muscles (Fig. 10.53).

Radiographic examination at the time of the first few hemarthroses, reveals only soft tissue swelling. However, after repeated episodes of bleeding into a given joint, there is radiographic evidence of regional osteoporosis, subchondral defects in the bone and narrowing of the cartilage space (Fig. 10.54).

Laboratory examination reveals a normal bleeding time but a prolonged partial thromboplastin time. The exact diagnosis is established by hematological assay of factor VIII (classical hemophilia) and factor IX (Christmas disease).

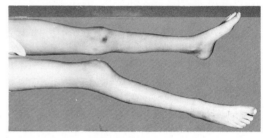

Figure 10.53. Hemophilic arthritis in the right knee of a 10-year-old boy. Note the gross swelling of the right knee joint and the atrophy of the quadriceps muscle. Note also a recent bruise over the medial aspect of the left knee.

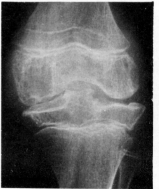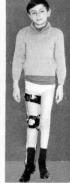

Figure 10.54. (*left*). Chronic hemophilic arthritis. Note the regional osteoporosis, subchondral defects in the bone and narrowing of the cartilage space.

Figure 10.55. (*right*). A boy with chronic hemophilic arthritis involving the right knee. He is wearing a brace to protect the badly damaged right knee joint from further hemarthroses.

TREATMENT

Hemarthrosis in a hemophilic patient constitutes an emergency since immediate treatment can prevent many of the late sequelae. The over-all management should ideally be under the supervision of a hematologist. As soon as the patient experiences the forewarning symptoms of a joint hemorrhage, he should be given intravenous therapy with either fresh frozen plasma or the appropriate concentrate of human factor (VIII or IX depending on the diagnosis) in order to prevent the development of a massive hemarthrosis.

One of the most important advances in the management of hemophilics during the past decade—and especially in the prevention of major hemarthroses—has been the development of "home care programs." Hemophilics are taught to recognize the previously mentioned "vague feeling of joint discomfort that heralds a major hemarthrosis." The appropriate factor as well as sterile needles and syringes are kept in the patient's home, and as soon as this warning signal is felt either the patient immediately gives himself an intravenous injection of the factor or one of his relatives does it for him. A hemarthrosis is thereby prevented. Many patients, as well as their relatives, master the management of home care, including the technique of intravenous injections, remarkably well.

If the patient is not seen until after the hemarthrosis has developed, his clotting mechanism should be corrected by the same measures and the affected joint splinted. Once the bleeding has stopped and the level of antihemophilic globulin has been adequately raised—and only then—the joint should be aspirated under sterile precautions to prevent the chronic synovial reaction to persistent blood in the joint.

Physiotherapy is necessary to improve joint motion and muscle strength and should be continued at least until previous motion is restored; during this time, the joint should be protected from weight bearing to prevent early recurrence of bleeding.

Chronic hemophilic arthritis in the lower limb may necessitate protective bracing to prevent recurrent hemarthroses (Fig. 10.55). Late reconstructive operations can be performed with relative safety provided the patient's clotting mechanism is corrected by appropriate treatment before, during and for a period of at least two weeks after the operation.

The future hope for hemophilic individuals lies in the continuing prevention of abnormal bleeding by means of daily prophylactic treatment with maintenance doses of the appropriate concentrate of human factor. At present the practical application of this form of prevention is limited by the fact that the human factor must be given intravenously each day; even so, as mentioned above, many patients have learned to master this technique of self treatment. Continued research is necessary to provide a more practical solution to this serious problem.

Suggested Additional Reading

Anastassiades, T. P., Dwosh, I. L. and Ford, P. M.: Intra-articular steroid injections: a benefit or a hazard? Can. Med. Assoc. J. 122: 389–390, 1980.

Anderson, F., and Hughes, S.: Bone and joint infection. In *The Basis and Practice of Orthopaedics*, edited by Hughes, S. and Sweetnam, R. London, William Heinemann Medical Books, 1980.

Anderson, J. R., Orr, J. D. MacLean, A. and Scobie, W. G.: Acute haematogenous osteitis. Arch. Dis. Child. 55: 953–957, 1980.

Ansell, B. M.: Chronic arthritis in childhood. Ann. Rheum. Dis. 37: 107–120, 1978.

Ansell, B. M.: *Rheumatic Disorders in Childhood. (Postgraduate Pediatric Series).* London, Butterworth, 1980.

Blockey, N. J.: Management of Bone and Joint Infections. In *Scientific Foundations of Orthopaedics and Traumatology*, edited by Owen, R., Goodfellow, J. and Bullough, P. London, William Heinemann Medical Books, 1980.

Boyd, W., and Sheldon, H.: *Introduction to the Study of Disease*, 8th ed. Philadelphia, Lea & Febiger, 1980.

Boyer, A. S.: Gonococcal arthritis syndromes. An update on diagnosis and management. Postgrad. Med. 67: 200–208, 1980.

Brewer, E. J., Giannini, E. H. and Person, D. A.: *Juvenile Rheumatoid Arthritis*, 2nd ed. Philadelphia, W. B. Saunders, 1982, vol. 6 in *Major Problems in Clinical Pediatrics*.

Buchanan, W. W.: Rheumatoid arthritis: modern medicine's major enigma. Ann. R. Coll. Phys. Surg. Can. 15: 93–97, 1982.

Cole, W. G., Dalziel, R. E., and Leith, S.: Treatment of

acute osteomyelitis in children. J. Bone Joint Surg. 64B: 218–223, 1982.

Curtiss, P. H.: Cartilage damage in septic arthritis. Clin. Orthop. 64: 87, 1969.

Duthie, J. J. R., Brown, P. E., Truelove, L. R., Barager, F. D., Lawrie, A. J.: Course and prognosis in rheumatoid arthritis. *Ann. Rheum. Dis.* 23: 193–204, 1964

Fam, A. G., Topp, J. R., Stein, H. B. and Little, A. H.: Clinical and roentgenographic aspects of pseudogout: a study of 50 cases and a review. Can. Med. Assoc. J. 124: 545–549, 1981.

Gilday, D. L., Paul, D. J. and Paterson, J.: Diagnosis of osteomyelitis in children by combined blood pool and blood imaging. Radiology 117: 331–335, 1975.

Gillespie, R.: Septic arthritis of childhood. Clin. Orthop. 96: 152–159, 1973.

Gillespie, W. J. and Mayo, K. M.: The management of acute haematogenous osteomyelitis in the antibiotic era. J. Bone Joint Surg. 63B: 126–131, 1981.

Gordon, D. A. (ed.): *Rheumatoid arthritis. In Discussions in Patient Management.* New York, Excerpta Medica, 1981.

Hastings, D. E. and Welsh, R. P.: *Surgical Reconstruction of the Rheumatoid Hand.* Toronto, Medisport and Orthomedic Management Corp., 1979.

Hodgson, A. R.: Anterior spinal fusion. The operative approach and pathological findings in 412 patients with Pott's disease of the spine. Br. J. Surg. 48: 172–178, 1960.

Houghton, G. R., and Duthie. R. B.: Orthopaedic problems in hemophilia. Clin. Orthop. 138: 197–216, 1979.

Kelley, W. H., Harris, E. J. Jr., Ruddy, S. and Sledge, C. B.: *Textbook of Rheumatology.* Philadelphia, W. B. Saunders, 1981.

Kuo, K. H., Lloyd-Roberts, G. C., Orme, I. M. and Soothill, J. F.: Immunodeficiency and infantile bone and joint infection. Arch. Dis. Child. 50: 51, 1975.

Lightfoot, R. W. Jr.: Treatment of rheumatoid arthritis. In *Arthritis and Allied Conditions*: A Textbook of Rheumatology, 9th ed., edited by McCarty, D. J. Philadelphia, Lea & Febiger, 1979, pp. 517–718.

Little, A. H.: Coping with rheumatoid arthritis (editorial). Can. Med. Assoc. J. 127: 190–191, 1982.

McCarty, D. J. (ed.): *Arthritis and Allied Conditions: A Textbook of Rheumatology*, 9th ed. Philadelphia, Lea & Febiger, 1979.

Miller, J. J. (eds.): *Juvenile Rheumatoid Arthritis.* Littleton, Mass., P. S. G. Publishing Co. Inc., 1979.

M.R.C. working party on tuberculosis of the spine. J. Bone Joint Surg. 60: 163–178, 1978.

New, H. C.: The place of cephalosporins in antibacterial treatment of infectious diseases. J. Antimicrob. Chemother. 6 (Suppl. A): 1–11, 1980.

Ogryzlo, M. A.: The rheumatic disease unit (RDU) concept. Arthritis Rheum. 10: 479–485, 1967.

Post, M. and Telfer, M. C.: Surgery in hemophilic patients. J. Bone Joint Surg. 57A: 1136–1145, 1975.

Prober, C. G.: Oral antibiotic therapy for bone and joint infections. Pediatr. Infect. Dis. 1: 8–10, 1982.

Rodnan, G. P. (ed.): *Primer on the Rheumatic Diseases*, 7th ed. J.A.M.A. 224 (Suppl.): 662–812, 1973.

Rudowski, W. J.: Major surgery in hemophilia (Moynihan Lecture). Ann. R. Coll. Surg. Engl. 63: 111–117, 1981.

Salter, R. B., Bell, R. S. and Keeley, F. W.: The protective effect of continuous passive motion on living articular cartilage in acute septic arthritis. An experimental investigation in the rabbit. Clin. Orthop. 159: 223–247, 1981.

Salter, R. B., Gross, A., and Hall, J. H.: Hydrocortisone arthropathy—an experiment investigation. Can. Med. Assoc. 97: 374–377, 1967.

Seddon, H. J.: The choice of treatment in Pott's disease (editorial). J. Bone Joint Surg. 58B: 395–397, 1976.

Shore, A. and Boone, J. E.: *You, Your Child and Arthritis. An Arthritis Society Fact Book.* Toronto, The Arthritis Society of Canada, June 1982.

Simmons, E. H.: Kyphotic deformity of the spine in ankylosing spondylitis. Clin. Orthop. 128: 74–76, 1977.

Smythe, H. A.: Therapy of the spondyloarthropathies. Clin. Orthop. 143:84–89, 1979.

Smythe, H. A.: *Assessment of Joint Disease*, 2nd ed. Teaching Handbook. Toronto, University of Toronto, 1980.

Smythe, H. A. and Moldofsky, H.: Two contributions to understand the "fibrositis syndrome." Bull. Rheum. Dis. 28: 928–931, 1977.

Stein, H. and Duthie, R.: The pathogenesis of chronic hemophilic arthropathy. J. Bone Joint Surg. 63B: 601–609, 1981.

Urowitz, M. B.: Immunosuppressive therapy in rheumatoid arthritis. J. Rheumatol. 1: 364–373, 1974.

Wenger, D. R., Bobechko, W. P. and Gilday, D. L.: The spectrum intervertebral disc-space infection in children. J. Bone Joint Surg. 60A: 100–108, 1978.

Wiley, J. J. and Fraser, G. A.: Septic arthritis in childhood. Can. J. Surg. 22: 326–330, 1979.

CHAPTER 11

Degenerative Disorders of Joints and Related Tissues

The various "rheumatic diseases" discussed in the the preceding chapter are predominantly *inflammatory*; by contrast, those rheumatic diseases discussed in the present chapter are predominantly *degen-*

erative. You will appreciate, however, that the division is somewhat arbitrary since some inflammatory reaction is incited in soft tissues even by the degenerative types of disorders of joints and related structures. This chapter includes a discussion of the degenerative types of arthritis (*degenerative joint disease* or *chronic articular rheumatism*) and also various rheumatic diseases of extra-articular, or nonarticular, structures such as tendons, muscles and bursae (*nonarticular rheumatism*). Many aspects of these diseases are related to normal aging, a process which merits separate consideration.

NORMAL AGING OF ARTICULAR CARTILAGE

Though most joints may be expected to last a lifetime, at least as far as reasonable function is concerned, the normal aging process, which begins in early adult life and slowly progresses throughout the remainder of life, gradually changes the smooth, glistening surface of youthful articular cartilage to a granular, dull surface in old age. Furthermore, because of the limited ability of articular cartilage to regenerate, the degenerative changes tend to be irreversible and progressive.

Biochemically, there is a gradual loss of proteoglycan, a basic component of the cartilage matrix; as the matrix deteriorates the collagen fibrils lose their support and the cartilage tends to become shredded (*fibrillation*). Thus, with advancing years articular cartilage becomes less effective, not only as a "shock absorber," but also as a lubricated surface; consequently it becomes more vulnerable to the repeated friction of normal function.

These changes of age in articular cartilage are present to some degree in all adults; however, since they do not usually cause significant symptoms, they may be considered a variation of normal. When these changes are either premature or excessive and cause pain, however, the condition becomes of clinical significance, and is known as *degenerative joint disease*.

DEGENERATIVE JOINT DISEASE

Degenerative joint disease, a common disorder of one or more joints, is initiated by a local deterioration of articular cartilage and is characterized by progressive degeneration of the cartilage, hypertrophy and remodeling of the subchondral bone, and secondary inflammation of the synovial membrane. It is a localized disorder with no systemic effects.

The currently accepted term *degenerative joint disease* is synonymous with the terms "osteoarthritis," "osteoarthrosis," "degenerative arthritis," "senescent arthritis" and "hypertrophic arthritis."

Incidence

Degenerative joint disease is by far the commonest type of arthritis, much commoner than the more dramatic condition of rheumatoid arthritis. It has been estimated, indeed, that after the age of 60 years, 25% of women and 15% of men have symptoms related to degenerative joint disease.

The *primary* type, which is somewhat more common in females, develops spontaneously in middle age and progresses slowly as an exaggeration of the normal aging process of joints. The *secondary* type, which is more common in males, develops at any age as a result of any injury, deformity or disease that damages articular cartilage. Since the "wear and tear" of continuing friction aggravates the underlying pathological process, degenerative joint disease is most common in weight-bearing synovial joints, such as the hip and knee, as well as the intervertebral disc joints of the lower lumbar spine. However, degenerative joint disease frequently involves joints of the hands as well as of the cervical spine, and all joints are susceptible.

Etiology

PRIMARY DEGENERATIVE JOINT DISEASE

The normal aging process in cartilage, just as the normal greying of hair, may be premature and accelerated in some individuals on a genetic basis; there may even be some unknown constitutional factor. In such individuals the resultant degenerative joint disease involves many joints without any known pre-existing abnormality and is said to be *primary*. Continued use—and especially abuse—of a given joint accelerates the local degenerative process. Obesity, although not an initiating factor, aggravates any existing degeneration in weight-bearing joints.

SECONDARY DEGENERATIVE JOINT DISEASE

Many types of injury, deformity and disease are capable of producing the initial cartilage lesion that leads to the development of progressive secondary degenerative joint disease. It will be obvious to you that such etiological factors will have a greater effect on aging cartilage than on young cartilage; however, any age group may be affected.

The following conditions are all capable of initiating the progressive degeneration in this secondary type of chronic arthritis:

1. Congenital abnormalities of joints: congenital dislocation of the hip, clubfeet.
2. Infections of joints: septic (pyogenic) arthritis, tuberculous arthritis.
3. Nonspecific inflammatory disorders of joints: rheumatoid arthritis, ankylosing spondylitis.
4. Metabolic arthritis: gout, ochronosis.
5. Repeated hemarthroses: hemophilia.
6. Injury: (a) Major trauma—intra-articular fractures, torn menisci. (b) Microtrauma—occupational stresses.
7. Acquired incongruity of joint surfaces: avascular necrosis, slipped epiphysis.
8. Extra-articular deformities with malalignment of joints: genu valgum, genu varum.
9. Joint instability: lax ligaments, stretched capsule, subluxation.
10. Iatrogenic damage to cartilage: continuous compression of joint surfaces during orthopaedic treatment of deformities.

Pathogenesis and Pathology in Synovial Joints

Whether degenerative joint disease is primary, secondary or a combination of the two, the pathological process in the early stages is similar and represents a marked exaggeration of the previously described aging process. The local pathological process is best considered in relation to the various tissue components of the joint.

ARTICULAR CARTILAGE

The earliest biochemical change of degenerative joint disease is always in the articular cartilage and consists of a loss of proteoglycan from the matrix. The resultant change in the physical, or biomechanical properties of the cartilage is softening (*chondromalacia*) and loss of the normal elastic resilience. Thus, the collagen fibrils of the cartilage, having lost some of their support and having become "unmasked," are rendered more susceptible to the friction of joint function; as a result, shedding of the tangential surface layers of cartilage is accelerated and the deeper vertical layers split with consequent *fissuring* and *fibrillation* (Fig. 11.1). The joint surface, which is normally bluish-

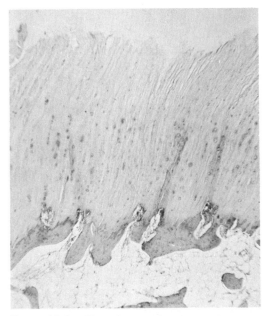

Figure 11.1. Fissuring and fibrillation of articular cartilage. This articular cartilage from a human arthritic joint exhibits a decreased number of chondrocytes in superficial layers, several deep vertical splits (fissuring) and innumerable superficial vertical splits (fibrillation).

white, smooth and glistening, becomes yellowish, granular and dull (Fig. 11.2).

As Mankin has stressed, the pathogenesis of osteoarthritis, far from being a passive "wear and tear" phenomenon, is characterized by much cellular and metabolic activity within the articular cartilage. Not only does the cartilage become more cellular but the chondrocytes synthesize proteoglycans and collagen at a greatly accelerated rate. Despite this valiant effort, however, the proteoglycan content is diminished because of the progressive destruction by lysosomal enzymes. Vascular invasion of the abnormal cartilage by vessels from the subchondral bone exposes the normally avascular cartilage to the systemic circulation for the first time and may lead to a type of self-perpetuating autoimmune disease which causes even further damage.

In the central area of the joint surface which is exposed to the most friction, the softened, fibrillated cartilage is gradually abraded down to subchondral bone which then serves as the articulating surface and gradually becomes as smooth as polished ivory (*eburnation*) (Fig. 11.3). The loss of articular cartilage is evidenced radiographically by a narrowing of the cartilage space (Fig. 11.4).

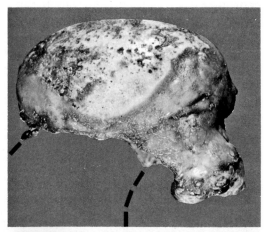

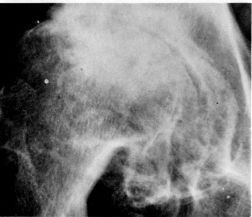

Figure 11.3 (*top*). Advanced degenerative arthritis of the right hip as seen in the femoral head. The articular cartilage over the weight-bearing area has been abraded down to subchondral bone which, in turn, has become eburnated to resemble polished ivory. The multiple pits in the eburnated surface represent arthritic cysts. The mass of bone growing out from the under surface of the medial margin of the femoral head is a large osteophyte. This femoral head was excised at the time of replacement arthroplasty in a 60-year-old man who had experienced increasing pain and loss of motion in the hip for 12 years.

Figure 11.4 (*bottom*). Pre-operative radiograph of the same hip as that from which the femoral head shown above was excised. Narrowing of the cartilage space indicates loss of articular cartilage. Note the increased radiographic density (sclerosis) in the weight-bearing area on both sides of the joint; note also the large osteophyte growing out from the under surface of the medial margin of the femoral head.

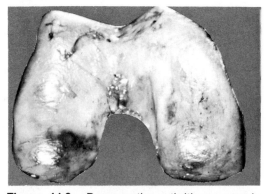

Figure 11.2. Degenerative arthritis as seen in the cartilage of the articular surface of the lower end of the femur (axial view from below). The cartilage was yellowish, granular and dull; in some areas it felt soft rather than rubbery. These abnormalities are most marked over the pressure areas—the weight bearing surfaces of the femoral condyles and also the patellar groove.

In the peripheral areas of the joint, the cartilage responds by hypertrophy and hyperplasia to form a thickened rim of cartilage around the joint margin. This outgrowth of cartilage (*chondrophyte*) subsequently undergoes endochondral ossification to become a bony outgrowth (*osteophyte*), also referred to as "osteoarthritic lipping" or "a bony spur." Osteophytes may become sufficiently large that they actually restrict joint motion (Figs. 11.3 and 11.4).

The loss of cartilage centrally and the building up of cartilage and bone peripherally produce incongruity of the joint surfaces which, in turn, alters both the distribution and the magnitude of the biomechanical stresses on the joint. Some areas are subjected to much more stress than normal while others are subjected to less than normal. Thus, the pathological process is self-perpetuating and a vicious cycle is established.

SUBCHONDRAL BONE

The striking reaction of the subchondral bone in degenerative joint disease accounts for the synonyms *osteoarthritis* and *osteoarthrosis*. In the central area of maximum stress and friction, the subchondral bone, in addition to becoming eburnated, hypertrophies to the extent that it becomes radiographically dense (*sclerotic*) (Fig. 11.5). In the peripheral areas, however, where there is minimal stress, the subchondral bone atrophies and becomes radiographically less dense (*rarefied*) (Fig. 11.6). Excessive pressure, particularly in weight bearing joints such as the hip, leads to the development of *cystic lesions* within the subchondral bone marrow, possibly because of mucoid and fibrinous degeneration in the local tissues secondary to microfractures of trabeculae. These "cysts" may even communicate with the joint surface through defects in the subchondral bone in which case they contain synovial fluid (Fig. 11.7). The increased vascularity associated with these bony reactions may be a factor in the production of pain.

The redistribution of biomechanical stresses on the joint leads to a *remodeling*

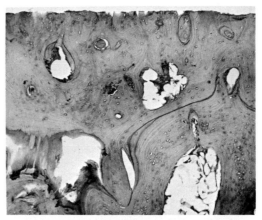

Figure 11.5. Hypertrophy of subchondral bone in an area of eburnation. This dense (sclerotic) bone has come to be the articulating surface and resembles cortical bone. A similar type of bone is seen at the site labeled *B* in Figure 11.6.

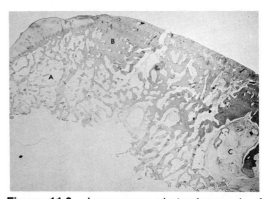

Figure 11.6. Low power photomicrograph of part of a femoral head excised at operation. In the peripheral, non-weight-bearing area (*A*) the cancellous bone has atrophied. In the weight-bearing area (*B*) the cancellous bone has responded to excessive pressures by becoming hypertrophied. Note also the large cystic lesion (*C*) under an area of weight-bearing. This arthritic "cyst" contains fibrous tissue.

of the subchondral bone; bone is worn away centrally but deposited (by endochondral ossification of the deep layer of cartilage) peripherally. Such remodeling accentuates the previously mentioned joint incongruity and contributes to the vicious cycle of degeneration (Fig. 11.8).

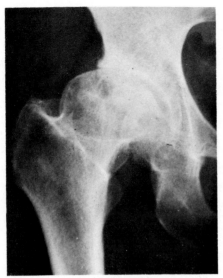

Figure 11.7. Right hip of a 65-year-old woman with degenerative arthritis. Note the large cystic lesion under the weight-bearing area of the femoral head. At operation this cyst was found to communicate with the joint cavity; it contained synovial fluid.

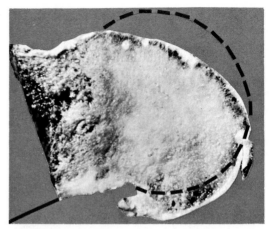

Figure 11.8. Cut surface of the femoral head from the arthritic hip of a 54-year-old man. The present shape of the femoral head is the result of gradual remodeling from the original shape (*dotted lines*). Such remodeling accentuates incongruity of the joint and contributes to the vicious cycle of degeneration.

SYNOVIAL MEMBRANE AND FIBROUS CAPSULE

Small fragments of abraded dead cartilage may float in the synovial fluid as loose bodies but tend to become incorporated in the synovial membrane which, in turn, reacts by undergoing hypertrophy and producing a moderate synovial effusion. The synovial fluid of such an effusion has an increased mucin content and consequently exhibits increased viscosity.

The fibrous capsule becomes greatly thickened and fibrotic, thereby further limiting joint motion. In the joints of the fingers, especially the distal interphalangeal joints, small areas of mucoid degeneration in the fibrous capsule at the joint margin form small subcutaneous protruberances which subsequently ossify and are known as *Heberden's nodes* (Fig. 11.9). Nevertheless, Heberden's nodes are not necessarily a manifestation of degenerative joint disease since the cartilage of the subjacent joint is usually normal.

MUSCLES

The muscles controlling the affected joint demonstrate spasm in response to pain and

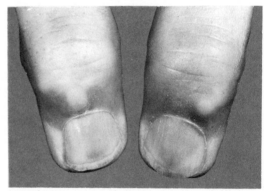

Figure 11.9. Heberden's nodes, which arise from the fibrous capsule at the margin of the distal interphalangeal joints.

eventually the stronger muscles (usually the flexors) undergo *contracture* with resultant joint deformity and further restriction of joint motion. With limited joint motion the excessive stresses are applied to a limited area of joint cartilage and this is another factor in the process of degeneration. The late result may be a *fibrous ankylosis* of the joint, but bony ankylosis seldom occurs spontaneously in degenerative joint disease.

Clinical Features and Diagnosis

Since there are no systemic manifestations of degenerative joint disease, the symptoms and signs are confined to individual joints.

The predominant symptom is *pain* which arises from bone as well as from the synovial membrane, fibrous capsule and the spasm of surrounding muscles. At first a dull ache and later more severe, the pain is intermittent; it is aggravated by joint movement ("friction effect") and relieved by rest. Eventually, however, the patient may even experience "*resting pain*" which is probably related to the hyperemia in the subchondral bone. Characteristically, the pain is worse when the barometric pressure falls just before a period of inclement weather. Paradoxically, the severity of the patients's pain is not necessarily related to the severity of the degenerative joint disease as evidenced by radiographic changes, but this may be due to individual differences in pain threshold as well as to differences in joint motion and the amount the joint is being used. Injuries, such as sudden strains or sprains, in an arthritic joint always aggravate the pre-existing symptoms.

The patient may become aware that the joint motion is no longer smooth and that it is associated with various types of *joint crepitus* such as squeaking, creaking and grating. The joint tends to become stiff after a period of rest, a phenomenon referred to as "*articular gelling.*" Gradually the involved joint loses more and more motion and eventually may even become so stiff that the pain (which is associated with motion) is decreased.

Physical examination reveals swelling of the joint due to a moderate effusion but there is relatively little synovial thickening; the joint swelling is more obvious because of the atrophy of surrounding muscles. Both active and passive joint motion are restricted and associated with joint crepitus, as well as pain and muscle spasm at the extremes of the existing range of motion. In the primary type of degenerative joint disease, Heberden's nodes are frequently seen at the distal interphalangeal joints (Fig. 11.8); they are more common in females but their exact relationship to degenerative joint disease is not clearly understood.

Radiographic examination reveals changes that are readily correlated with the pathological process. These include narrowing of the cartilage space, subchondral sclerosis and cysts, osteophyte formation, joint remodeling and incongruity (Fig. 11.10).

Laboratory examination does not reveal any evidence of systemic disease, but the synovial fluid exhibits an increased mucin content.

In each individual patient with degenerative joint disease, you should attempt to determine whether the disease is primary or secondary; if it is secondary you should diagnose the underlying condition.

Prognosis

While virtually every person who reaches old age has some degree of degenerative disease in one or more joints, many experience only mild, annoying discomfort which they ascribe, quite rightly, to "getting old" or to "a touch of rheumatism." When a given joint is severely involved, however, and the patient continues to use that joint, the course is one of progressive deterioration with increasing pain and loss of motion, unless the joint eventually becomes so stiff that the pain is decreased. Such stiffness is more likely to develop in the joints of the upper limb and spine; indeed, low back pain due to degenerative joint disease is much less common in the elderly than in middle age, presumably because the arthritic spine eventually becomes relatively stiff and stable and fewer demands are made on it.

In the lower limbs, degenerative joint disease has a relatively bad prognosis because of the continuing demands put on the affected joint with ordinary walking. This is particularly true in the hip joint, and when both hip joints are arthritic, the disability is very severe indeed.

Treatment

Although there is, as yet, no specific cure for degenerative joint disease and although the pathological lesions, being related to the aging process, tend to be permanent and progressive, much can be accomplished therapeutically for afflicted patients provided the treatment, both general and local, is

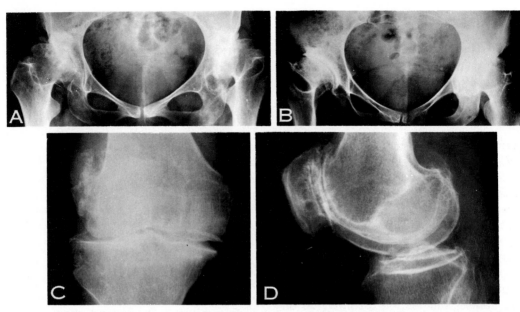

Figure 11.10. Radiographic changes of degenerative arthritis. *A,* Bilateral degenerative arthritis of the hips of a 36-year-old woman who had been treated for congenital dislocation of the hips at the age of 3 years. Both hips are subluxated, the left more so than the right. Note the joint incongruity, sclerosis, osteophytes, cysts, and narrowing of the cartilage space in both hip joints. *B,* bilateral degenerative arthritis of the hips in a 40-year-old woman who had been treated for congenital dislocation of the hips at the age of 4 years. The right femoral head had undergone avascular necrosis. Note the joint incongruity, subchondral sclerosis and remodeling. *C* and *D,* degenerative arthritis of the knee of a 75-year-old man. Note the large osteophytes, subchondral sclerosis and narrowing of the cartilage space.

tailored to fit the needs of each involved joint and each patient. Indeed, by means of local treatment, there is some hope of at least retarding, if not reversing, the pathological process.

AIMS OF TREATMENT

The over-all management of a patient with degenerative joint disease is based on the same general aims as outlined in the preceding chapter for rheumatoid arthritis, though the methods used to achieve these aims are somewhat different. The aims are as follows: (1) to help the patient understand the nature of the disease; (2) to provide psychological support; (3) to alleviate pain; (4) to suppress the inflammatory reaction (in the synovial membrane); (5) to maintain joint function and prevent deformity; (6) to correct existing deformity; (7) to improve function; (8) to rehabilitate the individual patient.

METHODS OF TREATMENT

1. Psychological Considerations

The patient with degenerative joint disease needs to be reassured that the local condition of his joint, or joints, is simply an exaggeration of the normal aging process, or "wearing out" of joints, with increasing age and furthermore that he does not have a generalized disease (such as the generalized rheumatoid disease associated with rheumatoid arthritis). The patient is then better prepared to live within the limits imposed by the painful joints. This implies a combination of rest and exercise with avoidance of long periods of either. Overweight patients with degenerative disease in a weight-bearing joint must be encouraged to lose weight with the understanding that this will decrease the load on the affected joint and thereby help to retard the arthritic process.

2. Therapeutic Drugs

Salicylates, either in the form of aspirin or sodium salicylate, are the most useful drugs in the treatment of degenerative joint disease, not only because they relieve pain in moderate doses but also because they may inhibit cartilage deterioration and may even exert a beneficial effect on the regeneration of cartilage. More powerful—and more dangerous—non-steroidal, anti-inflammatory drugs such as indomethacin and phenylbutazone are effective in relieving severe pain for some patients, but their toxic effects tend to outweigh their beneficial effects. Nevertheless, phenylbutazone and related drugs can often be administered by experienced physicians with much benefit to the patient. Narcotics should not be prescribed. The systemic administration of adrenocorticosteroids is of no value. Local intraarticular injections of corticosteroids, such as hydrocortisone, may produce temporary relief of joint pain but should not be repeated at frequent intervals in a given joint because of harmful effects on articular cartilage ("steroid arthropathy").

3. Orthopaedic Appliances

In addition to adequate periods of general rest, local rest of degenerated joints by removable splints is of value, not only in relieving pain but also in preventing deformity. Day braces are of limited value. When the hip is affected, the patient can take much weight off the joint by walking with a cane held in the hand of the opposite side (Fig. 11.11). When both hips are affected, the patient may need to use two canes or even crutches (Fig. 11.12).

4. Physical Therapy

Active movements of involved joints within the limits of pain are important in an attempt to preserve joint motion and maintain muscle strength; excessive exercising, however, tends to aggravate the condition. Local heat by any means, including heating pads and infrared lamps, frequently provide temporary relief of pain.

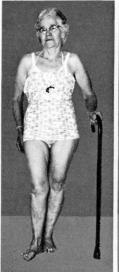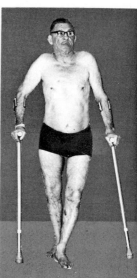

Figure 11.11. Woman with degenerative arthritis of the right hip taking weight off the hip joint by taking some weight on a cane on the opposite side. Note the adduction, external rotation contracture of the right hip.

Figure 11.12. Man with bilateral degenerative arthritis of the hips taking weight off both hip joints by taking some weight on two crutches. Note the adduction, external rotation contracture of both hips.

5. Orthopaedic Surgical Operations

A. Prophylactic. Degenerative changes can often be prevented, or at least delayed and sometimes even reversed, by surgical correction of joint conditions that are destined to cause the secondary type of degenerative joint disease—conditions such as subluxation of the hip, marked genu valgum (knock knee) and marked genu varum (bow leg).

B. Therapeutic. Surgical operations for the treatment of degenerative joint disease should not be considered as a last resort because once the degenerative changes become severe, only destructive operations can be expected to improve the situation. Nevertheless, considerable surgical judgment is required to assess the needs of each patient accurately and to choose the most effective method of surgical treatment as well as the optimum timing for such intervention. (For illustrations of the various operations, please see Chapter 6, Figures 6.14 to 6.23.)

Surgical operations that are effective for one joint may not be practical for another, but in general the types of operation that are performed for degenerative joint disease are the following:

(1) *Osteotomy* near the joint: to improve the biomechanics of the joint, especially the alignment, and to bring a different area of joint cartilage into function.

(2) *Arthroplasty* (reconstruction of a joint): *resection arthroplasty*, *interposition arthroplasty*, and replacement arthroplasty (prosthetic joint replacement of either one or both sides of the joint).

(3) *Arthrodesis* (fusion of a joint): to provide permanent relief of pain but at the expense of losing all motion.

(4) *Soft tissue operations:* release of tight muscles, excision of contracted capsule, neurectomy (denervation) of the joint; these operations tend to provide only temporary relief of pain.

(5) *Transplantation of whole joints:* still in the experimental stage but will be of great value once the immunological rejection phenomenon has been overcome.

Surgical Treatment of Degenerative Joint Disease in Specific Synovial Joints

FOOT AND ANKLE

Degenerative joint disease in the metatarsophalangeal joint of the great toe, without deformity, is called *hallux rigidus* (Fig. 11.13). Local treatment is either arthrodesis or resection arthroplasty (usually resection of the proximal half of the proximal phalanx). Degenerative changes can also develop secondary to a long standing deformity such as *hallux valgus* (Fig. 11.14, 15), in which case the treatment is similar to that of hallux rigidus.

Involvement of the tarsal joints, which is usually secondary, may require arthrodesis of the involved joints. Likewise, degenerative joint disease of the ankle, which is most frequently secondary to trauma (Fig. 11.16), is usually treated by arthrodesis, although prosthetic joint replacement is recommended by some.

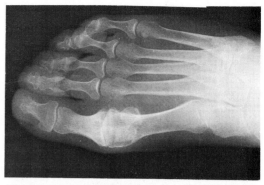

Figure 11.13. Hallux rigidus—degenerative arthritis in the metacarpophalangeal joint of the great toe. Note the narrowed cartilage space, cyst formation and sclerosis.

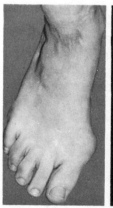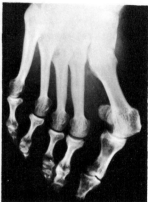

Figure 11.14 (*left*).   Hallus valgus of long duration in a 52-year-old woman who complained of increasing pain in the toe.
Figure 11.15 (*right*).   The same foot as shown at left; note the narrowing of the metatarsophalangeal joint.

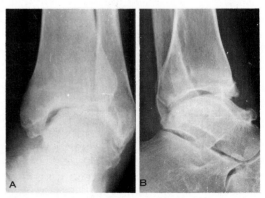

Figure 11.16.   Traumatic arthritis of the left ankle of a 57-year-old man who had injured his ankle 25 years previously.

KNEE

The initial site of degenerative joint disease in the knee is frequently the articular cartilage of the posterior surface of the patella, which is a sesamoid bone in the quadriceps mechanism. Characterized by softening (malacia), fissuring and fibrillation of the cartilage, this common disorder is referred to as "chondromalacia patellae" (Fig. 11.17). The most typical symptom is retropatellar pain that is aggravated by going up or down stairs and by running. Although the patella is certainly the most frequent site of chondromalacia, this disorder tends to be over-diagnosed, especially in adolescent girls. Non-operative treatment includes regular quadriceps exercise and salicylates. When true chondromalacia has been diagnosed by arthroscopic examination and when there is definite evidence of patellar malalignment (usually lateral "tracking") a surgical release of the tight lateral retinaculum may provide relief of symptoms—at least for a few years. Surgical elevation of the tibial tubercle (i.e. the insertion of the patellar tendon) as recommended by Maquet may also relieve pain by decreasing the pressure and friction between the cartilage surface of the patella and that of the patellar groove of the femur.

Although surgical "shaving" or "abrasion chondroplasty" of the cartilage—either at open operation or through the arthroscope—smoothes the joint surface and often decreases the patient's symptoms, mature hyaline articular cartilage is unable to regenerate unless the subchondral bone is entered (to provide access to the pluripotential mesenchymal cells). In the middle-aged and the elderly, chondromalacia of the patella may lead to patellofemoral arthritis of sufficient severity that excision of the patella (patellectomy) is required.

Degenerative joint disease of the lateral compartment of the knee joint, secondary to long standing genu valgum (Fig. 11.18) or of the medial compartment secondary to long standing genu varum (Fig. 11.19), can often be improved by corrective osteotomy of the upper end of the tibia to improve the joint alignment and redistribute the biomechanical forces to the more normal side of the joint. When cartilage destruction is severe, partial replacement arthroplasty (metallic prosthesis of the MacIntosh type for one or both tibial plateaus) or an osteocartilaginous allograft is frequently of value; but when the joint is irreparably damaged, prosthetic knee joint replacement or even arthrodesis may be required (as discussed in Chapter 6).

HIP

Degenerative joint disease of the hip represents one of the most challenging clinical

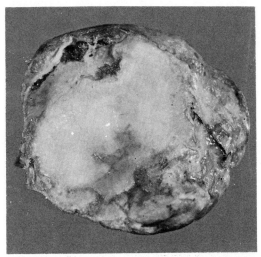

Figure 11.17. Articular surface of a patella with chondromalacia. The cartilage is not only irregular, but also soft.

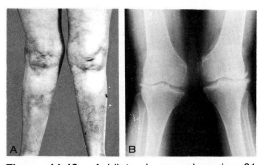

Figure 11.18. *A,* bilateral genu valgum in a 61-year-old woman who complained of pain on the lateral aspect of both kees. *B,* the radiograph reveals degenerative arthritis of the lateral compartment of both knees secondary to the excessive pressures related to genu valgum.

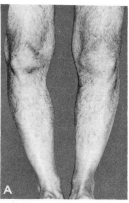
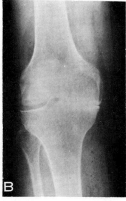

Figure 11.19. *A,* genu varum of the right knee in a 65-year-old man who complained of pain on the medial aspect of the knee. *B,* the radiograph reveals degenerative arthritis of the medial compartment of the knee secondary to the excessive pressures related to the genu varum.

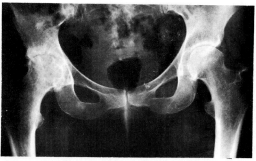

Figure 11.20. Primary degenerative arthritis of the right hip (malum coxae senilis) in 60-year-old woman who had no known pre-existing abnormality of the hip.

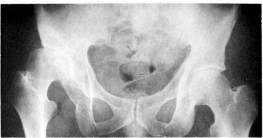

Figure 11.21. Degenerative arthritis of the right hip in a 32-year-old woman secondary to treated congenital dislocation.

problems for even the most experienced orthopaedic surgeon and taxes both his judgment and his skill. The disease may be *primary*, in which case it is sometimes referred to as *malum coxae senilis* (Fig. 11.20). Much more often, however the disease is *secondary* to the sequelae of such conditions as avascular necrosis, slipped femoral epiphysis and congenital dislocation of the hip (Fig. 11.21). Because of the complex biomechanics of the hip joint and the magnitude of stresses and forces to which it is subjected, degenerative hip joint disease is relentlessly progressive and disabling (Fig. 11.22). The previously mentioned operations of osteotomy (of either the femur or the innominate bone), resection arthroplasty, interposition arthroplasty, prosthetic joint replacement of either the conventional type ("total hip") or the surface replacement type, arthrodesis and soft tissue operations, all have their indications as well as their contraindications. In general, however, it may be stated that an osteotomy should be done before the disease is far advanced, that prosthetic joint replacement is better restricted to the older patient (preferably over 60 years) and that arthrodesis is most useful when only one hip is affected in a relatively young adult.

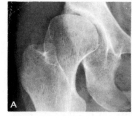
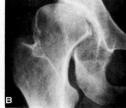

Figure 11.22. *A,* early degenerative arthritis of the right hip secondary to residual subluxation of the hip in a 43-year-old woman. Symptoms at this stage were minimal. *B,* the same hip only 2 years later reveals that the degenerative joint disease has been relentlessly progressive. Note that the subluxation has increased. The symptoms at this time were more severe.

HAND AND WRIST

Despite the obvious deformity caused by Heberden's nodes (Fig. 11.9), surgical treatment is seldom required. However, degenerative joint disease of the first carpometacarpal joint at the base of the thumb (Fig.

11.23) may be sufficiently disabling to require arthrodesis.

Involvement of the wrist is usually secondary to trauma and less commonly to avascular necrosis of the lunate (Kienbock's disease) (Fig. 11.24). If the arthritis does not respond to non-operative methods of treatment, it is best treated by arthrodesis of the wrist in the functional position of slight dorsiflexion.

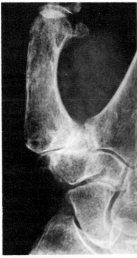

Figure 11.23. Degenerative arthritis of the carpometacarpal joint at the base of the thumb in a 33-year-old man who had sustained a fracture dislocation of this joint 10 years earlier.

ELBOW

Degenerative joint disease of the elbow is almost always of the secondary type, frequently traumatic (Fig. 11.25). When the disease is limited to the radiohumeral joint, excision of the radial head is effective. When the entire joint is destroyed, arthrodesis, resection arthroplasty or prosthetic joint replacement may be necessary.

SHOULDER

Osteoarthritis of the shoulder (glenohumeral) joint is not common but it can be quite disabling. In the early stages, a soft tissue operation consisting of division of the coracoacromial ligament, transection of the subscapularis muscle and capsulotomy of the joint often suffices to restore painless mobility of the shoulder. For more severe degrees of osteoarthritis, a prosthetic joint replacement may be required—either the unipolar (humeral component only) type of Neer or a bipolar type as devised by Macnab. Involvement of the acromioclavicular joint responds well to excision arthroplasty.

DEGENERATIVE JOINT DISEASE IN THE SPINE

Degenerative joint disease is even more common in the spinal column than in the limbs. This is not surprising when you consider the magnitude of the stresses and strains, partly related to man's upright po-

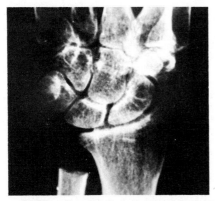

Figure 11.24. Traumatic arthritis of the wrist in a 50-year-old man who had sustained a fracture of the distal end of the radius and ulna 8 years earlier. The distal end of the ulna has already been resected to relieve pain.

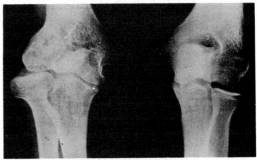

Figure 11.25. Traumatic arthritis of the radiohumeral joint in a 16-year-old boy who had sustained a fracture of the lateral condyle of the humerus at the age of 5 with a subsequent growth disturbance and secondary overgrowth of the radial head.

sition, that are applied to the spine during both work and play throughout a lifetime. Furthermore, the number of spinal joints is large, 23 intervertebral disc joints and 46 posterior facet joints. In addition, the intervertebral disc is the first structure in the musculoskeletal system to become affected by the degenerative changes of the normal aging process. Understandably, the incidence of such changes is higher in the more mobile lordotic segments of the lumbar and cervical spine than in the less mobile kyphotic segments of the thoracic spine (Fig. 11.26).

Form and Function of the Spinal Joints

The spine is an articulated column of vertebrae, each "couplet" of which is able to move through an intervertebral disc joint and two posterior facet joints. An abnormality of either type of joint will obviously have a deleterious effect on the other, a point of great importance in understanding the development of degenerative joint disease in the spine.

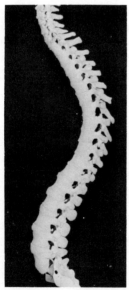

Figure 11.26. Lateral view of the human spinal column. The lumbar and cervical segments of the spine are lordotic and mobile, whereas the thoracic segment is kyphotic and relatively immobile.

THE INTERVERTEBRAL DISC JOINTS

Each intervertebral disc joint is a *symphysis* which forms a "coupling unit" between two vertebral bodies; it is comprised of three parts: the *nucleus pulposus*, the *annulus fibrosis* and the *hyaline cartilage end plates* of the opposing surfaces of each vertebral body (Fig. 11.27).

In youth the obliquely interlacing bands of fibrous tissue in the annulus fibrosus provide the annulus with *elasticity* which opposes the *turgor* of the nucleus pulposus, an incompressible gel containing proteoglycans. Normally with flexion, extension and lateral bending, the vertebral bodies roll over the turgid nucleus pulposus which thus behaves like a ball bearing. The normal nucleus pulposus contains neither nerves nor blood vessels and is nourished by diffusion of tissue fluids through minute channels in the cartilage endplates of the vertebral bodies. The nucleus is much more resilient, and therefore more resistant to injury, than the subchondral cancellous bone of the vertebral body.

THE POSTERIOR FACET JOINTS

The posterior facet (apophyseal) joints are of the *diarthrodial*, or *synovial* type; they serve to guide, steady and limit the movements of the vertebral bodies on one another. Being true synovial joints, they are comprised of a *fibrous capsule, synovial membrane* and *articular cartilage surfaces* (Fig. 11.28).

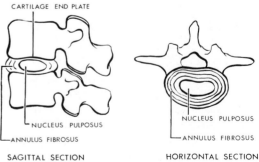

CARTILAGE END PLATE

NUCLEUS PULPOSUS

ANNULUS FIBROSUS

SAGITTAL SECTION

NUCLEUS PULPOSUS

ANNULUS FIBROSUS

HORIZONTAL SECTION

Figure 11.27. Components of the normal intervertebral disc joint in the human.

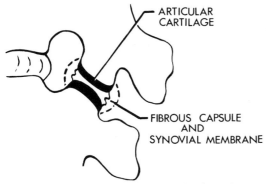

Figure 11.28. A normal posterior facet joint.

DEGENERATIVE JOINT DISEASE IN THE LUMBAR SPINE

Degenerative disease in the lumbar spine includes two interrelated conditions; the one involves the intervertebral disc joints (*degenerative disc disease*), the other, the posterior facet joints (*degenerative joint disease, osteoarthritis*). The latter condition is comparable to the degenerative disease of synovial joints in the limbs already described in this chapter. Both degenerative disc disease and degenerative joint disease represent an exaggeration of the normal aging process and may be aggravated by injury, deformity and pre-existing disease of the spine.

Pathogenesis and Pathology

The interrelated degenerative processes of disc disease and joint disease in the lumbar spine are best considered under the headings of *disc degeneration*, *segmental instability*, *segmental hyperextension*, *segmental narrowing* and *herniation of the intervertebral disc*.

DISC DEGENERATION

The initial degeneration in the spinal column of man occurs in the nucleus pulposus. Beginning in early adult life and progressing slowly thereafter, this degeneration is characterized by a gradual loss of chondroitin sulfate and water content with resultant loss of turgor and resilience as well as loss of actual height, or thickness, of the disc space. As the nucleus pulposus becomes inspissated, its gelatinous ground substance loses its homogeneous texture and becomes somewhat lumpy. While all of these degenerative changes may be considered within normal limits in an individual over the age of 60, they are considered abnormal if they develop to an advanced stage prematurely in a young person.

With increasing age, the annulus fibrosus gradually loses some of its elasticity, particularly posteriorly where it is relatively thin. Thus, its posterior fibers become more easily separated, or even torn, and this is one site of weakness in the annulus through which the nucleus pulposus may protrude or herniate. A second site of weakness is the thin cartilage end plate through which nuclear material may protrude into the underlying cancellous bone of the vertebral body and thereby form a *Schmorl's node* (Fig. 11.29). Schmorl's nodes are common

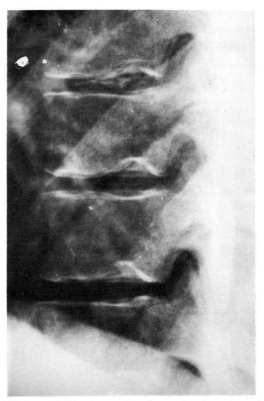

Figure 11.29. Lateral radiograph of portion of the thoracic spine showing Schmorl's nodes in three vertebral bodies.

radiographic findings but are of little clinical significance. Protrusion of the nucleus pulposus and annulus into the spinal canal occurs more readily in relatively young individuals in whom the nucleus still exhibits considerable turgor; it is rare in persons over the age of 50.

SEGMENTAL INSTABILITY

As a result of degenerative changes in the intervertebral disc joints, smooth motion in each involved segment of the spine is lost and is replaced by motion that is not only uneven, but also excessive. In this stage of segmental instability, the joint margins react by forming small traction spurs which are a form of osteophyte (Fig. 11.30). The unstable segments become more susceptible to injury which, in turn, may produce a sprain, or even a subluxation of the posterior facet joints.

SEGMENTAL HYPEREXTENSION

Normal extension of the lumbar spine is limited by the anterior fibers of the annulus fibrosus as well as by the abdominal muscles. However, the combination of degenerative changes in the annulus fibrosis, flabbiness of the abdominal muscles and obesity, all leads to persistent hyperextension of the lumbar spine through the intervertebral joints. Consequently, the posterior facet joints are chronically strained and may even subluxate with overriding (Fig. 11.31). Such malalignment causes degenerative joint disease (osteoarthritis) in these synovial joints with loss of articular cartilage, eburnation of subchondral bone and formation of osteophytes.

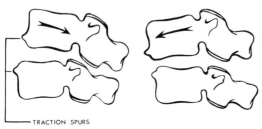

TRACTION SPURS

Figure 11.30. Segmental instability at an intervertebral disc joint with resultant traction spurs.

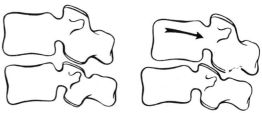

Figure 11.31. Segmental hyperextension at an intervertebral disc joint with resultant subluxation of the posterior facet joint.

SEGMENTAL NARROWING

Progressive narrowing of the intervertebral disc space with increasing age leads not only to degenerative changes in the posterior facet joints, but also to bulging of the annulus fibrosus which causes large osteophytes to develop from the bony margins of the adjoining vertebral bodies (*spondylosis, spinal osteophytosis*) (Fig. 11.32). Such osteophytes are detectable radiographically in 90% of individuals over the age of 60. At this stage the narrowed intervertebral joint has lost much of its motion; thus, the joint, having become relatively stiff, is less likely to be painful. This explains the high incidence of low back pain in early adult life and middle age, when radiographic changes are minimal, and the low incidence of low back pain in the elderly, when radiographic changes are maximal.

HERNIATION OF THE INTERVERTEBRAL DISC

Herniation (prolapse, protrusion, extrusion, rupture) of the intervertebral disc is not synonymous with degeneration of the disc; rather, it is a specific event that occurs as a complication of disc degeneration. The layman refers to it as a "slipped disc." Disc herniation is most frequent in relatively young individuals, particularly males, and the commonest sites in the lumbar region are L-4/5, L-5/S-1 and L-3/4, in that order.

The nucleus pulposus, having no nerves, is insensitive; but as it begins to herniate posteriorly, it stretches the sensitive annulus fibrosus and causes pain. Subsequently, the stretched and degenerated fibers of the an-

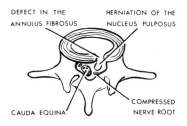

HORIZONTAL SECTION

Figure 11.33. Posterolateral herniation of the intervertebral disc.

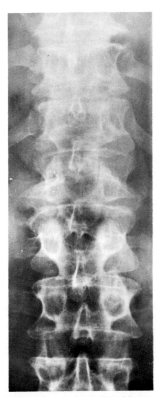

Figure 11.32. The spine of a 63-year-old man showing segmental narrowing at the intervertebral disc between the first and second lumbar vertebrae. Note the osteophytes arising from the bony margins of the adjoining vertebrae.

nulus separate and part of the nucleus herniates; since the posterior longitudinal ligament covers the annulus in the midline, the herniation tends to be posterolateral (Fig. 11.33). A posterolateral herniation either compresses or stretches the nerve root that leaves the intervertebral foramen distal to the disc; thus, a herniation of the L-4/5 disc affects the fifth lumbar nerve root, whereas a herniation of the L-5/S-1 disc affects the first sacral nerve root. The clinical manifestation of such nerve root irritation is *sciatica*, pain that radiates down the lower limb in the distribution of the sciatic nerve. A large herniation in the midline compresses the cauda equina.

The herniated portion of the nucleus pulposus becomes dehydrated and firm. Previously avascular, it may even become vas-

cularized, in which case the reaction to it might be in the nature of an autoimmune response. Eventually, several weeks after the event, the herniated portion of the nucleus undergoes fibrosis, shrinks and thereby relieves the pressure on the nerve root. Occasionally, however, the herniated portion becomes separated, or sequestrated, and may migrate either proximally or distally.

SPINAL STENOSIS

A bony narrowing of the spinal canal either centrally or in its lateral recesses (including the intervertebral foramina) is referred to as *spinal stenosis*. When the stenosis is central, the cauda equina is compressed, whereas when the stenosis is lateral, it is the emerging nerve roots and their blood supply that are compressed. In either case, the collective synonym "bony nerve root entrapment syndromes" is frequently used. Spinal stenosis may be congenital (as seen in association with achondroplastic dwarfism) or it may be acquired (as seen secondary to advanced disc degeneration, segmental narrowing, subluxation of the posterior facet joints or even secondary to a previous spinal fusion).

Clinical Features and Diagnosis of Various Syndromes in the Lumbar Spine

The various clinical manifestations of degenerative joint disease in the lumbar spine are best considered in relation to the phases of its pathogenesis described above. Disc degeneration, by itself, causes neither symptoms nor signs; indeed, the clinical syndromes in the lumbar spine are due to the secondary effects of disc degeneration; namely, segmental instability, segmental hyperextension, segmental narrowing and disc herniation.

SEGMENTAL INSTABILITY

The patient with instability of one or more lumbar segments is often aware of a chronic and intermittent backache that is aggravated by excessive activity and relieved by rest. The ache, which is deep, may be felt locally over the unstable segment, or it may be referred to the buttocks; there may be protective muscle spasm in the lumbar region.

Radiographic examination of the spine in both flexion and extension (after the pain has been controlled) provides evidence of the segmental instability, or hypermobility, as well as the associated traction spurs (Fig. 11.30).

SEGMENTAL HYPEREXTENSION

Chronic, persistent segmental hyperextension causes chronic and intermittent low back pain (lumbago) which may be felt locally, or may be referred over the buttocks and occasionally down the back of the thigh, but never below the knee. The low back pain is aggravated by any activity that involves active extension of the lumbar spine, such as lifting an object from the floor with the spine in a flexed position. During the painful episode, protective muscle spasm is apparent in the lumbar region. The patient obtains relief of the back pain by resting with the lumbar spine in flexion.

Radiographic examination of the spine in the standing position reveals overriding of the posterior facet joints (Fig. 11.31). Radiographic examination after injection of a radio-opaque material into the involved disc (discography) reveals evidence of degenerative changes and, in addition, reproduces the patient's symptoms.

SEGMENTAL NARROWING

Permanent narrowing of the intervertebral disc space represents a late stage in degenerative disc disease; the involved segment, being relatively stiff and stable, is less likely to be a source of acute pain. The patient, usually beyond middle age, is aware of stiff-

ness in the back, but complains of pain only after excessive activity. Loss of the normal mobility in the lumbar spine is detectable clinically.

Radiographic examination reveals spinal osteophytes in addition to narrowing of the involved disc space (Fig. 11.32).

HERNIATION OF THE INTERVERTEBRAL DISC

When the nucleus pulposus suddenly herniates as a complication of degenerative disc disease, the symptoms are often dramatic. For reasons already mentioned, this complication is most common during early adult life and middle age. The patient frequently gives the history that a few days after some excessive activity, or mild injury, he experiences the sudden onset of severe, agonizing low back pain (acute lumbago) during some simple act such as sneezing, coughing, twisting, reaching or stooping. Indeed, the pain may be so severe that even a stoical person is unable to move and has to be helped to a bed. Usually within a short time, a completely different type of pain is superimposed, severe pain radiating down one lower limb in the distribution of the sciatic nerve (acute sciatica).

Physical examination reveals muscle spasm in the lumbar region with loss of the normal lumbar lordosis; in addition, the patient may stand with his trunk shifted to one side (sciatic scoliosis) in a subconscious effort to relieve pressure of the herniated disc on the nerve root (Fig. 11.34). Active flexion and extension of the spine are markedly restricted.

The diagnosis of disc herniation with compression of a nerve root is dependent upon the clinical demonstration of nerve root irritation and, to a lesser extent, of impaired nerve root conduction. Limitation of straight leg raising (Lasegue's sign) is not sufficient evidence of nerve root irritation; more accurate is a positive bowstring test which specifically increases tension on the sciatic nerve (Fig. 11.35). Evidence of impaired conduction in the nerve root is provided by decreased skin sensation and muscle weakness in the distribution of the involved nerve root. For example, impaired conduction in the fifth lumbar nerve root is evidenced by sensory loss over the dorsum of the foot and weakness of the dorsiflexor muscles of the ankles and toes; impaired conduction in

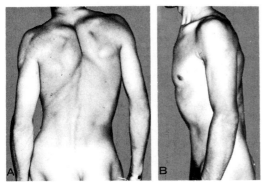

Figure 11.34. Sciatic scoliosis in a 30-year-old man who has an acute intervertebral disc protrusion. The longitudinal muscles are in spasm. In the lateral view there is loss of the normal lumbar lordosis as a result of the muscle spasm.

the first sacral nerve root is accompanied by sensory loss over the lateral aspect of the foot, a decreased or absent ankle reflex and weakness of the plantar flexor muscles of the ankle and toes. Accurate localization of the level of a disc herniation is usually possible by clinical examination alone.

Routine radiographic examination does not contribute to the diagnosis of disc herniation, but does help to exclude other causes of low back pain and sciatica. A disc herniation may be present with a radiographically normal disc space, whereas there may be radiographic narrowing of the disc space without a disc herniation. Radiographic examination after injection of a radio-opaque material into the spinal canal (*myelography*) is indicated if a spinal cord neoplasm is suspected, or if operative treatment is planned for a clinically diagnosed disc herniation (Fig. 11.36).

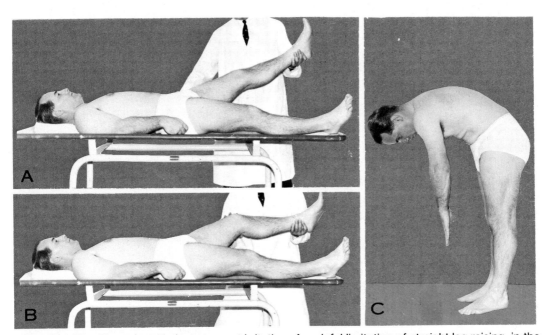

Figure 11.35. Tests for sciatic nerve root irritation. *A,* painful limitation of straight leg raising, in the absence of hip disease (Lasegue's sign), suggests irritation of the sciatic nerve root since this test increases the tension on the sciatic nerve and thereby aggravates the pain from any lesion, such as a herniated intervertebral disc, that is already stretching the nerve root. The normal range of passive straight leg raising is almost 90°. *B,* further evidence of sciatic nerve root pain is then provided by the bowstring test. After reaching the limitation of straight leg raising, the knee is flexed slightly to take tension off the sciatic nerve. At this point, pressure of the examiner's thumb on the medial popliteal nerve as it "bowstrings" across the popliteal fossa increases the tension on the sciatic nerve and reproduces the pain. *C,* forward bending with knees kept straight may be limited by sciatic nerve tension, spasm in the longitudinal muscles of the lumbar region, or a combination of the two.

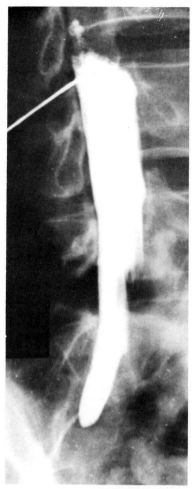

Figure 11.36. Myelogram. In this oblique projection, indentation of the column of contrast medium at the level of the L-5, S-1 intervertebral disc indicates a space-occupying lesion such as a herniated intervertebral disc. The diagnosis of herniated disc was confirmed at the time of laminectomy.

SPINAL STENOSIS

The central type of spinal stenosis that compresses the cauda equina may produce diffuse back pain whereas the lateral type of spinal stenosis causes nerve root compression and hence radicular pain (such as sciatica). The radicular pain from spinal stenosis, however, differs from that caused by herniation of the intervertebral disc in that it mimics the lower limb intermittent claudication type of pain associated with muscle ischemia. Thus, the pain, which is in part due to nerve

root ischemia, is likely to be brought on by walking. Unlike intermittent claudication, however, the claudication type of pain associated with spinal stenosis is not relieved by cessation of walking; it is relieved only by sitting or lying down. You will appreciate that the various forms of spinal stenosis are best seen in cross-section and hence are best demonstrated radiographically by means of computed tomography combined with metrizamide myelography.

Differential Diagnosis of Low Back Pain

Pain in the lower part of the back is experienced at some time by virtually every adult and is therefore the commonest symptom related to the musculoskeletal system. By no means, however, is all low back pain caused by degenerative joint disease or by degenerative disc disease, let alone disc herniation. Therefore, each patient who complains of low back pain, with or without sciatica, merits careful assessment on the basis of the history, physical examination, radiographic examination and laboratory investigation. You should be aware of the many possible sources of low back pain lest you fall into the ever present trap of erroneous diagnosis.

The following *classification of the causes of low back pain*, developed by Macnab, is most helpful:

1. *Viscerogenic.* Lesions of the genitourinary tract and pelvic organs as well as lesions, either intraperitoneal or retroperitoneal, that irritate the posterior peritoneum may cause low back pain. Characteristically, however, pain from such conditions is neither aggravated by activity nor relieved by rest.

2. *Vasculogenic.* Abnormalities of the descending aorta and iliac arteries, such as vascular occlusion and expanding or dissecting aneurysms, may cause pain that is referred to the back.

3. *Neurogenic.* Infections and neoplasms that involve either the spinal cord or the cauda equina may mimic disc herniation.

4. *Spondylogenic.* The commonest causes of low back pain, with or without sciatica, are disorders of the bony compo-

nents of the vertebral column (*osseous lesions*) and related structures (*soft tissue lesions*).

(a) *Osseous lesions*

Trauma: residual effects of fractures and dislocations

Infection: pyogenic osteomyelitis, tuberculous osteomyelitis

Non-specific inflammation: ankylosing spondylitis

Neoplasm: primary and secondary

Disseminated bone disorders: eosinophilic granuloma,Paget's disease

Metabolic bone disease: osteoporosis, osteomalacia, ochronosis

Bony deformities: spondylolysis, spondylolisthesis, scoliosis, adolescent kyphosis

(b) *Soft tissue lesions*

Myofascial lesions: muscle strains, tendinitis

Sacroiliac strain: usually related to childbirth

Intervertebral disc lesions: segmental instability, segmental hyperextension, segmental narrowing, disc herniation

Facet joint lesions: degenerative joint disease (osteoarthritis)

5. *Psychogenic.* The fact that a given patient who complains of low back pain is emotionally unstable or "neurotic" does not mean that his pain is imagined; indeed, in such a patient there is often an underlying organic basis for the pain, combined with a psychogenic exaggeration of its severity and significance (*functional overlay*). Thus, although low back pain is sometimes a manifestation of psychosomatic illness, an underlying organic cause of the pain must always be sought. The psychological needs of the patient, however, must always be met as well.

Treatment of Degenerative Joint Disease in the Lumbar Spine

AIMS OF TREATMENT

As with degenerative joint disease in the limbs, so also in the spine there is as yet no specific cure. Nevertheless, much can be accomplished therapeutically for afflicted patients provided the treatment is tailored to meet the specific needs of each patient. The overall treatment of patients with degenerative joint disease in the lumbar spine is based on the following aims: (1) to help the patient understand the nature of the disease (this aim has been met more effectively in recent years by the establishment of "Back Education Units" as recommended by Hall and others); (2) to provide psychological support; (3) to alleviate pain; (4) to improve function; (5) to rehabilitate the individual patient.

METHODS OF TREATMENT

1. Psychological Considerations

The patient needs to be reassured that the condition in his back represents an exaggeration of the normal aging process and that with non-operative methods of treatment, 90% of patients are relieved of their pain within six weeks. He must be prepared to live within the limits imposed by the disorder in his back. Since in a large percentage of patients with low back pain no organic cause can be readily detected, it is important to ascertain not only what kind of back disorder the person has, but also what kind of person has the back disorder.

2. Therapeutic Drugs

For the symptomatic relief of either severe or acute back pain (lumbago) or sciatica, the patient requires strong analgesics over a relatively short period; the continued use of narcotics, however, should be avoided. Muscle relaxants are of little value and phenylbutazone should be used with caution because of its harmful side effects.

3. Orthopaedic Apparatus and Appliances

All patients with degenerative joint disease in the lumbar spine are helped, at least to some degree, by adequate local rest of the spine. Patients with segmental instability, segmental narrowing and intervertebral disc herniation should rest in bed on a firm mattress which is supported by rigid boards. For acute attacks of either lumbago or sciatica, complete bed rest should be continued until at least two or three days after the pain has been relieved. Patients with segmental hyperextension are much more comfortable lying on their back with the mattress elevated at each end to keep the lumbar spine flexed, or alternatively, lying curled up on either side.

After a period of bed rest, the patient may require a temporary spinal support such as a plaster of Paris body jacket, a firmly applied felt jacket (Fig. 11.37), a surgical cor-

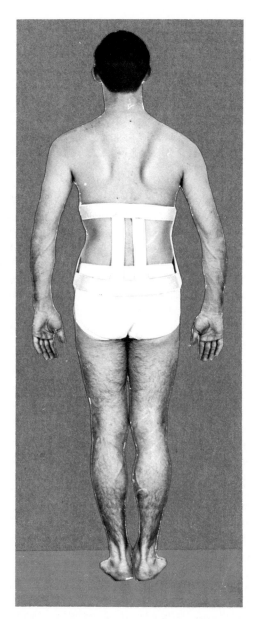

Figure 11.38 (*right*).   More permanent spinal support by means of a leather covered metallic back brace (Harris type).

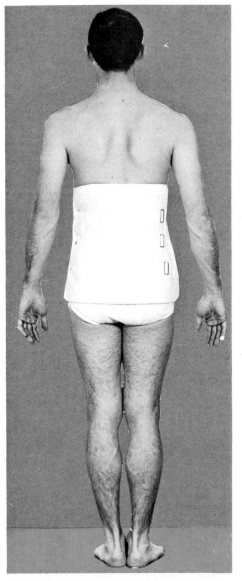

Figure 11.37. (*left*).   Temporary spinal support by means of a firmly applied felt jacket.

set, or a more permanent support such as a metal back brace (Fig. 11.38). The more permanent type of spinal support may have to be worn, at least during the day, for many months. Patients with segmental hyperextension require a spinal support that maintains their lumbar spine in flexion.

4. Physical Therapy

Local heat and massage may give temporary relief during an acute attack of pain, but the most important function of physical therapy is to strengthen spinal and abdominal muscles after the acute attack in an attempt to improve spinal posture and to prevent recurrence of pain.

5. Surgical Manipulation

Manipulation of the spine is a procedure which is very popular in some centers and one which should be performed only by an expert. Manipulation is probably best reserved for those patients with segmental instability and segmental hyperextension in whom an acute subluxation of a posterior facet joint is suspected. Spinal manipulation is potentially dangerous, however, in the presence of a suspected disc herniation because of the definite risk of aggravating the situation and increasing the neurological deficit.

6. Chemonucleolysis

The enzymatic dissolution of the nucleus pulposus by the transcutaneous intradiscal injection of chymopapain is known as *chemonucleolysis*, a relatively new and somewhat controversial form of treatment that is currently being used in many countries throughout the world. Chymopapain, a peptidase derived from papaya fruit, digests the polypeptide core of the proteoglycan molecules of the matrix of the nucleus pulposus. The resultant hydrolysis and shrinkage of the nucleus relieves the pressure of a protruded intervertebral disc on a nerve root and thereby relieves the pain. Thus, for patients with clear-cut evidence of herniation of an intervertebral disc in the lumbar region (the diagnostic features of which are outlined in an earlier section of this chapter), chemonucleolysis is a reasonable last step in the non-operative treatment when the other methods of non-operative treatment have failed and operative treatment seems indicated. McCulloch, from an experience with over 2000 such patients, has stated that when chemonucleolysis is used *only* for this particular and precisely diagnosed indica-

tion, 80% of the patients are relieved of their pain and are thereby spared surgical exploration and excision of the disc (discectomy) by laminectomy. If however, chemonucleolysis is used indiscriminately for spinal disorders other than nerve root irritation or compression from herniation of an intervertebral disc (such as spinal stenosis or psychogenic pain) the results are predictably disappointing. Chemonucleolysis, which is combined with discography, can be performed under local anesthesia; the procedure necessitates only a short stay in hospital and can even be done on an outpatient basis. The only serious complication is an anaphylactic reaction which fortunately is very rare, except in patients sensitized to chymopapain from a previous chemonucleolysis.

7. Surgical Operation

Approximately 90% of patients with degenerative joint disease and degenerative disc disease in the lumbar spine will recover without a surgical operation. Therefore, unless there is loss of bladder or bowel function (which represents a surgical emergency), the *initial* treatment should always be nonoperative. Myelography and discography should be reserved for those patients in whom surgical operation is deemed necessary (Fig. 11.36).

The indications for laminectomy and removal of a herniated disc are as follows:

(1) Loss of bladder and bowel control: a surgical emergency.

(2) Persistent, unbearable pain that is not relieved even by strong analgesics.

(3) Persistent, severe pain and evidence of persistent nerve root irritation or impairment of nerve conduction after three weeks of complete bed rest.

(4) Evidence of progression of neurological changes while the patient is in bed.

(5) Recurrent episodes of incapacitating back pain or sciatica.

(6) Spinal stenosis necessitates extensive laminectomy and excision of sufficient bone to decompress the compressed cauda equina or nerve root(s).

The operation of arthrodesis of one or more segments of the spine (spinal fusion) does not completely immobilize the intervertebral disc and cannot be expected to provide complete relief of pain. Furthermore, solid fusion is difficult to obtain, even in the hands of experienced orthopaedic surgeons. Modern methods of spinal fusion, including the bilateral intertransverse process fusion, have a higher percentage of success, but even with this technique, localized failure of fusion (pseudarthrosis) can still occur and can be a continuing source of pain. Spinal fusion is most effective for the treatment of segmental instability and segmental hyperextension with degenerative joint disease (osteoarthritis) in the posterior facet joints; however, spinal fusion should not be undertaken unless non-operative methods have failed to obtain relief of pain and unless the patient is willing to avoid heavy manual labor in the future.

8. Rehabilitation

Approximately 5% of all patients with degenerative joint disease in the lumbar spine remain severely disabled despite extensive treatment. For some of these unfortunate individuals the functional or emotional component of their disability is greater than the organic component: yet they need help. The future for this relatively small group of permanently disabled patients with degenerative joint disease in the lumbar spine, just as the future of other severely disabled persons, lies not so much in the development of better surgical operations, as in the development of more effective facilities for retraining them, and the development of more opportunities for gainful light work, either in sheltered workshops or in industry.

DEGENERATIVE JOINT DISEASE IN THE CERVICAL SPINE

Degenerative disease in the cervical spine (*cervical spondylosis*), which includes both degenerative disc disease and degenerative joint disease, though relatively common, is not so common as degenerative joint disease in the lumbar spine.

Pathogenesis and Pathology

Much of what has been written above concerning the pathogenesis and pathology of degenerative disc disease and degenerative joint disease in the lumbar spine is equally applicable to the cervical spine—the initial degeneration in the nucleus pulposus, the segmental instability, the segmental narrowing, the subsequent development of degenerative joint disease in the posterior facet joints with osteophyte formation and finally, herniation of the intervertebral disc. Thus, the details need not be repeated here.

The commonest segments to be affected by such degenerative changes in the cervical spine are C-5/6 and C-6/7 which, like the lower lumbar segments, are particularly mobile and in the area of maximum lordosis. In the cervical spine there is little room in the intervertebral foramina for exit of the nerve roots; consequently, subluxation and osteophyte formation in the posterior facet joints readily compress these roots, particularly after any injury with its associated soft tissue swelling.

Herniation of the intervertebral disc, though much less common in the cervical spine than in the lumbar spine, may occur as a dramatic event in the degenerative process for the same reasons and in the same manner as previously described for the lumbar segments. The more common type of herniation, which is posterolateral, compresses a nerve root; the relatively uncommon, but more serious central herniation compresses the spinal cord.

Clinical Features and Diagnosis

Most persons over the age of 60 exhibit radiographic evidence of degenerative disc disease and degenerative joint disease in the cervical spine, but in many the condition causes no symptoms apart from mild stiffness in the neck. When the cervical spondylosis is more severe, however, it may cause vague neck pain as well as pain that is referred to the shoulder even without nerve root compression.

Cervical nerve root irritation, either from encroachment of osteophytes in the intervertebral foramina, or from intervertebral disc herniation, produces a variety of clinical syndromes including pain in the neck and shoulder as well as pain radiating down the arm in the distribution of the involved nerve root (*brachialgia*). This radicular type of pain may be accompanied by paresthesia in the form of numbness or tingling. The onset of symptoms is often insidious, but can be acute, particularly when an injury is added to the pre-existing degenerative changes.

Compression of the sixth cervical nerve root (from either osteophytes or disc herniation at the C-5/6 level) produces weakness of the deltoid and biceps muscles, diminished biceps reflex and diminished skin sensation in the thumb and index finger. Compression of the seventh cervical nerve root (from either osteophytes or disc herniation at the C-6/7 level) produces weakness of the triceps muscle, diminished triceps reflex and diminished skin sensation in the index and middle fingers. When the spinal cord is compressed by a central herniation of the disc, the clinical picture is indistinguishable from a spinal cord neoplasm and requires immediate investigation. A neurosurgeon should always be consulted forthwith.

Examination of the neck in the presence of pain may reveal limitation of motion, particularly lateral flexion, but there is relatively little muscle spasm; in a quiescent phase, there may be few clinical findings other than crepitus in the cervical spine during active movement. Complete neurological examination of the upper limbs is always indicated.

Radiographic examination reveals disc space narrowing and osteophyte formation, both of which are best seen in the lateral projection (Fig. 11.39). Because of the oblique direction of the intervertebral foramina, however, an oblique projection is required to demonstrate the osteophytic encroachment (Fig. 11.40). If a central herniation of the disc is suspected, a myelogram is indicated.

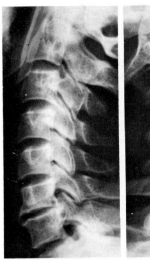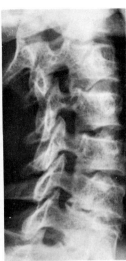

Figure 11.39 (*left*). Lateral radiograph of the cervical spine in a 60-year-old man with cervical degenerative joint disease (cervical spondylosis). Note the narrowing of the C-6/7 intervertebral disc space and the associated osteophytes arising from the adjoining vertebral bodies.

Figure 11.40 (*right*). Oblique radiograph of the cervical spine in the same patient whose lateral radiograph is shown at left. Note the osteophytic encroachment on the intervertebral foramen.

Differential Diagnosis of Neck and Arm Pain

As with low back pain and sciatica, so also with neck and arm pain (brachialgia), each of the many possible causes must be considered in a given patient. The following general classification developed by Macnab is equally applicable in the cervical and lumbar region—only the specific details differ.

1. *Viscerogenic.* Lesions of the pharynx, larynx and the upper part of the trachea and esophagus may cause neck pain.

2. *Vasculogenic.* Angina pectoris and the pain of myocardial infarction from coronary artery occlusion may be referred to the neck as well as to the shoulder and down one or both arms. Likewise, occlusion of a carotid artery may produce neck pain.

3. *Neurogenic.* A spinal cord neoplasm mimics central herniation of a cervical disc. A neoplasm at the apex of the lung (*Pan-*

coast tumor), or a cervical rib, can cause pressure on the brachial plexus with resulting radicular pain and can therefore mimic nerve root compression from cervical spondylosis with nerve root compression. Even involvement of peripheral nerves, such as irritation of the ulnar nerve at the level of a deformed elbow, and compression of the median nerve in the carpal tunnel, must be differentiated from cervical spondylosis and cervical disc herniation.

    4. *Spondylogenic*

    (a) *Osseous lesions*

        Trauma: residual effects of fractures and dislocations

        Infection: pyogenic osteomyelitis, tuberculous osteomyelitis

        Non-specific inflammation: ankylosing spondylitis

        Neoplasm: primary and secondary

        Disseminated bone disorders: eosinophilic granuloma

        Metabolic bone disease: osteoporosis, osteomalacia, ochronosis

    (b) *Soft tissue lesions*

        Myofascial lesions: muscle strains, tendinitis

        Intervertebral disc lesions: segmental instability, segmental narrowing

        Facet joint lesions: degenerative joint disease (cervical spondylosis)

    5. *Psychogenic.* The fact that a given patient who complains of neck and arm pain is emotionally unstable, or "neurotic," does not mean that his pain is imagined; indeed, in such a patient there is nearly always an underlying organic basis for the pain combined with a psychogenic exaggeration of its severity and significance (*functional overlay*). Thus, although neck pain, with or without arm pain, is sometimes a manifestation of psychosomatic illness, the underlying organic cause of the pain must always be sought. In addition, however, the psychological needs of the patient must also be met.

Treatment of Degenerative Joint Disease in the Cervical Spine

The aims and methods of treatment for degenerative joint disease in the cervical spine are comparable to those already described in relation to the lumbar spine with only a few minor differences. Therefore, only the differences will be discussed here.

Local rest for the neck, which helps to relieve pain, is achieved by means of a cervical "ruff" (Fig. 11.41) or, when the symptoms are more protracted, a cervical brace or collar (Fig. 11.42). Intermittent traction on the cervical spine through a halter may also provide considerable relief of pain. The majority of patients can be managed effectively by non-operative methods of treatment.

Surgical arthrodesis (fusion) of one or more segments of the cervical spine anteriorly (*anterior interbody fusion*) may be necessary to control the persistent pain of cervical spondylosis; the rate of successful spinal fusion is much higher in the cervical

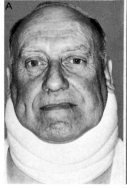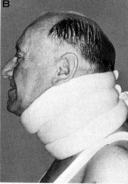

Figure 11.41. Local rest for the cervical spine by means of a firmly applied cervical "ruff," a series of three rolls of stockinette filled with cotton wool.

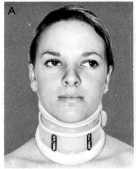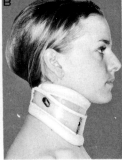

Figure 11.42. Local rest for the cervical spine by means of an adjustable plastic cervical collar.

spine than in the lumbar spine. Laminectomy and removal of a herniated cervical disc is seldom necessary for a posterolateral herniation, but is always indicated for a central herniation with compression of the spinal cord. Under these circumstances, laminectomy and decompression of the cord should be performed by a neurosurgeon; subsequently, it may be necessary for an orthopaedic surgeon to stabilize the decompressed segments by means of an anterior interbody fusion.

NONARTICULAR RHEUMATISM

A variety of "rheumatic diseases" affect musculoskeletal tissues other than joints; these include disorders of muscles, fascia, tendons, ligaments, synovial sheaths and bursae, all of which may be grouped under the general heading of nonarticular rheumatism (extra-articular rheumatism).

Myofascial Pain Syndrome ("Fibrositis")

The number of different terms applied to this common but poorly understood clinical disorder ("fibrositis syndrome," "sensitive deposits," "muscular rheumatism," "tension rheumatism," "psychogenic rheumatism") reflect the lack of scientific knowledge concerning both its etiology and its pathology. Of the many theories proposed to explain this syndrome, none has been proven. Nevertheless, the lack of understanding does not deny the existence of a clinical syndrome which is not only common and characteristic, but also very troublesome to those afflicted.

CLINICAL FEATURES

Myofascial pain syndrome is characterized by deep pain in the region of various muscles and their fascial attachment to bone, most commonly in the neck and back; it is both chronic and recurrent but does not necessarily remain confined to one muscle group. Involved muscles and fascia may be hypersensitive to direct pressure and squeezing, particularly at certain fairly constant "trigger points"; in these sites, small areas of induration in the muscle or fascia ("fibrositic nodules") may or may not be palpable. Pain may be felt locally but more often it is a referred type of pain and is thus felt elsewhere. Characteristically, the pain is aggravated by emotional tension, immobility and chilling; it is relieved by equanimity, activity and local heat. There is a plethora of symptoms but a paucity of physical signs. Studies by Smythe and Moldofsky have revealed a definite relationship between "fibrositis syndrome" and disturbed sleep patterns with particular reference to non-REM (rapid eye movement) sleep. The patient complains of weariness and yet there is neither clinical nor laboratory evidence of systemic disease; the patient complains of joint stiffness and yet there is neither clinical nor radiographic evidence of joint disease.

The psychogenic aspects of myofascial pain syndrome are apparent in these patients, most of whom exhibit a chronic anxiety state as well as a low pain threshold. Nevertheless, the pain, though exaggerated, is not imaginary. Indeed, the excessive muscle tension that accompanies the chronic emotional tension of a chronic anxiety state may, in itself, be a cause of pain either in the muscles or in their fascial attachment to bone. Unlike the complaints of purely psychogenic origin, which tend to vary with the patient's emotional state, or "internal climate," the complaints of myofascial pain syndrome (like those of many other rheumatic diseases) tend to be aggravated by changes in the weather, or "external environment."

The diagnosis of myofascial pain syndrome can be suspected on the basis of the characteristic clinical features but it can be established only after other, more serious, causes of musculoskeletal pain have been excluded.

TREATMENT

Patients who suffer from myofascial pain syndrome present a challenge to the physician because their condition represents a curious combination of psychological and somatic manifestations. Reassurance that the pain is related to tension, both emotional and muscular, is most helpful. Local pain and tenderness may be relieved, at least temporarily, by heat, massage, mild analgesics and, if necessary, local injections of hydrocortisone and a local anesthetic agent. From a long term point of view, however, these anxious patients need sound advice concerning a more appropriate way of life with less tension and more equanimity.

Degenerative Tendon and Capsule Disease

Whereas the weight bearing joints of the lower limb are frequently afflicted by degenerative joint disease, the nonweight bearing joints of the upper limb are more frequently afflicted by degenerative disease in the periarticular tissues such as tendon and capsule, *degenerative tendon and capsule disease*.

INCIDENCE AND ETIOLOGY

The periarticular tissues of the shoulder are particularly prone to develop this type of nonarticular rheumatism. As with degenerative joint disease, so also with degenerative tendon and capsule disease, many etiological factors are superimposed upon the progressive changes of the normal aging process in these tissues. With aging, the blood supply of tendons and joint capsules becomes less adequate; as a result of decreased diffusion of nutrients through the intercellular tissues, local degenerative changes are inevitable.

PATHOGENESIS AND PATHOLOGY

The basic underlying pathological change in degenerative tendon and capsule disease is *local necrosis* of varying extent in a tendon. Subsequently, these areas of necrosis tend to become calcified (*dystrophic calcification*) and this can cause a chemical as well as a physical inflammation (*calcific tendinitis*). Furthermore, local areas of degeneration in tendons so weaken their structure that they may rupture, or tear, with little trauma (*pathological tear*).

DEGENERATIVE TENDON AND CAPSULE DISEASE IN THE SHOULDER

The wide range of circumduction motion between the arm and the trunk occurs at several sites: (1) the glenohumeral (shoulder) joint; (2) the acromioclavicular joint; (3) the sternoclavicular joint; (4) between the scapula and the thorax. Normally, smooth motion is possible between the under surface of the acromion and the upper surface of the musculotendinous cuff because of the large intervening subacromial (subdeltoid) bursa. The musculotendinous cuff ("rotator cuff") is composed of the conjoined tendinous attachments of four muscles (subscapularis, supraspinatus, infraspinatus and teres minor) and the capsular attachment into the upper end of the humerus.

Degenerative disease in the musculotendinous cuff of the shoulder is usually most marked in the supraspinatus portion, possibly because the blood supply in this area is least adequate and, hence, most vulnerable to pressure. Frequently, the degenerative changes and their sequelae produce either an acute or a chronic inflammatory reaction in the tissues, hence the clinical terms, tendinitis, bursitis and capsulitis. The more common clinical syndromes, all of which represent complications of degenerative tendon and capsule disease, are the following: *calcific tendinitis*, *subacromial bursitis*, *bicipital tendinitis*, *tear of the musculotendinous cuff* and *adhesive capsulitis*.

Shoulder pain is a common symptom but it is not always a manifestation of intrinsic shoulder disease. The pain, though felt in the shoulder, may be either referred or radiating from a variety of extrinsic disorders including cervical spondylosis, cervical disc herniation, angina pectoris, myocardial infarction, basal pleurisy and subphrenic (subdiaphragmatic) inflammation from such conditions as cholecystitis, abscess and even a ruptured spleen.

Calcific Supraspinatus Tendinitis

Dystrophic calcification in the supraspinatus portion of the musculotendinous cuff is common (3% of the adult population). Such calcium deposits may cause no symptoms; when symptoms do arise however, the clinical condition is *calcific supraspinatus tendinitis* which may be either acute or chronic.

Acute Calcific Supraspinatus Tendinitis. Rapid deposition of calcium in a closed space within the substance of the supraspinatus tendon causes excruciating pain which, being due to increased local pressure, is throbbing in nature and is not relieved by rest. At this stage the calcium deposit has the consistency of toothpaste and behaves like a "chemical boil"; as it expands, it irritates the undersurface of the subacromial bursa and produces a secondary *subacromial bursitis* with aggravation of the pain. If, however, the calcium deposit bursts into the subacromial bursa, which has a good blood supply, the calcium is gradually absorbed and the symptoms subside.

The clinical picture is characteristic. The patient, more often a male and usually of middle age or older, may previously have experienced mild symptoms due to degenerative changes in the musculotendinous cuff with, or without, calcium deposits. After unusual or excessive use of the shoulder, he experiences the rapid onset of extremely severe shoulder pain that drives him to seek

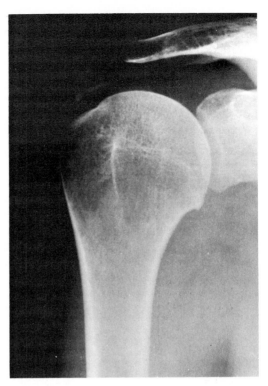

Figure 11.44. Chronic calcific supraspinatus tendinitis. Note the calcium deposits in the region of the musculotendinous cuff close to its insertion into the humerus.

immediate relief; the pain may radiate distally as far as the hand. The patient maintains the shoulder in an adducted position which keeps the painful lesion away from the undersurface of the acromion; there is exquisite local tenderness just lateral to the acromion. Abduction of the shoulder, both active and passive, is most painful during one arc of the normal range of motion, the arc from approximately 50° to 130°; this is an example of the *painful arc syndrome*, which is explained by the anatomical fact that during this arc of abduction, the involved area of the supraspinatus tendon is in intimate contact with the undersurface of the acromion (Fig. 11.43). Radiographic examination reveals deposits of calcium in the region of the musculotendinous cuff close to its insertion into the humerus (Fig. 11.44).

Treatment depends upon the severity and duration of the acute episode. Local rest with an arm sling, combined with analgesics

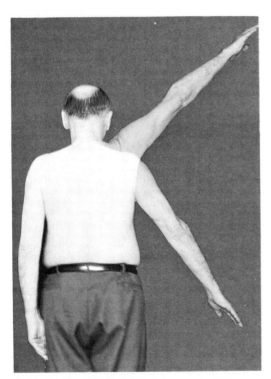

Figure 11.43. Painful arc syndrome. This double exposure photograph demonstrates the limits of the painful arc of abduction (approximately 50° to 130°).

and adrenocorticosteroid therapy, bring relief of pain for some patients. In others, however, the pain is so severe and so disabling that these measures are inadequate. Under such circumstances, attempts at *aspiration* of the semi-fluid calcium in the "chemical boil" are justified; the aspiration, which is performed under local anesthesia and accompanied by local injection of hydrocortisone, does not always yield calcium, but usually the multiple punctures in the deposit allow the calcium to be dispersed into the subacromial bursa where it can be absorbed. Occasionally, aspiration may have to be repeated. If these methods of treatment fail to relieve the severe pain, surgical removal of the calcium is indicated. After the acute symptoms have subsided, active exercises help to prevent prolonged stiffness of the shoulder.

Chronic Calcific Supraspinatus Tendinitis. Even when calcium is deposited slowly in degenerated areas of the supraspinatus tendon, the lesion may become sufficiently large that it causes symptoms. Deposits of long duration tend to become semi-solid and to have a gritty sensation because of dessication.

The clinical picture is less dramatic than that described for the acute episode. The patient experiences chronic pain which, though not severe, is annoying during the day and interferes with sleep at night. Examination reveals mild local tenderness just lateral to the acromion; the *painful arc syndrome* can also be demonstrated (Fig. 11.43).

Treatment by attempts at aspiration of chronic, dessicated calcium deposits is usually unsuccessful and even surgical removal of the deposit may be followed by recurrence. For patients with persistent pain, it may become necessary to eliminate friction between the degenerated area of the tendon and the acromion, either by excising the acromion, or by lowering the glenoid cavity through an osteotomy of the neck of the scapula.

Tears of the Musculotendinous Cuff

Pre-existing changes of aging in the musculotendinous cuff weaken it sufficiently that with a superimposed injury it is prone to tear (rupture). Thus, tears of the musculotendinous cuff are most common during middle age and beyond; they may be either *partial* or *complete.*

Partial Tear of the Musculotendinous Cuff. The supraspinatus component of the musculotendinous cuff, being the commonest site of degenerative changes and also being subjected to the greatest strains, is the most frequent site of a tear. Indeed, in postmortem studies of the shoulder, such tears are seen as an incidental finding in one quarter of elderly persons, most of whom had not complained of the shoulder.

The patient is usually able to initiate abduction, but experiences pain in so doing; the *painful arc syndrome* can be demonstrated (Fig. 11.43). After injection of a local anesthetic agent, active abduction becomes more comfortable. These observations help to differentiate between a *partial* tear and a *complete* tear.

Treatment consists of active exercises to prevent prolonged stiffness in the shoulder joint. Occasionally division of the coracoacromial ligament and excision arthroplasty of the acromioclavicular joint are necessary.

Complete Tear of the Musculotendinous Cuff. An injury such as a fall on the shoulder, may completely tear a previously degenerated musculotendinous cuff including the capsule. The proximal part of the cuff retracts and the glenohumeral (shoulder) joint then communicates with the subacromial bursa.

The patient with a complete tear of the musculotendinous cuff, usually a male over the age of 60, cannot initiate abduction of the arm and on attempting to do so, merely shrugs the shoulder (Fig. 11.45). If, however, his arm is passively abuducted to 90°, he is able to maintain this position of abduction by means of the deltoid muscle.

Radiographic examination, after injection of radio-opaque material into the shoulder joint (arthrography), reveals that the material spreads from the joint into the bursa and confirms the presence of a complete tear. Arthroscopy of the shoulder may also be of help in determining the extent of the tear.

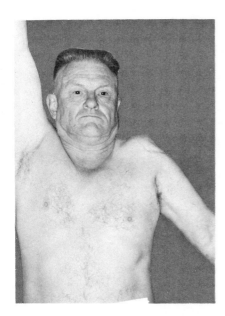

Figure 11.45. Complete tear of the musculotendinous cuff of the left shoulder in a 65-year-old man who is attempting to abduct the shoulder. He is able to obtain only slight abduction as he shrugs his shoulder and rotates the scapula. If, however, his arm were passively abducted to 90°, he would be able to maintain this position with his deltoid muscle.

Treatment of complete tears of the musculotendinous cuff by surgical repair is somewhat unsatisfactory because of degenerative changes in the torn edges. Thus, in the elderly, the best treatment consists of simple exercises to prevent shoulder stiffness. In more active persons, however, extensive surgical repair of the completely torn cuff is justified; postoperatively, the patient's shoulder is immobilized in a position of abduction for three weeks after which active exercises are begun.

Bicipital Tendinitis and Tenosynovitis

Degenerative changes in the tendon of the long head of the biceps muscle, combined with chronic inflammation of its enveloping synovial sheath within the bicipital groove of the humerus, can be a source of shoulder pain, particularly in the female. The pain, which is felt anteriorly, is aggravated by active supination of the forearm against resistance with the elbow flexed and with the shoulder moving; this phenomenon is sometimes referred to as the "*palm-up pain syndrome.*" There are no radiographic signs of the disorder.

Treatment of this relatively mild but irritating condition consists of local rest with an arm sling. One or more local injections of hydrocortisone may be required to relieve the pain. Occasionally, the symptoms are sufficiently severe and persistent that operative treatment is indicated; the degenerated tendon is divided and the distal stump is sutured to the bicipital groove.

Rupture of the Biceps Tendon

Pre-existing degenerative changes in the tendon of the long head of the biceps muscle may weaken it sufficiently that it may rupture during active flexion of the elbow against resistance as in lifting a heavy object.

The patient experiences immediate pain and is aware that something has "given way." Examination reveals that when the patient flexes the elbow (using the short head of biceps, brachialis and brachioradialis muscles), the muscle belly of the long head of biceps contracts into a "ball" which is more distal than normally (Fig. 11.46).

The resultant disability is not particularly severe in an elderly person, but for a man who requires strong elbow flexion for his work, it may be necessary to suture the distal stump of the ruptured tendon into the bicipital groove.

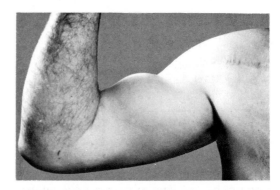

Figure 11.46. Rupture of the long head of the biceps tendon in a 52-year-old man who is flexing his elbow. The muscle belly of the long head of the biceps can be seen in a position that is more distal than normal.

Adhesive Capsulitis of the Shoulder (Frozen Shoulder)

A variety of disorders, not only in the shoulder (intrinsic) but also outside the shoulder (extrinsic) may lead to the development of diffuse capsulitis of the glenohumeral joint, particularly in older persons. Subsequently, the inflamed capsule becomes adherent to the humeral head rather like adhesive tape (*adhesive capsulitis*) and undergoes contracture: the adherent, shrunken capsule prevents motion in the glenohumeral joint which becomes "frozen" in one position (*frozen shoulder*).

Intrinsic disorders that may initiate this process include calcific supraspinatus tendinitis, partial tear of the musculotendinous cuff, bicipital tendinitis. Even prolonged immobilization of the shoulder in a cast or a sling may lead to adhesive capsulitis. Extrinsic disorders capable of producing this condition are those which cause pain in the region of the shoulder and which therefore cause the patient to keep the shoulder still. These disorders include cervical spondylosis, cervical disc herniation, myocardial infarction, basal pleurisy and subphrenic inflammation.

The onset of adhesive capsulitis is usually gradual. Initially, in the inflammatory phase, the patient experiences shoulder pain, and examination reveals muscle spasm in all the muscles about the shoulder. After a few weeks the inflammation becomes subacute, the shoulder becomes stiff or "frozen" and the acute pain subsides. Thus, when the patient attempts to abduct the arm he does so by elevating and rotating the scapula (Fig. 11.47). Because of the lack of motion in the glenohumeral joint, additional strain is applied to the acromioclavicular joint which may become painful; the pain radiates proximally from the shoulder and may be felt as high as the ear.

The prognosis for adhesive capsulitis is quite good in that the pathological process tends to be self-limiting. It may take several months, however, for the shrunken, adherent capsule to become separated from the humeral head and for reasonable motion to

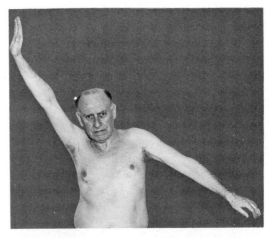

Figure 11.47. Adhesive capsulitis of the left shoulder (frozen shoulder) in a 63-year-old man who is attempting to abduct his shoulder. He can obtain 45° of apparent abduction by elevating and rotating his scapula.

return; the frozen shoulder usually "thaws" slowly.

Treatment of adhesive capsulitis in the early, painful stage includes local rest with the arm in a sling, local heat and analgesics. Forcing motion at this stage aggravates the situation. Approximately half of the patients are improved significantly by the systemic administration of adrenocorticosteroids. Inflation of the glenohumeral joint with saline injected through a needle is sometimes successful in separating the adherent capsule from the humeral head.

In the later stages, if motion is not returning at a reasonable rate, surgical manipulation, or even operative treatment, is occasionally required to release the contracture of the subscapularis muscle and to separate the adherent capsule from the articular cartilage of the humeral head.

Shoulder-Hand Syndrome

A distressing, but poorly understood, disorder affecting the upper limb, particularly the shoulder and hand, is the *shoulder-hand syndrome*, which is an example of *reflex sympathetic dystrophy*.

Although the etiology of the shoulder-hand syndrome is not known, it can be initiated by any disorder, either intrinsic or extrinsic, which is associated with pain in the upper limb.

This syndrome usually afflicts persons over the age of 50, especially those who have a low pain threshold. It is characterized by disabling pain in the shoulder and hand accompanied by local neurovascular disturbances, moisture and hyperesthesia of the skin, atrophy of subcutaneous tissues, chronic edema and eventually regional disease atrophy of bone (disuse osteoporosis) (Fig. 11.48).

Since the limb is painful, the fearful patient refuses to use it; absence of muscle action in the dependent limb results in chronic edema of the hand which, in turn, makes joint motion in the fingers more painful. Eventually joint contractures develop, disuse atrophy becomes progressive and a vicious cycle is established.

Treatment of the shoulder-hand syndrome includes psychological measures to support and encourage the patient, analgesics, systemic adrenocorticosteroids, local heat and active exercises. Injection of the stellate ganglion with a local anesthetic agent to produce a sympathetic nerve block may improve the local blood supply and help to reverse the process.

Degenerative Tendon Disease in the Elbow

As in the shoulder, so also in the elbow, the tendinous and fascial attachments of

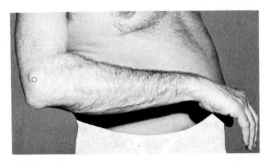

Figure 11.49. Tennis elbow (lateral epicondylitis). The circle marks the discrete point of local tenderness.

muscles may degenerate with subsequent local necrosis, dystrophic calcification and pathological rupture. Many etiological factors, including local trauma and excessive activity, are superimposed upon the progressive degenerative changes of the normal aging process.

Tennis Elbow (Lateral Epicondylitis). The commonest example of degenerative tendon disease in the elbow is "tennis elbow," also called *lateral epicondylitis*. Although proof of the pathogenesis of this disorder is lacking, it is thought to be a premature degeneration in the flat tendinous origin of the *forearm extensor muscles* from the lateral epicondyle of the humerus.

Tennis elbow is by no means limited to those who play tennis; it can develop as a sequel to local injury as well as to any activity that involves the forearm extensor muscles. Patients with cervical spondylosis may exhibit referred hyperesthesia and tenderness just distal to the lateral epicondyle, a phenomenon which is easily confused with tennis elbow.

Clinically, tennis elbow is characterized by pain over the lateral aspect of the elbow and radiation of the pain down the forearm. The pain is aggravated by any activity that puts tension on the forearm extensor muscle origin, such as active dorsiflexion of the wrist while grasping an object, and passive flexion of the wrist against resistance. A discrete point of local tenderness is detectable just distal to the lateral epicondyle (Fig. 11.49).

Radiographic examination may reveal

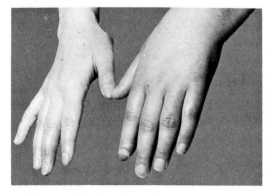

Figure 11.48. Shoulder-hand syndrome, a form of reflex sympathetic dystrophy. The left hand of this 54-year-old woman is swollen, cool and moist.

dystrophic calcification in the area of degeneration in the extensor muscle origin, but the elbow joint itself appears normal.

Treatment of this chronic and recurrent form of nonarticular rheumatism includes local rest, heat, and one or more injections of hydrocortisone and a local anesthetic agent into the precise area of local tenderness. For those patients in whom troublesome symptoms persist despite these measures, it may become necessary to immobilize the wrist in a cast for several weeks (to rest the wrist extensor muscles); on rare occasions, it is necessary to resort to operative treatment in which the fascial attachment of the extensor muscles to the lateral epicondyle is divided and allowed to retract distally

Degenerative Tendon Disease in the Wrist and Hand

The commonest form of nonarticular rheumatism in the wrist and hand is that associated with thickening of the fibrous sheath of a tendon with resultant narrowing of the tunnel (*tenovaginitis stenosans*). Two definite clinical entities are readily recognized, one at the wrist, the other in the fingers. Although tenovaginitis stenosans usually develops in otherwise normal persons, it occasionally is a manifestation of early rheumatoid arthritis.

De Quervain's Tenovaginitis Stenosans. At the level of the lower end of the radius, the tendons of the abductor policis longus and extensor pollicis brevis share a common fibrous sheath. Excessive friction between those tendons and their common sheath, due to repeated forceful use of the hands in gripping or wringing, probably account for the abnormal thickening of the fibrous sheath and the resultant constriction, or stenosis, of the tunnel.

This fairly common clinical disorder, which is seen most frequently in the female, is characterized by wrist pain which radiates proximally up the forearm and distally toward the thumb. Examination reveals local tenderness in the area of the common fibrous sheath (Fig. 11.50). Forceful passive adduction (ulnar deviation) of the patient's

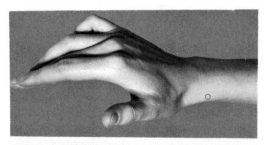

Figure 11.50. De Quervain's tenovaginitis stenosans. The circle marks the site of local tenderness over the common fibrous sheath for the tendons of the abductor pollicis longus and extensor pollicis brevis.

wrist with the thumb held completely flexed puts tension on the involved tendons and reproduces the pain (Finklestein's test).

Treatment of de Quervain's tenovaginitis stenosans by local injection of hydrocortisone into the tendon sheath usually brings temporary relief but frequently, operative division of the stenosed tendon sheath is required to provide permanent relief of pain.

Digital Tenovaginitis Stenosans (Trigger Finger) (Snapping Finger). In the palm of the hand the flexor tendons to each finger are enclosed by a common fibrous sheath. Excessive thickening of this fibrous sheath may develop spontaneously for no apparent reason, particularly in middle-aged females. It may also occur, however, as a complication of rheumatoid synovitis in the hand.

Thickening of the fibrous sheath produces a stenosis, or constriction, in the tunnel and as a result, free gliding of the flexor tendons is impeded. The tendons become secondarily enlarged proximal to the tunnel, presumably because of repeated friction. The patient is unable to actively extend the involved finger (Fig. 11.51). The finger can be extended passively and the extension occurs with a "snapping" motion. The patient is then able to flex the finger actively, but again with a "snapping" action similar to the action of a trigger. The nodular enlargement in the flexor tendons can be palpated just proximal to the base of the finger.

Treatment by means of local rest for the finger and one or more injections of hydro-

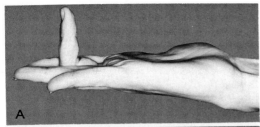
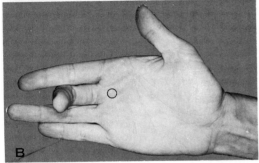

Figure 11.51. Tenovaginitis stenosans involving the right middle finger in a 43-year-old woman. *A*, the patient is attempting to extend the finger but is unable to do so. The finger can be extended passively and the extension occurs with a "snapping" motion. The patient is then able to flex the finger actively, but again with a snapping action similar to the action of a trigger. *B*, the circle marks the site of the palpable nodular enlargement in the flexor tendons.

cortisone may relieve the snapping phenomenon. Sometimes, however, operative division of the fibrous sheath is required to provide permanent relief of the symptoms.

A congenital type of fibrous tunnel stenosis involving the thumb of young children (trigger thumb) is discussed in Chapter 8.

Dupuytren's Contracture of the Palmar Fascia

Progressive fibrous tissue contracture of the palmar fascia (*Dupuytren's contracture*) on the medial (ulnar) side of the hand is not uncommon in men over the age of 50. The etiology is unknown but there is evidence of an hereditary predisposition. The disorder is frequently bilateral; it may even involve the plantar fascia of the feet.

The initial manifestation of this insidious and painless process is nodular thickening in the palmar fascia which becomes adher-

ent to the overlying skin. Over the ensuing years a slowly progressive contracture of the palmar fascia gradually pulls the ring and little fingers into flexion at the metacarpophalangeal and proximal interphalangeal joints (Fig. 11.52). Although the synovial joints are not involved primarily, they eventually develop secondary capsular contractures and degeneration of articular cartilage secondary to the persistent restriction of motion.

Treatment of Dupuytren's contracture involves surgical excision of all the abnormal palmar fascia; less complete operations, such as multiple subcutaneous division of fibrous bands, are frequently followed by recurrence of the contracture.

Ganglion

A *ganglion* is a thin walled cystic lesion containing thick, clear mucinous fluid; its origin is as yet unknown, but it arises in relation to periarticular tissues, joint capsules and tendon sheaths, possibly due to mucoid degeneration. Ganglia are limited to the hands and feet, by far the commonest site being the dorsum of the hand (Fig. 11.53).

The patient notices a soft swelling which tends to enlarge gradually, but which may vary in size from time to time. Occasionally, the ganglion causes local discomfort but usually the patient is more concerned about its appearance. A ganglion on the palmar

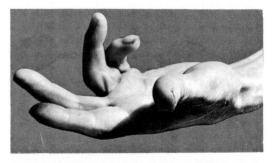

Figure 11.52. Dupuytren's contracture of the palmar fascia involving the ring and little fingers of the hand of a 56-year-old man. Note the flexion deformity of the metacarpophalangeal and proximal interphalangeal joints and the local adherence of the puckered skin to the palmar fascia.

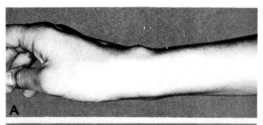

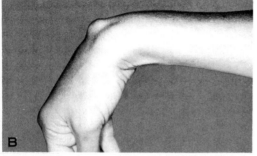

Figure 11.53. *A,* ganglion on the dorsum of the hand of a 26-year-old woman. *B,* the cystic swelling is more apparent when the wrist is flexed.

aspect of the hand may even cause pressure on either the median or ulnar nerve with resultant disturbance of nerve function.

Ganglia tend to regress spontaneously over a long period of time, but usually the patient wishes to be rid of the unsightly swelling. If a ganglion is deliberately ruptured by firm pressure, with or without needling, it tends to recur. Some ganglia respond to aspiration, but frequently complete operative excision of the ganglion is necessary in order to achieve a permanently satisfactory result.

Popliteal Cyst (Baker's Cyst)

A cyst that is somewhat similar to a ganglion may develop in the popliteal region, usually in relation to the semimembranous bursa. Such popliteal cysts (Baker's cysts) are common in childhood but seldom cause symptoms (Fig. 11.54). A popliteal cyst usually regresses spontaneously during childhood.

In adults, popliteal cysts usually communicate with the knee joint through a hollow stalk and in a sense represent a "synovial hernia." Thus, in the presence of a synovial effusion in the knee, due to either rheumatoid arthritis or degenerative joint disease,

the popliteal cyst becomes distended by the effusion and may extend distally even as far as the mid-calf.

If a popliteal cyst becomes sufficiently enlarged that it interferes with knee function, operative excision of the cyst and exploration of the joint are indicated.

Meniscal Cyst

A fluid-filled cyst of a meniscus may develop in childhood and produce a tender swelling at the joint line; it is more often the lateral meniscus that is involved. Barrie has demonstrated that such cysts usually communicate with a meniscal tear and are "fueled" by synovial fluid. When causing symptoms, such menisci may have to be excised.

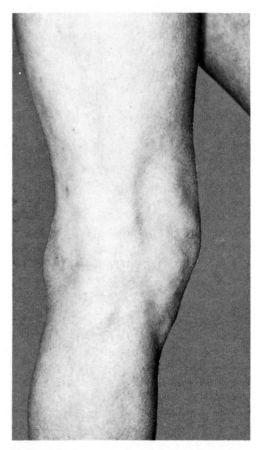

Figure 11.54. Popliteal cyst (Baker's cyst) behind the right knee of a 10-year-old child. The cyst caused no symptoms.

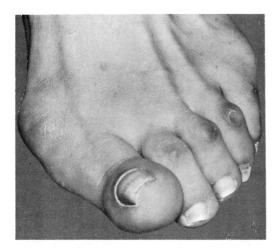

Figure 11.55. Bunion, an example of friction bursitis over the head of the first metatarsal in association over a hallux valgus deformity. Note also the corns overlying the proximal interphalangeal joints of the 4 small toes.

Bursitis

Bursae are synovial lined and synovial fluid containing sacs which exist normally at sites of friction between tendons and bone as well as between these structures and the overlying skin. In addition, pluripotential connective tissue cells are capable of creating "adventitious bursae" at sites of friction caused by such abnormalities as pathological bony prominences and protruding parts of metallic inserts.

As a result of repeated excessive friction, a bursa may become inflamed (*friction bursitis*); the wall of the bursa thickens and a bursal effusion develops. The commonest example of friction bursitis is that caused by the pressure and friction of tight shoes over the prominence of the first metatarsal head, especially in the presence of a hallux valgus deformity; this particular example of friction bursitis is referred to as a *bunion* (Fig. 11.55). The friction type of bursitis may be related to excessive friction associated with specific occupations. The following are examples of such bursitis: *prepatellar bursitis* ("housemaid's knee") (Fig. 11.56); ischial bursitis (*weaver's bottom*); olecranon bursitis ("student's elbow") (Fig. 11.57).

Degenerative changes and calcification in a subjacent tendon may irritate the overlying bursa and cause a *chemical bursitis;* subacromial bursitis secondary to calcific supraspinatus tendinitis is an example of chemical bursitis. In addition, chemical bursitis may develop secondary to the tophaceous deposits of urate crystals in gout.

Infection of a bursa, by either pyogenic or

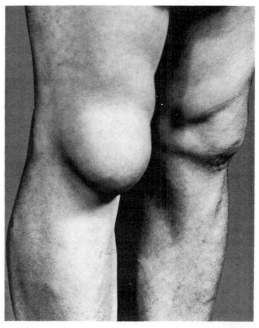

Figure 11.56. Prepatellar bursitis (housemaid's knee), an example of friction bursitis in a 45-year-old woman. In this patient the amount of fluid in the bursa is greater than is usually seen in prepatellar brusitis.

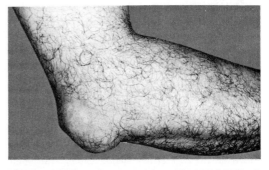

Figure 11.57. Olecranon bursitis (student's elbow), an example of bursitis that may be caused either by the repeated microtrauma of friction (as against a desk top) or by single direct trauma.

granulomatous organisms, results in an *infective*, or *septic*, *bursitis*, which though initially acute, may later become chronic.

Treatment of bursitis is directed toward the underlying cause. Friction bursitis usually resolves after cessation of the friction, but if the bursa has become sufficiently large, it may require excision. Chemical bursitis responds to removal of the responsible irritant (calcium or urate crystals) and the local injection of hydrocortisone. Acute septic bursitis requires surgical drainage, but chronic septic bursitis necessitates operative excision of the bursa.

Suggested Additional Reading

Amstutz, H. C., Graff-Radford, A., Mai, L. L. and Thomas, B. J.: Surface replacement of the hip with the Thaires system. J. Bone Joint Surg. 63A: 1069–1077, 1981.

Anastassiades, T. P., Dwosh, I. L. and Ford, P. M.: Intra-articular steroid injections: a benefit or a hazard? Can. Med. Assoc. J. 122: 389–390, 1980.

Barrie, H. J.: The pathogenesis and significance of meniscal cysts. J. Bone Joint Surg. 61B: 184–189, 1979.

Bentley, G.: Surgical treatment of chondromalacia patellae. J. Bone Joint Surg. 60B: 74–81, 1978.

Bombelli, R.: *Osteoarthritis of the Hip. Pathogenesis and Consequent Therapy*. Berlin, Springer-Verlag. 1976.

Charnley, J.: *Low Friction Arthroplasty of the Hip—Theory and Practice*. Berlin, Springer-Verlag, 1979.

Charnley, J.: Trends in arthroplasty of the hip. In *Clinical Trends in Orthopaedics*, edited by Straub, L. R. and Wilson, P. D. Jr. New York, Thieme-Stratton, 1982.

Chrisman, O. D., Laudenbauer-Bellis, I. M. and Penjabi, M.: The relationship of mechanical trauma and the biochemical reactions of osteoarthritic cartilage. Clin. Orthop. 161: 275–284, 1981.

Coventry, M. B.: Upper tibial osteotomy for gonarthrosis. The evolution of the operation in the last 18 years and long term results. Orthop. Clin. North Am. 10(1): 191–210, 1979.

Cruess, R. L. and Mitchell, N. S. (eds.): *Surgical Management of Degenerative Arthritis of the Lower Limb*. Philadelphia, Lea & Febiger, 1975.

Dinham, J. M.: Popliteal cysts in children: the case against surgery. J. Bone Joint Surg. 57B: 69–71, 1975.

Edmonson, A. S. and Crenshaw, A. H. (eds.): *Campbell's Operative Orthopaedics*, 6th ed. St. Louis, C. V. Mosby, 1980.

Ferguson, A. B. Jr.: Elevation of the insertion of the patellar ligament for patellofemoral pain. J. Bone Joint Surg. 64A: 766–771, 1982.

Freeman, M. A. R.: The fatigue of cartilage in the pathogenesis of osteoarthrosis. Acta Orthop. Scand. 46: 323–328, 1975.

Freeman, M. A. R.: Trends in arthroplasty of the knee. In *Clinical Trends in Orthopaedics*, edited by Straub, L. R. and Wilson, P. D. Jr. New York, Thieme-Stratton, 1982.

Freeman, M. A. R., Swanson, S. A. V., Day, W. H. and Thomas, R. J.: Conservative total replacement of the hip. J. Bone Joint Surg. 57B: 114, 1975.

Friedman, D. M. and Moore, M. E. : The efficacy of intra-articular steroids in osteoarthritis: a double-blind study. J. Rheumatol. 7(6): 850–856, 1980.

Goodfellow, J., Hungerford, D. S., Woods, C.: Patello-femoral joint mechanics and pathology. Chondromalacia patellae. J. Bone Joint Surg. 58B: 291–299, 1976.

Grabius, S.: The treatment of spinal stenosis. Current concepts review. J. Bone Joint Surg. 62A: 308–313, 1980.

Gordon, D. A. (ed.): Rheumatoid arthritis. In *Discussions in Patient Management*. New York, Excerpta Medica, 1981.

Gross, A. E., Silverstein, E. A., Falk, J., Falk, R. and Langer, F.: The allotransplantation of partial joints in the treatment of osteoarthritis of the knee. Clin. Orthop. 108: 7–14, 1975.

Gunston, F. and McKenzie, R. I.: Complications of polycentric arthroplasty. Clin. Orthop. 120: 11, 1976.

Hall, J. H.: The Canadian Back Education Units. Physiotherapy 66: 115–117, April 1980.

Harris, W. H.: Total joint replacement. N. Engl. J. Med. 297: 650, 1977.

Hunter, G. A., Welsh, R. P., Cameron, H. U. and Bailey, W. H.: The results of revision of total hip arthroplasty. J. Bone Joint Surg. 61B: 419–421, 1979.

Kelley, W. H., Harris, E. D. Jr., Ruddy, S., Sledge, C. B.: *Textbook of Rheumatology*. Philadelphia, W. B. Saunders, 1981.

Lord, G. A., Hardy, J. R. and Kummer, F. J.: An uncemented total hip replacement. Clin. Orthop. 141: 2–16, 1979.

MacIntosh, D. L.: Arthroplasty of the knee. J. Bone Joint Surg. 48B: 179, 1966.

Macnab, I.: *Backache*. Baltimore, Williams & Wilkins, 1977.

Macnab, I.: The surgical management of degenerative changes of the shoulder. Mod. Med. Can. 33: 994–1000, 1978.

Macnab, I., McCulloch, J. A., Weiner, D. S., Hugo, E. P., Galway, R. D. and Dall, D.: Chemonucleolysis. Can. J. Surg. 14: 280–289, 1971.

Mankin, H. J.: The reaction of articular cartilage to injury and to osteoarthritis. Part I. N. Engl. J. Med. 291: 1285, 1974.

Mankin, H. J.: The reaction of articular cartilage to injury and to osteoarthritis. Part II. N. Engl. J. Med. 291–1335, 1974.

Maquet, P.: The biomechanics of the knee and surgical possibilities of healing osteoarthritic knee joints. Clin. Orthop. 146: 102, 1980.

McCarty, D. J.: *Arthritis and Allied Conditions: A Textbook of Rheumatology*, 9th ed. Philadelphia, Lea & Febiger, 1979.

McCulloch, J. A. : Chemonucleolysis: experience with 2000 cases. Clin. Orthop. 146: 128–135, 1980.

McCulloch, J. A.: Chemonucleolysis for relief of sciatica due to a herniated intervertebral disc. Can. Med. Assoc. J. 124: 879–882, 1981.

Meyers, M. H. and Chatterjee, S. N.: Osteochondral transplantation. Surg. Clin. North Am. 58: 429–434, 1978.

Mitchell, N. S. and Cruess, R. L.: Classification of degenerative arthritis. Can. Med. Assoc. J. 117: 763–765, 1977.

Naylor, A.: Factors in the development of the spinal stenosis syndrome. J. Bone Joint Surg. 61B: 306–309, 1979.

Neer, C.: Articular replacement of the humeral head. J. Bone Joint Surg. 37A: 215–228, 1955.

Osborne, A. H. and Fulford, P. C.: Lateral release for chondromalacia patellae. J. Bone Joint Surg. 64B: 203–205, 1982.

Price, C. T. and Lovell, W. W.: Thompson arthrodesis of the hip in children. J. Bone Joint Surg. 62A: 1118–1123, 1980.

Radin, E. L.: Aetiology of osteoarthrosis. Clin. Rheum. Dis. 2: 509, 1976.

Salter, R. B. and Field, P.: The effects of continuous compression on living articular cartilage. An experimental investigation. J. Bone Joint Surg. 42A: 31–49, 1960.

Salter, R. B., Gross, A., and Hall, J. H.: Hydrocortisone arthropathy—an experimental investigation. Can. Med. Assoc. J. 97: 374–377, 1967.

Salter, R. B., McNeill, O. R. and Carbin, R.: The pathological changes in articular cartilage associated with persistent joint deformity. An experimental investigation. In *Studies of Rheumatoid Disease*, Proceedings of the Third Canadian Conference in the Rheumatic Diseases, p. 33–47. University of Toronto Press, Toronto, 1965.

Salter, R. B. and Thompson, G.: The role of innominate osteotomy in young adults. In *The Hip*, edited by Sledge, C. Proceedings of the Annual Meeting of the Hip Society. St. Louis, C. V. Mosby, 1979, pp. 278–311.

Smythe, H. A., and Moldofsky, H.: Two contributions to understanding of the "fibrositis syndrome." Bull. Rheum. Dis. 28: 929–931, 1977.

Sokoloff, L.: *The Biology of Degenerative Joint Disease.* Chicago, University of Chicago Press, 1969.

Swanson, A. B.: Flexible implant arthroplasty for arthritic finger joints; rationale, technique and results of treatment. J. Bone Joint Surg. 54A: 435–455, 1972.

Swanson, S. A. V. and Freeman, M. A. R.: *The Scientific Basis of Joint Replacement.* Tunbridge Wells, Putnam Medical, 1977.

Verbiest, H.: Results of surgical treatment of idiopathic development stenosis of the lumbar vertebral canal. A review of 27 years' experience. J. Bone Joint Surg. 59B: 181–188, 1977.

Wadsworth, T. G.: *The Elbow.* Edinburgh, Churchill-Livingstone, 1982.

Wagner, H.: Surface replacement arthroplasty of the hip. Clin. Orthop. 134: 102–130, 1978.

Walldius, P.: Arthroplasty of the knee joint using endo-prosthesis. Acta Orthop. Scand. (Suppl.) 24: 19, 1957.

Zenni, E. J. Jr. and Carothers, T. A.: Total knee arthroplasty: current state of the art. Orthop. Rev. 19: 51–60, 1980.

CHAPTER 12

Neuromuscular Disorders

In other chapters of this textbook concerning the *musculoskeletal* system, most of the emphasis is placed upon the *skeletal* components, i.e., the *bones* which provide a rigid framework for the body, and the *joints* which permit movement between the bones. The musculoskeletal system (sometimes called the *motorskeletal* or *locomotor* system), however, depends upon its voluntary muscles, or *motors* to provide active coordinated movement. The muscles, in turn, depend upon the *nervous* system for their innervation that provides the stimulus for contraction. Indeed, the interrelationship between the nervous system and the musculoskeletal system is so close that we must think of them together as the *neuromusculoskeletal* system.

A wide variety of clinical disorders and injuries of the nervous system are manifest by disturbances of both form and function of the musculoskeletal system and, therefore, the more significant of these are considered in this textbook. You will learn much about these neurological disorders and injuries from your neurological and neurosurgical teachers; the purpose of the present chapter, however, is to emphasize their musculoskeletal manifestations as well as the principles of their orthopaedic treatment and the rehabilitation of patients so afflicted.

CLINICAL MANIFESTATIONS OF NEUROLOGICAL DISORDERS AND INJURIES

Despite the complexity of the human brain, spinal cord and peripheral nerves, the clinical manifestations of neurological disorders and injuries are such that their diagnosis is an example of precise detective work. The data, or clues, obtained from a detailed history and a complete neurological examination usually permit the clinician to narrow the possible diagnoses down to a few suspects, or differential diagnoses, and often provide sufficient evidence to establish an exact diagnosis; these methods of investigation, of course, are available to *every* physician. Radiographic and laboratory investigations are sometimes necessary, however, to determine the precise localization of a lesion as well as its pathological nature.

In order to appreciate the *significance* of the clinical manifestations of neurological disorders and injuries, you must be aware of certain pathological, anatomical and physiological factors underlying these manifestations.

Pathological Factors

Nervous tissue is affected by disease and injury in only four ways and, therefore, all neurological symptoms and signs are manifestations of one or more of these four modes of disturbed function:

1. Destruction of nerve cells with permanent loss of their function, as in destruction of motor cells (anterior horn cells) in poliomyelitis.

2. Transient disturbance of nerve cells with temporary loss of their function, as in cerebral shock and spinal shock which are seen only in lesions of sudden development such as acute injury.

3. Unlimited action (usually over-action) of intact mechanisms of the nervous system that have been "released" from the normal inhibitory control of higher centers. An example of this phenomenon is the spasticity that develops after a lesion in the cerebral motor cortex.

4. Irritation phenomena caused by a lesion that stimulates nerve cells to excessive activity. Examples are excessive pain that may follow a peripheral nerve injury (*causalgia*) and also epilepsy.

Clinical Manifestations of Lesions in Specific Systems of Neurons

Equipped with the foregoing knowledge of the normal functions of the major neuron systems of the central and peripheral nervous system, you will readily understand the following clinical manifestations of neurological lesions.

UPPER MOTOR NEURON LESIONS

In man the pyramidal and extrapyramidal systems are so closely related anatomically throughout most of their respective courses that, in most sites, a given lesion tends to affect both systems. A cerebrovascular lesion involving the internal capsule, for example, affects both pyramidal and extrapyramidal tracts. Nevertheless, for clarity, it is wise to consider these two systems separately.

Pyramidal System Lesions

1. *Weakness (paresis) of voluntary movements.* The paresis, which initially is flaccid in type because of cerebral shock, involves *patterns of movement* rather than movement by individual muscles. Paresis is not a true paralysis of all movement because the pyramidal system is not the only mediator of movement. The remaining intact part of the motor cerebral cortex can compensate to a remarkable degree.

2. *Increased muscle tone.* Several weeks after the loss of initiating impulses from the pyramidal system, other reflexes, having been "released" from higher control, take over and produce increased muscle tone which, in turn, is manifest by spasticity, increased stretch reflex, exaggerated deep tendon reflexes and clonus.

3. *Muscle contractures.* The spastic muscles develop permanent shortening (contracture) due to increased fibrosis.

4. *Loss of abdominal cutaneous reflexes.*

5. *Extensor type of plantar cutaneous reflex* (Babinski response).

Extrapyramidal System Lesions

1. *Increased muscle tone.* Loss of the inhibitory, or relaxing, function of the extrapyramidal system leads to the development of increased muscle tone with manifestations similar to those of pyramidal system lesions described above.

2. *Muscle contractures.* The spastic muscles develop permanent shortening.

3. *Involuntary movements.* Lesions of the basal ganglia may lead to uncontrolled, purposeless movements that are aggravated by emotional tension and attempts at voluntary control. These "mobile spasms," which are referred to as *athetosis*, are seen in the athetoid type of cerebral palsy. Another type of involuntary movement due to lesions of certain basal ganglia is the *tremor* seen in paralysis agitans (Parkinson's disease).

4. *Rigidity.* Lesions of certain basal ganglia may cause rigidity of a limb as a result of uninhibited simultaneous stimulation of all muscles which move a given part.

CEREBELLAR LESIONS

1. *Loss of coordination of muscle action.* The resultant jerky, halting, uncoordinated movements of a limb are manifest by inability to perform the finger-to-nose test accurately.

2. *Disturbed sense of balance.* As a result, the gait is unsteady and stumbling (cerebellar ataxia).

3. *Decreased muscle tone.* The loss of cerebellar regulation of posture results in decreased muscle tone with resultant diminution of deep tendon reflexes. Muscle contractures do not develop with pure cerebellar lesions.

4. *Slow speech.*

5. *Nystagmus.*

SPINAL CORD LESIONS

Lesions of the spinal cord often produce a combined upper and lower motor deficit since damage to the upper motor neurons at a given level in the cord may also affect the lower motor neurons in the spinal nerve roots arising from a higher level. A lesion that develops suddenly, such as a spinal cord injury or hemorrhage, is followed by a transient state of "spinal shock" in which the innervated muscles demonstrate a flaccid paralysis. This state of flaccidity, however, is superseded within a few weeks by a state of *spasticity* of the paralyzed muscles since the spinal cord reflexes take over in the absence of the normal inhibitory impulses from higher centers. The paralysis may involve both lower limbs (*paraplegia, diplegia*) or all four limbs (*quadriplegia, tetraplegia*).

The reflex response to any stimulation is greatly exaggerated and, indeed, mass reflexes may occur in the paralyzed segments with total flexion of the limbs and trunk (paraplegia-in-flexion). These troublesome spasms may even cause the bladder to empty. When the responsible lesion is in the brain stem rather than in the spinal cord, the paralysis is associated with rigidity of all muscle groups (akin to decerebrate rigidity). The attitude of the limbs and trunk under these circumstances is one of persistent extension (*paraplegia-in-extension*).

LOWER MOTOR NEURON LESIONS

1. *Flaccid paralysis.* There is complete loss of contraction in some or all of the fibers of the affected muscle or muscles, depending on the number of lower motor neurons involved by the lesion.

2. *Absence of muscle tone* and therefore absence of deep tendon reflexes.

3. *Progressive atrophy of muscle.* This type of neurogenic atrophy of muscle is referred to as a *myotrophy*. During the period of atrophy there may be twitching of muscle fascicles (fasciculation) within the paralyzed muscle, particularly if the lesion is due to a subacute or chronic process.

4. *Muscle contracture.* Permanent shortening (contracture) may develop in the unopposed normal muscles which are no longer being passively extended to their full length.

5. *Sensory loss.* A lesion involving the spinal nerve root or the peripheral nerve, both of which carry sensory as well as motor fibers, will produce a corresponding loss of sensation in addition to the flaccid paralysis.

Examples of lower motor neuron lesions at various levels in the final common pathway are as follows: (1) destruction of motor cells (anterior horn cells) of the motor cortex by a virus as in poliomyelitis; (2) compression of a spinal nerve root by a herniated intervertebral disc; (3) traumatic division of a peripheral nerve; (4) chemical disturbance of the myoneural junction as in myasthenia gravis.

THE PATHOGENESIS OF NEUROGENIC DEFORMITIES OF THE MUSCULOSKELETAL SYSTEM

A serious sequel to many disorders and injuries of the nervous system is the development of progressive *musculoskeletal deformities* over a period of time, particularly during the growing years. These secondary deformities, which frequently add significantly to the patient's disability, are caused by the following factors:

1. *Muscle imbalance*. The continuing unequal pull of muscles in the presence of paralysis, whether it be due to the excessive pull of spastic muscles or to the inadequate pull of flaccid muscles, leads eventually to the development of a persistent joint deformity.

2. *Muscle contracture*. In any muscle that is not repeatedly extended to its full length many times a day, as in spastic muscles and in normal muscles lacking opposition from flaccid partners, fibrosis of the muscle leads to permanent shortening (contracture). Thus, muscle imbalance and muscle contracture are equally important in the pathogenesis of paralytic joint deformities. Examples of such deformities include paralytic equinus at the ankle, paralytic hip flexion deformity and paralytic scoliosis. The combination of muscle imbalance and contracture can even cause a major joint such as the hip to dislocate (paralytic dislocation).

3. *Muscle atrophy*. Neurogenic atrophy of muscle (amyotrophy) leads to an obvious deformity by altering the normal contour of a limb.

4. *Retardation of bone growth*. The combination of paralysis, disuse and decreased blood supply in an involved limb causes a retardation of longitudinal bone growth. When the paralysis involves either the lower or upper pair of limbs unequally, during childhood, the inevitable result is a progressive limb length discrepancy.

THE PRINCIPLES OF ORTHOPAEDIC TREATMENT OF NEUROLOGICAL DISORDERS AND INJURIES

The orthopaedic treatment of the residual sequelae of neurological disorders and injuries is based upon the following aims or principles.

1. *Prevention of musculoskeletal deformity*. Paralytic deformities of joints can be prevented to some extent by passively moving each involved joint through a full range of motion for at least several minutes each day. Other means of preventing paralytic deformity include the use of removable splints (Fig. 12.1) and day braces (Fig. 12.2). Correction of the underlying muscle

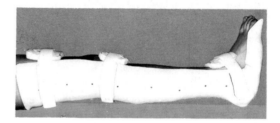

Figure 12.1. Removable splint to maintain the joints of a paralyzed limb in the optimal position in an attempt to prevent paralytic deformity.

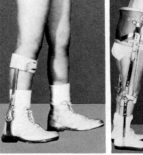
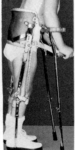
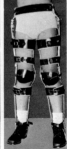

Figure 12.2. Lower limb braces which prevent unwanted motion while permitting desired motion in weak or unstable limbs.

imbalance is often possible by means of tendon transfer (Fig. 12.3).

2. *Correction of existing musculoskeletal deformity.* Passive stretching of a muscle contracture may suffice to correct an existing deformity. More often, however, permanent correction of a paralytic deformity requires such surgical operations as tendon lengthening (Fig. 12.4), tenodesis (Fig. 12.5), osteotomy (Fig. 12.6) or arthrodesis (Fig. 12.7).

3. *Improvement of muscle balance.* This requires the judicious use of muscle and tendon transfers (Fig. 12.3).

4. *Improvement of function.* Even when function in a limb cannot be helped by surgical operations, functional braces may be useful (Fig. 12.8).

5. *Improvement of appearance.* A lower

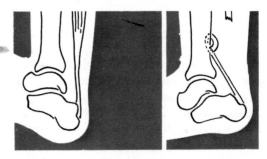

Figure 12.5. Tenodesis. In this example, the Achilles tendon of the paralyzed calf muscle is separated from the muscle and transplanted into the tibia so that it will serve as a check rein, or ligament, and thereby limit passive dorsiflexion.

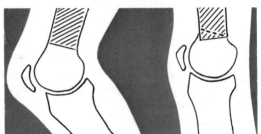

Figure 12.6. Osteotomy to deal with a joint deformity by producing a compensatory bony deformity near the joint. In this example the knee flexion deformity persists, but the limb is made straight by the compensatory osteotomy in the supracondylar region of the femur.

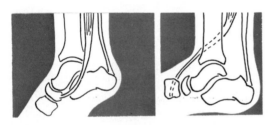

Figure 12.3. Tendon transfer. In this example the tendon of the tibialis posterior muscle has been rerouted through the interosseous membrane and transferred to the lateral cuneiform bone on the dorsum of the foot. In its new position, it will serve as a dorsiflexor of the ankle and an evertor of the foot.

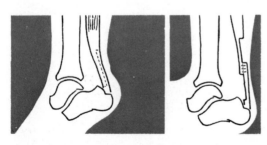

Figure 12.4. Tendon lengthening. Following the long step-cut in this Achilles tendon, the ends are allowed to shift in relation to each other and are then sutured in the elongated position.

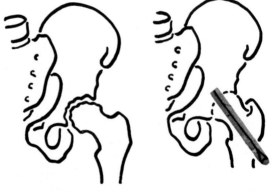

Figure 12.7. Arthrodesis. In this example the cartilaginous joint surfaces are excised from each joint surface and the raw bony surfaces are encouraged to unite to each other (fuse). Internal fixation and bone grafts may be required. The completely fused (arthrodesed) joint is immobile, but stable and painless.

limb length discrepancy may require an operation on the shorter leg (surgical stimulation, surgical lengthening) or on the longer leg (epiphyseal arrest, surgical shortening). The appearance of an atrophied limb can be improved by a suitably designed cosmetic prosthesis (Fig. 12.9).

6. *Rehabilitation.* A *philosophy in action*—the philosophy of total care *of* your patient as well as continuing care *for* him is vital—as outlined at the end of Chapter 6.

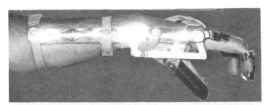
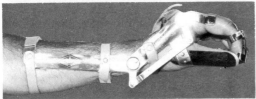

Figure 12.8. Functional brace, used to compensate for loss of power in the finger flexors. It is so designed that active dorsiflexion of the wrist causes the paralyzed fingers to flex and the thumb to oppose them.

DISORDERS OF THE BRAIN
Cerebral Palsy

The broad term *cerebral palsy* ("spastic paralysis," "brain damage") encompasses the various types and degrees of non-progressive brain disorders that develop shortly before, during or shortly after birth. These disorders, which become clinically apparent in early childhood and persist throughout the patient's life, are manifest by disturbances of voluntary muscle function and perception; there is often some associated impairment of mental acuity.

Since the effective prevention of musculoskeletal tuberculosis and paralytic poliomyelitis in recent years, cerebral palsy has become one of the foremost causes of crippling in childhood. Furthermore, because of its persistent nature, cerebral palsy presents serious social, psychological and educational problems.

INCIDENCE AND ETIOLOGY

Cerebral palsy is relatively common throughout the world. It has been estimated that every year for each 100,000 population, 6 children with cerebral palsy will be born and will survive while a 7th will succumb at birth. Thus, in a country with a population of 100,000,000 there will be 6,000 new cerebral palsied children each year.

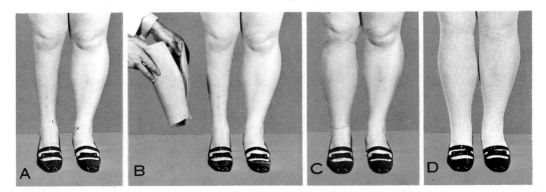

Figure 12.9. Cosmetic prosthesis for atrophy of the leg. *A*, marked residual atrophy in the leg of a 19-year-old girl from poliomyelitis. The girl was embarrassed by the appearance of her leg. *B*, a custom-made foam prosthesis (produced from a reverse mold of the normal leg) is about to be applied. *C*, the flesh-colored prosthesis in place; it closes with a hidden zipper on the inner side. The patient then puts on a flesh colored stocking on both legs prior to putting on dress stockings. *D*, the appearance is greatly improved.

There are many causes of cerebral palsy; indeed, any condition that leads to an abnormality of the brain can be responsible. The more common causes are:

1. Congenital maldevelopment of the brain, particularly of the cerebellum.

2. Cerebral anoxia in the perinatal period, especially when associated with prematurity.

3. Birth injury to the brain—prolonged labor, injury from forceps, precipitous delivery.

4. Erythroblastosis due to Rh incompatability with jaundice (icterus) that may affect the basal ganglia (kernicterus)—a less common cause since the development of early treatment by exchange transfusions.

5. Cerebral infections (encephalitis) in early postnatal life.

Nevertheless, since cerebral palsy is seldom diagnosed until at least several months after birth, the precise cause of the brain lesion in a given child is frequently speculative.

POSSIBLE PREVENTION

From extensive retrospective studies of children afflicted by cerebral palsy, it has been estimated that in at least one-third of these children the cerebral palsy could have been prevented by the following three measures: referral of the mother with a high-risk pregnancy to a perinatal center for her confinement; fetal monitoring and resuscitation at delivery; and early transfer of compromised infants to a neonatal care unit.

PATHOGENESIS AND PATHOLOGY

The underlying brain lesion in cerebral palsy, though irreparable, is not progressive. The loss of function in one neuron system of the brain results in the release of normal control over interdependent systems which, in turn, tend to overact; this is an example of the previously mentioned "release phenomenon."

The manifestations of the brain lesion in an afflicted child are determined by the extent of the lesion and by the area of the brain involved, cerebral motor cortex, basal ganglia or cerebellum. Three main types of cerebral palsy which comprise 90% of the total are:

1. *Spastic type,* 65%: pyramidal system lesion in the cerebral motor cortex.

2. *Athetoid type,* 20%: extrapyramidal system lesion in the basal ganglia.

3. *Ataxic type,* 5%: cerebellar and brain stem lesion.

Three additional types, *tremor, rigidity* and *atonia,* are rare and make up the remaining 10% of the total.

CLINICAL FEATURES AND DIAGNOSIS

The various types of cerebral palsy are not obvious clinically during the early months of postnatal development because the previously mentioned "release phenomena" tend to appear slowly over a period of months; furthermore, during these early months there is relatively little cerebral activity even in the normal brain. Cerebral palsy can be *suspected,* however, when an infant fails to achieve the milestones of motor development at the appropriate ages; (an average normal infant turns over at 5 months, sits up at 7 months, pulls himself to a standing position at 10 months, stands alone at 14 months and walks unaided at 15 months).

In addition to retarded motor development, many children with cerebral palsy exhibit some degree of retarded mental development; 40% are seriously retarded mentally and considered uneducable, another 40% are less retarded but still below average and the remaining 20% are average or above. Assessment of intelligence is particularly difficult in children with cerebral palsy because of the associated motor and sensory deficits, as well as their short attention span.

The severity of all types of cerebral palsy varies greatly. In the mildest forms the patient is capable of leading an almost normal life; in the severe forms the patient is almost completely incapacitated. The clinical manifestations of the three commonest types of cerebral palsy are sufficiently distinctive that they merit separate consideration.

Spastic Type of Cerebral Palsy, 65%

The characteristic features of spastic paralysis, or paresis, are paralysis of patterns of voluntary movement (rather than of individual muscles) and increased muscle tone (hypertonicity, spasticity, increased deep tendon reflexes and clonus).

In early life the disturbance of voluntary movements is manifest by difficulty in achieving fine, coordinated muscle action. When the infant or child attempts to carry out even simple movements, many muscles contract at the same time so that movement is restricted and laborious. The increased

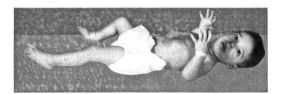

Figure 12.10. Startle reflex in an infant with cerebral palsy. The infant was startled by a sudden noise immediately before this photograph was taken. Note the mass muscle spasm in the limbs.

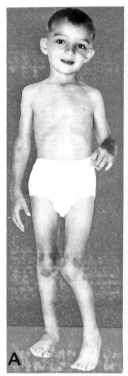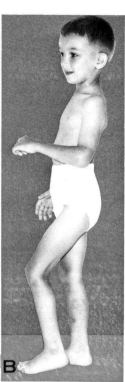

Figure 12.12. Spastic hemiplegia involving the left upper and lower limbs. This boy is just starting to take a step with his left foot. Note the internal rotation of the arm and the flexion deformities of the elbow and fingers; note also the flexion, adduction, internal rotation of the left hip, flexion of the knee and equinus of the ankle.

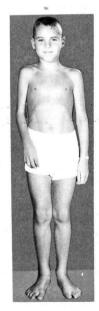

Figure 12.11. Spastic monoplegia involving the right upper limb. Note the internal rotation of the arm and the flexion deformity of the elbow, wrist and fingers.

muscle tone can be detected in fairly young infants by the "startle reflex," a mass muscle spasm elicited by any sudden noise (Fig. 12.10). The spastic limbs seem stiff and exhibit an increased stretch reflex (sudden contraction of a muscle when stretched). The deep tendon reflexes in the involved limbs are hyperactive and after the first year the plantar cutaneous reflex becomes extensor in type (Babinski response).

Depending on the extent of the lesion in the cerebral cortex, the spastic paralysis may involve only one limb, *monoplegia* (Fig. 12.11), upper and lower limb on one side, *hemiplegia* (Fig. 12.12), both lower limbs, *diplegia*, *paraplegia* (Fig. 12.13), or all four limbs, *tetraplegia*, *quadriplegia*, "*bilateral hemiplegia*" (Fig. 12.14). The muscles of the throat may also be affected.

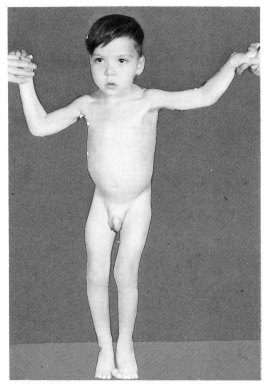

Figure 12.13. Spastic diplegia involving both lower limbs. This boy's upper limbs are normal. Note the flexion, adduction deformities of the hips, flexion of the knees and equinus of the ankles.

Although the paralysis affects movements more than individual muscles, some muscles are more spastic than others and some are weaker than others; consequently, there is serious muscle imbalance in the involved limbs. In general, muscles that cross two joints, such as the biceps in the arm and the gastrocnemius in the leg, tend to be more spastic than those that cross only one joint. Furthermore, flexor muscles tend to outpull extensor muscles, adductors outpull abductors and internal rotators outpull external rotators. Thus, the neurogenic deformities in affected limbs secondary to spastic muscle imbalance are predictable—flexion, adduction and internal rotation (Figs. 12.11-15).

The spastic gait is characteristically stiff, clumsy and jerky with the affected limbs held in the above-mentioned position of deformity. Rapid walking or running accentuate the abnormality of the gait and thereby make it more obvious. The child may also exhibit evidence of a central (cortical) type of sensory deficit.

Spastic paralysis of the muscles of speech is reflected in the child's difficulty in learning to speak clearly. Spastic paralysis of the muscles of swallowing interferes with the normally subconscious function of swallowing saliva and accounts for the clinical problem of drooling.

Athetoid Type of Cerebral Palsy, 20%

The characteristic feature of athetosis is the involuntary, uncontrollable movements ("mobile spasms") in muscle groups of the face and all four limbs. This purposeless athetotic muscle activity produces twisting,

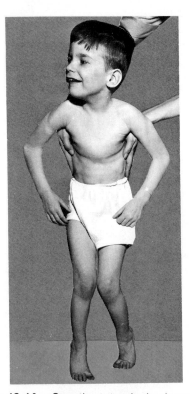

Figure 12.14. Spastic tetraplegia (paraplegia) involving all 4 limbs. Note the internal rotation of the arms and flexion deformity of the elbows; note also the flexion, adduction and internal rotation of the hips, flexion of the knees and equinus of the ankles. When this boy tried to walk, his knees crossed, one in front of the other (scissors gait).

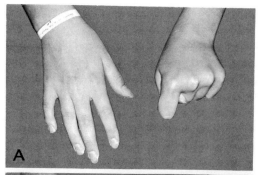

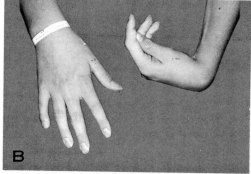

phenomenon of athetosis is exaggerated by attempts at voluntary movement as well as by emotional tension, but is absent during sleep. The deep tendon reflexes and the plantar cutaneous reflexes are usually normal.

Ataxic Type of Cerebral Palsy, 5%

The characteristic features of cerebellar ataxia are disturbed coordination of muscle groups and a relative lack of equilibrium, or balance. The gait is unsteady and the child frequently appears about to fall, though this is usually prevented by using the arms to maintain balance (Fig. 12.17). There is neither spasticity nor athetosis and, since the lesion is primarily cerebellar, the intelligence is usually unaffected.

Figure 12.15. *A,* thumb-clutched hand in cerebral palsy due to flexion and adduction of the thumb. *B,* the thumb is released only when the wrist is flexed.

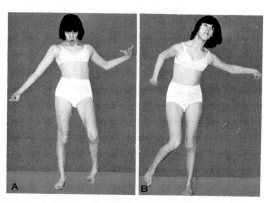

Figure 12.16. Athetosis in a girl with the athetoid type of cerebral palsy. These photographs were taken two seconds apart and give some indication of the twisting, writhing contortions in the limbs and the meaningless grimaces in the face.

writhing contortions in the limbs and meaningless grimaces in the face (Fig. 12.16). It also causes difficulty with speech and with swallowing. The distressing and humiliating

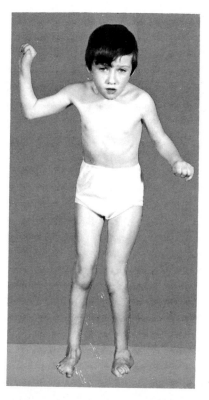

Figure 12.17. Ataxia and disturbed coordination of muscles in a girl with the ataxic type of cerebral palsy. Note that the child stands with a wide stance and uses her arms to help maintain her balance.

PROGNOSIS

Repeated mental and physical assessment of a given child with cerebral palsy over many months is necessary to establish a realistic prognosis. Despite the permanent nature of the underlying brain lesion, every cerebral palsied child exhibits some improvement in the motor skills during the growing years through natural maturation of the remaining intact part of the brain. This improvement, though delayed, is comparable to the improvement of motor skills in a normal child who sits up at 6 months and walks at 15 months.

Cerebral palsy may be so mild that the child is but a few months or a year behind in his milestones of development. It may, however, be so severe that at 5 years of age the child is still unable to sit up and is functioning at the level of a 5-month-old infant; or at 14 years of age is still unable to walk and is functioning at the level of a 14-month-old child.

Approximately one-third of all children with cerebral palsy have such a severe brain lesion that treatment is ineffectual and institutional care may be required; one-sixth have such a mild lesion that treatment is unnecessary; the remaining half can definitely be helped by realistic treatment.

TREATMENT OF CEREBRAL PALSY

The over-all management of children with cerebral palsy requires the combined skills of the family physician, rehabilitation physician, neurologist, orthopaedic surgeon, psychologist, physical, occupational and speech therapists, medical social worker, and teacher. Ideally, assessment and treatment of these children is carried out in a special treatment center with facilities for both inpatient and outpatient care. Management of the child's physical problem alone, however, is not sufficient; professional staff who care for children with cerebral palsy require an abundance of compassion, understanding and patience. The pervading attitude must be one of kindly realism.

Psychological Considerations

The parents of a cerebral palsied child need special consideration. Because the diagnosis is seldom made during the early months, the parents have assumed that their child is normal; their disappointment is extreme when they finally come to the painful realization that their child will, in fact, never be normal. Indeed, some parents have great difficulty accepting the reality of this tragic situation.

The psychological needs of the child depend on the age and the degree of mental development. Many have a labile temperament and a short attention span, both of which render training and teaching difficult. Understandably, most children with cerebral palsy experience psychological problems of adjustment, particularly during adolescence.

Therapeutic Drugs

No type of drug can affect the brain lesion itself and in general, the drugs that have been used to help control the effects of the brain lesion have been disappointing. Epilepsy, which may accompany cerebral palsy, can be controlled to a large extent by drugs.

Physical and Occupational Therapy

The aims are to encourage muscle relaxation, improve muscle coordination and develop voluntary muscle control so that purposeful patterns of movement can be achieved. Simple activities that a normal child can learn by himself, such as standing, walking, eating and dressing, must be taught the cerebral palsied child by painstaking and repetitive training (Fig. 12.18).

Daily passive stretching of spastic muscles in an attempt to prevent deformity is of limited value in children with marked spasticity and muscle imbalance. Hand skills are difficult to develop, particularly in the presence of a central (cortical) sensory deficit; nevertheless, many cerebral palsied children can become relatively independent through repeated training.

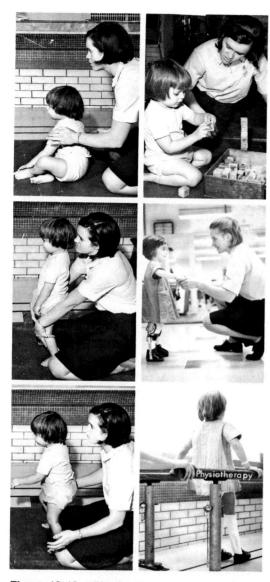

Figure 12.18. Physical and occupational therapy for children with cerebral palsy involves painstaking and repetitive training by cheerful and dedicated therapists.

Speech Therapy

By means of prolonged speech therapy, the defective speech in many afflicted children can be improved to the point of being reasonably intelligible.

Orthopaedic Appliances

Removable splints are of value in helping to prevent deformity as well as in preventing recurrence of a deformity that has been corrected. During the early years, braces for the lower limbs are often necessary to enable a child to stand and to walk with the help of crutches. Efforts should be made, however, to correct deformities and to improve function by physical therapy and surgical operations so that the child can be freed from cumbersome bracing as soon as is feasible.

Surgical Manipulation

Correction of fixed deformities by stretching of muscle contractures under general anesthesia is helpful in milder forms of spastic paralysis; the correction must be maintained by removable splints for many years to prevent recurrence. This method of treatment is of little value, however, for children with severe contractures secondary to marked spasticity.

Surgical Operations

The operative treatment of children with cerebral palsy is but one facet, albeit an important one, in the multifaceted approach to management. Operations are based on the first four of the six previously outlined *principles of orthopaedic treatment of neurological disorders and injuries*. In general, operative treatment is of value primarily in the spastic type of cerebral palsy, but is not indicated until the child has at least developed kneeling balance. Much clinical judgement is required in planning any operations for a cerebral palsied child; after an operation the child will still have cerebral palsy and unless the surgical decision has been sound, the child will not be any better after operation—just different. Parents must be made aware that well chosen operations can improve function, but cannot make spastic limbs function normally.

One or more of the following operations may be required for a given child with the spastic type of cerebral palsy: (1) *tendon lengthening* (Fig. 12.4), lengthening of the Achilles' tendon for equinus deformity; of the hamstring tendons for knee flexion deformity; of the iliopsoas tendon for hip flexion

deformity; (2) *tendon transfer* (Fig. 12.3), of the tibialis posterior tendon from the medial side of the foot to the dorsum; of the flexor carpi ulnaris from the medial side of the wrist to the dorsum; (3) *arthrodesis* (Fig. 12.7), of the three posterior joints of the foot (triple arthrodesis); of the wrist; of the metacarpo-phalangeal joint of the thumb.

Provision of special seating devices combined with surgical correction of deformities enables children with even the most disabling forms of cerebral palsy to sit comfortably.

Very few patients with the athetoid type of cerebral palsy can be helped by orthopaedic operations; occasionally, a particularly troublesome pattern of athetoid movement can be diminished by selective neurectomy. Neurosurgical operations on the globus pallidus to diminish athetosis have been only partially successful.

The ataxic type of cerebral palsy is not amenable to surgical treatment.

Rehabilitation

For cerebral palsied children, who have never been normal and hence, never "habilitated," the philosophy of rehabilitation is, in this sense, one of habilitation. This unfortunate group of children and their anxious parents represent one of the most important challenges to the whole concept of rehabilitation as described at the end of Chapter 6. No group is more deserving of compassionate consideration and kindly realism in relation to rehabilitation.

Cerebral Palsy in the Adult

The philosophy and principles of treatment described above for children with cerebral palsy must be carried on to meet the continuing needs of adolescents and adults whose cerebral palsy has been with them throughout their past, is with them in their present and will continue to be with them throughout their future. Although the cerebral palsied adult has outgrown the phase of being considered, particularly by the public, as "a cute little crippled kid," his needs are nonetheless just as worthy of our consideration in adulthood as in childhood.

Hopefully, the adult has at least reached his potential, however limited that may be, but he may still not be capable of taking a normal role in society. Under these circumstances, employment in a sheltered workshop, or better still in a modified area within industry, is of great importance. If we cannot change the cerebral palsied adult to fit his environment, then we must change his environment to fit the cerebral palsied adult.

Cerebrovascular Disease and Hemiplegia

The commonest of all neurological disorders is *cerebrovascular disease*, which includes all vascular disorders of the brain. The most catastrophic complication of the various types of cerebrovascular disease is sudden and irreversible ischemia of the brain which produces the familiar syndrome of *stroke* (*apoplexy*, *cerebrovascular accident*). This complication, which occurs most frequently in the elderly, may be caused by hemorrhage, thrombosis or embolism; it is particularly serious since brain tissue dies after relatively few minutes of complete ischemia.

The residual effects of a stroke are extremely variable, depending as they do on both the site and the extent of the area of cerebral ischemia. For the purpose of this textbook, however, we are concerned with the patient who develops a complete *hemiplegia* (Fig. 12.19). At the onset the paralysis is flaccid but within a few weeks it becomes spastic as evidenced by hypertonicity, increased deep tendon reflexes and clonus. The plantar cutaneous response becomes extensor in type (Babinski response).

Until recent years most victims of a stroke received only token therapy designed to improve their musculoskeletal function. It is now appreciated, however, that this large group of patients can be rehabilitated much more efficiently if they are vigorously treated in accordance with the previously outlined *principles of orthopaedic treatment of neurological disorders and injuries.*

The most important aspects of orthopaedic treatment for stroke victims with residual hemiplegia are psychotherapy, physi-

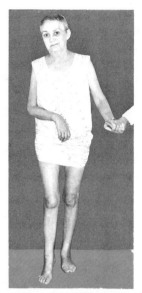

Figure 12.19. Right spastic hemiplegia in a 63-year-old woman who is recovering from a stroke due to a cerebrovascular accident involving the left cerebral hemisphere. Note the internal rotation of the shoulder, flexion of the elbow and wrist, flexion and adduction of the hip, flexion of the knee and equinus of the ankle. Note also the right facial weakness.

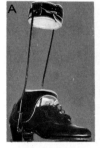
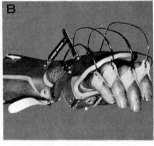

Figure 12.20. A, light spring brace with outside T strap to help overcome a paralytic foot drop and varus deformity for a patient with a spastic hemiplegia from a stroke. B, spring assisted hand splint to prevent deformities and improve hand function.

cal and occupational therapy, light braces (Fig. 12.20), selective nerve blocks to relieve spasticity and, occasionally, tendon transfers to restore muscle balance and improve function (e.g. transfer of the tibialis posterior tendon to the dorsum of the foot and transfer of the flexor carpi ulnaris tendon to the dorsum of the hand).

In recent years much progress has been made in the rehabilitation of stroke victims by means of selective electrical stimulation of weak muscles to improve function significantly in both the upper limb and the lower limb.

DISORDERS AND INJURIES OF THE SPINAL CORD

Congenital Myelodysplasia

Congenital defects of the spinal cord (*myelodysplasia*) and nerve roots associated with spina bifida are fully discussed along with other congenital abnormalities in Chapter 8.

Diastematomyelia

The term *diastematomyelia* refers to a rare but important congenital defect of the spinal column in which either the lower part of the spinal cord or the upper part of the cauda equina is split into two vertical components by a spur that passes backward from the posterior surface of a vertebral body and traverses the spinal canal. This congenital spur, which may be fibrous, cartilaginous, or even bony, interferes with the normal upward migration of the conus of the spinal cord during growth; consequently, during childhood the spur produces a progressive neurological deficit usually of the lower motor neuron type involving the lower limbs, bladder or bowel.

There is nearly always an associated congenital anomaly, either of the overlying skin, such as hairy patch, hemangioma or dermal sinus, or of the regional vertebral bodies. The diagnosis can be suspected on clinical grounds, but is confirmed by myelographic evidence of a midline split in the contrast medium (Fig. 12.21).

Neurosurgical treatment, which involves laminectomy and excision of the congenital spur, prevents further progression of the neurological deficit and may even result in some improvement.

Poliomyelitis

The disease *poliomyelitis* ("*polio,*" "*infantile paralysis*"), a viral infection affecting the motor cells (anterior horn cells) of the spinal

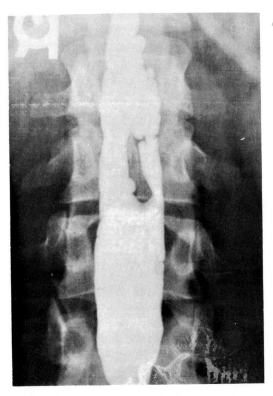

Figure 12.21. Myelogram in the upper lumbar region showing a midline split in the contrast medium at the level of the second lumbar vertebra due to the spur of diastematomyelia.

cord capable of producing permanent paralysis, is now an almost completely preventable disease as a result of the development of effective vaccines by both Salk and Sabin. It may be many years, however, before this disease is completely controlled, particularly in the developing countries of the world. For this reason, poliomyelitis still merits consideration in a textbook related to the musculoskeletal system.

INCIDENCE AND ETIOLOGY

Prior to the discovery of effective poliomyelitis vaccines, this dread disease was the most frequent cause of crippling in children and to a lesser extent in adults. In highly developed countries where the vaccination programs have been extensive, poliomyelitis is fortunately rare; in some of the developing countries, however, for a variety of reasons, poliomyelitis continues to pose a threat to both life and limb. It affects boys more often than girls and the lower limbs more often than the upper limbs or trunk.

The poliomyelitis virus, of which there are three types, is a member of the enterovirus group. Characteristically, it enters the body via the gastrointestinal tract whence it spreads through the bloodstream to its target, the anterior horn cells of the spinal cord and brain stem. Usually occurring in epidemics, particularly during late summer, poliomyelitis may also occur sporadically.

PREVENTION

The development of a killed virus vaccine by Salk, and of an attenuated living virus vaccine by Sabin, are among the most significant medical advances in the present century. Both vaccines are highly effective as well as safe.

PATHOGENESIS AND PATHOLOGY

Poliomyelitis may be *abortive* with no symptoms, *non-paralytic* with systemic symptoms, or *paralytic* with systemic symptoms and paralysis. After an incubation period of two weeks, the virus attacks anterior horn cells and may destroy them thereby producing a permanent lower motor neuron type of paralysis of muscle fibers which they innervate. Alternatively, the infection in the cord can produce a temporary inflammatory edema in the anterior horn, or even reversible damage to the cells, with resultant transient paralysis. The remainder of the discussion concerns only *paralytic* poliomyelitis.

CLINICAL FEATURES AND DIAGNOSIS

During the *prodromal phase*, which lasts two days, the patient experiences nonspecific systemic symptoms common to many viral infections—headache, malaise and generalized muscular aches.

During the *acute phase* of paralytic poliomyelitis, the patient develops a fever, severe headache, neck rigidity (indicating meningeal irritation), painful spasm and tenderness in affected muscles. At this time the cerebrospinal fluid contains large numbers of lymphocytes. It is during the acute phase, which lasts approximately two months, that a flaccid paralysis develops in those muscles innervated by the damaged anterior horn

cells. The extent of the paralysis varies from weakness of one muscle, or muscle group, to complete paralysis of all the muscles of all four limbs and the trunk; if the brainstem is affected as well (bulbar poliomyelitis) the muscles of respiration become paralyzed, and assisted (mechanical) respiration is necessary to preserve life.

The *recovery phase* (*convalescent phase*), which lasts up to two years, is the period during which there is gradual recovery of any transient paralysis; most of this recovery occurs within the first six months. Approximately one third of the patients will make a complete recovery during this phase.

The *phase of residual paralysis* persists for the rest of the patient's life and no further recovery can be expected. Approximately half of the patients with residual paralysis have only moderate involvement, but the remainder are left with extensive paralysis. The causes of paralytic deformity include muscle imbalance, muscle contracture, muscle atrophy and, during childhood, retarded longitudinal bone growth in an involved limb. A variety of typical post-poliomyelitis deformities develop, depending on the extent and distribution of the paralysis (Figs. 12.22–24).

No form of treatment affects the extent of the paralysis or the degree of its recovery. During the acute phase, the patient is kept in bed and treated symptomatically. Removable splints are used to prevent contractures in involved limbs and, after muscle spasm has subsided, the joints of a paralyzed limb are gently put through a full range of motion for several minutes each day.

Treatment during the recovery, or convalescent phase, includes active exercises to strengthen recovering muscles and suitable braces to stabilize weak limbs, prevent contractures and improve function (Fig. 12.2).

Treatment of patients with residual paralysis is selected in accordance with the six previously outlined *principles of orthopaedic treatment of neurological disorders and injuries*. Operative treatment is deferred until there is no further hope of muscle recovery. The most efficacious surgical operations for patients with flaccid paralysis in the residual phase of poliomyelitis include: (1) *tendon lengthening* (Fig. 12.4); (2) *tendon transfer* (Fig. 12.3); (3) *tenodesis* (Fig. 12.5); (4) *osteotomy near a joint* (Fig. 12.6); (5) *arthrodesis* (Fig. 12.7); (6) *leg length equalization* (either epiphyseal arrest or surgical shortening of the longer leg or, alternatively, either epiphyseal stimulation or surgical lengthening of the shorter leg). The choice of the many available operations for specific combinations of residual paralysis is not discussed here but some examples are cited in relation to a group of post-poliomyelitic deformities shown in Figs. 12.22–24.

For some patients the residual paralysis in a lower limb is so extensive that permanent bracing is required to provide stability for standing and walking. For others, with obvious atrophy of a lower limb, the appearance of the limbs can be effectively matched by wearing a cosmetic prosthesis over the atrophied segment of the limb (Fig 12.9).

Patients with extensive residual paralysis, particularly when it involves both upper limbs, require *rehabilitation*, the philosophy of which is described at the end of Chapter 6.

The Spinocerebellar Degenerations

A group of genetically related disorders, the *spinocerebellar degenerations*, is characterized by degeneration of ascending and descending tracts in the spinal cord, and sometimes of the peripheral nerves, cerebellum, and even the cerebral cortex. The two commonest disorders of this group are peroneal muscular atrophy and Friedreich's ataxia, which are described below. The two disorders may develop in different members of the same family, or the features of both may appear in a given patient.

PERONEAL MUSCULAR ATROPHY (CHARCOT-MARIE-TOOTH DISEASE)

Although this disease is one of the spinocerebellar degenerations, one of the early features is symmetrical degeneration in peripheral nerves, particularly the peroneal (lateral popliteal) nerves. Degenerative changes in the spinal cord are seen in the later stages. This form of hereditary motor and sensory neuropathy (HMSN) is usually inherited as

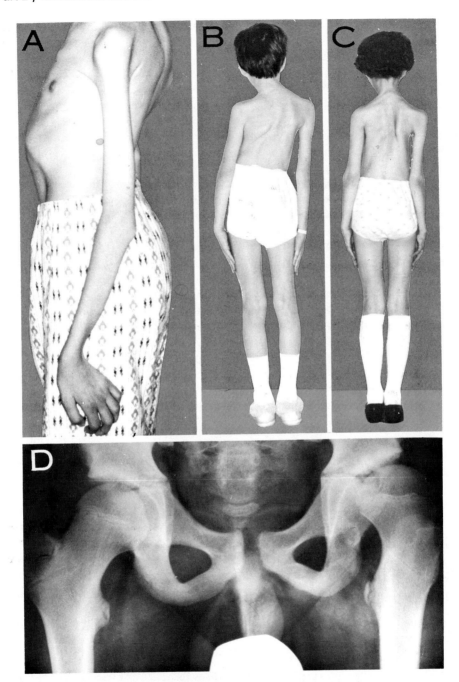

Figure 12.22.   Post-poliomyelitis deformities. *A,* extensive paralysis involving the left upper limb and spine. Note the paralytic thoracic kyphosis and the marked atrophy of the entire upper limb. This boy's function can be improved by arthrodesis of the wrist, tendon transfers in the hand and elbow, arthrodesis of the shoulder. *B,* paralytic scoliosis. Note the shift of the trunk to the right (decompensation). *C,* same child 6 months after correction of the scoliosis by Harrington type of instrumentation and spinal fusion. *D,* paralytic subluxation of the left hip; the acetabulum has become abnormal secondarily. This problem can be improved by the combination of transfer of the iliopsoas muscle (to make it an abductor instead of a flexor) and innominate osteotomy to redirect the acetabulum.

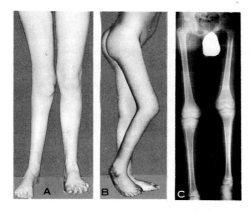

Figure 12.23. Post-poliomyelitis deformities. *A*, valgus deformity of the right knee, varus deformity of the foot, atrophy and leg length discrepancy. This combination of deformities can be improved by supracondylar osteotomy of the femur, triple arthrodesis of the foot and surgical lengthening of the tibia. *B*, hip flexion deformity, knee flexion deformity, equinovarus deformity of the foot. This child could be helped by soft tissue release and muscle transfer about the hip, supracondylar osteotomy of the femur, triple arthrodesis of the foot and tendon transfer (tibialis posterior tendon to the dorsum of the foot). *C*, leg length discrepancy. This can be improved by either surgically stimulating growth in shorter leg or surgical lengthening or both. Alternatively, the discrepancy could be decreased by epiphyseal arrest of the longer leg or surgical shortening.

an autosomal dominant but occasionally as a recessive and is more common in boys than in girls.

The disease becomes manifest in childhood or early adult life by the development of bilateral pes cavus, a paralytic deformity of the feet due to muscle imbalance. As the disease progresses, symmetrical muscular atrophy and weakness become apparent in the peroneal muscles and toe extensors. Subsequently, the disease may advance to involve the tibialis anterior muscles, in which case there is a bilateral drop foot gait. The upper limbs may also become involved, but the muscle atrophy and weakness are primarily peripheral and seldom extend above the knees or above the elbows (Fig. 12.25). The disease is characterized by low motor nerve conduction velocities. Sensory changes are slight but there is usually loss of vibration sense below the knee.

This disorder does not shorten the patient's life expectancy; and since muscular control of the hips and knees is always preserved, the patient can usually retain his ability to walk. Surgical operations, such as lengthening of the Achilles tendon, transfer of the tibialis posterior tendon from the medial side of the foot to the dorsum, and

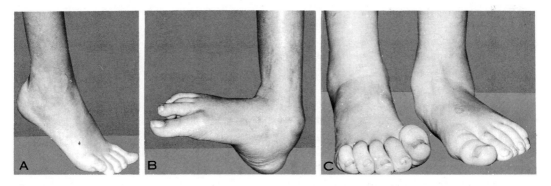

Figure 12.24. Post-poliomyelitis deformities. *A*, paralytic equinus of the ankle. This can be improved by lengthening of the Achilles tendon and tendon transfer (peroneal tendons to the dorsum of the foot). *B*, paralytic calcaneus deformity of the ankle. Tenodesis of the Achilles tendon and tendon transfer (tibialis anterior to the heel) would improve the function of this child's foot. *C*, paralytic varus deformity of the right foot and claw toe deformities. Paralytic deformity of the left foot. This child's feet can be improved by triple arthrodesis of both feet and tendon transfer in the right foot (Extensor hallucis longus to the first metatarsal).

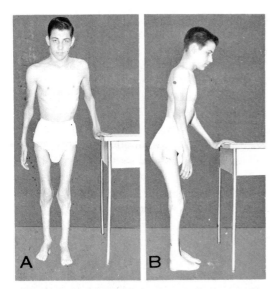

Figure 12.25. Peroneal muscular atrophy (Charcot-Marie-Tooth disease) in a 16-year-old boy. Note the bilateral pes cavus deformities, marked and symmetrical muscular atrophy of the calves, paralytic deformities of the hands and muscular atrophy of the forearms. This boy walks with a bilateral drop foot gait and requires braces.

arthrodesis of the posterior joints of the foot (triple arthrodesis), may be required.

FRIEDREICH'S ATAXIA

A more serious form of spinocerebellar degeneration, *Friedreich's ataxia*, is characterized by degenerative changes in the posterior and lateral tracts of the spinal cord and cerebellum with resultant loss of position sense, poor balance and ataxia. It may be inherited either as an autosomal dominant or as a recessive, but more often the latter.

The disease becomes manifest in early childhood by the development of bilateral pes cavus with claw toes (Fig. 12.26) and a progressive cerebellar ataxia with a swaying, staggering, irregular gait. Scoliosis develops in approximately 75% of the patients. Nystagmus and dysarthria indicate further cerebellar degeneration. The deep tendon reflexes disappear at the ankle and the plantar cutaneous reflexes become extensor in type (Babinski response). In addition, there is a profound loss of position sense and vibration sense.

Friedreich's ataxia is slowly but relentlessly progressive, rendering most victims wheelchair-bound by the age of 40; occasionally, however, the degenerative process becomes arrested. The cause of premature death (usually in the third or fourth decade) is progressive cardiomyopathy.

Surgical operations to correct foot deformities are similar to those described above for peroneal muscular atrophy but are of less permanent value because of the progressive ataxia.

Spinal Paraplegia and Quadriplegia

Disorders and injuries that damage the spinal cord are particularly serious, not only because of its limited power of regeneration but also because of the associated compli-

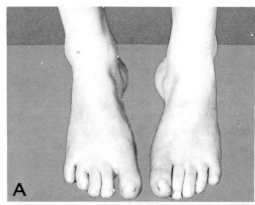

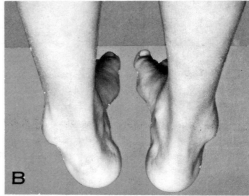

Figure 12.26. Friedreich's ataxia in a 10-year-old boy showing the bilateral pes cavus deformity and varus of the heels. At a later stage, his toes will become hyperextended at the metatarsophalangeal joints and flexed at the interphalangeal joints (claw toes).

cations. Indeed, prior to World War II, 80% of all spinal paraplegics were dead within a few years. Fortunately, at present, as a result of better understanding and more vigorous treatment, the mortality figures have been reversed and 80% of spinal paraplegics are *alive* even after 10 years.

INCIDENCE AND ETIOLOGY

The commonest cause of spinal paraplegia is *acute injury*, either *indirect* in association with fractures or dislocations of the spine (Fig. 12.27) and central herniations of

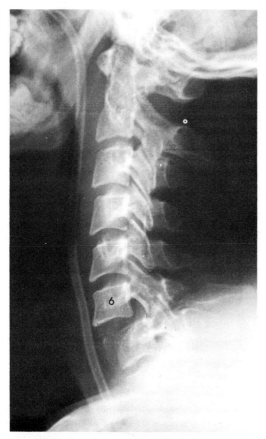

Figure 12.27. Fracture-dislocation of the cervical spine at the C-6-7 level in a 34-year-old man as the result of an automobile accident. Note that the inferior facet of C-6 has been dislocated to a position in front of the superior facet of C-7 and that there is a fracture of the anterosuperior corner of the seventh cervical vertebra. The shadow in front of the vertebral bodies is a gastric suction tube. This man was immediately quadriplegic, complete in the lower limbs and partial in the upper limbs.

the intervertebral disc, or *direct* from penetrating injuries such as gunshot and stab wounds. The paraplegia is usually immediate. It has been estimated that during each year in Canada and the United States, 12,000 persons sustain a spinal cord injury.

Causes of more slowly developing spinal paraplegia include: (1) neoplasms involving the spinal cord (intramedullary and extramedullary, primary and secondary); (2) infection of the vertebral bodies (particularly tuberculosis) with either pressure on the cord or actual invasion by granulation tissue; (3) diseases of the spinal cord itself, such as multiple sclerosis.

CLINICAL FEATURES

The clinical picture in the early stages of spinal paraplegia depends on whether the paraplegia is of sudden onset, as with traumatic paraplegia, or whether it is of gradual onset.

Complete Paraplegia of Sudden Onset (Traumatic)

Initially, the patient exhibits a state of spinal shock which is characterized by complete *flaccid* paralysis of all muscles innervated by that part of the spinal cord below, or distal to the level of injury, and a comparable complete loss of sensation. Injuries below the level of the first thoracic vertebra produce a paralysis of both lower limbs (*paraplegia*) while those above this level produce a paralysis of all four limbs (*quadriplegia, tetraplegia*). In either case there is, in addition, a flaccid paralysis of the urinary bladder and rectal sphincter, and absence of deep tendon reflexes in affected muscles.

After a few weeks the state of flaccid paralysis is superseded by a state of residual *spastic* paralysis as the cord reflexes below the level of injury take over in the absence of inhibitory impulses from the upper motor neurons. Thus, the muscles in the area of paralysis exhibit hypertonicity, increased deep tendon reflexes and clonus; the plantar cutaneous reflexes are extensor in type. There is no voluntary power below the injury. Although the loss of sensation remains complete, painful stimuli in the paralyzed areas can cause a massive reflex spasm of muscles which may even cause the bladder to empty.

Incomplete Paraplegia of Sudden Onset (Traumatic)

With incomplete lesions, some tracts have escaped damage at the level of injury; consequently, there is a greater likelihood that the damage to the remaining tracts is not sufficiently severe to be permanent and that some recovery may be expected.

Paraplegia of Gradual Onset

When the disorder involving the spinal cord is slowly progressive, as with a neoplasm or infection, the phenomenon of spinal shock is not seen. The paralysis progresses slowly and is *spastic* from the beginning.

Early Treatment of Traumatic Spinal Paraplegia

In recent years, scientific investigations by Tator and his colleagues have demonstrated that the injured spinal cord, in addition to suffering from the physical effects of trauma, also suffers from secondary pathological processes including ischemia and edema, both of which are amenable to treatment in the first few hours after injury. Consequently the currently recommended immediate treatment includes administration of both corticosteroids and mannitol to minimize ischemia and edema.

To prevent distension and also to keep the skin dry, the bladder is kept empty by means of an indwelling catheter during the flaccid stage of the paraplegia. Surgical decompression is indicated if the paraplegia is incomplete at the onset, or if there is evidence of progression in the neurological deficit. If, however, the paraplegia is complete from the beginning, surgical decompression is of no value. In the presence of an unstable fracture-dislocation of the spine, however, early operative reduction and stabilization of the spine by metal devices and bone grafts may enhance neurologic recovery. Such stabilization certainly facilitates the subsequent nursing care and enables the patient to get up with safety and comfort at an early stage during his rehabilitation.

The prevention of pressure sores (decubitus ulcers) in the anesthetic areas of skin is of paramount importance from the beginning since this complication of paraplegia is the greatest single cause of morbidity. The patient must be turned every two hours initially.

With high spinal cord injuries the voluntary muscles of respiration are paralyzed and consequently respiratory complications, such as atelectasis, may require bronchoscopic suction even during the first few days after the injury.

Continuing Treatment of Paraplegia

As soon as is feasible, paraplegic patients should be transferred to a special paraplegic unit or center for long term care and rehabilitation. Indeed, the development of paraplegic centers has been one of the most significant factors in the improved results of treatment. The over-all management of paraplegic patients requires the combined skills and dedication of a very large team including a rehabilitation physician, neurosurgeon, orthopaedic surgeon, urological surgeon, plastic surgeon, nurses, orderlies, physical and occupational therapist, social worker, teacher and job placement counselor. The most suitable individual to serve as captain of this team is usually the rehabilitation physician, but the captain's qualities as a compassionate and understanding person are of more importance than his particular specialty.

The following are some of the more important aspects of the long term care of paraplegic patients:

1. *Care of the urinary tract.* Urological complications account for 40% of deaths in paraplegics and, hence, their prevention is of extreme importance. After the early period, in which continuous drainage of the bladder is necessary, most patients can learn to empty their bladder by suprapubic manual compression. The aim is to establish an "automatic bladder" which empties when the patient initiates a cutaneous reflex.

2. *Care of the skin.* Paraplegics must eventually take the responsibility for preventing decubitus ulcers by turning frequently

and by learning to inspect their own skin, with the help of a hand mirror. If a decubitus ulcer does develop, it may necessitate extensive plastic operations.

3. *Musculoskeletal function.* The combination of spasticity with muscle imbalance and dependent edema leads to the development of joint contractures which, in turn, may interfere with the patient's rehabilitation. These contractural deformities are to a large extent preventable, provided all joints in the area of paralysis are moved through a full range daily. Braces are of little value to the paraplegic who has no control of his pelvic muscles and no sensation in his lower limbs. Indeed, most paraplegics find that they are much more mobile in a wheelchair to which they can readily transfer from bed or toilet (Fig. 12.28). For quadriplegics, carefully chosen tendon transfers may permit more efficient use of the few remaining muscles controlling the hands.

4. *Rehabilitation.* The philosophy of rehabilitation outlined at the end of Chapter 6 is particularly applicable to spinal paraplegics and quadriplegics. Previous formal education is the most significant factor in employability and, hence, many paraplegics require further education before they can be-

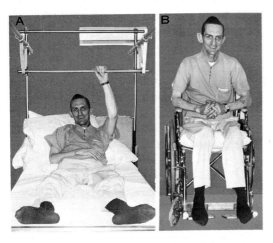

Figure 12.28. The paraplegic must have a bar over his bed in hospital and later in his home so that he may pull himself up and swing out of bed to a wheelchair. This young man, who prefers a wheelchair to full control braces and crutches, is well on his way to being rehabilitated.

come gainfully employed. The improved methods of overall management of spinal paraplegia and quadriplegia have made it possible for the majority of these patients to achieve reasonable independence and to lead useful, as well as rewarding, lives.

DISORDERS AND INJURIES OF THE SPINAL NERVE ROOTS AND PERIPHERAL NERVES

Polyneuritis

ACUTE POST-INFECTIVE POLYRADICULONEUROPATHY (GUILLAIN-BARRÉ SYNDROME)

This acute form of polyneuritis usually follows an infection, but its exact etiology is unknown. An affliction of young adults and occasionally of children, its clinical features are somewhat similar to those of poliomyelitis except that there is no fever and the lower motor neuron paralysis is almost always symmetrical; there may even be sensory changes. The cerebrospinal fluid changes are completely different from those of poliomyelitis in that the cell count is normal and the protein content is increased.

The prognosis of Guillain-Barré syndrome is good in that complete recovery is common. In the more severe forms, however, there may be residual paralysis, particularly in the lower limbs. Treatment is similar to that already described for poliomyelitis.

OTHER FORMS OF POLYNEURITIS

Peripheral polyneuritis is seen as a manifestation of toxic levels of arsenic, lead and other heavy metals. A common sign of lead poisoning, for example, is paralytic wrist drop. A nutritional form of polyneuritis may complicate such disorders as alcoholism and beri beri. Diabetic neuritis is seen as a complication in 5% of patients with severe diabetes. In leprosy (Hansen's disease), which is regrettably still common in many of the developing tropical countries, the most significant lesion is a peripheral neuritis with peripheral paralysis and loss of sensation, a combination which frequently necessitates tendon transfers and always requires precautions to prevent injuries to insensitive hands and feet.

Compression of Spinal Nerve Roots

Disorders of the spine including the intervertebral discs may cause either continuous, or intermittent, compression of associated nerve roots as discussed in Chapter 11. In the lumbar region the commonest cause is herniation of the intervertebral disc; in the cervical region the commonest cause is osteophytic narrowing of the intervertebral foramina. Many other disorders of the spine, however, may produce nerve root compression; these include spinal infections, primary and secondary neoplasms and spinal injuries.

The cardinal symptom of nerve root compression is pain that radiates in the nerve root distribution (radicular pain). Nerve root pain is increased by the following activities: (1) spinal movements that increase the nerve root compression; (2) coughing or sneezing, which raise the cerebrospinal fluid pressure; (3) straight leg raising, which increases the tension on the compressed nerve root. Paresthesia, such as numbness or tingling, in the nerve root distribution may also be experienced.

The motor signs of nerve root compression are those of a lower motor neuron lesion in the muscles innervated by that particular root. In considering nerve root lesions, it is important to appreciate that a given nerve root distributes fibers to more than one peripheral nerve, and a given peripheral nerve receives fibers from more than one nerve root.

The treatment of nerve root compression is that of the underlying causative condition. In addition to local rest and immobilization of the spine, surgical decompression of the nerve root is sometimes necessary.

Peripheral Nerve Entrapment Syndromes

Theoretically, any peripheral nerve could be subjected to continuous or intermittent compression. Certain nerves, however, course through specific anatomic regions in which they have less room to escape the effects of compression; in these regions, they are more easily "entrapped" by the internal pressure of an adjacent space-occupying lesion, such as edema, or by external pressure—hence the terms *nerve entrapment syndromes and entrapment neuropathies.*

The symptoms and signs vary with the degree of compression and whether it is continuous or intermittent. Pain and paresthesia in the sensory distribution of the nerve are common and may be associated with a sensory deficit. Muscle weakness (or even paralysis) and atrophy are commonly seen in the muscles innervated by the involved nerve at a later stage.

The more common nerve entrapment syndromes merit consideration as examples of this phenomenon.

MEDIAN NERVE AT THE WRIST (CARPAL TUNNEL SYNDROME)

At the wrist the median nerve and flexor tendons pass through a common tunnel whose rigid walls are formed by the carpal bones and joints and the transverse carpal ligament (flexor retinaculum). Any disorder that takes up space in this already crowded tunnel compresses the most vulnerable structure, the median nerve, and produces the *carpal tunnel syndrome.*

This fairly common syndrome can be caused by a variety of conditions including: (1) edema of acute and chronic trauma; (2) inflammatory edema associated with rheumatoid tenosynovitis; (3) osteophytes in the carpal joints; (4) ganglion; (5) lipoma.

Occurring most commonly in women of middle age or older, the syndrome produces pain and paresthesia in the sensory distribution of the median nerve in the hand; the patient may notice some clumsiness of finger function. The symptoms are aggravated by movements of the wrist. Subsequently, objective findings of sensory loss appear and eventually, there is weakness and atrophy of the thenar muscles (Fig. 12.29).

In the early stages of carpal tunnel syndrome, temporary immobilization of the wrist and the avoidance of strenuous work for a few weeks may be sufficient to relieve the pressure of edema on the median nerve. If the edema is inflammatory, a local injection of hydrocortisone may bring relief. Frequently, however, the problem persists and

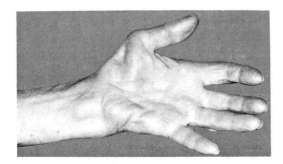

Figure 12.29. Atrophy of the thenar muscles in a 50-year-old woman due to longstanding compression of the median nerve at the wrist (carpal tunnel syndrome). Note the prominence on the anterior aspect of the wrist; this woman's median nerve compression was caused by a large ganglion in the carpal tunnel. Her condition should have been diagnosed at an earlier stage before muscle atrophy developed.

necessitates surgical decompression of the median nerve by longitudinal division of the transverse carpal ligament.

ULNAR NERVE AT THE ELBOW (DELAYED OR TARDY ULNAR PALSY)

At the elbow the ulnar nerve passes through a groove behind the medial epicondyle. In the presence of a valgus deformity of the elbow (increased carrying angle) the ulnar nerve is subjected to stretching, intermittent compression and friction during flexion and extension (Fig. 12.30).

The patient complains of pain and paresthesia in the sensory distribution of the ulnar nerve. Later, objective sensory changes can be detected. Paralysis, however, is usually delayed for many years (tardy paralysis), but eventually weakness and atrophy become apparent in the interosseous muscles of the hand. The only effective treatment is surgical transposition (relocation) of the ulnar nerve to the anterior aspect of the elbow.

RADIAL NERVE AT THE AXILLA (CRUTCH PALSY)

Prolonged and faulty use of the axillary type of crutch, taking weight through the axilla rather than through the hands, produces intermittent compression of the radial nerve in the axilla. After several months the patient experiences pain and paresthesia in

the distribution of the radial nerve. Subsequently, paralysis of the finger and wrist extensor muscles becomes apparent. This lesion is completely reversible, however, provided the cause is eliminated. The patient should be instructed in the proper use of crutches or better still, provided with elbow-length crutches.

BRACHIAL PLEXUS AT THE THORACIC OUTLET (SCALENUS SYNDROME)

The lower trunks of the brachial plexus may become entrapped as they cross over the first rib at the site of insertion of the scalenus muscles. Entrapment is more likely to occur if a congenital cervical rib is present. Persons with poor muscle tone and a long, thin thorax are most prone to develop this syndrome, which is manifest by radiating pain and muscular weakness in the upper limb; the precise distribution of the symptoms and signs depend on which trunks of the brachial plexus have become involved. The subclavian artery may also be com-

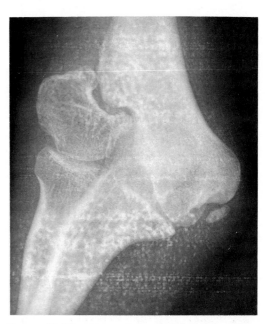

Figure 12.30. Non-union of a fracture of the lateral condyle of the humerus in a 21-year-old man. The fracture had occurred at the age of 5 years. The patient had a marked cubitus valgus deformity and a tardy ulnar palsy. Symptoms from the friction neuritis of the ulnar nerve did not develop until 10 years after the original injury.

pressed with resultant cyanosis of the arm and a weak radial pulse.

Exercises to strengthen the muscles that elevate the shoulder may be sufficient to relieve symptoms. Sometimes, however, it is necessary to explore the region surgically, to release the scalenus muscles and, if a cervical rib is present, to excise it.

DIGITAL NERVES IN THE FOOT (MORTON'S METATARSALGIA)

Women who wear excessively tight shoes run the risk of producing intermittent compression of their digital nerves in the forefoot—the folly of fashionable female footwear (Fig. 12.31). The digital nerve going to the space between the third and fourth toes is most commonly affected. Since the digital nerves are purely sensory, the only symptoms are pain and paresthesia. The pain may be sufficiently severe that the patient must literally stop in her tracks and remove her shoe. As a result of the repeated compression, a painful neuroma develops in the digital nerve. Examination reveals decreased sensation in the adjacent sides of the affected toes; lateral compression of the forefoot reproduces the pain of which the patient complains.

Wearing larger shoes with a metatarsal pad to elevate the transverse (anterior) arch and separate the metatarsals may relieve

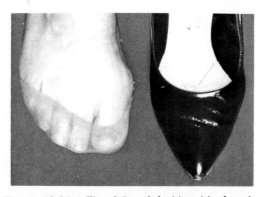

Figure 12.31. The folly of fashionable female footwear. This woman's foot is obviously much wider than her shoe. She had Morton's metatarsalgia due to intermittent compression of the digital nerve going to the space between the third and fourth toes.

the pain, but frequently the only form of treatment that brings permanent relief is surgical excision of a segment of the digital nerve with its neuroma.

Acute Injuries to Nerve Roots and Peripheral Nerves

Nerve roots and peripheral nerves may be injured by a blunt object which causes a *contusion*, by a sharp object that produces a *partial or complete laceration*, or by a severe stretch that results in a *traction injury* (a partial or complete tear). In addition, nerves are particularly vulnerable to prolonged ischemia which leads to *necrosis*.

CLASSIFICATION OF NERVE INJURIES

Seddon has developed the following classification of nerve injuries:

1. Neuropraxia

There is only slight damage to the nerve with transient loss of conductivity, particularly in its motor fibers. Wallerian degeneration (breakdown of the myelin sheaths into lipid material and fragmentation of the neurofibrils) does not ensue and complete recovery may be expected within a few days or weeks.

2. Axonotmesis

The injury damages the axons, which are prolongations of the cells in the spinal cord, but does not damage the structural framework of the nerve itself. The axons distal to the injury undergo Wallerian degeneration. Peripheral regeneration of the axons occurs along the intact neural tubes to the appropriate end organs but very slowly, approximately one millimeter each day, or three centimeters each month. Thus, if the axonotmesis in a given nerve occurred 9 cm proximal to its site of entrance into a given muscle it would take approximately three months for the regenerating axons to reinnervate that muscle.

3. Neurotmesis

In this type of injury the internal structural framework and the enclosed axons are divided, torn or destroyed. Wallerian degeneration occurs in the distal segment. Because the axons in the proximal segment have lost their neural tubes, natural regeneration is impossible. The neurofibrils and fibrous elements grow out of the divided end of the nerve to produce a bulbous *neuroma*. The only hope of recovery lies in surgical excision of the damaged section of the nerve and accurate suture of the freshened ends (preferably with the magnification provided by magnifying glasses or a dissecting microscope). Even under ideal circumstances for nerve suture, however, recovery is less than complete.

CLINICAL FEATURES AND DIAGNOSIS

Immediately after a nerve injury, there is complete loss of conductivity in the motor, sensory and autonomic fibers. The muscles supplied by the nerve root or peripheral nerve exhibit a flaccid paralysis and subsequently undergo atrophy. A loss of cutaneous sensations, deep sensation and position sense can be detected. The autonomic deficit is manifest by a lack of sweating (anhydrosis) in the cutaneous distribution of the nerve as well as a temporary vasodilation and resultant warm skin followed by a vasoconstriction and cold skin.

The precise diagnosis concerning both the type of injury and its location can be helped by appropriate electrical tests (nerve conduction tests, strength duration curves and electromyography).

PROGNOSIS AND RECOVERY

The prognosis depends on the type of injury (neuropraxia, axonotmesis or neurotmesis) as described above. If recovery does take place, it is evidenced first by return of muscle power in the most proximally supplied muscle. Return of sensation follows a definite pattern in that deep sensation returns first, followed by pain and position sense. As regeneration of axons proceeds along the nerve, the regenerated portion is hypersensitive so that finger tapping over it causes a tingling sensation (*Tinel's sign*). Thus, by assessing the distal limit of this phenomenon at intervals, it is possible to determine the progress of regeneration.

A disabling complication of *partial* nerve lesions during the recovery phase is severe burning pain (*causalgia*) in the sensory distribution of the nerve. The pain is sufficiently incapacitating in some patients that sympathetic denervation of the limb is required.

TREATMENT OF ACUTE NERVE INJURIES

Open Injuries

The open wound is explored and the nerve identified. If the division of the nerve is clean-cut, as by a piece of glass or a knife, immediate suture of the nerve is indicated (*primary repair*). If, however, the divided nerve ends are frayed, it is wiser to simply bring the two ends together with a single suture and defer definitive repair for two or three weeks (*secondary repair*), at which time it is possible to assess the extent of damaged portion that must be resected; furthermore, at this time the nerve sheath, having thickened, is more efficiently sutured.

Interfascicular repair of divided peripheral nerves under the high power magnification of microsurgery achieves the best alignment and coaptation of the neural elements.

Closed Injuries

In closed injuries that are complicated by loss of nerve function, it can usually, but not invariably, be assumed that the continuity of the injured nerve has not been lost (neuropraxia or axonotmesis). In over 75% of closed fractures complicated by a nerve injury for example, the nerve sheath is intact. Accordingly, it is reasonable to wait for the expected time of recovery (as described above for neuropraxia and axonotmesis). In the event that recovery has not occurred in the expected time, it can be assumed that the injury has been a neurotmesis, in which case surgical exploration and repair are indicated. In general, it is unwise to delay repair for longer than four months, by which time fibrotic changes in the distal segment of the nerve as well as in the paralyzed muscle militate against a good result.

Residual Paralysis

In some nerve injuries the damage is irreparable and the paralysis is permanent; in others, even following nerve repair there may be some residual paralysis. Under these circumstances the treatment is based on the *principles of orthopaedic treatment of neurological disorders and injuries* as stated earlier in this chapter.

TRACTION INJURIES OF THE BRACHIAL PLEXUS

The brachial plexus of nerves is much more vulnerable to traction injuries than is the lumbosacral plexus because the upper limb, being less firmly attached to the trunk than the lower limb, is more easily pulled away by forceful traction. Most traction injuries to the brachial plexus occur when the head and neck are forced laterally while, at the same time, the shoulder on the opposite side is either forced downward or kept from moving with the head and neck. Such injuries may result from a difficult delivery (birth injury) or from a road accident.

BIRTH INJURIES OF THE BRACHIAL PLEXUS (OBSTETRICAL PARALYSIS)

During the difficult delivery of a large baby as a vertex presentation, at the stage when the shoulders are still retained, strong lateral flexion of the head and neck may produce a traction injury of the brachial plexus. The same type of injury may occur during a breech delivery at the stage when the aftercoming head is still retained, if strong lateral flexion is applied to the trunk and cervical spine. The resultant brachial plexus injury may range from a mild stretch to complete tearing of one or more trunks, or even avulsion of nerve roots from the spinal cord. The result is a mixed sensory and lower motor neuron lesion.

Upper Arm Type (Erb's Palsy)

The commonest type of obstetrical palsy is a traction injury of upper trunks (C-5 and 6) with resultant paralysis of the shoulder and upper arm. The newborn infant exhibits no active movement in the affected arm, which, because of the distribution of muscle paralysis, lies by the side in a position of internal rotation (Fig. 12.32). Any recovery occurs most rapidly during the first six

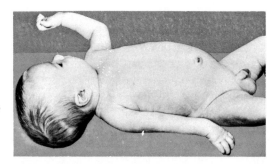

Figure 12.32. Obstetrical paralysis in an infant due to a traction injury of the brachial plexus at the time of a difficult delivery. From birth, the infant had not moved his right arm but had moved his hand. Note that the arm is adducted and internally rotated at the shoulder. This is the upper arm type of birth injury of the brachial plexus (Erb's palsy).

months. By the end of one year, 75% of the children will have made an almost complete recovery. During this year, all joints of the involved limb must be put through a full range of motion in an attempt to prevent contractures; a night splint is of doubtful value. Some paralysis persists in most children and the residual muscle imbalance produces the typical deformity of adduction and internal rotation at the shoulder and flexion at the elbow (Fig. 12.33). Surgical operations, such as muscle transfers about the shoulder or external rotation osteotomy of the humerus, may be required to permit the child to abduct the shoulder and to place the functioning hand in more useful positions.

Lower Arm Type (Klumpke's Paralysis)

In this rare type of obstetrical palsy the lower trunks of the brachial plexus (C-8, T-1) are injured and, consequently, the resultant paralysis involves the muscles of the forearm and hand (Fig. 12.34). The prognosis for recovery is unfavorable and operations, such as tendon transfer, may be necessary to improve hand function.

Whole Arm Type

An obstetrical traction injury that involves the entire brachial plexus is usually so severe that no recovery is to be expected. Indeed, it is likely that at least some of the

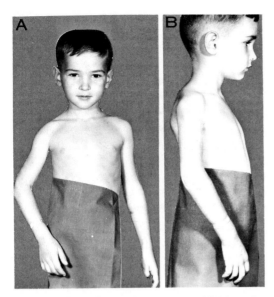

Figure 12.33. Residual paralysis of Erb's palsy in the right arm of a 6-year-old boy. Note the typical deformity of adduction and internal rotation of the shoulder and flexion of the elbow. This boy's appearance and function could be improved by an external rotation osteotomy of the humerus.

nerve roots are completely avulsed from the spinal cord. There is complete loss of sensation and complete paralysis of the entire upper limb; in addition there may be a Horner's syndrome on the side due to injury of the sympathetic fibers of the first thoracic root (Fig. 12.35). The completely flail, insensitive arm is not amenable to surgical treatment.

Psychological Consideration for the Parents

When a child has sustained a birth injury to the brachial plexus, the parents frequently bear some resentment toward the doctor who performed the delivery. This negative attitude, which is understandable but seldom justifiable, may persist for many years. Therefore, those who treat the child subsequently have a moral obligation to reassure the parents that had the doctor not acted as he did during this critical stage of the delivery, he might not have been able to save their child's life.

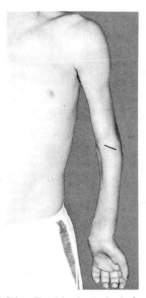

Figure 12.34. Residual paralysis from the lower arm type of birth injury of the brachial plexus (Klumpke's paralysis) in a 10-year-old boy. The hand and wrist are virtually flail and most of the forearm muscles are atrophied. This boy's hand function could be improved by arthrodesis of the wrist and tendon transfer to the fingers and thumb.

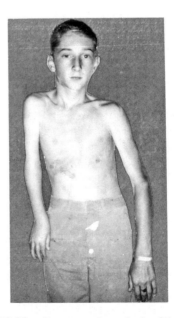

Figure 12.35. Permanent paralysis of the whole arm type of birth injury of the brachial plexus. The arm is completely paralyzed and completely insensitive. Did you notice the drooping of this boy's right eyelid indicating a Horner's syndrome?

BRACHIAL PLEXUS INJURIES
RESULTING FROM ACCIDENTS

Major accidents involving a severe fall or blow on the side of the head and simultaneous depression of the shoulder may produce a traction injury of the brachial plexus in both children and adults. Road accidents, particularly motorcycle accidents, are the most frequent cause of such injuries. Neurological examination of the limb reveals the extent and probable site of the injury. The traction force is so severe, however, that in more than half the patients, nerve roots have been avulsed from the spinal cord, in which case there is no hope of nerve regeneration. Avulsion of the roots can be detected by a myelogram, which reveals extravasation of the contrast medium along the nerve root sleeves (pseudomeningocele). If there is no radiographic evidence of root avulsion, exploration of the brachial plexus is justifiable in the hope that at least some of the nerves can be repaired.

Brachial plexus surgery including interfascicular nerve grafting under high power magnification has improved the results of surgical treatment of these devastating injuries.

Most brachial plexus injuries resulting from severe accidents are extensive and involve the entire plexus (whole arm type). Furthermore, the prognosis for recovery of function, particularly below the elbow, is poor. Persistent pain over a period of six months is a bad prognostic sign. Approximately one third of the patients recover sufficiently that hand function can be improved by surgical operations, such as tendon transfer and arthrodesis. When there is no recovery, a reasonable alternative to a flail, insensitive arm is amputation above the elbow and arthrodesis of the shoulder, after which the patient can obtain at least some function by means of a prosthetic limb.

ACUTE INJURIES TO SPECIFIC
PERIPHERAL NERVES

Although any peripheral nerve may be injured, some are injured more frequently than others. Examples of the more common peripheral nerve injuries are given below

without discussing details; the previously outlined general features of nerve injuries may be applied to each of the following specific injuries.

The *axillary nerve* may be injured in association with a traumatic anterior dislocation of the shoulder, or less commonly, a fracture of the proximal end of the humerus. The *radial nerve,* one of the most frequently injured, is usually involved at the time of a displaced fracture of the humeral shaft. The *ulnar nerve* at the elbow may sustain a mild traction injury at the time of a fracture-separation of the medial epicondyle, whereas the *median nerve* is more likely to be injured in association with a supracondylar fracture of the humerus. The median nerve at the wrist may also be injured by a severely displaced fracture of the distal end of the radius. At the wrist both the median and ulnar nerves are prone to being divided, since this is a common site of deep lacerations.

The *sciatic nerve* is frequently traumatized by a traumatic posterior dislocation of the hip, with or without an associated fracture of the acetabulum. The sciatic nerve may receive a direct injury from an inaccurately placed intramuscular injection of drug into the buttock. The *lateral popliteal (common peroneal) nerve* as it courses subcutaneously over the neck of the fibula is particularly vulnerable to laceration as well as to the pressure effects of tight bandages or casts.

DISORDERS OF MUSCLE

The majority of neuromuscular disorders are neurogenic rather than myogenic. Nevertheless, a variety of pure muscle disorders (*myopathies*) cause significant clinical disturbances of the musculoskeletal system and merit consideration.

The *congenital* disorders of muscle, *amyotonia congenita* and *amyoplasia congenita* are discussed in Chapter 8.

The most significant *acquired* disorders of muscle are the various types of *muscular dystrophy*.

Muscular Dystrophy

The term *muscular dystrophy* refers to a group of genetically determined disorders of muscle (*primary myopathies*). In recent years these tragic disorders have stimulated much interest, particularly in relation to their genetic and biochemical features.

DUCHENNE TYPE (PSEUDOHYPERTROPHIC MUSCULAR DYSTROPHY)

Two forms of the Duchenne type of muscular dystrophy exist. The commoner classical form is inherited as a sex-linked recessive trait; consequently, it afflicts males only, although non-afflicted female carriers can transmit the disease to their male offspring.

This form of muscular dystrophy becomes apparent in young children of preschool age but may develop in older children or even young adults. The boy is observed to tire easily and cannot keep up with his playmates. Symmetrical weakness of the pelvic muscles, particularly the gluteus maximus, develops early and accounts for the boy's difficulty in climbing stairs and standing up from a sitting or lying position. In getting up from the floor, he must "climb up his legs" and this is one of the most characteristic signs of muscular dystrophy (Gower's sign) (Fig. 12.36). Pseudohypertrophy develops most characteristically in the calf muscles, the increased bulk of the muscle being due to excessive fibrous tissue and fat rather than to muscular hypertrophy. Subsequently, the muscles of the trunk and shoulder girdle become weak. Deformities secondary to contractures are common.

Progression of the disease is relentless; most boys are physically incapacitated within 10 years of the onset and few survive beyond the age of 20; the commonest cause of death is cardiac failure due to associated cardiomyopathy.

Laboratory investigation reveals an elevation of certain cellular enzymes which probably arise from affected muscles. These enzymes include creatine phosphokinase, aldolase and alanine transaminase. Electromyography is helpful in differentiating neurogenic muscle weakness from myogenic weakness. Muscle biopsy is valuable in determining the exact type of muscular dystrophy.

The less common form of the Duchenne type of muscular dystrophy is inherited as an autosomal recessive trait and consequently afflicts girls as well as boys. Progression of the disease is less rapid than in the common form, but the clinical features are otherwise similar.

LIMB GIRDLE TYPE OF MUSCULAR DYSTROPHY

This rare type of muscular dystrophy, which begins in adult life, is inherited as an autosomal recessive trait; it affects muscles of both the shoulder girdle and the pelvic girdle. Muscle atrophy is characteristic of this type but pseudohypertrophy is seldom seen. The disease progresses slowly.

FACIO-SCAPULO-HUMERAL TYPE OF MUSCULAR DYSTROPHY

Commoner in adults than in children, this type of muscular dystrophy is inherited as an autosomal dominant trait and characteristically affects the muscles of the face, shoulders and arms. It may become arrested at any stage and does not shorten the patient's life expectancy.

TREATMENT OF MUSCULAR DYSTROPHY

In the past the inevitability of progressive muscular weakness and premature death in this pathetic group of children and young adults has led to an attitude of apathy in relation to treatment. Although there is, as yet, no specific cure for the various types of muscular dystrophy, much can be done through continuing overall management to make the remaining years of these patients, and of their parents, more bearable.

Ideally, patients with muscular dystrophy should be seen at regular intervals in combined or multidisciplinary outpatient clinics where their continuing care can be supervised by a team which includes a neurologist, rehabilitation physician, orthopaedic surgeon, physical and occupational thera-

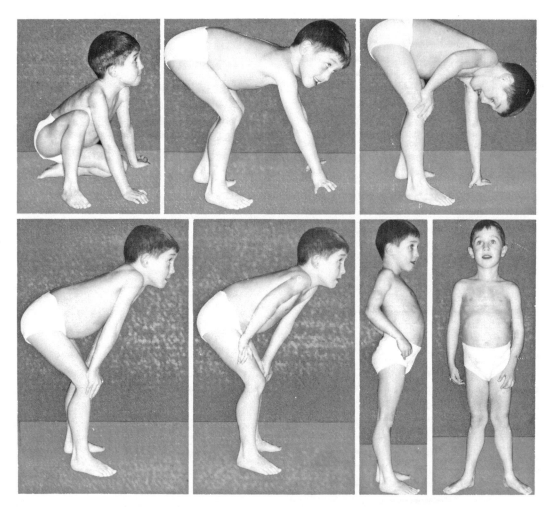

Figure 12.36. Gower's sign in muscular dystrophy. This series of photographs show how a boy with muscular dystrophy must get up from the floor by climbing up his legs with his hands because of weakness in the gluteus maximus and spinal muscles. Note the pseudohypertrophy of this boy's calf muscles and the lumbar lordosis in the standing position.

pist and medical social worker. Active exercises help to prevent the otherwise inevitable disuse atrophy of muscles that are not involved and minimize the patient's physical disability as well as improve his morale. Dietary supervision helps to reduce the obesity that accompanies relative inactivity and that accentuates the disability.

When the child can no longer walk unaided, he should be provided with light braces (Fig. 12.37). To overcome disabling contractures of the calf and thigh muscles, minor operations, such as subcutaneous tenotomies of the tendo achillis and fascio-

tomies of the fascia lata as well as transfer of the tibialis posterior tendon to the dorsum of the foot, are most helpful; the child is able to be up and walking the following day, thereby overcoming the ill effects that patients with muscular dystrophy suffer as a result of even a few weeks' confinement to bed.

The combination of light braces and orthopaedic operations will enable children with muscular dystrophy to keep on walking for an average of 25 additional months (which represents 10% of their life expectancy.

Even when these children become chair-

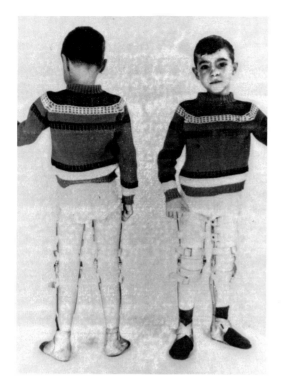

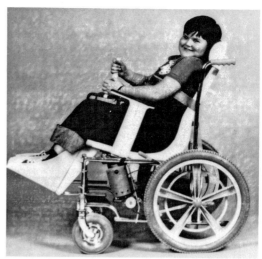

Figure 12.38. A boy with advanced muscular dystrophy reclining in a "spinal support system" that fits into his battery-powered wheelchair. Note the electric hand controls for forward and reverse motions as well as for right and left turns.

Figure 12.37. At first glance you may think that this is a composite photograph of a boy taken from the front and from the back. Actually, it is a photograph of *two* boys—identical twin brothers—both of whom have inherited muscular dystrophy. Note the modern light braces. Their disease had progressed to the point at which they were no longer able to walk unaided. With the help of orthopaedic operations and the support of these braces, the twin boys were able to continue walking for an additional two years.

bound, the provision of a custom-made "spinal support system" and a battery-powered wheelchair have proven to be of significant help to both the afflicted children and their distressed parents (Fig. 12.38).

Suggested Additional Reading

Adams, R. D. and Victor, M.: *Principles of Neurology*, 2nd ed. New York, McGraw-Hill, 1981.

Bateman, J. E.: *The Shoulder and Neck*, 2nd ed. (With special assistance of Fournasier, V. L.) Philadelphia, W. B. Saunders, 1978.

Bedbrook, G. M.: Spinal injuries with tetraplegia and paraplegia. J. Bone Joint Surg. 61B: 267–284, 1979.

Bedbrook, G. M.: *The Care and Management of Spinal Cord Injuries*. New York, Springer-Verlag, 1981.

Bennet, G. C. and Harrold, A. J.: Prognosis and early management of birth injuries to the brachial plexus. Br. Med. J. 1: 1520–1521, 1976.

Buxton, P. H.: Investigation of muscle dysfunction. In *Scientific Foundations of Orthopaedics and Traumatology*, edited by Owen, R., Goodfellow, J. and Bullough, P. London, William Heinemann Medical Books, 1980.

Edmonson, A. S. and Crenshaw, A. H. (eds). *Campbell's Operative Orthopaedics*, 6th ed. St. Louis, C. V. Mosby, 1980.

Hayter, R. R. P.: Stroke: the deficits, factors in rehabilitation and prevention of complications. Can. Fam. Phys. 25: 945–949, 1979.

Hoppenfeld, S.: *Orthopaedic Neurology. A Diagnostic Guide to Neurologic Levels*. Philadelphia, J. B. Lippincott, 1977.

Kutz, J. E., Shealy, G. and Lubbers, L.: Interfascicular nerve repair. Orthop. Clin. North Am. 12: 277–286, 1981.

MacEwen, G. D.: The management of neuromuscular imbalance in the growing child. In *Clinical Trends in Orthopaedics*, edited by Straub, L. R. and Wilson, P. D., Jr. New York, Thieme-Stratton, 1982.

Marakas, A.: Brachial plexus surgery. Orthop. Clin. North Am. 12: 303–323, 1981.

McManus, F., Rang, M., Chance, G. and Whittaker, J.: Is cerebral palsy a preventable disease? Obstet. Gynecol. 50: 71–77, 1977.

Millesi, H.: Interfascicular nerve grafting. Orthop. Clin. North Am. 12: 287–301, 1981.

Rang, M., Douglas, G., Bennet, G. C. and Koreska, J.: Seating for children with cerebral palsy. J. Pediatr. Orthop. 1: 279–287, 1981.

Rorabeck, C. H. and Harris, W. R.: Factors affecting the prognosis of brachial plexus injuries. J. Bone Joint Surg. 63B: 404–407, 1981.

Roy, L. and Gibson, D. A.: Pseudohypertrophic muscular dystrophy and its surgical management. Review of 30 patients. Can. J. Surg. 13: 13–21, 1970.

Samilson, R. L. (ed.): *Orthopaedic Aspects of Cerebral Palsy.* Philadelphia, J. B. Lippincott, 1975.

Shapiro, F. and Bresnan, M. J.: Orthopaedic management of childhood neuromuscular disease. Part I. Spinal muscular atrophy. J. Bone Joint Surg. 64A: 785–789, 1982.

Shapiro, F. and Bresnan, M. J.: Orthopaedic management of childhood neuromuscular disease. Part II. Peripheral neuropathies, Friedreich's ataxia, and arthrogryposis multiplex congenita. J. Bone Joint Surg. 64A: 949–954, 1982.

Sunderland, S.: *Nerves and Nerve Injuries*, 2nd ed. Edinburgh, Churchill-Livingstone, 1978.

Swaiman, K. F. and Wright, F. S. (eds.): *The Practice of Pediatric Neurology*, 2nd ed. St. Louis, C. V. Mosby, 1982.

Tator, C. H. and Rowed, D. W.: Current concepts in the immediate management of acute spinal cord injuries. Can. Med. Assoc. J. 121: 1453–1464, 1979.

Walton, J. N.: *Brain's Diseases of the Nervous System*, 8th ed., New York, Oxford University Press, 1977.

Walton, J. N. (ed.): *Disorders of Voluntary Muscle*, 4th ed. Edinburgh, Churchill-Livingstone, 1981.

Waters, R. L., Perry, J. and Garland, D.: Surgical correction of gait abnormalities following stroke. Clin. Orthop. 131: 54–63, 1978.

Wynn-Parry, C. B.: Electrodiagnosis. In *Scientific Foundations of Orthopaedics and Traumatology*, edited by Owen, R., Goodfellow, J. and Bullough, P. London, William Heinemann Medical Books, 1980.

CHAPTER 13

Disorders of Epiphyses and Epiphyseal Growth

The epiphyses and their epiphyseal plates constitute a captivating component of the skeletal system during the growing years of childhood. Since they are unique structural and functional units, it is not surprising that under abnormal circumstances they react differently from the rest of the skeleton; consequently, there exists a variety of unique disorders peculiar to epiphyses and epiphyseal growth.

The various *generalized* disorders of epiphyses and epiphyseal plates of *congenital* origin, such as achondroplasia, are discussed in the latter part of Chapter 8, whereas those that are *acquired*, such as rickets, are considered in Chapter 9. The present chapter is concerned with a discussion of the *localized* disorders of these unique units and, in particular, with the *pressure type* of epiphyses as opposed to the *traction type* (Fig. 13.1). Injuries involving the epiphyseal plate are considered in Chapter 16.

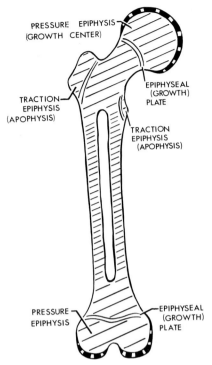

Figure 13.1. Types of epiphyses. A *pressure* epiphysis, situated at the end of a long bone, is subjected to pressures transmitted to the joint into which it enters. In this sense it may be considered an articular epiphysis; furthermore, its epiphyseal plate provides longitudinal growth of the bone. A *traction* epiphysis, by contrast, is the site of attachment of tendons and muscles; consequently, it is subjected to traction rather than to pressure. Since it does not enter into the formation of a joint, it is non-articular and it does not contribute to the longitudinal growth of the bone.

Epiphyses appear to be relatively resistant to many of the disorders seen in other parts of the skeleton. Hematogenous osteomyelitis, for example, never begins in an epiphysis and rarely spreads into it through the epiphyseal plate. Furthermore, during childhood nearly all bone neoplasms, both benign and malignant, avoid the epiphysis. By contrast, however, the epiphyses are particularly vulnerable to an idiopathic type of avascular necrosis (*osteochondrosis*). In addition, local epiphyseal growth is altered in a variety of childhood disorders such as idiopathic curvature of the spine (scoliosis);

consequently, such disorders are likely to be progressive throughout the growing years.

NUTRITION OF THE EPIPHYSIS AND ITS EPIPHYSEAL PLATE

A knowledge of the unique blood supply to epiphyses and their epiphyseal plates is pivotal in an understanding of their disorders. Most pressure epiphyses are covered to a considerable extent by articular cartilage and consequently receive blood vessels only through their "bare bone areas." Others, such as the femoral head, being com-

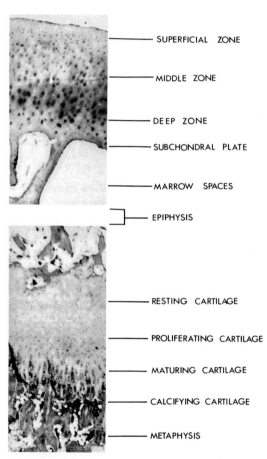

Figure 13.2. Sites of bone growth. The metaphysis grows in length from the epiphyseal plate (*below*) but the epiphysis itself grows in 3 dimensions from the deep zone of the articular cartilage (*above*). Small bones, such as the tarsal navicular and lunate, also grow from the deep zone of their articular cartilage.

pletely intra-articular and therefore completely covered by articular cartilage, receive their blood supply precariously from vessels that must penetrate the "cartilage clothing."

In addition to supplying the epiphyses, the epiphyseal blood vessels are also responsible for the nutrition of the growing cells of the epiphyseal plate; therefore, ischemia of the epiphysis is associated with ischemia of the epiphyseal plate and a subsequent disturbance of longitudinal growth of the bone.

Whereas the shaft of a long bone grows in length from the epiphyseal plate, the epiphysis itself grows in three dimensions from the deep zone of the articular cartilage; the same is true of the small bones such as the tarsal navicular (Fig. 13.2).

AVASCULAR NECROSIS OF BONE

Death of bone is by no means limited to epiphyses and, hence, the general subject of avascular necrosis merits consideration. Variously called avascular necrosis, aseptic necrosis and ischemic necrosis, this condition represents a series of pathological events from the initial loss of blood supply and resultant death of bone to the gradual replacement of the dead bone by living bone. It is a very common phenomenon indeed, since after every *fracture*, a minute area of each fracture surface undergoes avascular necrosis; furthermore, free *bone grafts*, which initially are both avascular and necrotic, eventually become replaced by living bone.

The present discussion, however, is concerned with avascular necrosis of *subchondral bone* that supports articular cartilage in synovial joints.

IDIOPATHIC AVASCULAR NECROSIS OF EPIPHYSES (THE OSTEOCHONDROSES)

A number of idiopathic clinical disorders of epiphyses in growing children share the common denominator of avascular necrosis and its sequelae; they are therefore considered as a group, *the osteochondroses*. To you, as a student, the multiple *synonyms* (epiphysitis, osteochondritis, aseptic necro-

sis, ischemic epiphyseal necrosis) may seem confusing; the confusion is not lessened by the multiple *eponyms* based on the name of the person, or persons, who have described the disorder in a given epiphysis (Kohler's disease, Osgood-Schlatter's disease, Legg-Calvé-Perthes' disease)—the "*osteochondroses eponymous.*" Some semblance of order out of this semantic chaos, however, comes from the realization that the underlying pathogenesis, if not the etiology, is similar in all of these entities and that the clinical manifestations in any given epiphysis are determined by the stresses and strains applied to it. The major source of concern in any of the osteochondroses is that during the pathological process the involved epiphysis may become permanently deformed.

Osteochondrosis usually involves a *secondary* epiphyseal center, or *pressure epiphysis*, at the end of a long bone (such as the femoral head) but may also involve the primary *epiphyseal* center of a small bone (such as the tarsal navicular). Understandably, the epiphyses that are most susceptible are those that are entirely covered by articular cartilage and therefore have a precarious blood supply. Somewhat similar lesions which affect *traction epiphyses* (such as the tibial tubercle) are sometimes considered as examples of idiopathic osteochondrosis, but are probably traumatic in origin and are therefore discussed separately.

General Features of the Osteochondroses

Many features of the various clinical entities of osteochondrosis are common to all and, hence, in order to avoid repetition are discussed as *general features* before proceeding to a consideration of the specific clinical entities.

INCIDENCE AND ETIOLOGY

The osteochondroses in general are most common during the middle years of growth, from the ages of 3 to 10. They generally affect boys more frequently than girls, and the lower limbs are more frequently involved than the upper limbs. Osteochondrosis of a given epiphysis is bilateral in approximately 15% of involved children.

As the adjective, *idiopathic*, implies, the precise *etiology* of the osteochondroses has so far escaped detection and remains an intriguing challenge. Despite the plethora of proposed theories, there has been a paucity of proven facts. Although it is generally agreed that the common denominator in the osteochondroses initially is avascular necrosis of the epiphyseal center, there is less agreement about the mechanism of the initial loss of blood supply.

Certain factors, such as genetically determined vascular configuration, may have a predisposing influence. Since boys sustain more injuries than girls and their lower limbs are injured more often than their upper limbs, the sex and site incidence of osteochondroses suggest that trauma may play a role. Trauma of sufficient severity to produce a fracture or a dislocation can definitely produce the well recognized traumatic type of avascular necrosis. In the idiopathic type, however, less severe trauma may produce a complication, such as a pathological fracture, in already necrotic bone and thereby aggravate the condition sufficiently to bring it to the physician's attention. A tense synovial effusion, either traumatic or inflammatory, may develop enough pressure to obliterate intra-articular vessels, such as those proceeding to the head of the femur.

PATHOGENESIS AND PATHOLOGY

The osteochondroses are self-limiting disorders that eventually heal spontaneously and, consequently, relatively little pathological tissue has been available for study. Nevertheless, the pathogenesis and pathology are more clearly understood than the etiology.

The pathological changes in the various phases of this process of events are well correlated with the radiographic changes and are best discussed in relation to a specific epiphysis as *an example*. Osteochondrosis of the femoral head (Legg-Perthes' disease) is most suitable for this purpose; its pathogenesis and pathology are presented as being representative of the

changes that take place in *all* the osteochondroses. The description that follows is based partly on clinical and radiographic observations in children, and partly on our experimental investigations in young pigs.

This fascinating pathological process is best considered in relation to four *phases*, even though the transition from one phase to another is both gradual and subtle. The whole process spans a long period, from two to eight years, depending on the age of onset and severity of the secondary changes.

1. Early Phase of Necrosis (the Phase of Avascularity)

After obliteration of the blood vessels to the epiphysis from whatever cause, the osteocytes and the bone marrow cells within the epiphysis die, but the bone remains unchanged for many months, neither harder nor softer than normal bone. The ossific nucleus of the epiphysis, however, ceases to grow because there is no blood supply for endochondral ossification. The articular cartilage, which is nourished by synovial fluid, remains alive and indeed continues to grow. Thus, over the ensuing months (sometimes up to a year or longer) the ossific nucleus of the involved epiphyseal center is smaller than that on the normal side, whereas the cartilage space is thicker (Fig. 13.3). During the avascular period, the radiographic density of the nucleus remains unchanged since neither bone deposition nor bone resorption can occur without a blood supply. Nevertheless, disuse atrophy (osteoporosis) and, hence, decreased radiographic density in the metaphysis, may give the appearance of a *relative* increase in density of the femoral head. This is the "quiet phase" of osteochondrosis during which the child is usually symptomless and during which no deformity takes place.

2. Phase of Revascularization with Bone Deposition and Resorption

This phase represents the vascular reaction of the surrounding tissues to dead bone; it is characterized by revascularization of the dead epiphysis, a process that brings about a series of changes that are detectable radiographically. Beginning peripherally around the rim of the epiphysis, ossification of the thickened pre-osseous cartilage resumes. At the same time new bone is laid down on dead trabeculae inside the original ossific nucleus; this *bone deposition* renders the original nucleus denser radiographically and gives the appearance of a "head-within-a-head" (Fig. 13.4). The new bone that forms, however, is primary woven bone comparable to that seen in a fracture callus; it is not soft in a physical sense but it has "*biological plasticity*" in that, as it grows, it is easily modeled, into either a normal, or an abnormal, shape depending on the forces to which it is subjected.

During the phase of revascularization, a *pathological fracture* occurs in the subchondral bone of the original ossific nucleus at the site of greatest stress (in the hip this is the anterosuperior portion of the femoral head) and this can be detected radiographically in at least one projection (Fig. 13.5).

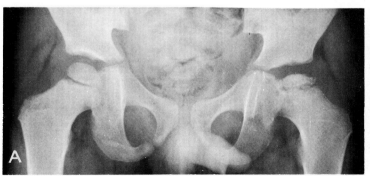

Figure 13.3. Osteochondrosis of the left femoral head (Legg-Perthes' disease) toward the end of the early phase of necrosis. Note that the left epiphyseal center of ossification is significantly smaller than the right, whereas the cartilage space of the left hip is thicker than that of the right. The apparent increase in density at this stage is only *relative* to the decreased density of the metaphysis.

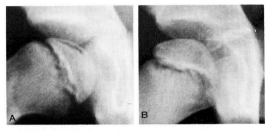

Figure 13.5. Osteochondrosis of the right femoral head (Legg-Perthes' disease) in the phase of revascularization. *A*, note the pathological fracture in the subchondral bone of the femoral head in this "frog position" view, which is a lateral projection of the femoral head and neck, but an anteroposterior projection of the pelvis. The fracture is pathological in the sense that it occurs through abnormal bone, in this case, dead bone. *B*, the fracture is difficult to see in the anteroposterior projection of the femoral head.

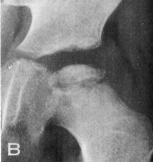

Figure 13.4. Osteochondrosis of the left femoral head (Legg-Perthes' disease) in the phase of revascularization with bone deposition and bone resorption. Note the small dense head (the size of the head when it stopped growing) and the new bone peripherally on either side of it; this is the "head-within-a-head" phenomenon. This is more clearly seen in the enlarged picture of the left hip. At this stage there is an *absolute* increase in radiographic density because of new bone laid down on dead trabeculae.

The fracture, which is almost certainly the result of superimposed trauma, is associated with pain and the development of a synovial effusion in the joint as well as synovial thickening with resultant limitation of motion. The overlying joint cartilage, however, remains intact. Continued micro-motion at the site of the pathological fracture incites a fibrous and granulation tissue reaction which results in excessive osteoclastic *bone resorption* and interferes with re-ossification. In the femoral head this resorption may involve only the anterior part (partial head type) or the entire head (whole head type) depending upon the extent of the subchondral fracture.

The combination of irregular areas of bone deposition and bone resorption provides the radiographic appearance of apparent "fragmentation" (Fig. 13.6). In the case of the femoral head, the hip may become *subluxated* with resultant abnormal forces being applied to it. During this most vulnerable

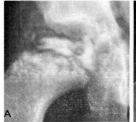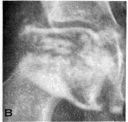

Figure 13.7. Osteochondrosis of the right femoral head (Legg-Perthes' disease) in the phase of revascularization. *A*, note that the femoral head is *subluxated* upward and outward in relation to the acetabulum. This complication has produced excessive forces on the femoral head and has resulted in a progressive deformity. *B*, the extent of the deformity in the femoral head at this stage is best appreciated in the arthrogram; part of the flattened head has extruded beyond the edge of the acetabulum.

phase of osteochondrosis, abnormal forces on the already weakened epiphysis may produce a progressive *deformity* due to biological plasticity of the new living bone, cartilage and fibrous tissue (Fig. 13.7). By the same token, suitable molding forces on the epiphysis during this phase can prevent deformity as will be seen later. The epiphyseal plate, having also suffered the effects of ischemia, may cease to grow normally and the metaphysis may become broadened. The phase of revascularization with bone deposition and bone resorption persists for varying periods, from one to four years, and during this phase, the epiphysis continues to be deformable.

3. Phase of Bone Healing

Eventually, bone resorption ceases and bone deposition continues so that the fibrous and granulation tissue are slowly replaced by new bone. The newly formed bone of the healing epiphysis, however, still exhibits "biological plasticity" and can still be molded to some extent, for better or for worse, by forces that are applied to it. The eventual contour of the epiphysis can be assessed only when re-ossification of the epiphysis is complete (Figs. 13.14 to 13.16).

4. Phase of Residual Deformity

Once bony healing of the epiphysis is complete, its contour remains relatively un-

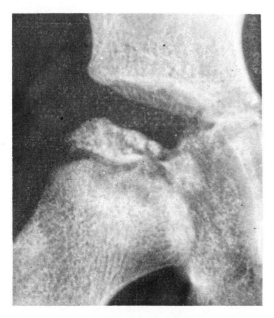

Figure 13.6. Osteochondrosis of the right femoral head (Legg-Perthes' disease) later in the phase of revascularization with bone deposition and bone resorption going on simultaneously in different areas of the head. Note the radiographic *appearance* of "fragmentation" (the overlying cartilage is still intact).

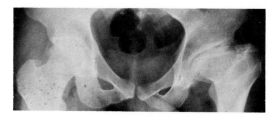

Figure 13.8. Late degenerative joint disease of the left hip in a 36-year-old man secondary to the residual joint deformity and incongruity of Legg-Perthes' disease which he developed at the age of 6 years. Note also the short, broad femoral neck. This man has pain on walking and painful limitation of motion; a reconstructive operation such as femoral osteotomy, arthroplasty, or even arthrodesis, will be required to relieve his symptoms.

changed. Thus, any residual deformity persists. Since the articular cartilage has remained reasonably normal, however, function in the joint can be fairly satisfactory for many years. Nevertheless, in weightbearing joints such as the hip, residual deformity and its associated joint incongruity and limitation of motion lead to the gradual development of degenerative joint disease in later life (Fig. 13.8).

CLINICAL FEATURES AND DIAGNOSIS

The osteochondroses produce neither symptoms nor clinical signs during the "quiet" early phase of necrosis. In the phase of revascularization, however, particularly if a pathological fracture develops in the subchondral bone, the child experiences pain. A synovial effusion develops and this accounts for local tenderness and painful limitation of motion in the joint. If the child is not treated, the symptoms and signs tend to be intermittent, but gradually the muscles controlling the joint exhibit some degree of disuse atrophy (Fig. 13.9). Occasionally, a child goes through all the phases of an osteochondrosis without any symptoms, In which case the diagnosis is made fortuitously on the basis of a radiograph taken for some other purpose.

The radiographic features of the various phases of osteochondrosis have been correlated with the pathogenesis and pathology (Figs. 13.3 to 13.7). The differential diagno-

sis radiographically includes irregular ossification in a normal epiphysis, and generalized disorders such as hypothyroidism and epiphyseal dysostosis in which abnormal findings are seen in multiple epiphyses.

COMPLICATIONS

The complications of osteochondrosis include: subchondral fracture in the epiphysis, subluxation of the involved joint, deformity of the epiphysis with resultant joint incongruity, and late degenerative joint disease.

AIMS AND PRINCIPLES OF TREATMENT

Osteochondrosis is a self-limiting disease either with or without treatment. Furthermore, the diagnosis is almost never made before the phase of revascularization and neither drugs, nor any other form of treatment, can reverse the process. The *aims* of treatment, therefore, must be to prevent deformity of the epiphysis and thereby preserve congruity of the joint.

The *principles* of treatment are concerned

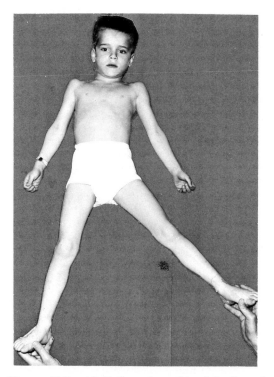

Figure 13.9. Limitation of passive abduction of the hip and disuse atrophy of the thigh due to Legg-Perthes' disease of the right hip in a 5-year-old boy.

with the prevention of abnormal forces on the epiphysis during its vulnerable phases of revascularization and healing; for osteochondrosis involving an epiphysis of the lower limb, this involves prevention of the complication of subluxation of the joint. From our experimental investigations we have learned that the time-honored practice of prolonged relief of weight bearing over a period of years, either by means of bed rest, or by weight-relieving braces, is neither necessary nor desirable. It has now been shown in the hip joint, for example, that weight bearing can be permitted with impunity, provided the femoral head is kept from subluxating and the hip maintains a good range of movement. Once significant deformity has developed, however, treatment has little effect on the final outcome. The specific methods of treatment are outlined in relation to the various clinical entities.

SPECIFIC OSTEOCHONDROSES OF SECONDARY CENTERS OF OSSIFICATION (PRESSURE EPIPHYSES)

The foregoing discussion of *general features* of the osteochondroses is applicable to each of the clinical entities to be described and should serve to make a discussion of these *specific* entities both interesting and meaningful.

Osteochondrosis of the Femoral Head (Legg-Perthes' Disease)

Easily the most important of the osteochondroses is Legg-Perthes' disease, not only because it is more common than the others, but also because it is more serious. Its numerous synonyms include the following; coxa plana (flat hip), pseudocoxalgia, osteochondritis deformans coxae juvenilis, Legg-Calvé-Perthes' syndrome.

INCIDENCE AND ETIOLOGY

Legg-Perthes' disease is most frequent between the ages of 3 and 11 years and is 4 times more common in boys (particularly physically active boys) than in girls. It is bilateral in approximately 15% of affected children and there may be a familial incidence. Of the many proposed theories of etiology, the one which seems most likely, and for which there is some experimental proof, is that the original occlusion of the precarious blood supply to the femoral head is caused by the excessive fluid pressure of a synovial effusion in the hip joint, either inflammatory or traumatic. As mentioned in Chapter 10, approximately 5% of children with transient synovitis of the hip and an associated synovial effusion in the joint develop the complication of Legg-Perthes' disease.

PATHOGENESIS AND PATHOLOGY

Legg-Perthes' disease was used as an example of all the osteochondroses in discussing their pathogenesis and pathology in the preceding general section of this chapter and need not be repeated here. It is well to emphasize, however, the specific importance of the pathological subchondral fracture and of secondary subluxation of the hip as harmful factors in the pathogenesis of deformity in Legg-Perthes' disease.

CLINICAL FEATURES AND DIAGNOSIS

The symptoms and signs in the various phases of Legg-Perthes' disease are similar to those described in the general section but a few specific points merit further discussion. The absence of clinical manifestations of the disease during the "quiet" early phase of necrosis accounts for the fact that the child is seldom brought to a physician until the phase of revascularization, or even later. The pain in this disease may be felt in the region of the hip, but can also be referred to the knee. The specific limitation of hip joint motion involves abduction and internal rotation; the disuse atrophy is most noticeable in the upper part of the thigh (Fig. 13.9). The child walks with a limp of the antalgic or protective type (protects the hip "against pain" by rapidly taking weight off the foot on the involved side with each step).

The diagnosis can be *suspected* clinically but can be *confirmed* only by radiographic examination, the findings of which are well correlated with the pathogenesis and pathology (Figs. 13.3 to 13.7).

COMPLICATIONS

Legg-Perthes' disease may be complicated by subchondral fracture in the epiphysis (Fig. 13.5), subluxation of the joint (Fig. 13.7), flattening of the epiphysis (coxa plana) with resultant incongruity (Fig. 13.7), and late degenerative joint disease (Fig. 13.8).

Treatment

The aim of treatment in Legg-Perthes' disease is to prevent deformity of the femoral head and thereby to prevent degenerative changes in the hip in adult life. The principle of treatment is prevention of *abnormal* forces on the femoral head during its vulnerable phases of revascularization and bony healing. In the hip particularly, this involves prevention of a secondary subluxation.

The methods of treatment of Legg-Perthes' disease in the past (all of which have been based on the avoidance of weight bearing) have varied from enforced and continuous confinement to bed in an institution for several years, through various types of weight-relieving braces to a sling and crutches (Fig. 13.11). Some surgeons have even adopted the nihilistic attitude that no treatment affects the final outcome of the disease and that consequently, no treatment is indicated.

Catterall's radiographic classification of four degrees of involvement of the femoral head is widely used but the essential point is simply whether less than half or more than half of the head is involved. Catterall has wisely pointed out that unless there is subluxation, only those children with more than half of the head involved require treatment and this means that approximately half of the children with Legg-Perthes' disease require regular observation only.

For those children who do require treatment the underlying principle (which we have proven in experimental investigations) is "containment" of the femoral head plus motion and weight bearing in order that the involved femoral head may be protected from becoming flattened.

An effective form of containment is weight bearing in abduction plaster casts (Fig. 13.10) or in some type of abduction brace (Figs. 13.11 and 13.12) both of which pre-

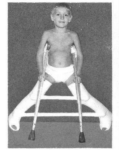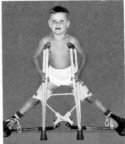

Figure 13.10. (*left*). Abduction plaster casts (Petrie) for Legg-Perthes' disease. The abducted position effectively prevents subluxation of the hip.

Figure 13.11. (*right*). Abduction brace (Bobechko) for Legg-Perthes' disease. This brace has the advantage of permitting knee motion and also of being removable for bathing and sleeping.

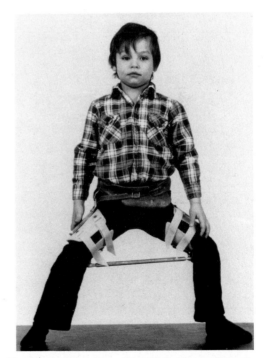

Figure 13.12. The "Scottish Rite" abduction brace for Legg-Perthes' disease. This brace is less restrictive than the Toronto brace but may not prove to be as effective in keeping the femoral head contained.

vent subluxation and enable the acetabulum to mold the "biologically plastic" healing femoral head in such a way that it does not become deformed. An inexpensive alternative method of containment treatment is the stirrup crutch (Fig. 13.13).

Surgical operations, such as femoral osteotomy and innominate osteotomy, designed to prevent or overcome subluxation, have been used successfully for older children who have a bad prognosis, provided the operation is done *before* any deformity has developed; after the osteotomy has united, the child is allowed to walk and run unhampered by braces or crutches. In the late stages of the disease when marked deformity of the femoral head has developed, the salvage operation of excision of the extruded portion of the head may improve motion.

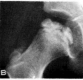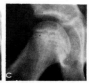

Figure 13.14. Good prognosis. *A*, at the age of 4 years near the end of the early stage of recovery. *B*, two years later. *C*, four years later the femoral head is round, a good result.

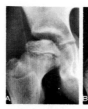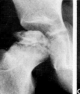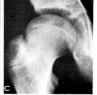

Figure 13.15. Fair prognosis. *A*, at age 6 years, early in the revascularization phase. *B*, one year later. *C*, five years later the femoral head is large (coxa magna) but reasonably round, a fair result.

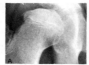

Figure 13.16. Poor prognosis. *A*, at age 8 years early in the revascularization phase. *B*, one year later there is marked subluxation. *C*, five years later the femoral head is not only large but also flat (coxa plana), a poor result.

PROGNOSIS

In Legg-Perthes' disease more than in any of the other osteochondroses, the prognosis, even with treatment, is extremely variable. The age of onset is an important factor; in general, the prognosis is *good* in children whose onset is under the age of five years (Fig. 13.14), *fair* in children with an onset from five to seven years of age (Fig. 13.15) and *poor* in children with an onset over the age of seven years (Fig. 13.16). The prognosis is definitely worse in the whole head type and in the presence of subluxation. In the older child, failure to treat Legg-Perthes' disease may lead to severe residual deformity (Fig. 13.17).

Other important factors in worsening the

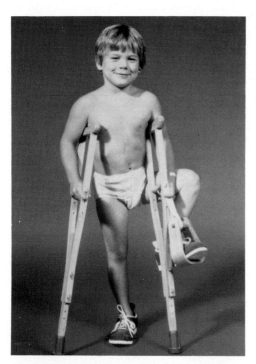

Figure 13.13. The stirrup crutch method of treating Legg-Perthes' disease. The abducted and flexed position of the hip ensures containment of the femoral head and yet the child is able to bear weight through the stirrup (as in riding a horse). This is an inexpensive alternative to an abduction brace but it requires complete co-operation of the child and his parents.

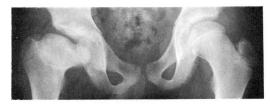

Figure 13.17. Severe residual deformity in the femoral head due to *untreated* Legg-Perthes' disease in a 14-year-old boy whose parents had refused treatment for him when he first had symptoms at the age of 8 years.

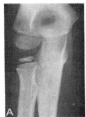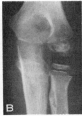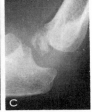

Figure 13.18. Osteochondrosis of the left capitellum (Panner's disease) in a 6-year-old boy. *A*, the normal right elbow for comparison. *B*, and *C*, note the combination of rarefaction due to bone resorption, and sclerosis due to bone deposition giving the *appearance* of "fragmentation." Note also the phenomenon of a "capitellum-within-in-a-capitellum."

prognosis for a given child are extensive involvement (more than half the head), subluxation and loss of hip joint motion.

Osteochondrosis of the Capitellum (Panner's Disease)

The capitellum of the humerus is only rarely the site of avascular necrosis. Afflicting children between the ages of 3 and 11 years, its pathogenesis and pathology are those of all osteochondroses (described in an earlier section of this chapter).

Panner's disease is manifest by pain and slight swelling in the elbow as well as by restriction of joint motion. The radiographic appearance is typical of osteochondrosis in other pressure epiphyses (Fig. 13.18). Since the elbow joint is non-weight-bearing, and excessive and abnormal forces are not normally applied to the capitellum, deformity is unlikely and the prognosis is good. Treatment consists of providing the child with a sling during periods of discomfort.

Osteochondrosis of a Metatarsal Head (Freiberg's Disease)

Unlike other osteochondroses, Freiberg's disease begins during adolescence and is more common in girls. Most of those afflicted have a congenitally long second metatarsal, or a short first metatarsal, both of which cause excessive pressures on the head of the second metatarsal, particularly when wearing high-heeled shoes; this may be a predisposing factor. Although the second metatarsal is the common site, Freiberg's disease occasionally affects the third metatarsal.

The pathogenesis and pathology are those of all osteochondroses (described in an early section of this chapter) except that an osteochondral fragment may become loose as in osteochondritis dissecans. The most significant complication is residual deformity with resultant degenerative disease of the metatarsophalangeal joint after the deformity has been present for several years.

The patient complains of pain in the forefoot on standing and walking. Examination reveals local thickening and tenderness as well as painful restriction of motion in the metatarsophalangeal joint. The radiographic appearance is typical of all osteochondroses (Fig. 13.19).

Non-operative treatment by means of low-heeled shoes and a stiff "rocker-bottom" sole may relieve the symptoms from the complication of degenerative joint disease. Frequently, however, excision arthroplasty (which is accomplished by removal of the distorted metatarsal head, or of the base of the phalanx) is necessary for permanent relief.

Osteochondrosis of Secondary Centers of Ossification in the Spine (Scheuermann's Disease)

Each vertebral body increases in height from two epiphyseal plates, one covering the upper surface, the other covering its lower surface. The so-called "ring epiphysis" is, in effect, a traction epiphysis, or apophysis, and does not contribute to the

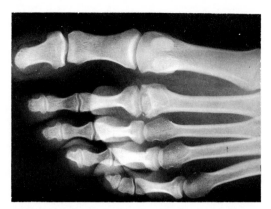

Figure 13.19. Osteochondrosis of the second metatarsal head (Freiberg's disease) in a 19-year-old girl. The normally domed-shaped head has become flattened, broad and irregular with resultant joint incongruity and early degenerative joint disease. Originally, this metatarsal would have been longer than the first; the hypertrophy of the shaft suggests that it has been bearing excessive weight for many years.

height of the vertebral body. In the thoracic spine a growth disturbance of the epiphyseal plates anteriorly, with a resultant accentuation of the normal kyphotic curve, is variously known as osteochondrosis of the spine, *Scheuermann's disease*, vertebral epiphysitis, adolescent kyphosis or adolescent round back (Fig. 13.20).

INCIDENCE AND ETIOLOGY

This fairly common but poorly understood disorder, which affects both boys and girls, usually begins at puberty and progresses during adolescence until vertebral growth has ceased in the late teens. In at least some of the patients the disorder is inherited with an autosomal dominant pattern. It commonly involves the epiphyseal plates of three or four adjoining vertebral bodies in the mid-thoracic region.

Persistent anterior vascular grooves in the vertebral bodies may be a predisposing factor. Multiple minor injuries to the epiphyses and their epiphyseal plates have also been incriminated. Whatever the cause, there would seem to be an element of avascular necrosis affecting the anterior portion of the

involved epiphyseal plate, but whether this is primary or secondary is not known.

PATHOGENESIS AND PATHOLOGY

A consistent finding in the involved vertebral bodies is the presence of herniation of the intervertebral disc through the anterior portion of the epiphyseal plate into the body of the vertebra (Schmorl's node). As a result, there is less disc material between the vertebral bodies and the intervertebral disc space narrows. Such a herniation may interfere with the epiphyseal plate growth directly; or by disturbing the blood supply to the plate, it may interfere with growth indirectly. Ossification in the anterior portion of the vertebral epiphysis becomes irregular and, in this sense, is typical of osteochondrosis. Deficient growth anteriorly, in the

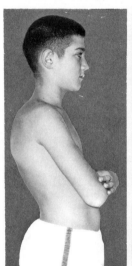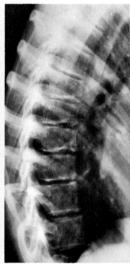

Figure 13.20 (*left*). Osteochondrosis of the secondary centers of ossification in the spine (Scheuermann's disease) in a 14-year-old boy. Note the exaggerated kyphosis in the thoracic region (round back) and the compensatory exaggerated lordosis in the lumbar region.

Figure 13.21 (*right*). The thoracic spine of the same boy as shown at left. The 4 middle vertebrae are involved. Note the irregular ossification of the anterior portion of the epiphyses of these 4 vertebrae. The indentations into the bodies of the vertebrae represent Schmorl's nodes. The intervertebral disc spaces are uniformly narrow and the kyphosis is accounted for by the anterior wedging of the involved vertebral bodies.

presence of continuing growth posteriorly, inevitably produces a wedge-shaped vertebral body that is shorter in front than behind; a series of three or four such wedge-shaped vertebral bodies accounts for the increased kyphosis.

CLINICAL FEATURES AND DIAGNOSIS

The child is usually noticed by the parents, or by a school physician, to have "poor posture" or "round shoulders" at about the time of puberty. At this stage the disorder is symptomless. During the ensuing few years, however, the round back appearance becomes progressively more noticeable and the patient complains of moderate back pain, particularly at the end of an active day. Examination reveals an exaggerated kyphosis in the thoracic region and a compensatory exaggerated lordosis in the lumbar region (Fig. 13.20). There may be local tenderness over the spinous processes of the involved thoracic vertebrae. The hamstring muscles are always tight. The symptoms subside spontaneously when growth ceases, but the spinal deformity persists.

Radiographic examination of the thoracic spine reveals irregular ossification in the anterior portion of the epiphyses of several adjoining vertebrae, as well as indentations through their epiphyseal plates at the site of the Schmorl's nodes. The intervertebral disc spaces are uniformly narrow but the involved vertebral bodies are wedge-shaped (Fig. 13.21).

Treatment

Since Scheuermann's disease is self-limiting and the symptoms are mild, the aim of treatment is to prevent a progressive thoracic kyphosis. In the early stages, spinal exercises are beneficial. An effective method of treatment during growth is the Milwaukee brace (Fig. 13.38), which is normally used for scoliosis (lateral curvature), but which can be modified for the treatment of kyphosis.

Once growth is completed, a brace is no longer effective. Thus in older adolescents and adults with an unsightly kyphosis and back pain, surgical correction and spinal instrumentation may be required.

SPECIFIC OSTEOCHONDROSES OF PRIMARY CENTERS OF OSSIFICATION

Short bones, such as the tarsal navicular and the lunate, form as primary centers of ossification and, having no epiphyseal plates, they grow from the deep zone of their articular cartilage. These bones are to a large extent covered by articular cartilage and, consequently, have a precarious blood supply that reaches them only through their "bare areas of bone." Two of the short bones that are prone to develop osteochondrosis are the tarsal navicular and the lunate.

Osteochondrosis of the Tarsal Navicular (Kohler's Disease)

In young children the tarsal navicular bone normally develops from more than one center of ossification, and this should not be confused with true osteochondrosis (which is relatively uncommon).

In children, particularly boys, between the ages of four and eight years, true osteochondrosis may develop in the navicular and initiate the series of events outlined in the pathogenesis and pathology of all osteochondroses early in this chapter. In this particular osteochondrosis, however, healing is usually complete in two years and there is seldom a residual deformity. Occasionally the disorder is bilateral.

During the early phase of necrosis, Kohler's disease is symptomless, but in the phase of revascularization, the child usually complains of mild pain in the mid-foot and tends to walk with an antalgic (protective) limp. Examination reveals local tenderness and swelling due to a synovial effusion in the region of the navicular. The radiographic findings are comparable to those already described for all osteochondroses earlier in this chapter (Fig. 13.22).

The prognosis of Kohler's disease is excellent in that regardless of the type of treatment, the lesion heals with no significant sequelae. Treatment therefore is aimed at relief of the transient local symptoms and

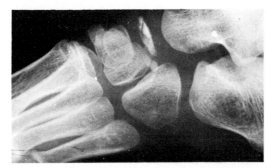

Figure 13.22. Osteochondrosis of the tarsal navicular (Kohler's disease) in a 5-year-old boy. The process is in the phase of revascularization with areas of bone deposition and bone resorption. The ossific nucleus is thin but the cartilage space is thicker than normal, which means that the overall size of the navicular is not diminished. This explains the eventual normal appearance of the navicular at the end of the healing process.

usually consists of providing the child with a sponge rubber arch support during the active phases of the osteochondrosis. A walking cast may be required for a few weeks to relieve an episode of acute pain, but this is unusual.

Osteochondrosis of the Lunate (Kienbock's Disease)

The lunate bone is occasionally involved by a process that would seem to represent avascular necrosis. Occurring most frequently in young adults, Kienbock's disease may be secondary to trauma, either major or minor. Workmen such as carpenters and riveters, who sustain repeated micro-trauma to their wrists, are much more often afflicted than others, and it may be significant that the right hand is involved more frequently than the left. It is possible that micro-fractures within the lunate disturb its already precarious blood supply and initiate the necrosis.

The pathogenesis and pathology are similar to those described for all osteochondroses in an earlier section of this chapter, with two exceptions. The healing process is much slower in the adult than in the child and indeed, it is unlikely that the lunate in Kienbock's disease ever reaches complete healing; furthermore, in the adult, the arti-

cular cartilage is likely to be affected. For these two reasons, degenerative joint disease in the wrist is an almost inevitable complication of Kienbock's disease.

The patient initially complains of mild aching in the wrist, but this tends to become progressive over a period of years secondary to degenerative joint disease. It may cause considerable disability, particularly in a workman. Examination reveals local tenderness over the lunate but little swelling; wrist motion is restricted by pain and the grip is weaker than on the normal side. The radiographic appearance is characteristic of avascular necrosis depending on the phase of the process at the time (Fig. 13.23).

Since in this disorder the pathological process is irreversible, the aim of treatment is relief of pain. In the early phases, immobilization of the wrist may bring temporary relief, but the most reasonable treatment is excision of the lunate (with or without the insertion of a carved plastic spacer) before degenerative changes develop in the carpal joint. In the presence of advanced degener-

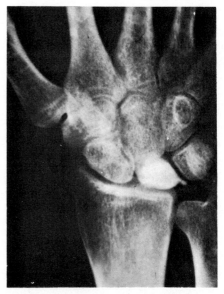

Figure 13.23. Osteochondrosis of the lunate (Kienbock's disease) in a 30-year-old workman who had complained of pain in his wrist for 2 years. Note the marked sclerosis and irregularity of the lunate as well as the disuse osteoporosis in the surrounding bones.

ative joint disease, the only form of treatment that is likely to bring permanent relief is arthrodesis of the wrist.

Osteochondrosis of a Primary Center of Ossification in the Spine (Calvé's Disease)

The primary center of ossification of a vertebral body is occasionally the site of osteochondrosis (*Calvé's disease*, vertebral osteochondrosis, vertebra plana) but less commonly than the previously described disorder of Scheuermann's disease which affects the secondary centers. Calvé's disease occurs in children between the ages of two and eight years and is almost always limited to one vertebral body.

Once thought to be an idiopathic type of osteochondrosis, Calvé's disease probably represents avascular necrosis secondary to a local *eosinophilic granuloma*, (which is one form of skeletal reticulosis, Chapter 9). Since both osteochondrosis and eosinophilic granuloma are self-limiting disorders, however, the prognosis is good.

The child may complain of mild back pain but is otherwise healthy. Examination reveals a slight kyphosis and, occasionally, muscle spasm. Radiographic examination reveals a striking change in the vertebral body, the ossified part of which becomes wafer-thin and sclerotic (Fig. 13.24) A radiographic study of other bones (skeletal survey) should be carried out to seek other evidence of a skeletal reticulosis, such as eosinophilic granuloma or Hand-Schüller-Christian disease. Needle biopsy, or punch biopsy, of the vertebral body may be required to establish the diagnosis. Within two or three years, re-ossification of the cartilage model of the vertebral body and the continued growth from its secondary centers of ossification results in an almost complete restoration of the vertebra, which is only slightly thinner than normal.

Since this disorder is self-limiting, treatment is aimed at relieving symptoms. A temporary spinal brace usually suffices for this purpose.

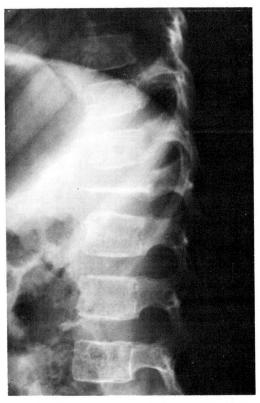

Figure 13.24. Osteochondrosis of the primary center of ossification of a vertebral body (Calvé's disease) in a 7-year-old boy. The ossified portion of the vertebral body is wafer-thin and sclerotic, but the cartilage spaces above and below are thicker than those in the rest of the spine. This means that the cartilage model of the vertebra has not flattened completely and explains the almost complete restoration in the thickness of the vertebral body after healing of the lesion by ossification of the cartilage model.

TANGENTIAL AVASCULAR NECROSIS OF A PRESSURE EPIPHYSIS (OSTEOCHONDRITIS DISSECANS)

The convex surfaces of certain pressure epiphyses are susceptible to avascular necrosis of a small tangential segment of subchondral bone which may become separated, or "dissected," from the remaining portion of the epiphysis by reactive fibrous and granulation tissue—hence the name, *osteochondrosis dissecans*. This relatively uncommon disorder is entirely different from the more common phenomenon of irregular epiphyseal ossification, or a separate center of ossification, both of which are variations of normal.

Incidence and Etiology

Osteochondritis dissecans usually occurs in older children and young adults; boys are afflicted more frequently than girls. The most frequently involved epiphyses are the medial femoral condyle, patella, capitellum, femoral head and talus.

The etiology of the initial avascular necrosis in osteochondritis dissecans is not known. The observations that this disease is sometimes familial and, in some patients, is associated with osteochondrosis elsewhere, suggest that there may be a pre-existing abnormality in the epiphysis which plays a predisposing role. In the adult, however, trauma is probably responsible for aggravating the lesion and may even initiate the necrosis.

Pathogenesis and Pathology

The tangential area of avascular necrosis on the convex surface of the epiphysis is usually no larger than 2 cms. in diameter and often smaller. Whatever the cause of the necrosis, the osteocytes die, but the overlying articular cartilage, which is nourished by synovial fluid, remains alive. An ingrowth of fibrous and granulation tissue (from the marrow spaces of the remaining healthy part of the epiphysis) "dissects" in a plane between living and dead bone thereby isolating the necrotic segment.

As the necrotic segment becomes revascularized, a combination of bone deposition and bone resorption occur and, consequently, the convex surface of the epiphysis may flatten. Provided the overlying articular cartilage remains intact, bony healing eventually takes place.

Superimposed trauma at this stage, however, may tear the overlying cartilage, in which case the necrotic fragment is forced out of its concave soft tissue bed and becomes an osteo-cartilaginous loose body (sometimes referred to as "joint mouse" since it is free to flit elusively from place to place within the synovial cavity).

Clinical Features and Diagnosis

There are usually neither symptoms nor clinical signs during the "quiet" early phase of necrosis, but during the revascularization phase, the patient may experience intermittent local pain with relatively little disturbance of joint function. Examination reveals a moderate synovial effusion in the joint and slight disuse atrophy of surrounding muscles, but little restriction of joint motion. Should the necrotic segment become partially detached, however, the symptoms and signs are more marked; should it become completely detached, the patient complains of intermittent catching, or locking, of the joint due to the presence of the loose body.

Radiographically, the lesion is characterized by a small isolated segment of subchondral bone separated from its bed by a radiolucent line which represents soft tissue (Figs. 13.25 and 13.26). Since the lesion is tangential, its radiographic detection may necessitate special tangential projections.

Arthrography is helpful in determining whether or not the overlying cartilage is intact; in the knee joint, arthroscopy is particularly appropriate for this purpose.

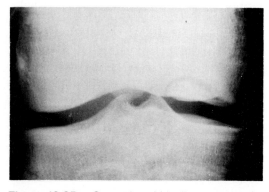

Figure 13.25. Osteochondritis dissecans on the convex surface of the medial femoral condyle in a 19-year-old boy. Note the small subchondral segment of bone separated from the remainder of the epiphysis by a radiolucent line which represents fibrous tissue. In the knee joint the necrotic segment and its overlying cartilage may become detached and move freely about the joint as a loose body; the same complication is known to occur in the elbow joint when the osteochondritis dissecans involves the capitellum.

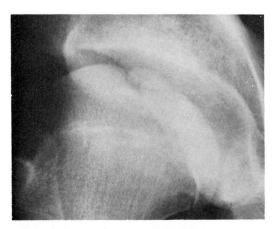

Figure 13.26. Osteochondritis dissecans on the convex surface of the femoral head in a 15-year-old boy. The small subchondral segment of necrotic bone is clearly seen. This segment, however, is unlikely to become separated since it is well protected by the opposing congruous joint surface of the acetabulum.

Prognosis

Many lesions of osteochondritis dissecans heal spontaneously over a period of two or three years without leaving any residual joint incongruity, especially in the juvenile type in which the epiphyseal plates are still open. In the *knee* and in the *elbow*, however, the process is more likely to be complicated by complete separation of the necrotic fragment with its overlying cartilage, thereby forming a loose body and leaving a residual and permanent defect in the joint surface of the epiphysis. If the defect is small, or is on a non-weight-bearing surface of the joint, the consequences are not significant; but if it is large and involves a weight-bearing surface, degenerative disease of the joint may ensue over a period of years.

Treatment

The aims of treatment depend on the phase of the pathological process at the time. If the cartilage overlying the tangential segment of dead bone is still intact, the aim of treatment is to prevent its detachment; this involves restriction of activity and may even necessitate temporary relief of weight bearing from the joint to encourage healing. If the segment is large and involves a weight

bearing surface of the joint, particularly in the knee, arthrotomy of the joint and insertion of peg-shaped bone grafts accelerate healing of the fragment to its bed and therefore prevent its separation. Once the overlying cartilage has been torn and the fragment has become either partially or totally separated, it should be removed unless it is large (more than 2 cm. in diameter), in which case it should be replaced and held in its bed either by metal pins or bone pegs.

IDIOPATHIC AVASCULAR NECROSIS OF THE FEMORAL HEAD IN ADULTS (CHANDLER'S DISEASE)

Avascular necrosis may develop in one or both femoral heads in adults without a preceding injury and from no apparent cause. This idiopathic type of femoral head necrosis in adults, which seems to have become more prevalent in recent years, is more often seen, however, in middle-aged persons who have a history of some generalized disorder such as alcoholism, or who have received systemic adrenocorticosteroids for an unrelated condition. It is possible, though not proven, that a pathological fracture in osteoporotic cancellous bone may even initiate the avascular necrosis.

The pathogenesis and pathology of avascular necrosis of the mature femoral head differ markedly from those of osteochondrosis of the immature femoral head (Legg-Perthes' disease). The entire process extends over a period of many years and indeed, never heals spontaneously. A large segment of the weight-bearing area may collapse; furthermore, the articular cartilage frequently fails to survive and may even become lifted off the underlying bone. The joint is eventually irreparably destroyed.

The patient complains of pain, either in the hip or referred to the knee, and notices a slowly progressive stiffening of the joint. The pain and joint stiffness increase gradually until sudden collapse of a major weight-bearing area of the femoral head causes severe pain. Examination at this time reveals painful limitation of hip joint movement which is associated with muscle spasm. Function in the hip deteriorates relentlessly and irreversibly.

Radiographic changes include marked sclerosis of a major segment of the femoral head that includes the weight-bearing area. The sclerotic segment may be indefinitely demarcated from the rest of the head by irregular areas of rarefaction and sclerosis; it may have collapsed, or have become impacted, with resultant incongruity of the joint (Fig. 13.27).

The prognosis of idiopathic avascular necrosis of the adult femoral head is very poor indeed because of the irreparable damage to the joint. Consequently, treatment frequently involves surgical operations such as a varus osteotomy of the femur or a Sugioka type of osteotomy that turns the femoral head "upside down" so that the uninvolved part of the femoral head comes to bear weight. If, however, the entire femoral head is involved, the patient will require a prosthetic hip joint replacement, either unipolar or bipolar depending on the state of the acetabulum. If the lesion is unilateral, arthrodesis of the hip may be indicated.

IDIOPATHIC AVASCULAR NECROSIS OF THE KNEE IN ADULTS

This disorder, also known as *spontaneous osteonecrosis of the knee*, has been recognized only in the past two decades. It is the medial femoral condyle that is usually involved and the average age of onset is over 60 years—more commonly in women than in men. Although acute pain in the knee may precede radiographic changes by six months, the diagnosis can be made earlier by scintigraphy because of increased uptake of the radionuclide in the medial femoral condyle, which indicates an attempt at revascularization of the necrotic bone. Eventual collapse of the medial femoral condyle can be managed by either an osteocartilaginous allograft or a high tibial osteotomy if the area of necrosis is not extensive; otherwise, a prosthetic knee joint replacement is indicated.

POST-TRAUMATIC AVASCULAR NECROSIS OF TRACTION EPIPHYSES (APOPHYSES)

Two disorders which were formerly considered to represent a form of osteochondrosis of traction epiphyses (apophyses) are presently thought to be caused by partial avulsion of the apophysis and its related tendon. These disorders, Osgood-Schlatter's disease and Sever's disease, are therefore discussed separately from the osteochondroses of pressure epiphyses.

Partial Avulsion of the Tibial Tubercle (Osgood-Schlatter's Disease)

In very young children the tibial tubercle is formed by a cartilaginous tongue-shaped downward prolongation of the upper tibial epiphysis. Toward the end of growth one or more centers of ossification appear in the tibial tubercle and at this stage it is most vulnerable to the effects of repeated, forceful traction through the attached patellar tendon.

Partial avulsion of the growing tibial tuber-

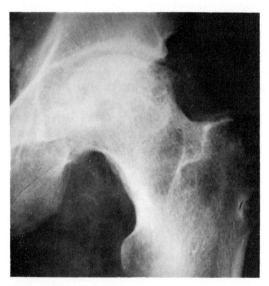

Figure 13.27. Idiopathic avascular necrosis of the femoral head in a 47-year-old man who had been receiving adrenocorticosteroid therapy for 2 years as treatment for an unrelated disorder. Note the sclerosis of a large segment of the femoral head. The convex weight-bearing area has collapsed with resultant incongruity of the joint surfaces. Irregular areas of bone resorption can be seen between the large sclerotic segment and the remainder of the femoral head. This man's hip joint is irreversibly damaged.

cle, with subsequent avascular necrosis of the avulsed portion, is probably the explanation for the clinical disorder known as *Osgood-Schlatter's disease*. Understandably, boys, particularly active boys, between the ages of 10 and 15 years are most frequently affected; the lesion may be bilateral.

The child complains of local pain which is aggravated by kneeling on the tibial tubercle, by direct blows and by running. Clinically, a prominent subcutaneous swelling, some of which is due to reaction in the soft tissues, is apparent in the region of the tibial tubercle (Fig. 13.28). The prominence is tender and the pain can usually be reproduced by having the patient extend the knee against resistance.

Radiographically, the proximal part of the tibial tubercle exhibits irregular areas of bone deposition and bone resorption when com-

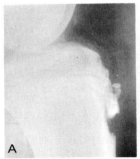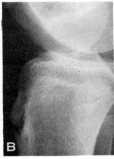

Figure 13.29. Osgood-Schlatter's disease due to partial avulsion of the tibial apophysis in a 14-year-old boy. Note the irregular areas of bone deposition and bone resorption in the proximal part of the traction epiphysis (apophysis). *B*, the normal tibial tubercle of the opposite knee is perfectly smooth and regular.

pared to the tubercle on the normal side (Fig. 13.29).

Osgood-Schlatter's disease is usually self-limiting, in which case the tibial tubercle becomes completely ossified over a period of about two years. In some children, however, a complication develops; a proximal segment fails to unite to the remainder of the tubercle, remains mobile and persists as a source of local pain and tenderness.

The aim of treatment in uncomplicated Osgood-Schlatter's disease is prevention of further irritation during the healing phase. This is accomplished by the avoidance of kneeling and jumping; it is not necessary to immobilize the knee nor to restrain the child from running. Residual non-union of a proximal fragment after the remainder of the tibial tubercle has healed will not improve spontaneously and will continue to cause symptoms; under these circumstances, excision of the ununited fragment is indicated.

Partial Avulsion of the Calcaneal Apophysis (Sever's Disease)

The traction epiphysis (apophysis), through which the Achilles tendon inserts into the os calcis, normally ossifies from multiple centers; furthermore, being broad and flat, it normally appears radiographically dense in a lateral projection. This combination may lead to an erroneus radiographic diagnosis of osteochondrosis. Nevertheless, a clinical disorder, which may represent

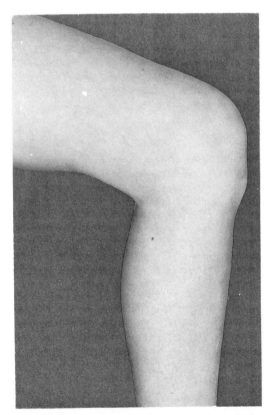

Figure 13.28. Osgood-Schlatter's disease due to partial avulsion of the tibial apophysis in a 14-year-old boy. Note the prominent subcutaneous swelling over the tibial tubercle; some of this swelling is due to reaction in the local soft tissues.

chronic strain, or even partial avulsion of the calcaneal apophysis, does exist and is seen in children, particularly active boys, between the ages of 8 and 15 years.

The child experiences pain behind the heel and walks with little spring in his step (calcaneus gait) in a subconscious effort to reduce the powerful pull of the Achilles tendon on the apophysis. Local tenderness and slight swelling are usually found over the posterior aspect of the heel. The radiographic findings are within the wide range of normal variations mentioned above.

This self-limiting disorder improves spontaneously in less than a year, but during this time the child's symptoms can be relieved by elevating the heel of the shoe one centimeter and thereby decreasing the pull of the Achilles tendon during walking.

POST-TRAUMATIC AVASCULAR NECROSIS OF SUBCHONDRAL BONE

The main blood vessels to a significant part of a bone may be torn at the time of a severe injury such as a fracture or a dislocation, or a combination of the two (which is referred to as a "fracture-dislocation"). Even if not torn initially, the blood vessels may be compressed by the displaced fragments or by the dislocated bone. In either event, resulting ischemia can lead to the serious complication of avascular necrosis, a complication which occurs most commonly after certain types of fractures and dislocations involving the femoral head and neck, the carpal scaphoid and the talus.

In children, post-traumatic avascular necrosis of a pressure epiphysis is most likely to occur after fracture-separation of the upper femoral epiphysis or after traumatic dislocation of the hip (Fig. 13.30). The course is similar in many ways to that of Legg-Perthes' disease (described in an earlier section of this chapter). The most important sequelae are incongruity of the joint and retardation of growth in the epiphyseal plate.

In adults, fractures of the neck of the femur and traumatic dislocation of the hip are the commonest causes of post-traumatic avascular necrosis. This complication

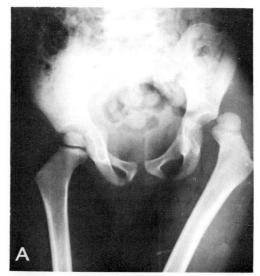

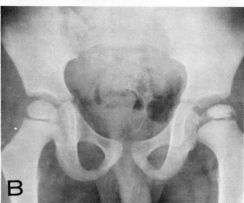

Figure 13.30. Post-traumatic avascular necrosis of the left femoral head. *A,* traumatic posterior dislocation of the left hip in a 4-year-old boy. *B,* the radiograph 16 months later reveals definite evidence of avascular necrosis of the femoral head. Note the increased density of the relatively small ossific nucleus of the left femoral head. This ossific nucleus is approximately the same size as it was at the time of the dislocation. Note also the evidence of bone deposition peripherally in the preosseous cartilage of the femoral head. This condition is comparable in many ways to Legg-Perthes' disease.

in adults delays, but does not prevent, healing of a fracture; frequently, however, it leads to the type of irreparable joint damage seen in idiopathic avascular necrosis of the femoral head in adults (described in an earlier section of this chapter) (Fig. 13.31).

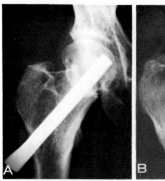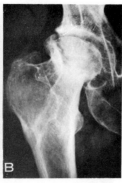

Figure 13.31. Post-traumatic avascular necrosis of the femoral head in a 65-year-old woman after fracture of the neck of the femur. *A*, the hip 2 months after internal fixation of the fracture with a Smith-Petersen nail reveals no significant change in the density of the femoral head. *B*, the radiograph 2 years later reveals evidence of extensive avascular necrosis of the femoral head. The fracture of the neck of the femur has healed and the nail has been removed. Proximal to the original fracture site, however, is a large segment of avascular necrosis. This triangular-shaped segment containing the weight-bearing surface has collapsed resulting in marked joint incongruity. Note the evidence of bone deposition and bone resorption in the femoral head demarcating the necrotic fragment from the remainder of the head. Note also that this patient's hip is now adducted due to an adduction contracture. This patient's hip is irreparably destroyed.

MISCELLANEOUS CAUSES OF AVASCULAR NECROSIS OF SUBCHONDRAL BONE

The blood supply to bone may be disturbed in a variety of ways; the subchondral bone at the end of long bones is most susceptible. In certain blood diseases, such as *polycythemia*, the likely cause is thrombosis. In certain metabolic disorders, such as *Gaucher's disease*, accumulation of abnormal cells may obliterate the blood supply (Chapter 9). Nitrogen emboli arising from fatty tissues, such as the fatty marrow, after atmospheric decompression in divers and underground construction workers (*decompression illness, caisson disease, "the bends"*), may cause avascular necrosis of bone with subsequent degenerative joint disease (Fig. 13.32). *Burns* and *frostbite* are likely to destroy blood supply to bone, par-

ticularly pressure epiphyses in children. In the past, *radiation therapy* was sometimes complicated by avascular necrosis of bone in the region, particularly the neck of the femur in women who were being radiated for malignant lesions of the uterus; fortunately, this complication has been reduced in recent years by improved methods of radiotherapy.

DISORDERS OF EPIPHYSEAL GROWTH

A variety of entirely different disorders of childhood share one thing in common; they are related, either directly or indirectly, to epiphyseal growth; consequently, they begin during the growing years and tend to be progressive as long as the child is still growing. For these reasons they are grouped together in this chapter as "disorders of epiphyseal growth." These disorders include *slipping of the upper femoral epiphysis* (*adolescent coxa vara*), *Blount's disease* (*tibia vara*), *Madelung's deformity*, and *idiopathic curvature of the spine* (*idiopathic scoliosis*).

Slipped Upper Femoral Epiphysis (Adolescent Coxa Vara)

The hip joint is probably subjected to greater physical forces than any other joint in the extremities; furthermore, the upper femoral epiphyseal plate is set obliquely in relation to the axis of the femoral shaft and, consequently, it is subjected to *shearing*

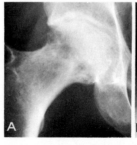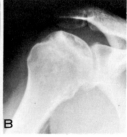

Figure 13.32. Avascular necrosis of: *A*, the femoral head, and *B*, the humeral head secondary to caisson disease. The patient is a 42-year-old underground construction worker. The infarcts of bone are due to nitrogen emboli released from the fatty bone marrow during excessively rapid decompression.

forces. It is not surprising, therefore, that in the presence of either a generalized or a localized weakness of the epiphyseal plate, the upper femoral epiphysis is particularly prone to slip off the femoral neck through its weakened plate.

In the disorder of *slipped upper femoral epiphysis* (*adolescent coxa vara*) the epiphysis either gradually, or suddenly, slips downward and backward in relation to the neck of the femur, or, if you prefer, the femoral neck slips upward and forward in relation to the epiphysis.

INCIDENCE AND ETIOLOGY

Slipping of the upper femoral epiphysis is most likely to develop in older children and adolescents, from the age of nine years to the end of growth, and is more common in boys than in girls. The slip first becomes apparent in one hip, but there is approximately a 30% chance of the second hip becoming involved subsequently.

Although the upper femoral epiphysis may slip in otherwise normal individuals, it is more likely to do so in the presence of some pre-existing endocrine imbalance, as evidenced by the high incidence in the very tall, thin, rapidly growing adolescent and the even higher incidence in the obese Fröhlich type of adolescent with a female distribution of fat and sexual underdevelopment (Fig. 13.33).

The etiology of slipped upper femoral epiphysis is not entirely understood; the experimental investigation of Harris, however, suggests that an imbalance between growth hormone and sex hormones (either excessive growth hormone or deficient sex hormones) weakens the epiphyseal plate and renders it more vulnerable to the shearing forces of both weight bearing and injury. From immunofluorescent staining of the synovial membrane, Morrissy has postulated that, at least in some patients, there is an underlying abnormality of the immune system.

PATHOGENESIS AND PATHOLOGY

The femoral epiphysis usually slips slowly and progressively and leads to a progressive coxa vara deformity with secondary remod-

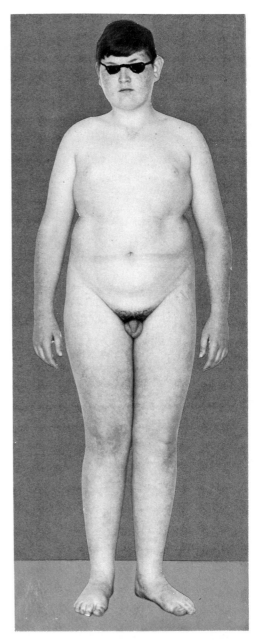

Figure 13.33. Slipped left upper femoral epiphysis in a 14-year-old boy of the Fröhlich type with a female distribution of subcutaneous fat and underdeveloped genitalia. Note that the boy's left lower limb is externally rotated. Radiographic examination confirmed the clinical suspicion of slipping of the left upper femoral epiphysis.

eling of the femoral neck; the posterior periosteal attachment remains intact. An acute injury superimposed upon this pathological process, however, may cause a sudden fur-

ther slip; indeed, the epiphysis may become completely separated from the femoral neck, in which case the precarious blood supply of the femoral head may be severely damaged with resultant avascular necrosis. Once the epiphyseal plate closes by bony union, no further slip occurs; but residual displacement of the femoral head alters the mechanics of the hip and leads to the development of degenerative disease of the hip in adult life.

CLINICAL FEATURES AND DIAGNOSIS

Early diagnosis is of extreme importance in order that surgical treatment may be instituted in the earliest possible stages of slipping. The commonest initial symptom is mild discomfort arising in the hip; the discomfort may be referred to the knee and indeed, at this stage the patient's knee may be examined clinically and radiographically with negative results, and the underlying slip of the upper femoral epiphysis, having escaped detection, progresses. In the early stages there is usually a slight limp, most noticeable when the patient is tired. As the slip progresses, there develops a Trendelenburg type of gait (the patient's trunk leans toward the affected side as weight is borne on the affected limb); the lower limb becomes externally rotated (Fig. 13.33). Further examination reveals limitation of internal rotation and abduction of the hip; as the hip is passively flexed, the thigh rotates externally.

The diagnosis can be *suspected* from the aforementioned symptoms and signs but it can be *confirmed* only by radiographic examination of the upper end of the femur in two projections; a minimal slip is always more obvious in the lateral projection than in the anteroposterior projection (Fig. 13.34). This is the stage at which the diagnosis should always be made.

If the femoral epiphysis continues to slip gradually, remodeling of the femoral neck becomes apparent (Fig. 13.35). The radiographic appearance of a complete separation of the epiphysis is striking; there is usually evidence of a preceding gradual slip (Fig. 13.36).

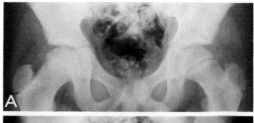
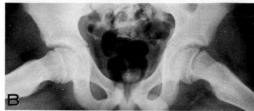

Figure 13.34. Minimal slip of the left upper femoral epiphysis in a 14-year-old boy. *A*, in the anteroposterior projection there is an abnormal relationship between the femoral head and the neck; the slip is not very obvious. *B*, in the lateral projection of the upper end of the femur ("frog position projection"), the slip of the left upper femoral epiphysis is much more obvious.

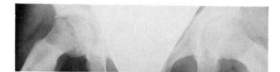

Figure 13.35. Gradual slipping of the right upper femoral epiphysis in a 15-year-old boy. Note the new bone formation in the angle between slipped femoral head and the posterior aspect of the femoral neck; this type of remodeling always indicates a chronic, slowly progressive slip.

TREATMENT

Since the precarious blood supply has already been threatened by the slipping through the epiphyseal plate, forceful manipulation should be avoided.

The aim of treatment in the early stages is to prevent further slip. If the femoral head has slipped minimally (less than 1 cm in the lateral projection), it should be surgically stabilized *in situ* by means of threaded pins following which weight bearing may be resumed (Fig. 13.37). A complete separation of the epiphysis can usually be reduced to a satisfactory position by means of gentle manipulation (provided it had not slipped too far prior to the acute slip) and then stabilized

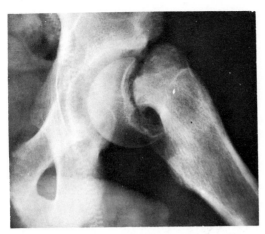

Figure 13.36. Complete separation of the left upper femoral epiphysis in a 13-year-old boy. The remodeling of the femoral neck provides evidence that the epiphysis had been slipping gradually prior to the complete separation; this is in keeping with the boy's history of pain in the left hip and a limp during the 4 months preceding the acute injury that caused the complete separation. The risk of avascular necrosis in this femoral head is high.

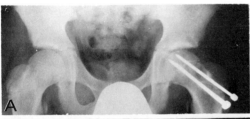

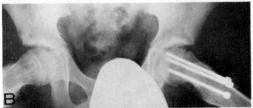

Figure 13.37. Surgical stabilization of a minimal slip of the left upper femoral epiphysis *in situ* by means of threaded pins; these post-operative radiographs are of the same 14-year-old boy whose pre-operative radiographs are shown in Figure 13.34. The illusion of only 2 pins in the anteroposterior projection of the femur is explained by superimposition of 2 of the 3 pins seen in the lateral projection; this serves to emphasize the limitations of a single radiographic projection.

surgically by threaded pins. After such treatment, weight bearing must be avoided until the epiphysis has healed to the neck, and this may require several months. More diffi-

cult to treat is the *chronic* slip that has progressed beyond 1 cm. and in which there has not been a superimposed acute slip (Fig. 13.35). Surgical correction of the residual deformity of the head and neck may become necessary if there is inadequate remodelling or if the gait remains unsatisfactory. Under these circumstances, the associated abnormal relationship between the femoral head and the acetabulum is most safely achieved by a compensatory subtrochanteric osteotomy of the femur. Operation in the region of the epiphyseal plate would seem more logical, but the risk of producing *iatrogenic avascular necrosis* is considerable; furthermore, the prognosis for future hip function after avascular necrosis of the femoral head in this age group is very bad indeed. Such an operation might be called "orthopaedic roulette" because the surgeon never knows which time the operation is going to kill the femoral head!

The follow-up care of patients treated for slipped upper femoral epiphysis must continue at least until the epiphyseal plate has closed; during this time, the opposite femoral epiphysis must also be assessed at regular intervals because of the 30% chance that it will begin to slip before growth is complete.

Tibia Vara (Blount's Disease)

The medial portion of the upper tibial epiphyseal plate may become the site of a localized epiphyseal growth disturbance known as *tibia vara* (*Blount's disease, osteochondrosis deformans tibiae*), which is characterized by a progressive bow leg (varus) deformity.

This disorder, which is more common in girls than in boys, usually becomes manifest at the age of about two years. The growth disturbance may involve only one tibia or both. Tibia vara is relatively uncommon in most areas of the world, but is unexplainably common in two completely different types of country, Finland and Jamaica.

Once considered to be the result of a localized osteochondrosis of the medial portion of the upper tibial epiphysis, tibia vara is now thought to represent a localized form

of *epiphyseal dysplasia*. The combination of diminished growth in the medial portion of the epiphyseal plate and continued normal growth in the lateral portion acounts for the progressive angulatory deformity of varus. After a number of years the medial portion of the epiphyseal plate closes prematurely.

In the early stages of tibia vara, there are no symptoms. Examination, however, reveals a characteristic varus deformity of the knee, a deformity that is particularly striking when it is unilateral (Fig. 13.38). Radiographically, there is defective ossification of the medial portion of the upper tibial epiphysis, a beaked appearance of the underlying metaphysis and obvious retardation of longitu-

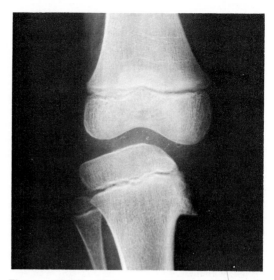

Figure 13.39. Tibia vara (Blount's disease). This is the radiograph of the girl shown in Figure 13.38. Note the defective ossification of the medial portion of the upper tibial epiphysis, the beaked appearance of the underlying metaphysis and the evidence of a growth disturbance in the medial portion of the epiphyseal plate.

dinal growth in the medial side of the tibia (Fig. 13.39).

Treatment in the early stages of tibia vara in young children is aimed at preventing progression of the varus deformity; this can sometimes be accomplished by means of a night splint of the type used for physiological bow legs (Chapter 7). In older children, however, the varus deformity progresses despite splinting; it can be corrected only by osteotomy of the tibia, which may have to be repeated on one or more occasions during the remaining period of growth.

Madelung's Deformity

An epiphyseal growth disturbance may develop on the medial (ulnar) side of the distal radial epiphysis as the result of a localized form of *epiphyseal dysplasia*. The resultant deformity of the wrist, which does not usually become apparent until adolescence, is known as *Madelung's deformity* and is characterized by prominence of the distal end of the ulna on the dorsum of the wrist and forward displacement of the hand in relation to the forearm. It is more common in girls than in boys and is usually bilateral (Fig. 13.40). Further examination reveals lim-

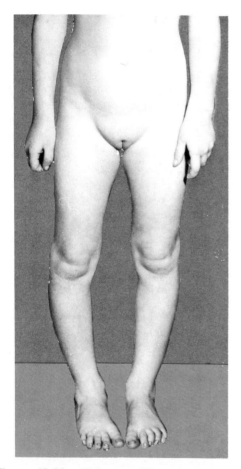

Figure 13.38. Tibia vara (Blount's disease) of the medial portion of the right upper tibial epiphyseal plate in a 6-year-old girl. Note the varus deformity as well as the internal tibial torsion in the right lower limb compared to the normal left lower limb.

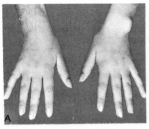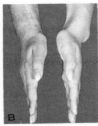

Figure 13.40.   Madelung's deformity in the left wrist of a 14-year-old girl. The distal end of the ulna is prominent on the dorsum of the wrist and the hand appears to be displaced forwards in relation to the forearm. In this girl the deformity had been bilateral, but the deformity in the right wrist has been corrected surgically.

itation of flexion of the wrist as well as limitation of supination of the forearm.

Treatment is aimed at correction of the rather ugly deformity as well as improvement of wrist function; this is best accomplished by excision of the distal portion of the ulna and osteotomy of the deformed distal end of the radius.

Scoliosis

When you consider the complexity and multiplicity of the intervertebral and apophyseal joints in the human spinal column, it is remarkable that in the vast majority of persons the spine grows straight during childhood and remains straight throughout adult life. It is not surprising, therefore, that a variety of disorders are capable of disturbing this normal growth pattern and can thereby lead to a progressive and serious spinal deformity.

The broad term *scoliosis* refers to *a lateral curvature of the spine;* thus, scoliosis is *a deformity* rather than a specific disease or disorder. As such, it takes many forms depending on its etiology and the age at which it begins. It is of the utmost importance for you to learn about the *nature* of scoliosis, its *early diagnosis* in childhood, its *prognosis* and, in a general way at least, what can and should be done for these deformed persons in the way of *preventive and corrective treatment.*

At the outset a few terms should be de-

fined. A *non-structural scoliosis* is a reversible lateral curvature of the spine *without* rotation; it can be reversed either voluntarily by the patient, or by correcting the underlying cause (Fig. 13.41). A *structural scoliosis*, by contrast, is an irreversible lateral curvature of the spine *with rotation* of the vertebral bodies in the abnormal area (major curve) (Fig. 13.46). (The term, *major* curve, is synonymous with the term *primary* curve, but the adjective *major* is presently preferred by members of the Scoliosis Research Society of North America). The scoliosis is said to be *compensated* when the shoulders are level and are directly above the pelvis; this is possible because of the development of *compensatory* curves above and below the *major* curve. When the major curve is greater than the sum of its compensatory curves, however, the scoliosis is said to be *decompensated* since the shoulders are not level and there is a lateral shift or "list" of the trunk to one side. The designations, *right* or *left* scoliosis, refer to the convex side of the major curve.

The following etiological classification should help to put the various types of scoliosis in reasonable perspective.

ETIOLOGICAL CLASSIFICATION OF SCOLIOSIS

I. *Non-Structural Scoliosis (Reversible)*
  1. Habitual Poor Posture (Postural Scoliosis)
  2. Pain and Muscle Spasm
      Painful lesion of a spinal nerve root (e.g. Sciatic scoliosis, Chapter 11)
      Painful lesion of the spine (inflammation, neoplasm)
      Painful lesion of the abdomen (appendicitis, perinephric abscess)
  3. Lower Limb Length Discrepancy
      a) Actual shortening of the lower limb (Fig. 13.41)
      b) Apparent shortening of the lower limb (pelvic obliquity)
          i) Adduction contracture of the hip on the shorter side
          ii) Abduction contracture of the hip on the opposite side

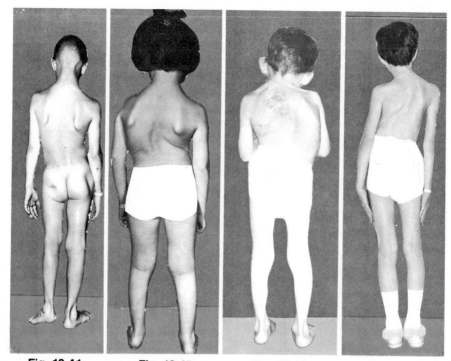

| Fig. 13.41 | Fig. 13.42 | Fig. 13.43 | Fig. 13.44 |

Figure 13.41. Non-structural scoliosis (functional scoliosis) secondary to lower limb length discrepancy in a 6-year-old boy. In the standing position the left side of this boy's pelvis is lower than the right and, consequently, his spine must compensate by curving to the right in order that he may remain upright; there is no rotational deformity in the spine. This compensatory type of scoliosis is completely reversible in that the spine straightens when an appropriate lift is put under the short limb and also when the individual either sits or lies down.

Figure 13.42. Congenital scoliosis due to failure of segmentation of the lateral components of the lower thoracic spine in a 5-year-old girl. This girl's deformity is rigid and her scoliosis is decompensated to the left.

Figure 13.43. Neuropathic scoliosis due to neurofibromatosis (von Recklinghausen's disease) in a 4-year-old boy. Note the large café-au-lait spot and the severe right thoracolumbar scoliosis. Scoliosis secondary to neurofibromatosis has an extremely bad prognosis concerning progression of deformity and, consequently, requires operative treatment as soon as it is recognized.

Figure 13.44. Neuropathic paralytic scoliosis secondary to extensive poliomyelitis involving trunk muscles in a 10-year-old girl. The curve pattern is right thoracic and the scoliosis is decompensated to the right. In the paralytic type of scoliosis the spine tends to sag, or collapse, in the standing position because of the associated muscle weakness.

II. *Structural Scoliosis (Irreversible)*
   1. *Idiopathic Scoliosis* (85% of all scoliosis)
      Infantile: appears from birth to 3 years
      Juvenile: appears from 4 years to 9 years
      Adolescent: appears from 10 years to the end of growth (Fig. 13.45)
   2. *Osteopathic Scoliosis*
     a) Congenital (Chapter 8)
       i) Localized; hemivertebrae, failure of segmentation (Fig. 13.42)
      ii) Generalized; osteogenesis imperfecta, arachnodactyly.
     b) Acquired
       i) Fractures and dislocations of the spine; traumatic and pathological
      ii) Rickets and osteomalacia (Chapter 9)

    iii) Thoracogenic; unilateral pulmonary disease (emphysema) and unilateral chest operations (thoracoplasty)

3. *Neuropathic Scoliosis*
  a) Congenital (Chapter 8)
    i) Spina bifida with myelodysplasia
    ii) Neurofibromatosis (von Recklinghausen's disease) (Fig. 13.43)
  b) Acquired (Paralytic Scoliosis) (Chapter 12)
    i) Poliomyelitis (Fig. 13.44)
    ii) Paraplegia
    iii) Friedreich's ataxia
    iv) Syringomyelia

4. *Myopathic Scoliosis*
  a) Congenital (Chapter 8)
    i) Amyotonia congenita
    ii) Amyoplasia congenita (arthrogryposis)

IDIOPATHIC SCOLIOSIS

All the aforementioned types of *structural* scoliosis are potentially serious and patients so afflicted merit continuing supervision by an orthopaedic surgeon. For the purpose of this textbook, however, the major emphasis is placed on the *idiopathic type* of structural scoliosis which comprises 85% of the total and which develops in otherwise normal, healthy children and adolescents.

Incidence and Etiology

Idiopathic scoliosis is a relatively common musculoskeletal deformity in that it is present to some degree in approximately 0.5% of the population; there is a definite familial incidence. The *infantile* type, which appears between birth and three years of age, is more common in boys and, for reasons unknown, is seen more frequently in some countries than in others. The *juvenile* type, which appears between the ages of four and nine years, and the more common *adolescent* type which first becomes apparent between the ages of ten years and the end of growth, are both much commoner in girls.

The pattern of the curve may be *lumbar*, *thoracolumbar*, *thoracic* or *combined* lumbar and thoracic (double major curve), but by far the most common pattern is a right thoracic scoliosis in adolescent girls (Fig. 13.45). Despite much investigation, both clinical and experimental, the precise etiology remains an unsolved and challenging problem.

Pathogenesis and Pathology

The most important aspect of the pathogenesis of deformity is its *progression* with skeletal *growth*. As the lateral curvature and the rotation of the spine increase, *secondary* changes develop in the vertebrae and ribs due to progressive *growth disturbance*. On the concave side of the curve, increased pressure on one side of the epiphyseal plates of the vertebral bodies produces wedge-shaped vertebrae. Such *structural* changes help to explain the irreversibility of

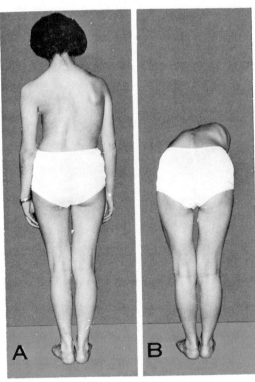

Figure 13.45. Idiopathic scoliosis in a 13-year-old girl. *A*, note that the right shoulder is higher than the left, the right scapula is more prominent than the left and that the left hip protrudes more than the right; the curvature in the thoracic spine is apparent. This girl's scoliosis is of the right thoracic pattern and is decompensated to the right. *B*, the rotation of the vertebrae and ribs is most readily detected as the girl bends forward.

structural scoliosis (Fig. 13.46). Persistent malalignment of the spinal joints may become worse very slowly (1° per year) even *after* growth is over especially when the curve is over 40°; such malalignment eventually leads to painful degenerative joint disease of the spine in adult life. Furthermore, very severe thoracic deformities seriously compromise cardiopulmonary function and may shorten the patient's life expectancy.

Clinical Features and Diagnosis

Idiopathic scoliosis begins slowly, insidiously and painlessly. Thus, in the early stage of its development, the patient is not aware of the curvature, and since it is well con-

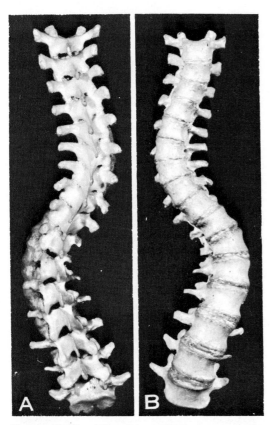

Figure 13.46.   Idiopathic scoliosis as seen in the postmortem specimen of a spine from an adolescent (who died from an unrelated cause). The curve pattern is a combined left lumbar and right thoracic scoliosis (double major curve). *A*, note in this view from behind, the rotation of the spine in both major curves. *B*, in this view from the front, note the secondary changes, particularly wedging in the vertebral bodies, due to a growth disturbance.

cealed by clothing at this stage, the parents are not aware of it either. Later, the parents may observe that one shoulder is higher than the other, one shoulder blade is more prominent than the other or that one hip protrudes more than the other. By the time a spinal curvature has progressed sufficiently to be readily detected clinically, it has already reached 30 degrees.

Examination of the otherwise healthy child or adolescent from behind reveals a *curvature* of the spine and *rotation* in the area of the major curve; the rotation of the spine is most noticeable when the patient is asked to bend forward (Fig. 13.45). Complete physical examination, including lower limb length measurement and neurological assessment, is necessary to exclude other causes of scoliosis.

Radiographic examination, which should include the full length of the spine in the *standing* position, reveals a curvature that is always more marked than would be expected from the external physical appearance (Figs. 13.49 and 13.50).

During the past decade widespread school screening programs to detect scoliosis in girls from 12 to 14 years of age have detected a curvature of 10° or more in 2% of such girls (a radiographic curve of less than 10° is considered to be a variation of normal). Of all girls screened in these programs only approximately 0.3% require treatment and the majority are mild curves which can be managed by bracing. Happily, scoliosis is thereby being detected early so that the incidence of severe curvatures (over 40°) and hence the need for major spinal operations is decreasing. An alternative to radiographic diagnosis of minimal scoliosis is moiré fringe photography by which ordinary light is projected through special grids; the major advantage is the avoidance of exposure to radiation.

Prognosis

Since the deformity of scoliosis increases with growth, it is obvious that an important factor in assessing the prognosis for a given child is the amount of growth that remains. In addition, the more severe the degree of curvature is at the time of assessment, the more likely it is to increase. For example, a mild curvature first noticed in a 14-year-old girl may not increase significantly, whereas the same degree of curvature, first noticed in a 10-year-old girl, is almost certain to increase, particularly during a period of rapid growth (Fig. 13.47).

Treatment

The patient with idiopathic scoliosis should be seen by an orthopaedic surgeon to determine the need for correction of the deformity, and thereafter should be assessed at regular intervals throughout the growing period.

The *aims* of treatment are to *prevent progression* of a mild scoliosis and to *correct* and *stabilize* a more severe deformity; the *indications* for treatment and the *methods* of treatment require the judgment and skills of an experienced orthopaedic surgeon.

Non-Operative Methods. Exercises designed to prevent the progression of idiopathic scoliosis have been proven ineffectual as have body casts.

For children with curves of 20° to 40° and with two years or more of anticipated

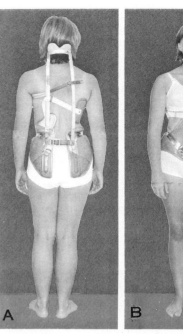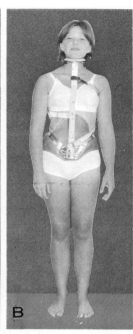

Figure 13.48. Milwaukee brace in the treatment of idiopathic scoliosis. This brace combines the forces of longitudinal traction and lateral pressure; it must be "tailor-made" to fit very accurately and requires careful continuing supervision to be effective.

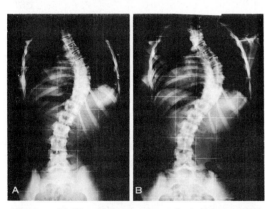

Figure 13.47. Progression of deformity with growth (viewed from behind). *A*, idiopathic scoliosis of the right thoracic type in a 12-year-old girl; the curve is relatively mild. The girl's parents declined treatment at this time. *B*, the same girl just one year later shows a considerable progression in the severity of the curve. The scoliosis has become decompensated and the curve has become relatively rigid. These radiographs emphasize how much progression of the curvature can take place in just one year of rapid growth.

skeletal growth, spinal braces can usually reduce the curve and prevent it from increasing; they may even provide some permanent correction. For many years the Milwaukee brace has been the standard orthosis for this form of non-operative management (Fig. 13.48). A more recent modification, proven to be effective for lumbar and thoracolumbar curves, is the Boston brace that eliminates the metal superstructure and is consequently hidden by ordinary clothes, a feature that is particularly appreciated by adolescent girls.

An alternative to bracing for children with curves of 20° to 40° and with two years or more of growth remaining is electrospinal instrumentation developed by Bobechko. At operation electrodes are inserted into the deep muscles on the convex side of the curve and their wires are attached to an implanted miniaturized radio receiver. During the remaining years of growth, the radio receiver is activated at night only by the application of an external radio antenna. The muscles are stimulated to contract every 10 seconds throughout the night as the child sleeps comfortably. During the day, unrestricted activities are permitted and the child is unencumbered by any brace. In an attempt to provide a non-invasive method of electrospinal stimulation, surface electrodes have been developed but they tend to produce stimulation of more superficial muscles and they may cause troublesome skin problems.

Operative Treatment. Idiopathic scoliosis with a curve of over 40° that is already producing an obvious clinical deformity, or that can be predicted to do so in the future, is best treated by the combination of correction of the curvature and surgical stabilization (fusion) of the involved area of the spine. Operative treatment is usually deferred until the child is at least ten years of age but, under certain circumstances, it is performed at an earlier age.

For severe scoliosis, i.e. over 40°, however, the most effective operative treatment

to date, is the combined operation of forceful, mechanical correction of the curvature by internal *spinal instrumentation* (designed by Harrington) and *spinal fusion* (Fig. 13.49). Following the operation of spinal fusion for scoliosis, the patient's spine must be protected by a body cast for at least three months, and sometimes longer, to allow the fusion area in the spine to become consolidated. Bobechko has developed a modified hook for the upper end of the Harrington rod that provides sufficient stability so that no external support is required post-operatively.

For adolescents with severe lumbar and thoracolumbar curves, especially those of paralytic origin and those in which the posterior elements are deficient, the Dwyer method of anterior correction and interbody fusion using cables has been useful.

For children with paralytic forms of scoliosis, the method of "segmental spinal instrumentation" without fusion, developed by Luque, provides good correction and an effective internal splint for the spine.

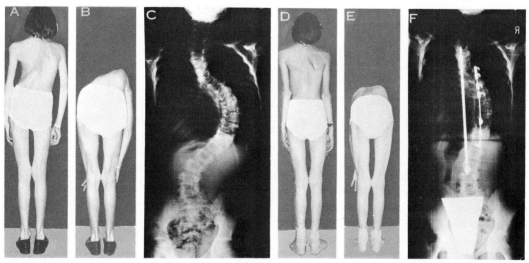

Figure 13.49. Severe idiopathic scoliosis of the right thoracic pattern in a 15-year-old girl. *A*, *B*, and *C*, before treatment; note the decompensation of this girl's scoliosis and the severe rotational rib deformity. This girl's scoliosis could have, and ideally should have, been treated earlier. *D*, *E*, and *F*, one year after mechanical correction of the scoliosis by means of the Harrington type of internal spinal instrumentation (distraction rod on the concave side, compression rod on the convex side); the operation included spinal fusion of the curved portion of the spine. This girl's spine is better compensated and the rib deformity has been well corrected. A completely different type of spinal instrumentation (involving staples, screws and a cable) applied to vertebral bodies—after excision of intervertebral discs—has been developed in Australia by Dwyer.

Very young children with progressive idiopathic scoliosis present a challenging problem, since bracing is usually inadequate to control their curves and spinal fusion is contraindicated because it stops vertical growth of the fused part of the spine. For these children, Gillespie has placed the end hooks of a Harrington rod in bone but has passed the rod subcutaneously and has avoided a fusion. Vertical growth continues, necessitating exchange of the rod for a longer one from time to time but the system (which is combined with bracing) has allowed these children to grow relatively straight and reach an age when definitive spinal fusion can be performed.

The development of more physiological methods of treatment must await the discovery of the precise etiology of idiopathic scoliosis—which conceivably might even be of a metabolic nature. In the meantime, early diagnosis and early, effective orthopaedic treatment can do much to prevent the dreadfully severe spinal curvatures and rib deformities that have been allowed to develop all too often in the past.

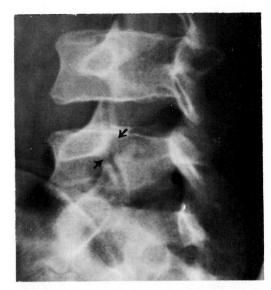

Figure 13.50. Spondylolysis of the pars interarticularis of the neural arch of the fifth lumbar vertebra as seen in an oblique radiograph (*arrows*). Note the intact pars interarticularis of the fourth lumbar vertebra above. The pars interarticularis in this projection may be likened to the narrow knot of an obliquely placed bow tie. The defect of spondylolysis is at the site of the knot.

SPONDYLOLYSIS

A mysterious defect occasionally develops in one or both sides of the neural arch of a lower lumbar vertebra for no apparent reason. Approximately 85% of such defects occur in the fifth lumbar vertebra and most of the remaining 15% occur in the fourth lumbar vertebra.

The defect, which consists of fibrous tissue, is known as *spondylolysis.* It always develops in the weakest part of the neural arch—the narrow isthmus (pars interarticularis) between the superior articular process and the inferior articular process. Being in the posterolateral part of the neural arch, the defect of spondylolysis is not readily detected in either anteroposterior or lateral radiographic projections; it is clearly seen, however, in an oblique projection (Fig. 13.50).

Incidence and Etiology

Once thought to be a congenital defect, spondylolysis is now known to develop during postnatal life. Moreover, the incidence of spondylolysis has been discovered to increase with age—not only during the growing years but also during adult life. Indeed, the defect can be demonstrated radiographically in approximately 10% of adults. Since the lower lumbar region of the human spine is subjected to much stress in the erect position, it is possible that spondylolysis represents either a stress fracture (fatigue fracture) from oft-repeated stresses or an ordinary fracture from a single injury. Nevertheless, the precise etiology remains obscure.

Clinical Features and Treatment

In the majority of individuals with spondylolysis the defect produces neither symptoms nor signs. After an injury or even chronic strain however, the fibrous tissue in the defect may be stretched; the resultant pain may persist for many months and necessitate the use of a lumbosacral type of brace. You must always rule out other causes of low back pain in a patient who has spondylolysis since the spondylolysis may be an incidental finding that is unrelated to the source of the patient's pain.

Complication

When spondylolysis is bilateral the vertebra is in a sense separated into two parts— the vertebral body, pedicles and superior articular processes anteriorly and the lamina and inferior articular processes posteriorly. Under these circumstances the anterior part may slip forward in relation to the posterior part and thereby produce one form of *spondylolisthesis.*

SPONDYLOLISTHESIS

Forward slipping of one vertebral body (and the remainder of the spinal column above it) in relation to the vertebral segment immediately below is referred to as *spondylolisthesis.* It occurs most commonly in the lower lumbar spine—particularly between the fifth lumbar vertebra and the sacrum. A normal lumbar vertebral body is prevented from slipping forward by an intact neural arch and the almost vertically inclined posterior facet joints on each side through which it articulates with the vertebral segment below. With loss of continuity of the pars interarticularis or an abnormality of the posterior facet joints the intervertebral disc is not sufficiently strong to prevent displacement of the vertebra.

Incidence and Etiology

Some degree of spondylolisthesis of a lower lumbar vertebra is detectable in approximately 2% of adults.

The commonest type is secondary to the aforementioned bilateral defect in the pars interarticularis of the neural arch (spondylolysis). Consequently, the usual site is the fifth lumbar vertebra. In this type (*spondylolytic spondylolisthesis*) the vertebral body, its pedicles and superior articular processes—and the spinal column above—become progressively displaced forward leaving the inferior articular processes, the lamina and the spinous process behind as a separated neural arch (Fig. 13.51). Forward displacement is most likely to be progressive during the rapid growth spurt of early adolescence.

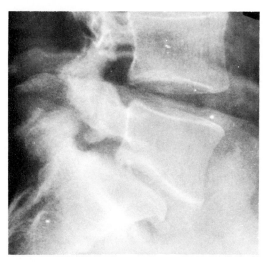

Figure 13.51. Spondylolisthesis of the fifth lumbar vertebra in relation to the sacrum. The body of the fifth lumbar vertebra, its pedicles and superior articular processes—and the spinal column above—have become displaced forward leaving the inferior articular processes, the lamina and the spinous process behind. There is a bilateral defect in the pars interarticularis through which the spondylolisthesis has occurred and hence this is the spondylolytic type of spondylolisthesis.

Less common is the type of spondylolisthesis secondary to degenerative disc disease and subluxation of the posterior facet joints. In this type (*degenerative spondylolisthesis*) the displacement may be either forward or backward; the usual site is the fourth lumbar vertebra.

In a third type (*congenital spondylolisthesis*) which is associated with either a congenital abnormality of the posterior facet joints or congenital elongation of the pars interarticularis, the anterior displacement of the fifth lumbar vertebra is severe.

Two rare types are *traumatic spondylolisthesis* secondary to a single injury and *pathological spondylolisthesis* secondary to a pathological weakness of bone.

Clinical Features and Diagnosis

Spondylolytic spondylolisthesis usually becomes manifest during childhood by the gradual onset of low back pain which is aggravated by standing, walking and running and relieved by lying down. The associated clinical deformity, which is related to the degree of forward slip, is characterized by a "step" in the lumbosacral region at the level of the spondylolisthesis and an increased lumbar lordosis above (Fig. 13.52). The hamstring muscles are tight with resultant limitation of straight leg raising. Significant involvement of the nerve roots is not common in this type of spondylolisthesis although nerve root irritation may produce sciatica. Radiographic examination reveals forward displacement of the affected vertebral body in the lateral projection (Fig. 13.51). Oblique radiographic projections are required to detect the underlying spondylolysis (Fig. 13.51).

In degenerative spondylolisthesis the displacement—either forward or backward (retrospondylolisthesis)—is relatively slight. Osteophyte formation in relation to the subluxated and degenerated posterior facet joints, however, may produce compression of the related nerve roots. The predominant symptom is chronic low back pain due to instability of the abnormal segment.

In congenital spondylolisthesis the forward displacement of the fifth lumbar vertebra in relation to the sacrum is severe. Consequently there may be pressure on the cauda equina as well as on the nerve roots. Such pressure may be increased during a period of rapid growth as in early adolescence and consequently may produce acute low back pain with or without sciatica.

Treatment

Spondylolisthesis may cause no symptoms, in which case the patient should be examined clinically and radiographically at regular intervals to detect any progression of the forward slip of the affected vertebral body. Progressive forward slip is an indication for stabilization of the unstable segment by means of a local spinal fusion which may be achieved posteriorly, anteriorly (interbody fusion) or laterally (intertransverse process fusion). The latter is the most effective type of fusion for spondylolisthesis.

Mild low back pain in the absence of a progressive slip can usually be relieved by wearing a lumbosacral type of brace. Severe back pain and nerve root irritation, however, usually necessitate surgical decompression of the nerve roots and local spinal fusion—preferably of the lateral intertransverse process type. In a patient with spondylolisthesis who has either back pain or nerve root irritation, however, you must look for other causes of the symptoms because their

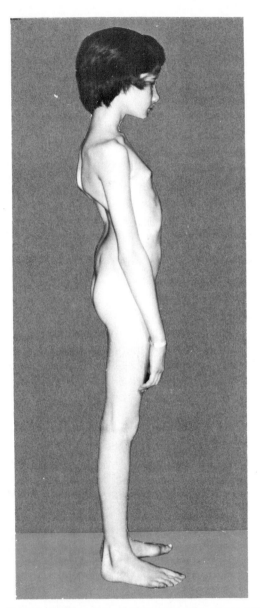

Figure 13.52. The clinical deformity of severe spondylolisthesis of the fifth lumbar vertebra in an 11-year-old girl. Note the vertical inclination of the sacrum, the step in the lumbosacral region and the increased lumbar lordosis above. Chronic low back pain and a progressive anterior displacement of the fifth lumbar vertebra in this girl necessitated a local spinal fusion.

source may be at a level other than that of the spondylolisthesis.

Complications

Severe forward displacement of the fifth lumbar vertebra (which was first described by an obstetrician) may narrow the pelvic inlet sufficiently in the female that normal delivery is impossible and Caesarean section becomes necessary. This is particularly true of the congenital type of spondylolisthesis.

Suggested Additional Reading

Blount, W. P.: The virtue of early treatment of idiopathic scoliosis (editorial). J. Bone Joint Surg. 63A: 335–336, 1981.

Bobechko, W. P., Herbert, M. A., and Friedman, H. G.: Electrospinal instrumentation for scoliosis: current status. Orthop. Clin. North Am. 10: 927–941, 1979.

Bradford, D. W.: Vertebral osteochondrosis (Scheuermann's kyphosis). Clin. Orthop. 158: 83–90, 1981.

Catterall, A.: Legg-Calvé-Perthes' syndrome. Clin. Orthop. 158: 41–52, 1981.

Cruess, R. L.: Steroid-induced osteonecrosis: a review. Can. J. Surg. 24: 567–588, 1981.

Dwyer, A. F.: Experience of anterior correction of scoliosis. Clin. Orthop. 93: 191, 1973.

Edmonson, A. S. and Crenshaw, A. H. (eds.): Campbell's Operative Orthopaedics. St. Louis, C. V. Mosby, 1980.

Gillespie, H. S. and Day, B.: Bone peg fixation in the treatment of osteochondritis dissecans of the knee joint. Clin. Orthop. 143: 125–130, 1979.

Glimcher, M. J. and Kenzora, J. E.: The biology of osteonecrosis of the human femoral head and its clinical implications. III. Discussion of the etiology and genesis of the pathological sequelae; comments on treatment. Clin. Orthop. 140: 273–312, 1979.

Goldblatt, J., Sacks, S. and Beighton, P.: The orthopaedic aspects of Gaucher disease. Clin. Orthop. 137: 208–214, 1978.

Halal, F., Gledhill, R. B. and Fraser, F. C.: Dominant inheritance of Scheuermann's juvenile kyphosis. Am. J. Dis. Child. 132: 1105–1107, 1978.

Hall, J. E.: Dwyer instrumentation in anterior fusion of the spine. Current concepts review. J. Bone Joint Surg. 63A: 1188–1190, 1981.

Harris, W. R.: The endocrine basis for slipping of the upper femoral epiphysis. J. Bone Joint Surg. 32B: 5, 1950.

King, A. G. and Blundell-Jones, G.: A surgical procedure for the Osgood-Schlatter lesion. Am. J. Sports Med. 9: 250, 1981.

Lovell, W. W. and Winter, R. B. (eds.): Pediatric Orthopaedics. Philadelphia, J. B. Lippincott, 1978.

Luque, E. R.: Segmental spinal instrumentation for correction of scoliosis. Clin. Orthop. 163: 192–198, 1982.

McManus, F. and Rang, M.: Preventive orthopaedics. Clin. Orthop. 125: 243–247, 1977.

Milgram, J. W.: Radiologic and pathologic manifestations of osteochondritis dissecans of distal femur: study of 50 cases. Radiology 126: 305–311, 1978.

Mital, M. A., Matza, R. A. and Cohen, J.: So-called unresolved Osgood-Schlatter lesion: a concept based on 15 surgically treated lesions. J. Bone Joint Surg. 62A: 732–739, 1980.

Moe, J. H., Winter, R. B., Bradford, D. and Lonstein, J. E.: Scoliosis and Other Spinal Deformities. Philadelphia, W. B. Saunders, 1978.

Morrissy, R. R., Kalderson, A. E. and Gerdes, M. H.: Synovial immunofluorescence in patients with slipped femoral capital epiphysis. J. Pediatr. Orthop. 1: 55–60, 1981.

Moseley, C. F.: A straight-line graph for leg-length discrepancies. J. Bone Joint Surg. 59A: 174–179, 1977.

Mubarak, S. J. and Carroll, N. C.: Juvenile osteochondritis dissecans of the knee: etiology. Clin. Orthop. 157: 200–211, 1981.

Rang, M. (ed.): The Growth Plate and Its Disorders. Edinburgh, E. & S. Livingstone, 1968.

Rogala, E. J., Drummond, D. S. and Garr, J.: Scoliosis: incidence and natural history—a prospective epidemiologic study. J. Bone Joint Surg. 60A: 173–176, 1978.

Rozing, P. M., Insall, J. and Bohne, W. H.: Spontaneous osteonecrosis of the knee. J. Bone Joint Surg. 62A: 2–7, 1980.

Salter, R. B.: Legg-Perthes' disease: the scientific basis for the methods of treatment and their indications. Clin. Orthop. 150: 8–11, 1980.

Salter, R. B.: Legg-Perthes' disease: relevant research and its application to treatment. Controversies in Orthopaedic Surgery, edited by Hoagland, F. Philadelphia, W. B. Saunders, 1981.

Sharrard, W. J. W.: Pediatric Orthopaedics and Fractures. Blackwell Scientific Publications, Oxford and Edinburgh, 1971.

Smith, C. F.: Tibia vara (Blount's disease). Current concepts review. J. Bone Joint Surg. 64A: 630–632, 1982.

Sugioka, Y.: Transtrochanteric anterior rotational osteotomy of the femoral head in the treatment of osteonecrosis affecting the hip. Clin. Orthop. 130: 191–201, 1978.

Suman, R. K. and Miller, R. H.: Panner's disease. Osteochondritis of the capitellum of the humerus. J. R. Coll. Surg. Edinb. 27: 62–63, 1982.

Tachdjian, M. O.: Pediatric Orthopaedics. Philadelphia, W. B. Saunders, 1972.

Taylor, T. C., Wenger, D. R., Stephen, J., Gillespie, R. and Bobechko, W. P.: Surgical management of thoracic kyphosis in adolescents. J. Bone Joint Surg. 61A: 496–503, 1979.

Torell, G., Nordwall, A. and Nachemson, A.: The changing pattern of scoliosis treatment due to effective screening. J. Bone Joint Surg. 63A: 337–341, 1981.

Wagner, H.: Operative lengthening of the femur. Clin. Orthop. 136: 125–142, 1978.

Watts, H. G., Hall, J. E. and Stanish, W.: The Boston Brace System for the treatment of low thoracic and lumbar scoliosis by the use of a girdle without superstructure. Clin. Orthop. 126, 87–92, 1977.

Weinstein, S. L., Zavala, D. C. and Ponseti, I. V.: Idiopathic scoliosis. Long term follow-up and prognosis in untreated patients. J. Bone Joint Surg. 63A: 702–712, 1981.

Willner, S.: Moiré topography for the diagnosis and documentation of scoliosis. Acta. Orthop. Scand. 50: 295–302, 1979.

CHAPTER 14

Neoplasms of Musculoskeletal Tissues

In the experience of a family physician in medical practice, *malignant* neoplasms, or new growths that develop as *primary* lesions in the musculoskeletal tissues are relatively rare. Indeed, they represent only 1% of malignant disease of all age groups and 5% in childhood. Less rare are *benign* neoplasms and *non-neoplastic* lesions that simulate neoplasms; *secondary* neoplasms that develop in bone as *metastases* from a primary neoplasm elsewhere (especially metastatic carcinoma) are common.

In the experience of certain types of specialists—orthopaedic surgeon, radiologist, pathologist, radiotherapist and medical oncologist—musculoskeletal neoplasms and lesions that simulate them are relatively common and constitute an extremely important, though incompletely understood, group of disorders.

From your point of view, as a medical doctor of the future, it is most important that you learn about the *general features* of this wide variety of lesions, their *clinical features* and *diagnosis*, their *prognosis* and, in a general way at least, the available *methods of treatment* for patients so afflicted. Of less importance to you at this stage of your career are the minute details of their microscopic changes, let alone the *interpretation* of these changes; indeed, even the most experienced bone pathologist may cavil about the interpretation of the microscopic minutiae of these perplexing lesions.

PRIMARY NEOPLASMS AND NEOPLASM-LIKE LESIONS OF BONE

Our limited understanding of neoplasms in general, and of neoplasms of bone in particular, makes it difficult even to arrive at a *classification* that is universally acceptable.

Probably the three best known classifications are those of the World Health Organization, of Lichtenstein and of Aegerter.

You need not, however, become confused by the wide divergence of opinions related to such classifications; suffice it that you learn *one* that is reasonable and that will help you in the organization of your knowledge. For this purpose the most recent classification by Aegerter (1975) is chosen. Before proceeding to the classification itself, however, you may find the following definition of terms useful.

Definition of Terms

The term *tumor* (which is often loosely used to describe any localized swelling, or lump) seems less precise than the term *neoplasm*, or new growth, which refers to a new and abnormal formation of cells, a process that *progresses* and continues to progress, throughout the life of the patient, unless some type of therapy intervenes. The hereditary mechanism of the neoplastic cells has been irreversibly altered in such a way that they and their "offspring cells" alike *do not reach maturity*. Thus, succeeding generations of neoplastic cells continue to divide by mitosis more rapidly than do normal cells of that particular tissue and consequently produce a *progressive* lesion; this explains the presence of excessive numbers of mitotic figures in rapidly growing neoplasms.

If, in addition, neoplastic cells demonstrate ability to initiate independent growth in distant sites (*metastases*), the neoplasm is *malignant* and is referred to as *cancer*. *Primary* neoplasms of a given structure arise from cells that are normally "local inhabitants" of that structure, whereas *secondary* neoplasms arise from cells that are "outside invaders" from elsewhere. Thus, one might speak of a primary neoplasm *of* bone and of a secondary neoplasm *in* bone.

It is more difficult to define a *benign* neoplasm, one which remains localized in its primary site. Indeed, many so-called "benign neoplasms" may not be *truly* neoplastic and may be more reasonably considered either as *reactive lesions* (constituting a self-limiting reaction to some other phenomenon) or as *hamartomas* (lesions in which cells normally present in a local area grow faster than others but *do* reach maturity just as do normal cells and, hence, exist as a useless but relatively harmless cell mass). On the basis of these definitions, neither *reactive lesions* nor *hamartomas* are progressive in the sense that true neoplasms are progressive; consequently, they have a much better *prognosis* than do neoplasms. Still other lesions of bone, such as *fibrous dysplasia* and *simple bone cyst*, do not fit any of these categories, but in some ways simulate neoplasms; they are, therefore, also considered in the present chapter. The various forms of *histiocytosis X*—particularly *eosinophilic granuloma*—may also simulate neoplasms; they are discussed in Chapter 9.

A CLASSIFICATION OF PRIMARY NEOPLASMS AND NEOPLASM-LIKE LESIONS OF BONE

The cells of the musculoskeletal tissues all share a common *mesodermal* origin but have differentiated along a variety of lines to become *osteoblasts*, *osteoclasts*, *chondroblasts*, *fibroblasts* (*collagenoblasts*) and *myeloblasts* (*of the bone marrow*). It seems reasonable, therefore, to use a classification that is based (insofar as is presently known) on the cell origin or *genesis* of the lesion. Thus, the primary lesions may be divided into the following groups: *osteogenic*, *chondrogenic*, *collagenic* and *myelogenic*. Furthermore, in each group there may be *reactive lesions* (which are *not* neoplasms), *hamartomas* (which many consider to be "benign neoplasms") and *true neoplasms* (some of which are *potentially* malignant and others of which are *frankly* malignant).

CLASSIFICATION (Aegerter, 1975)

I. Reactive Bone Lesions
   A. Osteogenic
      1. Osteoid osteoma
      2. Benign osteoblastoma
   B. Collagenic
      1. Subperiosteal cortical defect
      2. Non-osteogenic fibroma
II. Hamartomas Affecting Bone
   A. Osteogenic
      1. Osteoma
      2. Osteochondroma
   B. Chondrogenic
      1. Enchondroma
   C. Collagenic
      1. Angioma
      2. Aneurysmal bone cyst
III. True Neoplasms of Bone
   A. Osteogenic
      1. Osteosarcoma
      2. Parosteal sarcoma
   B. Chondrogenic
      1. Benign chondroblastoma
      2. Chondromyxoid fibroma
      3. Chondrosarcoma
   C. Collagenic
      1. Fibrosarcoma
      2. Angiosarcoma
   D. Myelogenic
      1. Plasma cell myeloma
      2. Ewing's tumor
      3. Reticulum cell sarcoma
      4. Hodgkin's disease
   E. Osteoclastoma (giant cell tumor of bone)

GENERAL CONSIDERATIONS

Although much remains to be discovered about the *nature* and the *etiology* of neoplasms and neoplasm-like lesions of bone, much knowledge has been accumulated concerning their *incidence*, *pathogenesis*, *clinical features*, *diagnosis* and the principles of their *treatment*. Some of this knowledge is most appropriately considered in a *general* way before discussing the various *specific* clinical entities themselves.

Incidence

The *age incidence* of some of these lesions is quite distinctive; for example, osteo-sarcoma occurs principally during childhood and adolescence, whereas osteoclastoma (giant cell tumor) occurs almost exclusively during adult life. The differences in *sex incidence* of the various lesions are less striking. The *site incidence* is of particular value since some of these lesions are common in certain bones but almost unknown in others. Even the *anatomical* site within a given bone is of significance; for example, many of the lesions that develop during childhood seem to be related to the rate of "bone turnover" or cellular activity and this is greatest in the flared-out *metaphyseal* regions of long bones at the most rapidly growing end (lower end of femur, upper end of tibia, upper end of humerus). The *epiphyses*, by contrast, are usually spared.

A knowledge of these various aspects of the incidence of the various lesions is often of considerable help in the differential diagnosis of a given lesion in a certain area of a certain bone in a patient of a certain age.

Correlation of Pathogenesis and Radiographic Features

Since the pathogenesis of bone neoplasms and neoplasm-like lesions is well reflected by changes in the radiographic appearance of the bone and soft tissues, a correlation of the two will make the study of each aspect more interesting and more meaningful.

Neoplastic cells do not destroy bone, but their presence incites local *osteoclastic resorption of bone.* The cells of certain neoplasms also incite local osteoblastic deposition of normal bone which is referred to as *reactive bone.* The neoplastic cells of the osteogenic group of neoplasms, however, are capable of producing osteoid and bone which is then referred to as *tumor bone*, or *neoplastic bone.* Thus, in a given lesion affecting bone, the radiographic appearance reflects varying proportions of bone resorption (osteolysis) and bone deposition (osteosclerosis), some of the latter being reactive bone.

Some slowly growing lesions incite a marked reaction in the surrounding bone; indeed, the reactive bone may almost obscure the underlying neoplasm (Fig. 14.1).

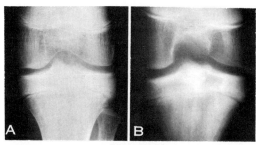

Figure 14.1. Reactive bone surrounding a slowly growing benign neoplasm, in this case a chondroblastoma of the upper tibial epiphysis in a 13-year-old boy. *A*, in the *plain radiograph*, the reactive bone almost obscures the neoplasm. *B*, in this *tomogram* the radiolucent neoplasm is clearly seen in the center of the reactive bone. By means of this special technique (tomography, laminography), many films are taken, each of which shows a different layer, or slice, of the tissue in focus.

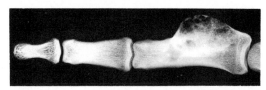

Figure 14.2. Expansion of a bone by a slowly growing lesion. The enchondroma in this proximal phalanx is slowly eroding the cortex from the inside; simultaneously, periosteal new bone is being deposited from the outside. When the rate of erosion exceeds that of periosteal bone formation, the bone expands.

In a slowly growing lesion within the bone, the deep surface of the cortex is gradually eroded from the inside, but at the same time the periosteum reacts by depositing bone on the outside; these combined phenomena explain *expansion* of a bone (Fig. 14.2).

When the periosteum is elevated by a neoplasm that has eroded the cortex, it produces reactive bone in the angle where it is still attached. This triangular-shaped area of reactive bone is often called *Codman's triangle* (Fig. 14.3).

Elevation of the periosteum in "stages" stimulates the formation of successive layers of periosteal reactive bone and this phenomenon explains the radiographic "onion-skin" appearance (Fig. 14.4).

As a malignant neoplasm grows rapidly beyond the confines of the cortex, its blood vessels keep pace and grow in a radial fashion from the cortex. Both neoplastic bone and reactive bone form along these radiating vessels and this explains the radiographic "sunburst" appearance (Fig. 14.5).

Bone that has been weakened by local destruction (osteoclastic resorption) from any cause is more readily fractured than normal bone. This complication is referred to as a *pathological fracture* since it occurs through an area of abnormal, or pathological bone (Fig. 14.6). If the regenerative process of fracture healing is more rapid than the destructive process of the neoplasm, the pathological fracture will eventually unite; but if the reverse be true, the pathological fracture will never unite.

In the presence of rapidly growing malignant neoplasms there may be little or no reactive bone, in which case the radi-

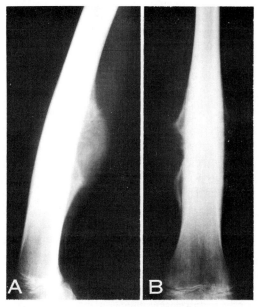

Figure 14.3. Triangular shaped areas of reactive bone (Codman's triangles) which have been deposited by the elevated periosteum. In these radiographs of the femur, a malignant neoplasm, osteosarcoma, has eroded the cortex and elevated the periosteum; the reactive new bone is laid down around the periphery of the neoplasm in the angle between the elevated periosteum and the cortex. Codman's triangle is not always so apparent; it is not pathognomonic of any one bone lesion.

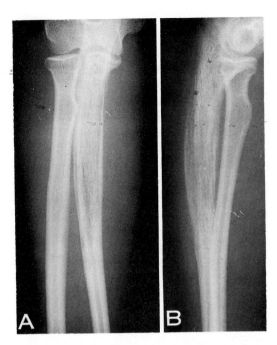

Figure 14.4. Successive layers of reactive bone which have been deposited by periosteum as it has been elevated in "stages." In these radiographs of the radius and ulna, the underlying neoplasm is a Ewing's sarcoma of the ulna. This radiographic "onion-skin" appearance is not pathognomonic of any one bone lesion.

ographic appearance is that of an osteolytic defect; this is particularly true of the *osteolytic* type of metastases in bone (Fig. 14.7). Certain primary neoplasms, however, particularly carcinoma of the prostate, incite a brisk osteoblastic reaction when they metastasize to bone and produce the osteoblastic, or *osteosclerotic* type of metastases (Fig. 14.8).

The only true *cyst* (a cavity containing gas or fluid) in bone is the *simple bone cyst*, which is not a neoplasm at all (Fig. 14.9). Other osteolytic lesions may *appear* to be cystic radiographically, but since they contain tumor tissue, they are, in fact, solid lesions (Fig. 14.10).

Certain of these radiographic signs are sometimes considered by the inexperienced to be pathognomonic of a given type of neoplasm (sunburst appearance indicates osteosarcoma, onion-skin appearance indicates Ewing's tumor). These signs, however, are by no means either specific or constant and, consequently, a "spot diagnosis" on the basis of a single radiograph is an example more of cleverness than of wisdom. Indeed, *all* available data must be correlated in order to reach a high standard of diagnostic accuracy.

Clinical Features

A history of recent local trauma is often given by patients with a neoplasm of the musculoskeletal tissues; such trauma, however, only brings the pre-existing neoplasm to the attention of the patient.

Slowly growing neoplasms and neoplasm-like lesions of bone seldom cause symptoms unless, because of their location, their mere

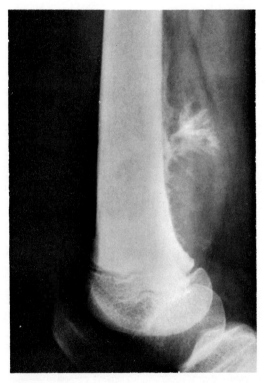

Figure 14.5. Neoplastic and reactive bone radiating out from the cortex into the radiolucent tumor mass. The bone is deposited along the course of blood vessels that radiate out from the cortex; this accounts for the radiographic "sunburst" appearance. In the lower end of this femur, the neoplasm is an osteosarcoma. The radiographic "sunburst" appearance may also be seen in other malignant neoplasms and is not invariably present in osteosarcoma.

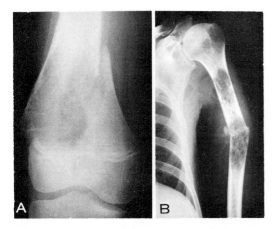

Figure 14.6. Pathological fractures through an abnormal area of bone that has been weakened by the local destruction (osteoclastic resorption) of a neoplasm. *A*, pathological fracture through an osteosarcoma of the lower end of the femur in a 14-year-old girl. *B*, pathological fracture through one of the two lesions of plasma cell myeloma (multiple myeloma) in the humerus of a 43-year-old man.

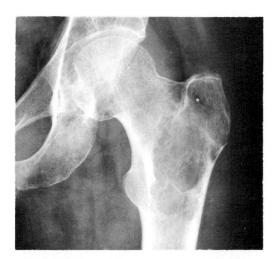

Figure 14.7. Osteolytic type of secondary (metastatic) neoplasm in the intertrochanteric region of the femur of a 62-year-old woman. The primary neoplasm was carcinoma of the breast.

physical presence interferes with function in surrounding tissues, or unless they have been complicated by a pathological fracture. The fact that pain is a characteristic feature of an osteoid osteoma suggests that it is a reactive lesion rather than a true neoplasm.

Pain is the most significant symptom of rapidly growing neoplasms. Initially mild and intermittent, the pain from such a neoplasm becomes progressively more severe and more constant. It is caused mostly by either tension or pressure on the sensitive periosteum and endosteum. A history of sudden

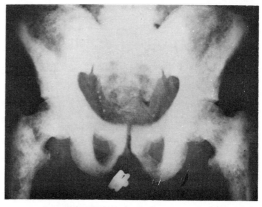

Figure 14.8. Osteosclerotic, or osteoblastic, type of secondary (metastatic) neoplasms in the pelvis and femora of a 75-year-old man. The primary neoplasm was carcinoma of the prostate; the metallic clamp is on an indwelling catheter.

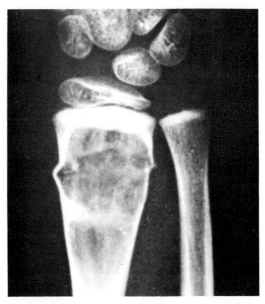

Figure 14.9. Simple (solitary) bone cyst of the lower end of the radius of a 10-year-old boy. This is a true cyst in that it is a lined cavity that contains fluid. Note also the transverse pathological fracture through the cyst.

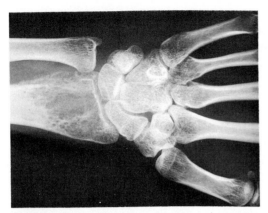

Figure 14.10. Osteolytic neoplasm which, radiographically, has a "cystic" appearance, but which is a solid lesion filled with neoplastic tissue; hence, it is not a true cyst. This neoplasm in the lower end of the radius in a 32-year-old man is an osteoclastoma (giant cell tumor).

onset of severe pain usually indicates the complication of a pathological fracture.

Local swelling can be detected when the lesion protrudes beyond the normal confines of the bone. The swelling of a benign lesion is usually firm and non-tender (Fig. 14.11). In the presence of a rapidly growing malignant neoplasm, however, the swelling is more diffuse and is frequently tender (Fig. 14.12). When the lesion is particularly vascular, the overlying skin may be warm and the superficial veins dilated; the latter are best seen under infrared light (Fig. 14.13).

If the lesion is close to a joint, function in that joint may be disturbed and there may also be painful restriction of joint motion.

Diagnosis

The aforementioned clinical history, physical signs and radiographic features are important components of the data required for the diagnosis of a neoplasm or neoplasm-like lesion of bone, but they are not enough in themselves. They must be correlated with the appropriate biochemical findings as well as with the gross appearance of the lesion at the time of biopsy and the microscopic appearance of the biopsy sample.

Recent advances that have made the diagnosis of musculoskeletal neoplasms progressively more sophisticated merit special consideration.

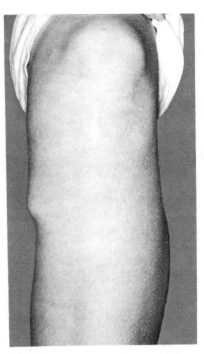

Figure 14.11. Local swelling, or lump, on the medial aspect of the left leg just below the knee in a 10-year-old boy. This local swelling, which was firm and non-tender, was due to an underlying osteochondroma (osteocartilaginous exostosis) arising from the medial aspect of the metaphysis of the tibia.

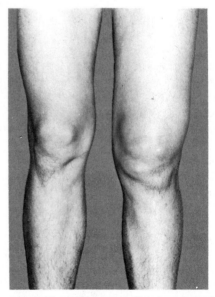

Figure 14.12. Diffuse swelling in the region of the knee of a 16-year-old boy. This swelling, which was warm and tender, was due to an underlying osteosarcoma.

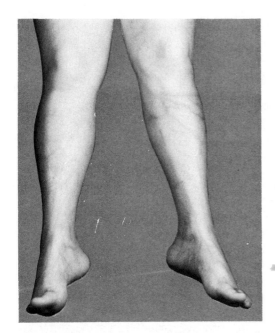

Figure 14.13.   Dilated superficial veins in the left leg just below the knee in a 10-year-old boy. This photograph was taken under infra-red light. The skin in the area of dilated veins was warm; the underlying lesion was a vascular, rapidly growing osteosarcoma.

Scintigraphy, or the *bone scan*, using radionuclides often reveals the site of a primary neoplasm—either benign or malignant—particularly when such neoplasms are associated with an increased blood flow or an increased rate of bone deposition as discussed in Chapter 5 (Figs. 5.28 and 5.29). High-resolution bone scans may also detect "skip" lesions of a malignant neoplasm proximal to the main lesion within the same bone. Furthermore, a skeletal survey by means of a "total body scan" may reveal skeletal metastases.

Computed tomography has made possible a three-dimensional visualization of musculoskeletal neoplasms (as discussed in Chapter 5). This is especially relevant to radiographically inaccessible sites such as the pelvis and spine (Fig. 5.30). Even in the limbs, computed tomography is of value in determining the extent of the lesion, not only within the bone (including "skip" lesions) but also within the surrounding soft tissues (Figs. 5.31 and 5.32). In addition, computed

tomography of the lungs makes possible the detection of very small pulmonary metastases not detectable by conventional radiography.

Arteriography, or *angiography*, provides useful information concerning the vascularity of a given neoplasm as well as the extent of any soft tissue extension.

Biochemical investigations include laboratory determinations of serum calcium, inorganic phosphate, alkaline phosphatase, acid phosphatase and serum proteins.

The serum calcium is elevated in any disorder (such as widespread osteolytic metastases) in which bone is being destroyed rapidly. The serum alkaline phosphatase reflects osteoblastic activity and, hence, is usually elevated in patients with osteogenic neoplasms such as osteosarcoma; nevertheless, a normal serum alkaline phosphatase does not exclude the possibility of a malignant neoplasm. Elevation of the serum acid phosphatase in the male nearly always indicates that a carcinoma of the prostate has spread beyond its capsule; thus, in the presence of skeletal metastases, this test is of considerable diagnostic significance. Elevation of the total protein concentration in the serum suggests the possibility of plasma cell myeloma (multiple myeloma), as does the detection of Bence-Jones protein in the urine.

SURGICAL BIOPSY

In the diagnosis of neoplasms and neoplasm-like lesions of the musculoskeletal tissues, biopsy is essential in order to avoid two serious errors in relation to treatment: (1) failure to recognize a malignant neoplasm (*underdiagnosis*), which results in inadequate treatment; (2) diagnosis of a nonmalignant lesion as a malignant neoplasm (*overdiagnosis*), which results in excessive treatment.

Recent multi-center investigations have revealed that one-quarter of the surgical biopsies of musculoskeletal neoplasms are either improperly performed or misinterpreted (or both), especially when the biopsy is performed in a referring hospital as opposed to a referral center. Frozen sections ("quick sections") may be adequate—depending on the experience of the pathologist—but if doubt exists, definitive treatment should await the interpretation of paraffin sections.

The biopsy samples must be adequate in size and must also be representative of the lesion. In general, open surgical biopsy is more reliable than aspiration biopsy (needle or punch biopsy), although in relatively inaccessible sites, such as vertebral bodies for which open biopsy would require an extensive operation, punch biopsy with radiographic control is often of value. In patients suspected of having a widespread neoplasm of the bone marrow, such as plasma cell myeloma (multiple myeloma), aspiration biopsy of the marrow in the sternum or the iliac crest is usually adequate.

Transmission electron microscopy has supplemented routine histology and histochemistry in the differentiation of neoplasms containing small round cells, e.g. Ewing's sarcoma and metastatic neuroblastoma. By using surface-marker antigens it is now possible to differentiate Hodgkin's lymphoma from other lymphomas.

All the available data are required to make an accurate diagnosis of a given lesion before definitive treatment is instituted. The final decision concerning both diagnosis and the optimal method of treatment is ideally reached from the combined opinions of the orthopaedic surgeon, radiologist, radiotherapist, medical oncologist and pathologist.

Principles of Treatment

During the investigation of a patient with an undiagnosed lesion in bone, the loose use of the words "cancer" and "malignancy" causes both patient and relatives unnecessary anxiety and anguish. Once the diagnosis of a malignant neoplasm is established beyond reasonable doubt, however, it becomes necessary to discuss the gravity of the situation with a close relative, or with the patient, depending on the circumstances. The attitude must always be one of *kindly realism* and both patient and relatives deserve the assurance that everything possible will be done to help. Even when, from a scientific point of view, the situation is hopeless, the patient must never be allowed to feel bereft of compassionate care.

In selecting forms of treatment for a given patient, an extremely important consideration is the anticipated duration, or *quantity*, of life remaining and equally important the anticipated *quality* of that life.

A most important principle in the treatment of patients with neoplasms and neoplasm-like lesions of the musculoskeletal tissues is that the treatment must be based on an accurate diagnosis; this is of particular importance when the contemplated treatment involves such major and irreversible operations as amputation. The prognosis of malignant musculoskeletal neoplasms is very poor regardless of treatment; hence, failure to treat a patient for a malignant lesion is serious enough—but needless amputation of a limb on the basis of a mistaken diagnosis is even more serious.

Benign neoplasms and other *non-malignant* lesions of bone are best treated surgically by such methods as excision or curettement and bone grafting (Fig. 14.14). It is basically unwise to treat by radiation any non-malignant lesion that can be managed satisfactorily by another form of treatment.

Malignant musculoskeletal primary neoplasms are generally best treated by surgical ablation, or eradication, with or without ra-

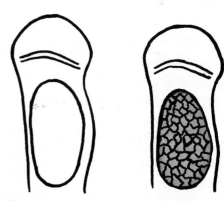

Figure 14.14. Bone grafting with fragments of cancellous bone to fill a defect after curettage (currettement) of a non-malignant lesion of bone.

diotherapy and adjuvant chemotherapy. The surgical eradication can vary in extent from excision with varying margins of surrounding tissue even up to amputation or disarticulation. Enneking has developed a useful system for "staging" of musculoskeletal sarcomas based on the histological grade of malignancy (low or high), the extent of the neoplasm within and without the bone (in relation to anatomic soft-tissue compartments) and the presence or absence of metastases. This staging system can be used in determining the extent of surgical excision required—intralesional or with a margin (marginal, wide or radical). Furthermore, the system is helpful in standardizing nationwide and international clinical investigations of the efficacy of various forms of treatment.

One of the most exciting recent advances in musculoskeletal cancer surgery is the development of *"limb-sparing" ("extremity-saving") ("limb-salvaging") procedures* as an attractive alternative to amputation or disarticulation—especially in the upper limb. These procedures involve a radical *en bloc* resection of the neoplasm and surrounding tissues in keeping with the established principles of cancer surgery. The awesome residual defect is then repaired or reconstructed in one of a variety of ways including autogenous bone grafting, arthrodesis of resected joints, osteocartilaginous allografts or custom-made endoprostheses including prosthetic joint replacement.

Radiotherapy continues to be an important form of treatment for musculoskeletal neoplasms, but such neoplasms exhibit varying degrees of radiosensitivity. For example, Ewing's sarcoma and reticulum cell sarcoma are relatively radiosensitive whereas chondrosarcoma is radio-resistant.

Adjuvant systemic chemotherapy has developed rapidly during the past decade and continues to develop as a means of either destroying microscopic metastases or, in a prophylactic sense, inhibiting their implantation. These powerful chemotherapeutic agents are cytotoxic—especially for rapidly growing malignant cells—but they are generally ineffective in destroying either the primary neoplasm or radiographically visible (macroscopic) metastases. Many chemotherapeutic agents have been used (often in various combinations) including methotrexate, vincristine, adriamycin, actinomycin D and cyclophosphamide. High-dose methotrexate, which interferes with the intracellular metabolism of folic acid, requires a subsequent "rescue" of the patient's folic acid metabolism by administration of a reduced form of folic acid known as "citrovorum factor." It is generally considered that when combined with surgical ablation of the primary neoplasm, adjuvant chemotherapy has increased the five-year survival rate of patients with osteosarcoma, for example, from approximately 10% to as high as 40%. Although chemotherapy is associated with various toxic side effects such as alopecia, leukopenia, nausea and impaired wound healing, these effects are reversible after the chemotherapy has been discontinued.

Immunotherapy of various types to enhance the patient's immunological response to a malignant neoplasm is still in the investigative stage.

Resection of solitary lung metastases has shown promising results when it can be demonstrated by computed tomography that a given pulmonary metastasis is, in fact, solitary and when the resection is combined with adjuvant chemotherapy.

Pathological fractures that occur through a *non-malignant* lesion of bone will usually heal, but the risk of repeated pathological fractures may necessitate *bone grafting* to reinforce the weakened area of bone. Pathological fractures that occur through a *malignant* neoplasm, however, will not heal spontaneously if the destructive process of the neoplasm exceeds the reparative process of fracture healing. Under these circumstances, *rigid intramedullary metallic fixation* of a fractured long bone may be required as palliative treatment to relieve persistent pain.

When the destruction of bone is extensive it may be necessary to use *bone cement (methylmethacrylate)* as an adjunct to the internal fixation in order that the patient may regain some effective use of the involved limb during the remaining months of his or her life.

SPECIFIC PRIMARY NEOPLASMS AND NEOPLASM-LIKE LESIONS OF BONE

Reactive Bone Lesions

OSTEOID OSTEOMA

Osteoid osteoma, which is probably a reactive bone lesion rather than a true neoplasm, is a relatively uncommon but distinctive clinical entity characterized by persistent pain. It usually develops in children and adolescents, particularly boys, but occasionally in young adults. Although an osteoid osteoma may occur in almost any bone, it has a predilection for bones of the lower limb, especially the femur and tibia. Its etiology remains a puzzle.

This curious lesion, which consists of a small round core of osteoid tissue surrounded by reactive bone, does not continue to grow in size and is seldom larger than 1 cm in diameter. When the core of osteoid (which is uncalcified and therefore radiolucent) develops in cancellous bone it incites very little reactive bone (Fig. 14.15). When it develops in cortical bone, however, the amount of reactive bone is strikingly out of

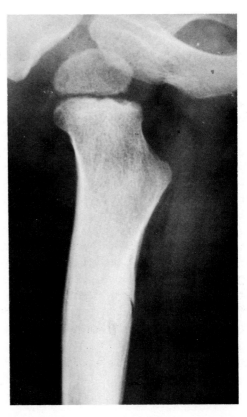

Figure 14.16. Osteoid osteoma in the cortical bone of the femoral shaft in a 5-year-old boy. The radiolucent lesion, which is less than 1 cm in diameter, is almost obscured by remarkably extensive reactive bone that is out of proportion to the size of the lesion.

proportion to the size of the central lesion (Fig. 14.16).

The predominant symptom of an osteoid osteoma is pain which is mild and nagging, more noticeable at night and characteristically relieved by mild analgesics such as aspirin. When the lesion is located near a joint, a synovial effusion develops and interferes slightly with joint function; local muscle atrophy may ensue. The radiographic features, which are well correlated with the pathology of the lesion, are almost pathognomonic (Figs. 14.15, 16). The lesion must be differentiated from a local area of chronic osteomyelitis. Scintigraphy is of special value in the diagnosis of an osteoid osteoma as discussed in Chapter 5 (Fig. 5.29).

Although osteoid osteomas are not pro-

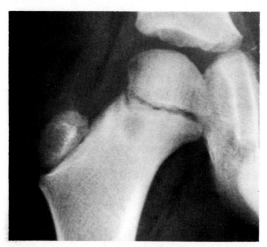

Figure 14.15. Osteoid osteoma in the cancellous bone of the right femoral neck in a 7-year-old boy. The round, radiolucent lesion, which is approximately 1 cm in diameter, has incited relatively little reactive bone formation. This boy complained of pain in the right knee (referred pain), but examination revealed painful limitation of motion in the right hip and atrophy of the muscles in the upper part of the right thigh.

gressive and, indeed, may even be self-limiting over a period of many years, the persistent pain necessitates their surgical excision. The central core of osteoid and a small margin of surrounding bone must be completely removed to prevent a recurrence; after excision of an osteoid osteoma in cortical bone, the residual reactive bone gradually disappears. The complete relief of pain and the return of normal function after adequate excision of an osteoid osteoma are gratifying to both the patient and the orthopaedic surgeon.

Another reactive bone lesion, which is similar in some ways to an osteoid osteoma, but much larger, is *benign osteoblastoma* ("giant osteoid osteoma"). This rare lesion, which tends to develop in vertebrae with little sclerosis is usually painful and is best treated by surgical excision.

SUBPERIOSTEAL CORTICAL DEFECT (METAPHYSEAL FIBROUS DEFECT)

By far the commonest radiographic lesion in bone is the *subperiosteal cortical defect*,

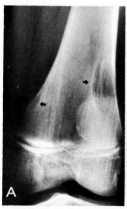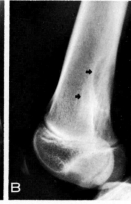

Figure 14.17. Subperiosteal cortical defects (metaphyseal fibrous defects) in the metaphysis of the lower end of the left femur in a 13-year-old boy. Both of these two small defects are just under the periosteum when viewed tangentially. This boy complained of pain in the left knee, which prompted his physician to obtain these radiographs. These lesions, however, could not account for the boy's pain. Examination revealed limitation of internal rotation and abduction of the left hip; radiographs of the hips revealed a minimal slip of the left upper femoral epiphysis which was the cause of the referred pain in the knee.

a small, eccentrically placed, superficial crater filled with fibrous tissue which seems to arise from the periosteum. It is estimated that these lesions can be detected in 10 to 20% of all children at some stage during skeletal growth; they are most commonly seen in the metaphyseal region of the lower end of the femur and usually represent an incidental finding (Fig. 14.17).

Subperiosteal cortical defects, which probably constitute a local area of defective endochondral ossification, tend to fill in with bone spontaneously after a number of years, having caused neither symptoms nor clinical signs. The clinical significance of these lesions, however, lies in the fact that they may be overdiagnosed as a more serious lesion that requires treatment; furthermore, their presence in a child who is complaining of local pain cannot explain such pain, the cause of which must be sought elsewhere. No treatment is required for subperiosteal cortical defects.

NON-OSTEOGENIC FIBROMA (NON-OSSIFYING FIBROMA)

Non-osteogenic fibroma is a relatively common fibrous lesion that is somewhat similar to the aforementioned subperiosteal cortical defect. Whether it is a reactive bone lesion or simply a local developmental disorder is not clear; but being self-limiting, it is not a true neoplasm. Although it may persist into early adult life, non-osteogenic fibroma is seen in children and adolescents. The commonest sites are the long bones, especially those of the lower limbs.

Non-osteogenic fibromas do not cause symptoms and are therefore usually seen as incidental findings. The fibrous lesion arises in the cortex and gradually replaces it from within. It grows only slowly to a maximum size of about 4 cms and incites a thin zone of reactive bone around it, thereby producing a characteristic radiographic appearance (Fig. 14.18). Pathological fractures may occur, but only after a fairly severe injury.

The clinical significance of non-osteogenic fibroma, like that of a subperiosteal defect, is that it may be overdiagnosed as a more

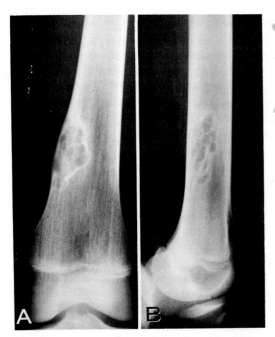

Figure 14.18. Non-osteogenic fibroma in the metaphyseal region of the femur in a 16-year-old boy. In the anteroposterior projection, which is tangential to the lesion, it can be seen to be eccentrically placed just under the periosteum; the lateral projection gives the impression that the lesion is centrally placed. Note the clearly defined edges and the zone of reactive bone around this slowly growing lesion. The non-osteogenic fibroma was an incidental finding in these radiographs which were taken because of a recent mild injury.

serious lesion and hence overtreated, or that it may be considered the explanation for local pain. Since most non-osteogenic fibromas fill in with bone spontaneously over a few years, no treatment is required.

Other Non-neoplastic Lesions of Bone

MONOSTOTIC FIBROUS DYSPLASIA

Although fibrous dysplasia of bone is not a neoplasm, it is included in this chapter because it simulates a neoplasm radiographically (Fig. 14.19). *Monostotic fibrous dysplasia* consists of a local lesion of fibrous tissue proliferation in the cancellous area of a single bone and occurs in children, adolescents and young adults. Histologically, the lesion is comparable to any given lesion in the multiple form known as polyostotic fibrous

dysplasia (Chapter 9). As a progressively larger area of bone is replaced by fibrous tissue, a pathological fracture may ensue.

The prognosis of monostotic fibrous dysplasia is excellent. Treatment consists of curettement of the lesion and reinforcement of the weakened area by bone grafts to prevent repeated pathological fractures.

SIMPLE BONE CYST (SOLITARY BONE CYST) (UNICAMERAL BONE CYST)

Simple, or solitary bone cyst, is not a neoplasm but, like fibrous dysplasia, can simulate a neoplasm. The only true cyst of bone, it develops most commonly in children and adolescents. The most frequent sites are the upper end of humerus, upper end of femur, upper end of tibia and lower end of radius, in that order.

For reasons unknown, the cyst develops

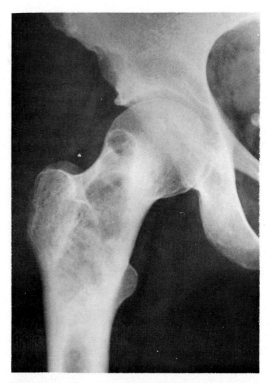

Figure 14.19. Monostotic fibrous dysplasia in the upper end of the femur of a 25-year-old woman. This lesion, which is not a neoplasm, but merely fibrous tissue proliferation in cancellous bone, simulates a neoplasm radiographically. Note the clearly defined margins and the surrounding zone of reactive bone.

subjacent to the epiphyseal plate and gradually expands to fill the entire metaphysis, and even part of the diaphysis. Cortical bone is resorbed from the inner surface, but periosteal reactive bone on the outer surface contains the lesion. The cavity is lined by non-neoplastic connective tissue cells and is filled with serous or serosanguinous fluid (reminiscent of the lining and contents of a chronic subdural hematoma). The overlying cortex becomes markedly thinned out and, consequently, pathological fractures are common (Fig. 14.20).

Simple bone cysts expand slowly and hence are painless. The most frequent event that brings them to the attention of a physician is a pathological fracture, resulting from a minor injury. The radiographic features of simple bone cysts are characteristic (Figs. 14.20, 21).

As the cyst becomes more mature, and hence, less "active," it stops enlarging, in which case the epiphyseal plate grows away from it. Since simple bone cysts are almost never seen in adults, they are obviously due to a self-limiting process. In the meantime, however, repeated pathological fractures are not only painful and inconvenient for the child, but may lead to progressive deformity, particularly when the cyst is in the upper end of the femur. Although pathological fractures through a simple bone cyst heal readily, the cyst usually persists. Until recently the most suitable treatment was thorough curettement of the cystic cavity and filling it with bone grafts (Fig. 14.14).

In the early 1970's, however, Scaglietti initiated the transcutaneous injection of corticosteroid (in the form of methylprednisolone acetate) into simple bone cysts as a means of not only arresting the osteolytic process but even reversing it so that the cyst could heal by bone deposition. Theoretically the corticosteroid inhibits the growth of the connective tissue cells in the lining of the cyst and hence favors progressive healing by new bone formation. The injection may have to be repeated on one or more occasions, but in growing children the results have been very satisfactory; 45% of the cysts have disappeared over a period of three years and in the majority of the remainder, the wall of the cyst has become sufficiently thick and strong that there have been no further pathological fractures. Thus, for many children with an immature and hence "active" bone cyst it is now possible to avoid the open surgical procedure of curettage with its attendant risk of damage to the adjacent epiphyseal plate.

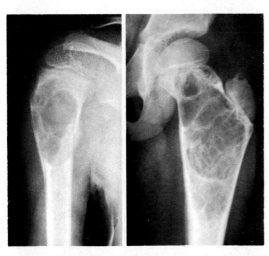

Figure 14.20 (*left*).   Simple (solitary) bone cyst in the metaphyseal region of the upper end of the humerus in a 10-year-old boy. Note the healing pathological fracture through the weakened cortex on the medial side. This boy had sustained a minor injury three weeks previously.

Figure 14.21 (*right*).   Simple (solitary) bone cyst in the upper end of the femur in an 8-year-old boy. There is only one cavity (unicameral); the radiographic appearance of several cavities (multilocular) is due to ridges of bone on the deep surface of the thin cortex. The proximal end of this cyst extends to the upper femoral epiphyseal plate.

Hamartomas Affecting Bone

OSTEOCHONDROMA (OSTEOCARTILAGINOUS EXOSTOSIS)

Although often considered to be a benign neoplasm, an *osteochondroma* is probably an abnormality of growth direction and remodeling in the metaphyseal region of long bones in growing children. As indicated by the synonym (osteocartilaginous exostosis), this lesion consists of an outgrowth of both bone and cartilage which forms a prominent "tumor," in the sense of a local swelling, or lump.

A single osteochondroma is seen most commonly in young persons, although if untreated, it persists into adult life. The lesion always arises from the metaphyseal region and the commonest sites are the lower end of femur, upper end of tibia and upper end of humerus, the most actively growing ends of long bones.

A given osteochondroma is comparable pathologically to each of the osteochondromas seen in the congenital condition of *diaphyseal aclasis* (multiple osteocartilaginous exostoses, Chapter 8). The protruding lesion, which always points away from the nearest epiphyseal plate, consists of normal bone and is capped by normal cartilage. Indeed, during the growing years an osteochondroma has its own epiphyseal plate from which it grows, but growth ceases about the same time as in the neighboring epiphyseal plates. A synovial bursa, of the friction type, develops between the protruding part of the osteochondroma and the surrounding soft tissues. Osteochondromas may be long with a narrow base (pedunculated, or stalked type) or they may be short with a broad base (sessile type). Malignant change (usually chondrosarcomatous) occurs in approximately 1% of single osteochondromas in adult life although the incidence is higher in the multiple form.

Osteochondromas are not painful lesions in themselves, but they may interfere with the function of surrounding soft tissues such as tendons and nerves. Usually the patient happens to become aware of the firm localized swelling incidentally; understandably, the parents are often concerned about the possibility of "bone cancer" (Fig. 14.22). Radiographic examination reveals only the bony part of the osteochondroma, which explains why the lesion is always larger clinically than it appears radiographically (Fig. 14.23).

Not all osteochondromas require treatment. If, however, the osteochondroma is producing an ugly lump, or if it is interfering with normal function of the limb in any way, it should be surgically excised.

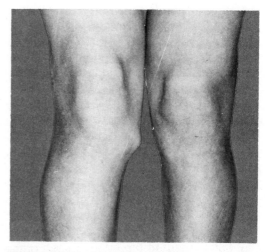

Figure 14.22.   Localized swelling just below the medial side of the right knee of a 13-year-old boy; the underlying lesion is an osteochondroma (osteocartilaginous exostosis) arising from the metaphyseal region of the tibia.

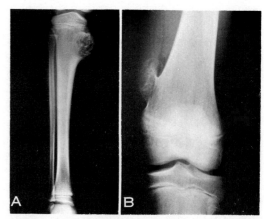

Figure 14.23.   Osteochondroma (osteocartilaginous exostosis). *A,* sessile type of osteochondroma arising from the metaphyseal region of the tibia in a 7-year-old boy. The radiolucent cartilage cap accounts for the lesion being larger clinically than is apparent radiographically. *B,* pedunculated, or stalked, type of osteochrondroma arising from the metaphyseal region of the femur in a 13-year-old girl. Note that the osteochondroma points away from the epiphyseal plate. It will continue to grow slowly from its cartilage cap until the lower femoral epiphyseal plate stops growing.

ENCHONDROMA

Enchondroma is a lesion comprising a mass of relatively normal cartilage cells within the interior of a single bone. Although sometimes considered to be a benign neoplasm, it probably develops as a local abnormality of growth from cartilage cells of the epiphyseal plate during childhood. The patient, however, may not become aware of the lesion until adolescence or early adult life. The most frequent sites are the tubular bones of the hands and feet (phalanges, metacarpals, metatarsals), usually near one end; a less common site is one of the larger long bones.

Pathologically, a given enchondroma is comparable to each of the individual enchondromas seen in the congenital condition of *enchondromatosis* (Ollier's dyschondroplasia). Its cells divide only slowly; and as the lesion grows, bone is slowly absorbed from the inner cortex and at the same time, periosteal reactive bone is deposited on the outer surface. Since resorption exceeds deposition, the involved bone slowly becomes expanded with a thinned-out overlying cortex. Histologically, an enchondroma may be difficult to differentiate from a slowly growing chondrosarcoma. Occasionally, a single enchondroma in a large long bone does, in fact, undergo malignant change to become a chondrosarcoma.

Since enchondromas are not painful lesions in themselves, the patient is usually unaware of the lesion until a firm swelling is noticed or until a local injury causes a pathological fracture in the thin cortex. The radiographic features are quite characteristic (Fig. 14.24). In long-standing enchondromas, particularly in large bones, irregular calcification may appear within the radiolucent cartilage.

Enchondromas are best treated by thorough curettement and packing of the residual cavity with bone grafts (Fig. 14.14).

ANGIOMA OF BONE

Hemangioma, a vascular type of hamartoma, is relatively common in many tissues. Occasionally, a hemangioma develops in bone, usually the vertebral bodies and the skull, but they seldom cause symptoms and consequently may remain undiagnosed.

Rarely a rapidly growing *lymphangioma* in bone causes alarming destruction ("massive

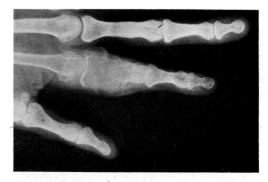

Figure 14.24. Enchondroma in the proximal phalanx of the index finger of a 21-year-old man. Note the central radiolucent lesion which has expanded the phalanx. There is a small pathological fracture through the thinned out cortex on both sides of the lesion.

osteolysis") in one or more bones and leads to the bizarre condition of "disappearing bone" or "phantom bone."

ANEURYSMAL BONE CYST

The curious lesion called *aneurysmal bone cyst* is not a true neoplasm, but its pathogenesis is not understood. It is a solitary vascular abnormality that begins within the marrow tissue of cancellous bone.

Aneurysmal bone cysts develop most frequently in adolescents and young adults, usually in the spine and less commonly in the metaphyseal region of a long bone such as the humerus. Locally destructive, it erodes cortical bone from the inner surface; at the same time periosteal reactive bone deposition on the outer surface contains the lesion, but allows it to expand to such a degree that it resembles an aneurysmal dilatation—hence the term, *aneurysmal* bone cyst. Since the lesion contains vascular tissue rather than mere fluid, however, it is not a true cyst. If left untreated, an aneurysmal bone cyst may reach an alarming size and may even rupture into the surrounding tissues thereby producing a hematoma. Histologically, aneurysmal bone cysts contain a sponge-like network of large vascular channels which carry circulating blood and which may represent some type of arteriovenous malformation.

Since aneurysmal bone cysts expand rapidly, they are usually painful; pathological

osteoblastic cells of the periosteum; it grows mostly *beside* the bone (parosteal) as a radiographically dense, osteoblastic lesion (Fig. 14.29).

Since parosteal sarcoma grows relatively slowly, at least in comparison with osteosarcoma, pain is not an early clinical feature; and since the cortex is seldom eroded, pathological fracture is rare. Parosteal sarcoma metastasizes relatively late to the lungs, and consequently, its prognosis is much better than that of osteosarcoma. Indeed, early

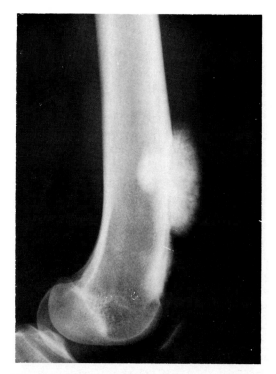

Figure 14.29. Parosteal sarcoma (periosteal sarcoma) arising from the anterior surface of the lower end of the femur in an 18-year-old girl. The major portion of the neoplasm is outside the confines of the bone; it is predominantly osteoblastic (osteosclerotic) and is consequently dense radiographically.

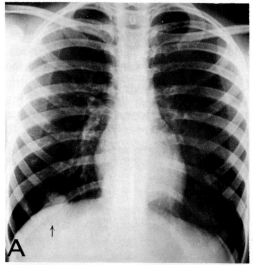

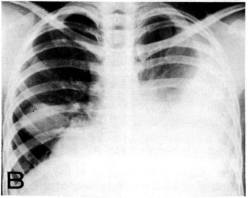

Figure 14.28. Pulmonary metastases secondary to osteosarcoma of the femur in a 9-year-old girl. *A*, note the round metastasis at the base of the right lung (*arrow*). *B*, the radiograph only two months later reveals a massive pleural effusion on the left side, a small pneumothorax on the right side and multiple metastases in both lungs.

total resection, either by limb-sparing procedures or by amputation can be expected to result in a permanent cure in 80% of patients.

CHONDROGENIC NEOPLASMS
BENIGN CHONDROBLASTOMA

A rare, benign neoplasm, *chondroblastoma* develops within the epiphysis of older children and adolescents, particularly at the upper end of tibia, lower end of femur and upper end of humerus; in this last site it is known as a Codman's tumor because he described it there. Because the lesion is subjacent to the articular cartilage, the patient complains of pain and experiences disturbed function in the nearby joint.

Chondroblastoma grows slowly and becomes surrounded by sclerotic reactive bone which may even obscure the underly-

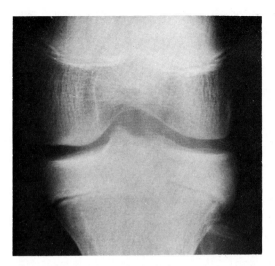

Figure 14.30. Chondroblastoma of the upper tibial epiphysis in a 13-year-old boy. The small benign neoplasm is almost obscured by the surrounding sclerosis which is due to reactive bone. A tomogram of this boy's lesion (shown in Fig. 14.1) reveals the radiolucent neoplasm much more clearly.

ing cartilaginous neoplasm radiographically (Fig. 14.30). Histologically, this lesion may be difficult to differentiate from a chondrosarcoma. Chondroblastomas are benign neoplasms, however, and consequently respond well to local curettement and bone grafting.

CHONDROMYXOID FIBROMA

Chondromyxoid fibroma is actually more of a chondroma than a fibroma since it is a noeplasm of chondroblastic origin. It develops in the metaphyseal region of long bones and also in the small bones of adolescents and young adults. Although usually benign, chondromyxoid fibroma is considered to be at least potentially malignant.

Chondromyxoid fibroma grows relatively slowly and tends to maintain an eccentric location in the bone. The overlying cortex is often expanded and the neoplasm is surrounded by a sclerotic zone of reactive bone (Fig. 14.31). Since chondromyxoid fibromas are at least potentially malignant neoplasms, they are more effectively treated by local excision that includes a zone of normal bone rather than by simple curettement.

CHONDROSARCOMA

Chondrosarcoma is usually a relatively slowly growing malignant neoplasm that arises either spontaneously in previously normal bone, or as the result of malignant change in a pre-existent non-malignant lesion, such as an osteochondroma or an enchondroma. Occurring mostly in adults over the age of 30, it tends to develop in the pelvic and shoulder girdles and proximal long bones. There is often radiographic evidence of patchy calcification within this cartilaginous neoplasm. Histologically, the lesion consists of poorly differentiated cartilage cells but relatively few mitotic figures. Nevertheless, varying degrees of malignity exist within this category.

Since chondrosarcoma grows relatively slowly, pain is not a prominent clinical feature. A large cartilaginous mass slowly develops. Metastases tend to develop late and consequently, the prognosis of chondrosarcoma is considerably better than that of osteosarcoma. Since chondrosarcomas are radio-resistant and exhibit only a limited response to chemotherapy, the optimum form of treatment is complete removal of the neoplasm and this usually necessitates either limb-sparing procedures or amputation. After such treatment, the patient has at least a 35% chance of cure.

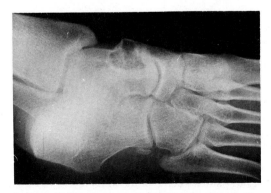

Figure 14.31. Chondromyxoid fibroma in the neck of the talus in a 25-year-old man. Note the eccentric location of the neoplasm in the bone, the expanded and thin overlying cortex and the surrounding sclerotic zone of reactive bone.

Collagenic Neoplasms

FIBROSARCOMA

Fibrosarcoma is an uncommon malignant neoplasm which may arise in a long bone in young adults. The principal sites are the femur, tibia and radius. Since it grows relatively slowly, it is seldom painful. Radiographically, fibrosarcoma produces a fairly well demarcated osteolytic defect with little reaction in the surrounding bone (Fig. 14.32).

The prognosis of fibrosarcoma is only slightly better than that of osteosarcoma because it metastasizes late. Its treatment, which involves complete removal of the lesion, frequently necessitates amputation.

Myelogenic Neoplasms

PLASMA CELL MYELOMA (MULTIPLE MYELOMA)

Plasma cell myeloma is a widespread, multicentric neoplasm that arises in the he-

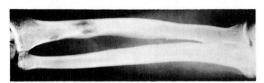

Figure 14.32. Fibrosarcoma in the radius of a 28-year-old woman. Note that there are several well demarcated osteolytic defects, all of which are part of the same neoplasm.

mopoietic tissue of the bone marrow in older persons, usually over the age of 50. It may occasionally remain localized as a solitary plasmacytoma for many years, but even then it usually becomes multicentric. This neoplasm is particularly fascinating since recent electrophoretic studies of the associated changes in specific fractions of the serum proteins suggest that the initial neoplastic change may start in a *single* cell, as opposed to a *group* of cells. Plasma cell myeloma is the commonest of all primary malignant neoplasms of bone. Since in older persons hemopoietic (red) marrow is most prevalent in the spine, pelvis, ribs, sternum and skull, these are the most frequently involved sites, but multiple bones may become riddled with rapidly destructive lesions which are painful (Fig. 14.33). The rapid destruction of bone with little reactive bone formation accounts for the high incidence of pathological fractures (Fig. 14.6b).

Since plasma cells of the bone marrow normally produce γ-globulin, the concentration of this protein in the serum is markedly elevated in patients with plasma cell myeloma. The excessive γ-globulin is excreted in the urine and may interfere with renal function; a specific protein—Bence-Jones protein—can be detected in the urine of approximately 50% of the patients.

Because this neoplasm is so widespread,

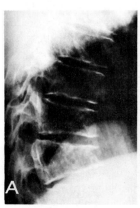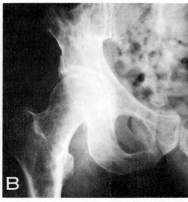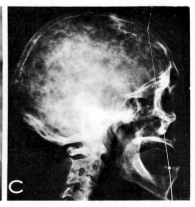

Figure 14.33. Plasma cell myeloma (multiple myeloma) in the spine, pelvis and skull of a 58-year-old man. *A,* note the pathological compression fracture through an osteolytic lesion in a thoracic vertebra. *B,* there are multiple lesions, not only in the innominate bone of the pelvis, but also in the femur. *C,* the skull is riddled with multiple, small, clearly defined osteolytic defects.

the diagnosis of plasma cell myeloma can often be confirmed by needle aspiration biopsy of the marrow from either the iliac crest or the sternum. Until recently the prognosis was extremely grave in that most patients succumbed within two years of the time of diagnosis. In recent years, however, encouraging results are being obtained with intensive chemotherapy. In the meantime, pathological fractures require palliative treatment for the relief of pain.

EWING'S TUMOR (EWING'S SARCOMA)

Ewing's tumor is a rapidly growing malignant neoplasm that arises from primitive cells of the bone marrow in young persons, usually in the medullary cavity of long bones. It is the third commonest primary malignant neoplasm of bone (being exceeded only by plasma cell myeloma and osteosarcoma). Like osteosarcoma, it develops in children, adolescents and young adults; the commonest sites are the femur, tibia, ulna and metatarsals.

Beginning within the medullary cavity, Ewing's tumor soon perforates the cortex of the shaft and elevates the periosteum; the repeated elevation of the periosteum and consequent reactive bone formation account for the laminated, or "onionskin" appearance seen radiographically (Fig. 14.4). Ewing's tumor metastasizes early, not only to the lungs, but also to other bones. Microscopically, this neoplasm is characterized by poorly differentiated round cells of marrow origin and containing intracellular glycogen as detected by means of a periodic acid-Schiff stain.

Ewing's tumor grows so rapidly that it often outgrows its blood supply and consequently, central areas of the neoplasm degenerate. The products of this degeneration enter the blood stream and produce systemic manifestations which include slight fever, moderate leucocytosis and an elevated sedimentation rate. In addition, the blood supply to local areas of bone may be compromised with resultant avascular necrosis of bone.

As with other rapidly growing malignant neoplasms, the principal symptom is pain of progressive severity. A diffuse soft tissue mass is usually palpable and is moderately tender. Initially, the neoplasm exhibits relatively little bone destruction but subsequently, there is considerable reactive bone from the periosteum (Fig. 14.34).

The pain, local tenderness, systemic manifestations and radiographic features raise the differential diagnoses of chronic osteomyelitis and eosinophilic granuloma; the only certain method of diagnosis of Ewing's tumor is surgical biopsy and histological ex-

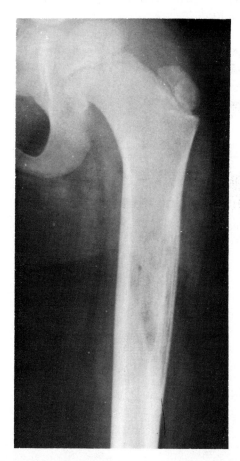

Figure 14.34. Ewing's tumor (Ewing's sarcoma) in the shaft of the femur in a 6-year-old girl. This neoplasm is in an early stage of its development and is only moderately destructive. Note the radiographic "onion-skin" appearance of periosteal reactive bone on the lateral aspect of the lesion. A more advanced stage of Ewing's tumor is shown in Figure 14.4.

amination of representative samples of the lesion.

The prognosis of Ewing's tumor, like that of osteosarcoma, is extremely grave. Until recently, regardless of whether the patient was treated surgically or by radiation, the mortality rate within the first few years after diagnosis was approximately 95%.

Since the primary lesion is relatively radiosensitive and may "melt away" after intensive radiotherapy, this has been the initial treatment of choice. Nevertheless, metastases were still very common and consequently in recent years there has been increasing emphasis on the combination of radiotherapy, adjuvant systemic chemotherapy and surgical eradication (especially for young children in whom the effects of radiotherapy on local epiphyseal growth would be devastating). The combination of radiotherapy and chemotherapy has already increased the success rate from approximately 5% to as high as 50%.

RETICULUM CELL SARCOMA (RETICULOSARCOMA)

Although an uncommon malignant neoplasm of the myelogenic group, *reticulum cell sarcoma* must be differentiated from Ewing's tumor because it has a better prognosis. Occurring mostly in adults, it grows more slowly than Ewing's tumor and consequently causes less pain. Reticulum cell sarcoma is more destructive locally, however, and may therefore be complicated by pathological fracture. The radiographic features, which include local destruction of bone and the presence of reactive bone, are non-specific (Fig. 14.35). Histologically reticulin fibers can be detected.

Reticulum cell sarcoma is more radiosensitive than other malignant neoplasms of bone. Consequently, radiation therapy, which provides a cure rate of approximately 50%, is considered the most appropriate form of treatment

OTHER MYELOGENIC NEOPLASMS

Hodgkin's disease, which is one of the lymphomas, may be complicated by local

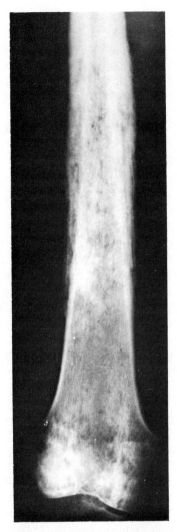

Figure 14.35. Reticulum cell sarcoma of the femur in a 29-year-old woman. Note the mottled appearance due to a combination of osteoclastic bone resorption (osteolysis) and osteoblastic bone deposition (osteosclerosis); the layers of subperiosteal reactive bone are somewhat similar to those seen in Ewing's sarcoma.

deposits in the bone as part of a generalized body involvement.

Leukemia is not usually considered in discussions of neoplasms of bone; nevertheless, *acute leukemia* in infants and children may be accompanied by widespread leukemic infiltrations in the bones giving rise to a characteristic radiographic appearance (Fig. 14.36).

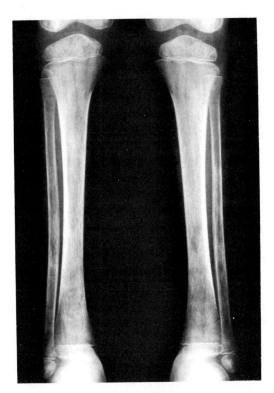

Figure 14.36. Acute leukemia in a 7-year-old boy. The multiple, ill-defined areas of rarefaction in the long bones represent leukemic infiltrations. This boy complained of deep pain in his legs and examination revealed bone tenderness.

OSTEOCLASTOMA (GIANT CELL TUMOR OF BONE)

A variable lesion, *osteoclastoma*, or *giant cell tumor of bone*, is a potentially malignant, and sometimes frankly malignant neoplasm that arises in the cancellous end of long bones in young adults.

Much confusion and divergence of opinion surround this neoplasm; the origin of the osteoclast is not known and there is not even general agreement that the osteoclast is the principal neoplastic cell of an osteoclastoma. Formerly, several benign neoplasms, and even non-neoplastic lesions that contained osteoclasts, or giant cells, were considered to be osteoclastomas. Now that these less serious "giant cell variants" have been excluded, what remains as a true osteoclastoma is a formidable neoplasm.

Osteoclastoma develops in the region of the former epiphysis of long bones after the epiphyseal plate has closed; hence, it is rare under the age of 20 years. The most common sites are the lower end of radius, upper end of tibia and lower end of femur; the neoplasm usually extends to the articular cartilage.

Osteoclastomas are locally destructive neoplasms; the cancellous and cortical bone are resorbed from the inside and simultaneously, the periosteum deposits bone on the outside so that the end of the bone eventually becomes expanded. Growth may be slow, or relatively rapid, depending on the aggressiveness of the particular lesion. Two-thirds of these neoplasms are benign in their behavior, one-sixth are locally aggressive and one-sixth become frankly malignant. Areas of hemorrhage within the lesion are common, and indeed, a phenomenon comparable to aneurysmal bone cyst may be superimposed upon the original lesion and cause it to expand at an alarming rate. Even those osteoclastomas that are frankly malignant, however, tend to metastasize late. Microscopically, osteoclastomas consist of a vascular network of stromal cells and large numbers of multinucleated giant cells.

The patient complains of local pain, the severity of which is related to the rate of growth of the neoplasm. Since the lesion abuts the articular cartilage, there is nearly always some disturbance of joint function. The radiographic appearance is variable, but reveals local bone destruction and eventually expansion of the end of the bone (Fig. 14.37).

Osteoclastomas have a disturbing tendency to recur after local surgical treatment such as curettement; hence, the original operation should be as extensive as necessary to remove all neoplastic tissue, and yet not sufficiently extensive to disturb function in the limb unnecessarily. A local recurrence after curettement is an indication for complete excision of the entire lesion and replacement of the resected part of the bone by an autogenous bone graft, an osteocar-

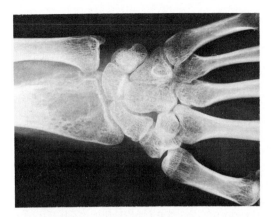

Figure 14.37. Osteoclastoma (giant cell tumor) in the lower end of the radius of a 32-year-old man. Note that the destructive (osteolytic) neoplasm includes the site of the epiphysis and extends to the subchondral bone. In this relatively early stage, the radius is just beginning to expand on the medial (ulnar) side.

tilaginous allograft or a custom-made endoprosthesis including prosthetic joint replacement. For the most aggressive osteoclastomas, the only reasonable form of treatment may be amputation.

METASTATIC NEOPLASMS IN BONE

By far the commonest malignant neoplasms *in* bone (rather than *of* bone) are *metastatic neoplasms* or "bone secondaries" that have invaded bone from a primary malignant neoplasm elsewhere. In adults, particularly the elderly, these "outside invaders" almost always originate from *carcinoma*, whereas in children their commonest source is *neuroblastoma.*

Metastatic Carcinoma

Metastatic carcinoma is common, as evidenced by the postmortem observation that at least one-quarter of all patients who have died from carcinoma have one or more metastases in bone. Viable neoplastic cells from a primary carcinoma may reach bone by the bloodstream, by the lymphatics or by direct extension. Hemopoietic (red) marrow seems to provide the most fertile "soil" for the "seeding" of carcinoma cells, and hence, the commonest sites for metastatic carci-

noma are the vertebrae, pelvis, ribs and proximal long bones of the limbs.

The most frequent *primary* sources for metastatic carcinoma in bone are breast, prostate, lung and kidney. Most of the metastatic neoplasms in bone are locally destructive and produce *osteolytic metastases* (Fig. 14.38). Others, particularly those from carcinoma of the prostate, incite a marked osteoblastic reaction in their metastatic site and produce *osteosclerotic metastases* (Fig. 14.39).

The most prominent symptom of metastatic carcinoma in bone is severe and unrelenting pain, some of which is due to the complication of pathological fracture (Fig. 14.40). Indeed, metastatic neoplasms in bone are the commonest cause of the pathetically painful demise of patients dying from cancer.

Osteoblastic resorption in multiple bones releases excessive amounts of calcium into the blood stream, and hence, in patients with multiple metastases, the serum calcium is usually elevated. The reactive bone formation stimulated by these lesions accounts for the elevation of serum alkaline phosphatase. A raised serum acid phosphatase is almost always an indication of advanced carcinoma of the prostate and is therefore detected in patients with prostatic metastases in bone.

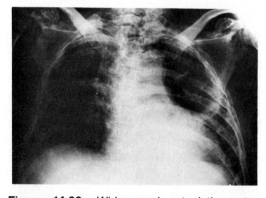

Figure 14.38. Widespread osteolytic metastases in the vertebrae, scapulae and ribs of a 49-year-old woman. The primary neoplasm was carcinoma of the breast. Another example of the osteolytic type of metastatic carcinoma in bone is shown in Figure 14.7.

The treatment of patients with metastatic carcinoma is palliative only. Local radiation therapy can retard the rate of growth of a metastasis and thereby help to relieve pain. Various forms of hormone therapy and even endocrine operations such as castration, adrenalectomy and hyophysectomy, depending on the source of the primary neoplasm, may help to retard the rate of progression of the metastases and thereby relieve pain, as well as prolong life somewhat. To relieve pain, pathological fractures in limb bones are stabilized by metallic internal fixation with or without bone cement (methylmethacrylate) whenever feasible; those in the vertebrae are immobilized in an appropriate spinal brace for the same purpose. The total care of a patient with metastatic carcinoma requires unending understanding and kindly compassion. The dignity of the dying must always be preserved.

Metastatic Neuroblastoma

In infants and young children, *neuroblastoma*, an extremely malignant neoplasm of the adrenal medulla, is the commonest primary source of multiple metastases in

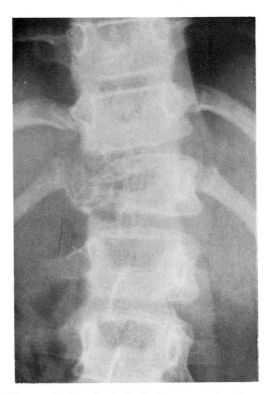

Figure 14.40. Pathological compression fracture through an osteolytic metastasis in the body of the 12th thoracic vertebrae in a 54-year-old man. Note the asymmetrical collapse of the vertebral body. The primary neoplasm was bronchogenic carcinoma of the lung.

bone which tend to develop in the vertebrae, skull and metaphysis of long bones (Fig. 14.41). There is usually a high urinary excretion of catecholamines. Cytotoxic drugs and local radiation therapy tend to retard the growth of these metastases and thereby relieve pain.

SPECIFIC PRIMARY NEOPLASMS AND NEOPLASM-LIKE LESIONS OF SYNOVIAL JOINTS, AND TENDON SHEATHS

The one tissue that is common to synovial joints, bursae and tendon sheaths is *synovial membrane*. Compared to bone, synovial membrane is the site of very few malignant neoplasms, the most significant of which is *synovial sarcoma*. Two additional lesions of synovial membrane (synovial

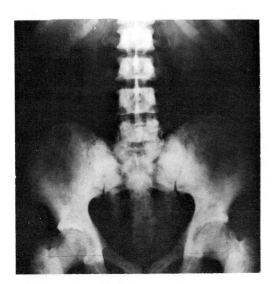

Figure 14.39. Widespread osteosclerotic (osteoblastic) metastases in the femora, pelvis and vertebrae of a 60-year-old man. The primary neoplasm was carcinoma of the prostate. Another example of the osteosclerotic type of metastatic carcinoma in bone is shown in Figure 14.8.

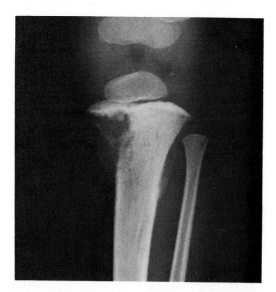

Figure 14.41. Osteolytic metastasis in the upper end of the tibia in a 2-year-old child. Note the marked bone destruction in the medial part of the metaphysis as well as the subperiosteal reactive bone on the lateral aspect. The primary neoplasm was a neuroblastoma of the adrenal medulla.

chondrometaplasia and pigmented villo-nodular synovitis), though not neoplasms, are neoplasm-like and also merit discussion.

Synovial Sarcoma (Synovioma)

Synovial sarcoma is a malignant neoplasm that arises from cells of synovial potential, often in tendon sheaths, near, but not actually in, a major joint in young adults. More common in the lower limbs than elsewhere, synovial sarcoma usually becomes manifest by the development of a painless, soft tissue swelling near a joint, most commonly the knee. Since the bone is not involved, radiographic examination reveals only a soft tissue mass which may exhibit calcification within it. Histologically, tissue spaces, or clefts, may be seen within the neoplasm.

Metastases may appear late, sometimes more than five years after the diagnosis and treatment of the primary lesion. Synovial sarcoma often recurs, even after extensive local excision and radiotherapy; indeed, amputation is usually necessary to eradicate this serious neoplasm and to achieve a success rate of 50%.

NON-NEOPLASTIC LESIONS OF SYNOVIAL MEMBRANE

Synovial Chondrometaplasia (Synovial Chondromatosis)

Metaplasia is a change in adult cells of a given tissue whereby they produce a different type of cell and consequently, a different type of tissue. On rare occasions in adults, and for reasons unknown, the cells of the synovial membrane may undergo metaplasia (*synovial chondrometaplasia*) whereby they come to resemble chondroblasts and subsequently produce deposits of cartilage tissue within the membrane. These cartilaginous deposits may become vascularized and develop centers of ossification, in which case, they become radio-opaque. As these osteochondral masses grow, they become pedunculated and may be torn loose from the synovial membrane to become free bodies in the synovial cavity (osteochondral loose bodies or "joint mice"). The ossific nucleus, having lost its blood supply, dies, but remains in its coffin of cartilage. The cartilaginous portion, however, being nourished by synovial fluid, survives and may even continue to grow. Arthroscopic examination is helpful in establishing the diagnosis.

Adults over the age of 40 are most prone to develop this unusual type of metaplasia; the commonest sites are the knee, hip and elbow. The patient complains of "grinding" in the joint and the sensation of something moving about inside the joint. The radiographic appearance of synovial chondrometaplasia, or synovial chondromatosis is characteristic (Fig. 14.42).

Simple removal of the multiple osteochondral loose bodies is inadequate, since more will form and therefore, in order to alleviate the condition, surgical synovectomy is required.

Pigmented Villonodular Synovitis

Definitely not a neoplasm, pigmented villonodular synovitis is probably a proliferative reaction to some type of inflammatory agent. This reaction, which is characterized by large numbers of giant cells, produces vil-

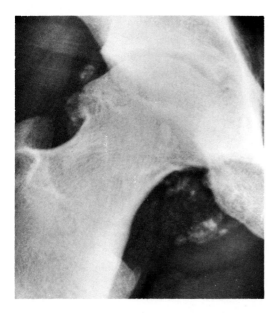

Figure 14.42. Synovial chondrometaplasia (synovial chondromatosis) in the hip joint of a 54-year-old man. Note the multiple radio-opaque loose bodies in the joint; each of these ossified bodies is encased in cartilage.

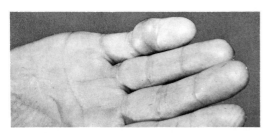

Figure 14.43. Pigmented villonodular synovitis in the flexor tendon sheath of the fifth finger in a 42-year-old woman; the nodular swelling was firm. This lesion, which is not a neoplasm, is sometimes referred to as a xanthoma, or giant cell tumor, of the tendon sheath.

lous and nodular masses that fuse together in the synovial membrane to form a single mass. Arthroscopy and biopsy through the arthoscope are of value in making the diagnosis. The pigment of pigmented villonodular synovitis is hemosiderin, which gives the lesion a yellowish color. Microscopically, these lesions contain lipid-filled histiocytes and giant cells.

Pigmented villonodular synovitis, which is relatively rare, occurs in adults and the knee is the commonest synovial joint affected; the lesion produces a bulky mass in the synovial membrane and may even erode bone. Involvement of the synovial sheath of tendons is most common in the flexor tendon sheaths of the hand where the lesion forms a solitary firm nodule (Fig. 14.43).

Pigmented villonodular synovitis, both in joints and in tendon sheaths, responds well to surgical excision of the involved area of synovial membrane. For diffuse and widespread intra-articular disease, however, extensive synovectomy is required.

Suggested Additional Reading

Aegerter, E. and Kirkpatric, J. A.: *Orthopaedic Diseases. Physiology, Pathology, Radiology*, 4th ed. Philadelphia, W.B. Saunders, 1975.

Bullimore, J. A. and Yeoman, P. M.: Modern concepts of the management of malignant bone tumours. In *Scientific Foundations of Orthopaedics and Traumatology*, edited by Owen, R., Goodfellow, J. and Bullough, P. London, William Heinemann Medical Books, 1980.

Cameron, H. U. and Kostuik, J. P.: Long-term follow-up of synovial sarcoma. J. Bone Joint Surg. 56B: 613–617, 1974.

Campbell, C. J.: Place of resection in management of primary bone tumours. Can. J. Surg. 20: 518–521, 1977.

Chang, P.: Progress in the treatment of osteosarcoma. Med. Clin. North Am. 61: 1027–1038, 1977.

Dahlin, D. C.: *Bone Tumours: General Aspects and Data on 6,221 Cases*, 3rd ed. Springfield, Ill., Charles C Thomas, 1978.

D'Aubigne, R. M. and Tomeno, B.: Treatment of giant cell tumours: analysis of 85 consecutive cases. Int. Orthop. 1: 159–164, 1977.

Enneking, W. F.: *Clinical Musculoskeletal Pathology*, 2nd ed. Gainesville, Fla., Storter Printing Co., 1977.

Enneking, W. F., Eady, J. L. and Burchardt, H.: Autogenous cortical bone grafts in reconstruction of segmental skeletal defects. J. Bone Joint Surg. 62A: 1039–1058, 1980.

Enneking, W. F., Spanier, S. S. and Goodman, M. A.: A system for the surgical grading of musculoskeletal sarcoma. Clin. Orthop. 153: 106–120, 1980.

Eriksson, A. I., Schiller, A. and Mankin, H. J.: The management of chondrosarcoma of bone. Clin. Orthop. 153: 44–66, 1980.

Graham-Pole, J.: Ewing's sarcoma: treatment with high dose radiation and adjuvant chemotherapy. Med. Pediatr. Oncol. 7: 1–8, 1979.

Harrington, K. D., Sim, F. H., Enis, J. E., Johnston, J. O., Dick, H. M. and Gristina, A. G.: Methylmethacrylate as adjunct in internal fixation of pathologic fractures: Experience with 375 cases. J. Bone Joint Surg. 58A: 1047–1055, 1976.

Huvos, A. G.: *Bone Tumours: Diagnosis, Treatment and Prognosis*. Philadelphia, W.B. Saunders, 1979.

Jenkin, R. D. T., Rider, W. D. and Sonley, M. J.: Ewing's sarcoma. Adjuvant total body irradiation, cyclophosphamide and vincristine. Int. J. Radiat. Oncol. Biol. Phys. 1: 407, 1976.

Johansson, J. E., Ajjoub, S., Coughlin, L. P., Wener, J. A. and Cruess, R. L.: Pigmented villonodular synovitis of joints. Clin. Orthop.. 163: 159–166, 1982.

Lichtenstein, L: *Bone Tumours*, 4th ed. St. Louis, C.V. Mosby, 1972.

Lisbona, R. and Rosenthal, L.: Role of radionuclide imaging in osteoid osteoma. Am. J. Roentgenol. 132: 77–80, 1979.

Luck, J. V. Jr., Luck, J. V. and Schwinn, C. P.: Parosteal osteosarcoma. A treatment-oriented study. Clin. Orthop. 153: 92–105, 1980.

Mankin, J. H.: Advances in diagnosis and treatment of bone tumours. N. Engl. J. Med. 300: 543–545, 1979.

Mankin, H. J., Cantley, K. P., Lippsiello, L. Schiller, A. L., and Campbell, C. J.: The biology of human chondrosarcoma. J. Bone Joint Surg. 62A: 160–194, 1980.

Mankin, H. J., Fogelson, F. S., Thrasher, A. Z. and Jaffe, F.: Massive resection and allograft transplantation in treatment of malignant bone tumours. N. Engl. J. Med. 294: 1247–1255, June 3, 1976.

Marcove, R. C.: En bloc resection for osteogenic sarcoma. Can. J. Surg. 20: 521–528, 1977.

Marcove, R. C. and Rosen, G.: Radical en bloc excision of Ewing's sarcoma. Clin. Orthop. 153: 86–91, 1980.

Miller, T. R.: Surgical management of malignant bone tumours. Am. J. Surg. 20:513–517, 1977.

Pritchard, D. J.: Indications for surgical treatment of localized Ewing's sarcoma of bone. Clin. Orthop. 153: 39–43, 1980.

Rosen, G.: Role of chemotherapy in the management of malignant bone tumours. In *Clinical Trends in Orthopaedics*, edited by Straub, L. R. and Wilson P. D. Jr. New York, Thieme-Stratton, 1982.

Rosen, G., Marcove, R. C., Caparros, B., Nirenberg, A., Kosloff, C. and Huvos, A. G.: Primary osteogenic sarcoma: Rationale for preoperative chemotherapy and delayed surgery. Cancer 43: 2163, 1979.

Salzer, M., Knahr, K., Kotz, R. and Salzer-Kuntschik, M.: Bone tumours—the role of comprehensive surgical management. In *Clinical Trends in Orthopaedics*, edited by Straub, L. R. and Wilson, P. D. Jr. New York, Thieme-Stratton, 1982.

Scaglietti, O., Marchetti, P. G. and Bartolozzi, P.: Final results obtained in the treatment of bone cysts with methylprednisalone acetate (depo-medrol) and a discussion of results obtained in other bone lesions. Clin. Orthop. 165: 34–42, 1982.

Schajowicz, F., Ackerman, L. V., and Sisson, H. A.: *International Histological Classification of Tumours, No. 6: Histological Typing of Bone Tumours*. World Health Organization, Geneva, 1972.

Smith, C. F. and Monsen, D. C. G.: Advances in bone tumours (editorial): Clin. Orthop. 153: 2–6, 1980.

Smith, F. W. and Gilday, D. L.: Scintigraphic appearances of osteoid osteoma. Radiology 137: 191–195, 1980.

Smith, R. J. and Mankin, H. J.: Allograft replacement of the distal radius for giant cell tumour. J. Hand Surg. 2: 299–309, 1977.

Swee, R. G., McLeod, R. A. and Beabout, J. W.: Osteoid osteoma: detection, diagnosis and localization. Radiology 130: 117–123, 1979.

Sweetnam, R.: Tumours of bone and soft tissues. In *The Basis and Practice of Orthopaedics*, edited by Hughes, S. and Sweetman, R. London, William Heinemann Medical Books Ltd., 1980.

Taylor, W. F., Ivins, J. C., Dahlin, D. C., Edmonson, J. H. and Pritchard, D. J.: Trends and variability in survival from osteosarcoma. Mayo Clin. Proc. 53: 695–700, 1978.

Tefft, M., Chabora, B. and Rosen, G.: Radiation in bone sarcomas: re-evaluation in the era of intensive systemic chemotherapy. Cancer 39: 806–816 (Suppl.), 1977.

Telander, R. L., Pairolero, P. C., Pirtchard, D. J., Sim, F. H. and Gilchrist, G. S.: Resection of pulmonary osteogenic sarcoma in children. Surgery 84: 335–341, 1978.

Unni, K. K.: Classification of bone tumours. Can. J. Surg. 20: 504–509, 1977.

Wallace, S., Chuang, V. P., Cohen, M. A., Zornoza, J., Benjamin, R. S., Jaffe, N., Murray, J. and Ayala, A.: Interventional radiology in skeletal lesions. In *Clinical Trends in Orthopaedics*, edited by Straub, L. R. and Wilson, P. D. Jr. New York, Thieme-Stratton, 1982.

Watts, H. G.: Introduction to resection of musculoskeletal sarcomas. Clin. Orthop. 153: 31–39, 1980.

PART 3

Musculoskeletal Injuries—General

"He who loves practice without theory is like a seafarer who boards a ship without wheel or compass and knows not whither he travels."
—LEONARDO DA VINCI (1495)

CHAPTER 15

Fractures and Joint Injuries—General Features

GENERAL INCIDENCE AND SIGNIFICANCE

The present age, which is characterized by increasing individual participation in high-speed travel, complex industry, competitive and recreational sports, might well be called the *age of injury*, or the *age of trauma*. The present incidence of injuries is disturbingly high—and continues to rise. Furthermore, of all the significant injuries that befall man, at least two-thirds involve the musculoskeletal system—fractures, dislocations and associated soft tissue injuries. Thus, musculoskeletal injuries have become increasingly common and important and will continue to be so throughout your professional life.

Although isolated musculoskeletal injuries in healthy individuals are seldom fatal, they are serious in that they cause much physical suffering, mental distress and loss of time for the victim; that is to say, they have a low mortality but a high morbidity. Multiple injuries involving other body systems as well, in a given individual, are even more serious since they endanger life as well as limb; that is, they have a high mortality as well as a high morbidity. Furthermore, as a result of our increasing life span, more persons are now reaching "old age," at which time decreasing coordination causes them to fall more frequently and senile weakening of their bones from osteoporosis renders them more susceptible to even minor injury. In this elderly age group, musculoskeletal injuries, particularly if treated by prolonged bed rest, may initiate a series of pathological processes that lead to the patient's progressive deterioration and even to his death.

The important *general features* of fractures, dislocations and soft tissue injuries are discussed in the present chapter in order that you will be better prepared to understand and appreciate the significance of the more common *specific* injuries in children and in adults as discussed in the subsequent two chapters. Indeed, your knowledge and understanding of the *general* features of musculoskeletal injuries, combined with your own good common sense, will enable you to deduce, and therefore to anticipate the appropriate methods of treatment for *specific* injuries under *specific* circumstances. As a medical student, you must learn much about musculoskeletal injuries including their *production*, *complications*, *diagno-*

sis, *healing process* and the *general principles and methods of their treatment*. At a later stage, during your intensive hospital training you will learn from your own clinical teachers of the specific *techniques* of the various methods of treatment through "live demonstrations," the most effective way to teach the *technical details* of treatment.

FRACTURES AND ASSOCIATED INJURIES

A *fracture*, whether of a bone, an epiphyseal plate or a cartilaginous joint surface, is simply a *structural break in its continuity*. Since bones are surrounded by soft tissue, however, the physical forces that produce a fracture, as well as the physical forces that result from sudden displacement of the fracture fragments, always produce some degree of soft tissue injury as well. When you think of a fracture, you quite naturally visualize a radiographic picture of a broken bone, since radiographs provide such graphic evidence of a fracture. Radiographs, however, seldom provide evidence of the extent of the associated soft tissue injury and consequently, you must constantly think in terms, not only of the fracture, but also of what has happened to the surrounding soft tissues. Indeed, under certain circumstances, the associated soft tissue injury, particularly if it involves brain, spinal cord, thoracic or abdominal viscera, a major artery or peripheral nerve, may assume much greater clinical significance than the fracture itself.

Physical Factors in the Production of Fractures

In order to understand *why* and *how* a bone breaks, you must appreciate the physical nature of bone itself, as well as the nature of the physical forces required to break it. Normal living bone, rather than being absolutely rigid, has a degree of elasticity and is capable of being bent slightly; it is more like wood in a living tree than it is like a non-living material such as a stick of chalk.

Cortical bone as a structure can withstand compression and shearing forces better than it can withstand tension forces and, in fact, the majority of fractures represent *tension failure* of bone in that bone is actually pulled apart, or torn apart by the tension forces of bending, twisting and straight pull. Thus, a bending (angulatory) force causes a long bone to bend slightly and then, if the force is sufficiently great, it suddenly causes an almost explosive tension failure of the bone on the *convex* side of the bend, a failure that usually then extends across the entire bone and produces either a *transverse* fracture or an *oblique* fracture (Fig. 15.1). In *young* children, cortical bone is like green wood in a living young tree; an angulatory force may produce tension failure on the convex side of the bend and only bending on the concave side of the *green-stick* fracture (Fig. 15.2). A twisting (torsional, rotational) force causes a spiralling type of tension failure in a long bone and produces a *spiral* fracture (Fig. 15.3). A sudden straight pulling (traction) force on a small bone (such as the patella) or part of a bone (such as the medial malleolus of the tibia) through at-

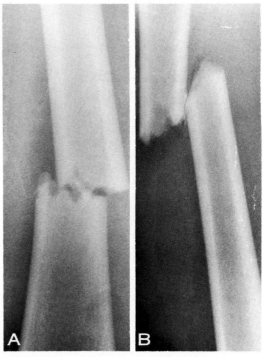

Figure 15.1. *A,* transverse fracture of the femoral shaft. *B,* oblique fracture of the femoral shaft.

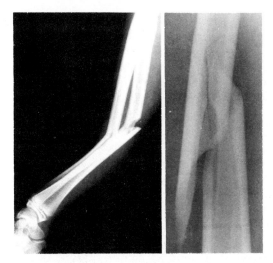

Figure 15.2 (*left*).   Green-stick fracture of the radius and ulna in a child.
Figure 15.3 (*right*).   Spiral fracture of the femoral shaft.

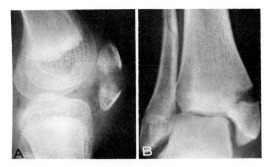

Figure 15.4.   Avulsion fractures. *A*, avulsion fracture of the patella which is a sesamoid bone in the quadriceps tendon; the fragments remain distracted because of quadriceps muscle pull. *B*, avulsion fracture of the medial malleolus which has been pulled off by the intact medial collateral ligament of the ankle at the time of a severe abduction, external rotation injury of the right ankle. Note also the slightly angulated fracture of the fibula and the lateral position of the talus. The attachment of normal ligaments to bone via Sharpey's fibers is so secure that the tendon does not pull out of bone; tension failure occurs either through the bone or through the ligament first.

tached ligaments or muscle attachments may also result in tension failure of bone and produce an *avulsion* fracture (Fig. 15.4).

Cancellous bone, having a sponge-like structure (spongiosa), is more susceptible to

crushing (compression) forces than is cortical bone and consequently, sudden compression may produce a *crush* fracture (*compression* fracture) in which one fracture surface is driven into, or *impacted* into its opposing fracture surface (Fig. 15.5). In young children a compression fracture may merely "buckle" the thin cortex surrounding the cancellous bone of the metaphysis and thereby produce a *buckle fracture*, sometimes referred to as a "torus fracture" (Fig. 15.6).

The causative force, producing a fracture may be a *direct injury*, or a blow to the bone by either a sharp, or a dull object which fractures the bone at the site of impact. More frequently the causative force is an *indirect injury* in which the initial force is transmitted indirectly through one or more joints to the involved bone which fractures at some distance from the site of impact.

Descriptive Terms Pertaining to Fractures

The infinite variety and varying significance of individual fractures necessitates the use of many qualifying terms, or adjectives, in order that a given fracture may be accurately described. These terms, as you

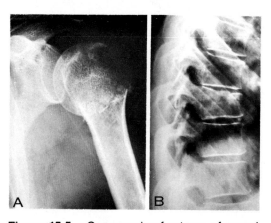

Figure 15.5.   Compression fractures of cancellous bone. *A*, compression fracture of the surgical neck of the humerus in an elderly adult. Note the impaction of the fracture on the medial side. *B*, compression fracture of a vertebral body in the mid-thoracic region of an adult. The vertebral body has lost height and has become wedge-shaped as a result of being compressed.

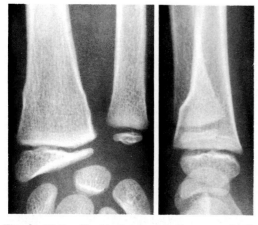

Figure 15.6. Buckle fracture in the metaphysis of the radius of a 7-year-old boy. The thin cortex has become buckled but not completely broken; in this child, the buckle fracture is more obvious in the lateral projection than in the anteroposterior projection.

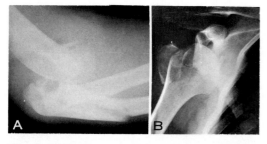

Figure 15.7. Fracture-dislocations. *A*, fracture-dislocation of the elbow in an adult. Note the fracture of the shaft of the ulna and the neck of the radius as well as the dislocation of the elbow joint. *B*, fracture-dislocation of the right shoulder in an adult. Note the fracture of the greater tuberosity of the humerus and the dislocation of the humeral head in relation to the glenoid cavity.

will see, are of great practical importance clinically since they indicate not only the nature of the clinical problem, but also the general type of treatment that will be required. Thus, a fracture is described according to its *site*, *extent*, *configuration*, the *relationship of the fracture fragments to each other*, *the relationship of the fracture to the external environment* and finally, *the presence or absence of complications*.

1. *Site*. A fracture may be *diaphyseal*, *metaphyseal*, *epiphyseal* or *intra-articular*; if

associated with a dislocation of the adjacent joint it is a fracture-dislocation (Fig. 15.7).

2. *Extent*. A fracture may be *complete*, or it may be *incomplete*. Incomplete fractures include *crack*, or *hairline* fractures (Fig. 15.8), *buckle* fractures (Fig. 15.6) and *greenstick* fractures (Fig. 15.2).

3. *Configuration*. A fracture may be *transverse*, *oblique* (Fig. 15.1) or *spiral* (Fig. 15.3). When there is more than one fracture line, and therefore, more than two fragments, it is a *comminuted* fracture (Fig. 15.9).

4. *Relationship of the Fracture Fragments to Each Other*. A fracture may be *undisplaced*, or it may be *displaced*, in which case, the fracture fragments may be displaced in one or more of the six following ways: (1) *shifted sideways*; (2) *angulated*; (3) *rotated*; (4) *distracted*; (5) *overriding*; (6) *impacted*. At the time the bone is fractured, the causative force usually "follows through" and consequently the degree of displacement of the fragments is maximal at

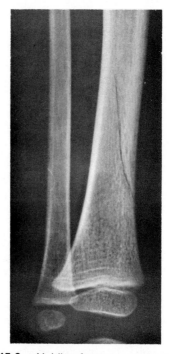

Figure 15.8. Hairline fracture, or crack fracture in the distal third of the tibia in a child. Since there is no displacement, the fracture line is apparent in only one projection.

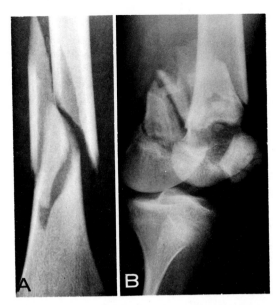

Figure 15.9. Comminuted fractures. A, comminuted fracture of the shaft of the femur in a child. There are 2 fracture lines and hence 3 fragments; because of its shape, the 3rd fragment in this type of comminuted fracture is referred to as a "butterfly fragment." B, severely comminuted fracture of the distal end of the femur in a young adult who had fallen from a 5th story window. The tremendous force of the impact has shattered the bone into many fragments. Note also in this oblique projection the comminuted fracture of the patella.

that precise moment. An immediate "recoil" of the surrounding soft tissues, including periosteum, reduces the displacement to some extent; furthermore, the efforts of attendants to "straighten the crooked limb" may further reduce the displacement at the fracture site before you see the patient. The relationship of the fracture fragments is also dependent on the effects of gravity, as well as on the effects of muscle pull on the fragments; these factors are of considerable importance in relation to the treatment of fractures as you will see later.

5. *Relationship of the Fracture to the External Environment.* A *closed* fracture is one in which the covering skin is intact. By contrast, an *open* fracture is one which has communicated with the external environment, either because a fracture fragment has penetrated the skin *from within* or because a sharp object has penetrated the skin to fracture the bone *from without* (Fig. 15.10). Open fractures, of course, carry the serious risk of becoming complicated by infection. Closed fractures were formerly referred to as "simple" and open fractures as "compound"; the terms, *closed* and *open*, however, are more accurate and are therefore preferable.

6. *Complications.* A fracture may be *uncomplicated* and remain uncomplicated; or it may either be *complicated* or become complicated. The complication may be local or systemic and it may be related either to the original injury or to its treatment.

Associated Injury to the Periosteum

Since the periosteum is an *osteogenic* sleeve surrounding bone, it is an important structure in relation to fracture healing. The periosteum is thicker, stronger and more osteogenic during the growing years of

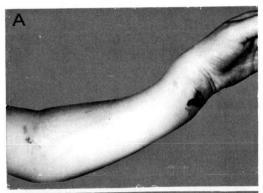

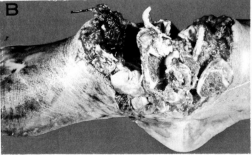

Figure 15.10. Open fractures. A, open fracture of the ulna; a sharp fracture fragment has penetrated the skin *from within*. B, open fractures of the foot; the blades of a hay mower have penetrated the skin *from without* and have produced multiple fractures.

childhood than it is in adult life. In all ages it is thicker over portions of bone that are surrounded by muscle (such as the diaphysis, or shaft of the femur) than it is over portions of bone that lie subcutaneously (such as the anteromedial surface of the tibia or portions of bone that lie within synovial joints, such as the neck of the femur).

The periosteum, being a close-fitting sleeve, is certain to be injured at the moment a bone fractures. In young children the thick periosteum is easily separated from the underlying bone and is not readily torn across; whereas in adults the thin periosteum is more firmly adherent to bone, is less easily separated and is more readily torn across. Except in severely displaced fractures in older children and adults, the periosteal sleeve usually remains intact on at least one side and this portion is referred to as the *intact periosteal hinge* (Fig. 15.11). If the periosteal sleeve is intact around most of its circumference, it can be used to advantage in *reducing* the fracture as well as in *maintaining* the reduction; furthermore, it serves as a relatively intact osteogenic sleeve across the fracture site and aids fracture healing. By contrast, a periosteal sleeve that is torn around most of its circumference is

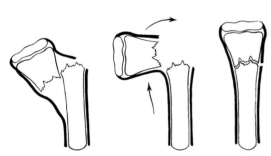

Figure 15.11. The intact periosteal hinge. In the left drawing the periosteum is intact on the concave side of the angulatory fracture deformity but is torn on the convex side. The middle drawing demonstrates how this type of fracture should be reduced; the fracture deformity is first increased after which the distal fragment is moved distally and only then is it possible to engage the fracture surfaces and correct the angulation. The right drawing shows how the intact periosteal hinge helps to prevent overcorrection of the deformity and helps to maintain the reduction of the fracture.

of little help in reducing the fracture, of little help in maintaining the reduction, and is ineffective as an aid to fracture healing.

These facts concerning the periosteum help to explain why fractures heal more rapidly and more certainly in childhood than in adult life; why relatively undisplaced fractures heal more rapidly than severely displaced fractures; and why fractures of some bones heal more rapidly than fractures of other bones at any age.

The Diagnosis of Fractures and Associated Injuries

Usually when a patient sustains a fracture, both he and those who bring him to you are well aware that he has "broken a bone." Under certain circumstances, however, the diagnosis is not at all apparent and careful investigation is necessary lest you make the serious error of allowing a fracture to go unrecognized. This is particularly true when the patient is unable to communicate clearly because of infancy, language barrier, unconsciousness, or mental confusion. Likewise, the fracture may not be obvious when it is either undisplaced, or is impacted and is consequently stable. Furthermore, even when the diagnosis of a fracture is obvious, you must be diligent in diagnosis lest you overlook an associated soft tissue injury, a visceral injury, a coexistent dislocation or even a second fracture (Fig. 15.12). Thus, methods of obtaining data (clues)—the investigation—as outlined in Chapter 5 are as important in the exact diagnosis of musculoskeletal injuries as in the diagnosis of other musculoskeletal conditions.

THE PATIENTS' HISTORY

The history of a fall, a twisting injury, a direct blow, or a road accident may be given but frequently the exact details of the *mechanism* of injury are lacking simply because "it all happened so suddenly." In addition one patient may suffer a severe injury without a fracture, while another may suffer a seemingly minor injury and sustain a significant fracture. The common symptoms of fracture are *localized pain*, which is aggravated by movement, and *decreased function*

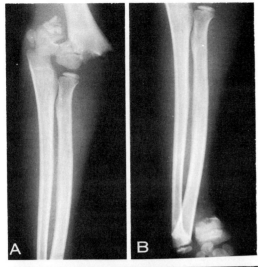

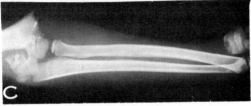

Figure 15.12. The danger of overlooking a second fracture. *A*, if your physical examination revealed an obvious fracture of the elbow and you failed to examine the wrist, you might obtain this radiograph, which demonstrates a severe supracondylar fracture of the humerus. *B*, if your physical examination revealed an obvious fracture of the wrist and you failed to examine the elbow, you might request this radiograph, which demonstrates a displaced fracture of the radius and an undisplaced fracture of the ulna. *C*, careful physical examination would have led you to obtain this radiograph, which provides clear evidence of all three fractures.

of the involved part. The patient may even have "heard the bone break" or may "feel the ends of the bone grating" (*crepitus*).

Not all fractures are equally painful or interfere equally with function; these manifestations are most severe when the fracture is unstable. Thus, when a patient has sustained a stable fracture of one bone in addition to an unstable fracture of another bone, the severe pain of the unstable fracture may mask the mild pain of the stable fracture initially until the more severe pain subsides as a result of treatment.

PHYSICAL EXAMINATION

By first *looking* (inspection), you will observe the evidence of pain in the patient's facial expression and also the way in which he is protecting the injured part. Local inspection may reveal *swelling* (unless the fractured bone is deep in the tissues, as in the neck of the femur or a vertebral body), *deformity* (angulation, rotation, shortening), or *abnormal movement* (occurring at the fracture site) (Fig. 15.13). Discoloration of the skin by subcutaneous extravasation of blood (*ecchymosis*) usually is apparent only after a few days (Fig. 15.14). By *feeling* (palpation) you will detect marked and *sharply localized tenderness* at the site of fracture as well as *aggravation of pain* and *muscle spasm* during even slight passive

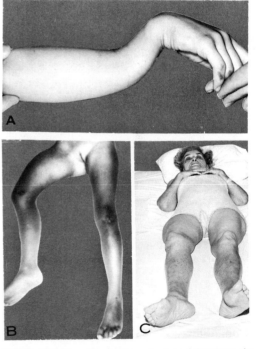

Figure 15.13. Examples of clinical fracture deformities. *A*, angulation deformity in the right forearm of a child with a green-stick fracture of the radius and ulna. *B*, angulation, external rotation and shortening deformities in the right thigh of a child with a completely displaced and overriding fracture of the femoral shaft. *C*, external rotation deformity of the entire right lower limb of an elderly lady with a displaced fracture of the femoral neck.

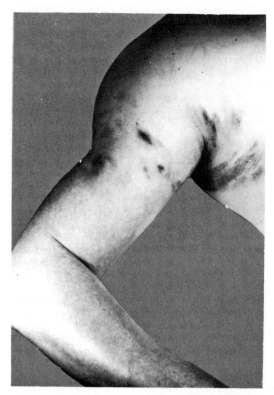

Figure 15.14. Ecchymosis in the skin of the axilla and upper arm of an adult 3 days after he had sustained a fracture-dislocation of the right shoulder. The hematoma in the deep tissues has gradually spread into the subcutaneous tissues.

movement of the injured part. Feeling for the grating of bone ends (crepitus) is neither necessary nor kind. You should always look and feel for other less apparent injuries not only in the same limb, but also elsewhere, bearing in mind that there may be more than one injury. Many fractures escape detection because of an inadequate physical examination which, in turn, results in failure to obtain the appropriate radiographic examination.

Physical examination must always include a careful assessment of the patient's general condition as well as a diligent search for any associated injuries to brain, spinal cord, peripheral nerves, major vessels, skin, thoracic and abdominal viscera.

RADIOGRAPHIC EXAMINATION

The presence of a fracture can usually be suspected and often established by physical

examination alone but radiographic examination is required to determine the exact nature and extent of the fracture.

In order to avoid causing the patient unnecessary pain, as well as further soft tissue injury, you should provide him with some type of radiolucent splint for immobilization before he is subjected to radiographic examination. The radiographic film should include the entire length of the injured bone and the joints at each end (Fig. 15.15). At least two projections at right angles to each other (*anteroposterior* and *lateral*) are essential for accurate diagnosis (Fig. 15.16). For certain fractures, particularly those of small bones and the vertebrae, special *oblique* projections are often required (Fig. 15.17).

For fractures of the spine and pelvis that may be difficult to visualize by conventional radiography, computed tomography (CT) scans can provide useful additional data (Fig. 15.18).

The radiographic features of a given fracture should provide you with a three-dimensional concept of where the fragments lie in relation to each other, and also how they came to be in that position (the mechanism of injury). As mentioned previously however, the fragments, at the precise moment that the fracture occurred, would have been more widely displaced than at the time of the radiographic examination.

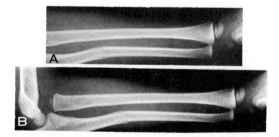

Figure 15.15. The importance of including the entire length of the fractured bone and the joints at each end in the radiographic examination. *A*, this inadequate radiographic examination reveals only an angulated fracture of the ulna. *B*, this radiograph reveals, in addition to the fracture of the ulna, a complete anterior dislocation of the proximal end of the radius in relation to the capitellum. (The combination is known as a Monteggia fracture-dislocation.)

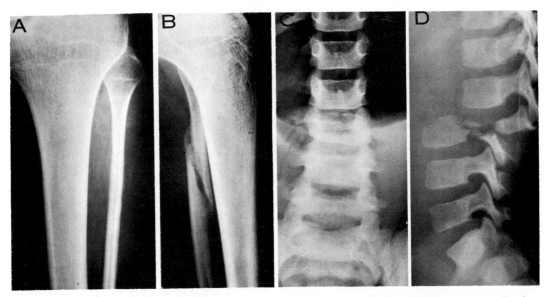

Figure 15.16. The importance of at least two radiographic projections at right angles to each other (anteroposterior and lateral). *A*, the anteroposterior projection reveals little evidence of disturbance of the tibia or fibula. The oblique fracture of the fibula, however, is obvious in the lateral projection (*B*). *C*, the anteroposterior projection of this severely injured boy reveals relatively little evidence of disturbance of the spine. The radiolucent area across the top half of this radiograph represents gas in a dilated stomach (acute gastric dilatation). The lateral projection (*D*), however, reveals a severe fracture-dislocation of the lumbar spine.

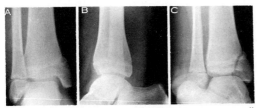

Figure 15.17. The importance of oblique radiographic projections. *A*, in the anteroposterior projection there is only slight evidence of a fracture of the medial malleolus. *B*, the lateral projection reveals no evidence of a fracture. *C*, this oblique projection clearly demonstrates a displaced intra-articular fracture of the medial malleolus and disruption of the joint surface as well as of the epiphyseal plate.

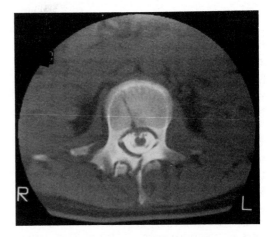

Figure 15.18. Computed tomography (CT) scan of the first lumbar vertebra of a young adult who had sustained a spinal injury from an automobile accident (a cross-sectional "slice" of the spine at this level as viewed from below). Note the fractures of the vertebral body, the lamina (in the midline) and the right transverse process (on the left of the computed tomograph). The fractures of the vertebral body and lamina were not readily detectable in the conventional anteroposterior and lateral radiographs.

When definite physical signs of a fracture are not confirmed even by additional radiographic projections, you would be wise to treat the patient as though a fracture were present since an undisplaced fracture, which may not be radiographically apparent at first, may become so after one or two weeks as a result of the healing process (Fig. 15.19).

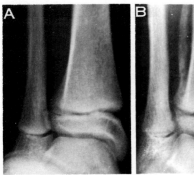
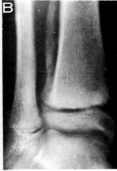

Figure 15.19. Late evidence of a fracture. *A*, the ankle of a 10-year-old boy on the day of injury. He was thought to have a sprained ankle and there is no radiographic evidence of a fracture. *B*, the same boy's ankle 2 weeks later reveals subperiosteal new bone formation along the lateral aspect of the tibia and this provides late evidence that the original injury was a fracture-separation of the distal tibial epiphysis with spontaneous reduction rather than a sprain.

The Normal Healing of Fractures

The normal healing of a fracture is a fascinating biological process, particularly when you realize that a *fractured bone*, unlike any other tissue that has been torn or divided, is capable of healing *without a scar*, i.e. of healing by *bone* rather than by fibrous tissue. An understanding of the response of living bone and periosteum during the healing of a fracture is pivotal in your appreciation of how fractures should be treated. While mechanical factors of treatment (such as physical immobilization of the fracture fragments) are very important for healing in certain types of fractures, the biological factors are *absolutely essential* to healing and must always be respected lest you make the error of treating fractures merely as a mechanic or as a carpenter, or of "treating the X-ray picture" at the risk of interfering seriously with the normal biological phenomenon of healing. Fractures are wounds of bone and as with all wounds, treatment must be designed to cooperate with the natural laws of biological healing.

The process of fracture healing is quite different in the dense cortical bone of the shaft of a long bone from the process of healing in the spongy cancellous bone of the metaphysis of a long bone or of the body of a short bone, as you might expect from looking at a cross-section of these two types of bony architecture (Fig. 15.20). These two types of fracture healing, therefore, will be considered separately.

HEALING OF A FRACTURE IN CORTICAL BONE (DIAPHYSEAL BONE)(TUBULAR BONE)

Initial Effects of the Fracture

At the moment of fracture in the shaft of a long bone, the tiny blood vessels coursing through the canaliculi in the Haversian systems are torn across at the fracture site. After a brief period of local internal bleeding, normal clotting occurs in these tiny vessels and extends for a short distance from the fracture site (to intact anastomosing vessels within bone). Thus the osteocytes in their lacunae for a distance of a few millimeters from the fracture site lose their blood supply and die; consequently there is always a "ring" of avascular, dead bone at each fracture surface shortly after the injury. These segments of dead bone are eventually replaced by living bone through the simultaneous process of bone resorption and new bone deposition, but it is obvious that initially the two surfaces of dead bone cannot contribute to the early stages of fracture healing.

In a relatively undisplaced fracture of a

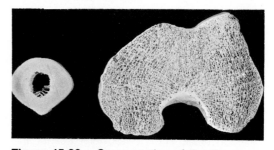

Figure 15.20. Cross-section of the dense cortical bone of the mid-shaft of an adult femur (*left*) and of the trabeculated sponge-like cancellous bone of the distal metaphyseal region of the same femur. You would expect that fracture healing would differ in these 2 completely different types of bony architecture.

long bone, most of the internal bleeding in and around the fresh fracture site comes from the torn nutrient artery or its branches and from the vessels of the periosteal sleeve so that the resultant *fracture hematoma* is well localized around the bone ends. When the fracture site has been severely displaced, however, and the periosteal sleeve severely disrupted, larger arteries in the surrounding muscle and fat are also torn with a resultant massive hematoma that spreads throughout the surrounding soft tissues.

Early Stages of Healing from Soft Tissues

The fracture hematoma is the medium in which the early stages of healing take place through the reactions of the *soft tissues around the fracture.* The "repair cells" of fracture healing are osteogenic cells which proliferate from the periosteum to form an *external callus*, and to a lesser extent from endosteum to form an *internal callus.* When the periosteum is severely torn, the healing cells must differentiate from the ingrowth of undifferentiated mesenchymal cells in the surrounding soft tissues. During the early stages of fracture healing, a "population explosion" of osteogenic cells results in an extremely rapid growth of osteogenic tissue, more rapid indeed than the rate of growth of the most malignant bone neoplasm. Indeed, by the end of the first few weeks, the *fracture callus* consists of a thick enveloping mass of osteogenic tissue.

At this stage the callus does not contain bone and therefore is radiolucent and not apparent radiographically. The fracture callus, initially soft and almost fluid in consistency, becomes progressively firmer like a slowly setting glue with the result that the fracture site becomes progressively "stickier" and less mobile. Histologically this stage of callus maturation is characterized by new bone formation in the osteogenic callus, first at a site away from the fracture (where the periosteum still has a good blood supply and where there is least movement). You will recall from Chapter 2 that whenever new bone is formed rapidly, it is the *primary woven type of bone*—and early fracture healing is a good example of this phenome-non. Thus, the osteogenic cells differentiate into osteoblasts, and primary woven bone is formed. Closer to the fracture site, where the blood supply is less adequate and where more movement is taking place, the osteogenic cells differentiate into chondroblasts and, therefore, cartilage is formed initially.

Stage of Clinical Union

A temporary external and internal callus, consisting of a mixture of primary woven bone and cartilage, comes to surround the fracture site forming a "biological glue" that gradually hardens as the cartilaginous components of the callus are replaced by bone through a process of endochrondral ossification. When fracture callus becomes sufficiently firm that movement no longer occurs at the fracture site, the fracture is said to be "clinically" united (*clinical union*), but it has by no means been restored to its original strength at this time. Radiographic examination reveals evidence of bone in the callus but the fracture line is still apparent. Histological examination at this stage reveals varying amounts of primary woven bone, as well as cartilage undergoing endochondral ossification.

Stage of Consolidation (Radiographic Union)

As time goes on the primary, or temporary callus, is gradually replaced by mature lamellar bone and the excess callus is gradually resorbed. Many months after the fracture, when all the immature bone and cartilage of the temporary callus have been replaced by mature lamellar bone, the fracture is said to be *consolidated* by sound bony union (*radiographic union*). Once bony union has been established, the now redundant mass of callus is gradually resorbed and the bone eventually returns to almost its normal diameter. Sharp corners of residual angulation, displacement, or overriding become smoothed off or remodeled by the process of simultaneous bone deposition and bone resorption—another example of *Wolff's law* (previously described in Chapter 2). Although the corners of a residual angulation deformity become rounded off, the actual

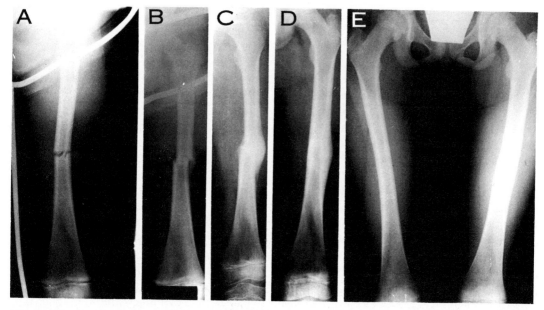

Figure 15.21. The stages of fracture healing in cortical bone. *A*, the day of injury a transverse fracture is seen in the mid-shaft of the left femur of this 8-year-old girl. The fracture has been aligned by means of continuous traction and a Thomas splint (part of which is seen in this radiograph). *B*, two weeks after injury callus, which is evident on the lateral aspect of the fracture, has "glued" the fragments together. At this stage the fracture was clinically "sticky" and, consequently, continuous traction was replaced by a hip spica cast. *C*, eight weeks after injury, callus is abundant and the fracture line is barely apparent. Clinical examination at this stage revealed no movement at the fracture site and no pain on attempting to move it. Thus the fracture had healed to the stage of clinical union. The cast was removed and full weight bearing was allowed. *D*, six months after injury the excess callus has been resorbed, the medullary cavity has been re-established and fracture healing has reached the stage of radiographic consolidation. *E*, eighteen months after injury the fractured femur has returned almost to its normal shape through the process of remodeling, which is an example of Wolff's law.

change in alignment tends to persist except under certain circumstances during childhood when subsequent epiphyseal growth may partially correct it spontaneously.

The various stages of fracture healing in cortical bone are illustrated in a series of radiographs of a diaphyseal (shaft) fracture (Fig. 15.21).

HEALING OF A FRACTURE IN CORTICAL BONE WITH RIGID INTERNAL FIXATION

When a fracture in cortical bone has been accurately reduced at open operation and when the fracture fragments have been compressed together and then held by rigid internal fixation by metallic devices, the fracture site is "stress protected" and indeed the bone hardly knows it has been fractured.

The AO/ASIF system of fracture treatment (which is described in a subsequent section of this chapter) achieves such reduction and fixation. Under these circumstances there is no stimulus for the production of either external callus from the periosteum or internal callus from the endosteum and consequently the fracture healing occurs directly between the cortex of one fracture fragment and the cortex of the other fracture fragment. This process is referred to by the AO/ASIF fracture surgeons as "primary" bone healing as opposed to the "secondary" bone healing involving external and internal fracture callus. In the areas of precise contact (that are under compression) osteoclastic "cutter heads" cross the microscopic fracture site and are followed by new bridging osteons. Even when there is a tiny gap,

the healing is direct by the formation of new osteons that become oriented through Haversian remodeling to the axis of the bone.

As long as the metallic device, such as a rigid plate, remains in place the bone underlying the plate continues to be "stress protected" since the normal stresses bypass the bone through the plate. Thus the bone in this region tends to develop disuse osteoporosis which is sometimes referred to as "stress-relief osteoporosis." For this reason, when the fracture has united, the plate and screws must be removed to allow reversal of this osteoporosis. During the ensuing few months the healed bone must be protected from excessive stress until it regains its normal strength.

HEALING OF A FRACTURE IN CANCELLOUS BONE (METAPHYSEAL BONE AND CUBOIDAL BONES)

Cancellous bone (sponge bone) in the flared out metaphysis of long bones and in the bodies of short bones, as well as in the flat bones such as the pelvis and ribs, consists of a sponge-like lattice of delicate interconnected trabeculae. The surrounding cortex, which is a relatively thin shell of cortical bone, represents only a small fraction of the cross-sectional area of these bones in contrast to the shafts of long bones, which may be considered as hollow tubes with thick walls of dense cortical bone (Fig. 15.20). Just as the structural arrangement of these two types of bone differs, so also does the process of healing after a fracture.

The healing of a fracture in cancellous bone occurs principally through the formation of an *internal* or *endosteal* callus, although the external or periosteal callus surrounding the thin shell of cortex does play an important role, particularly in children. Because of the rich blood supply to the thin trabeculae of cancellous bone, little necrosis of bone occurs at the fracture surfaces, and furthermore there is a large area of bony contact at the fracture site. Therefore, in relatively undisplaced fractures and also in well reduced fractures through cancellous bone, union of the fragments proceeds more rapidly than it does in dense cortical bone. The osteogenic "repair cells" of the endosteal covering of trabeculae proliferate to form primary woven bone in the internal fracture hematoma. The resultant *internal callus* readily fills the open spaces of the spongy cancellous fracture surfaces and rapidly spreads across the fracture site wherever there is good contact.

Thus, early fracture healing in cancellous bone occurs at sites of direct contact between the cancellous fracture surfaces by means of endosteal callus; but once union is established at a point of contact, the fracture is "clinically" united and union spreads across the entire width of the bone. Subsequently the woven bone is replaced by lamellar bone as the fracture becomes *consolidated*; eventually the trabecular pattern is re-established by "internal" remodeling of bone. You will recall that cancellous bone, unlike cortical bone, is particularly susceptible to compression forces which result in a compression, or crush type, of fracture. Impaction of cancellous fragments provides a broad surface contact for fracture healing. However, if the crushed surfaces are pulled apart (during reduction of the fracture), a space, or gap, is created, healing is delayed, and indeed, there may be subsequent collapse at the fracture site before bony union is consolidated.

The various stages of fracture healing in cancellous bone are illustrated in a series of radiographs of a metaphyseal fracture (Fig. 15.22).

HEALING OF A FRACTURE IN ARTICULAR CARTILAGE

In contrast to bone, the hyaline cartilage of joint surfaces is extremely limited in its ability to either heal or regenerate. Whereas a fracture through bone normally heals by bone, a fracture through articular cartilage either heals by fibrous scar tissue or fails to heal at all. If the fracture surfaces of the cartilage are perfectly reduced, the thin scar leads to local degenerative arthritis. If there is a gap, however, the fibrous tissue that comes to fill this gap will not withstand the normal wear and tear of joint function and

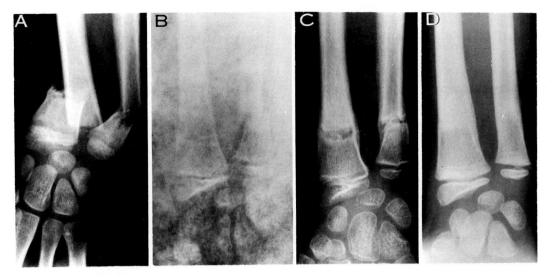

Figure 15.22.   The stages of fracture healing in cancellous bone. *A*, the day of injury a transverse, angulated overriding fracture of the metaphyseal region of the distal end of the radius and an angulated green-stick fracture of the same region of the ulna are seen in this radiograph of the wrist of a 10-year-old boy. *B*, the same day the post-reduction radiograph (taken through the plaster cast) reveals satisfactory reduction of both fractures. *C*, six weeks after injury, endosteal callus and periosteal callus are adequate although the fracture lines are still apparent. At this stage there was no movement at the fracture site and no pain on attempts to move it. This is the stage of clinical union and hence immobilization was discontinued. *D*, six months after injury radiographic examination reveals obliteration of the fracture line; the fracture healing has reached the stage of radiographic consolidation. Internal and external remodeling of bone at the fracture sites are also apparent. Note the amount of longitudinal bone growth that has taken place from the epiphyseal plates since the injury (the distance between the epiphyseal plate and the fine radio-opaque line just proximal to it).

more widespread degenerative changes ensue. Furthermore, any irregularity, such as a "step" in the fractured joint surface produces joint incongruity that leads inevitably to degenerative arthritis (Fig. 15.23).

We have investigated the biological effects of immobilization (cast), intermittent active motion (cage activity) and continuous passive motion (CPM) on the healing of the cartilage in an experimental model of an intra-articular fracture in the rabbit. The accurate reduction of the fracture was maintained by a metal screw. At four weeks postoperatively we found that in the casted knees the fracture in the cartilage had not healed by cartilage in any of the knees; it had healed by cartilage in only 20% of the cage activity group compared to 80% of the CPM group (Fig. 15.24). We then conducted a long term study at six months in another series of rabbits in which after a one- or three-week period of post-operative man-

agement by one of the three aforementioned methods, the animals were allowed to run freely for the remaining six months. From this investigation we found that degenerative arthritis had developed in 90% of the knees managed post-operatively by immobilization for one or three weeks, in 76% of the knees managed by cage activity throughout the six months compared to only 20% of the knees managed post-operatively by either one or three weeks of CPM. These experimental investigations are relevant to the immediate post-operative management of patients with intra-articular fractures after open reduction and internal fixation.

HEALING OF A FRACTURE INVOLVING THE EPIPHYSEAL PLATE

The inclusion of an epiphyseal plate in a fracture alters the picture of fracture healing considerably and adds the risk of local growth disturbance. The normal healing of

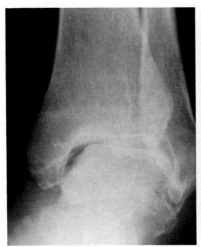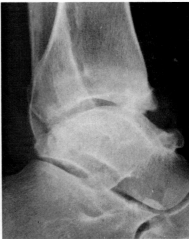

Figure 15.23.   Post-traumatic degenerative joint disease in the ankle of a 57-year-old man whose original ankle injury had occurred 25 years previously. Note the incongruity of the joint surfaces, subchondral sclerosis and osteophyte formation.

fractures that involve the epiphyseal plate is discussed, along with other important aspects of these special injuries of childhood, in Chapter 16.

THE TIME REQUIRED FOR UNCOMPLICATED FRACTURE HEALING

The healing time of fractures is extremely varied and yet, in relation to a given fracture in a given individual, it is possible to estimate the healing time by considering the following important factors: age of the patient, site and configuration of the fracture, initial displacement, and the blood supply to the fracture fragments.

1. Age of the Patient

The rate of healing in *bone* varies much more with age than it does in any other tissue in the body, particularly during childhood. At birth, fracture healing is remarkably rapid, but it becomes progressively less rapid with each year of childhood. From early adult life to old age, however, the rate of fracture healing remains relatively constant. It would seem that the rate of healing in bone is closely related to the osteogenic activity of periosteum and endosteum, which, in turn is related to the normal process of remodeling of bone, a process that is remarkably active at birth, becomes progressively less active with each year of child-

hood and remains relatively constant from early adult life to old age. Fractures of the shaft of the femur serve as a reasonable example of this phenomenon: a femoral shaft fracture occurring at birth will be united in three weeks; a comparable fracture at the age of eight years will be united in eight weeks; at the age of twelve years it will be united in twelve weeks; and from the age of twenty years to old age it will be united in approximately twenty weeks.

2. Site and Configuration of the Fracture

Fractures through bones that are surrounded by muscle heal more rapidly than fractures through portions of bones that lie subcutaneously or within joints. Fractures through cancellous bone heal more rapidly than fractures through cortical bone; epiphyseal separations heal approximately twice as rapidly as cancellous metaphyseal fractures of the same bone in the same age group. Long oblique fractures and spiral fractures of the shaft, having a large fracture surface, heal more readily than transverse fractures.

3. Initial Displacement of the Fracture

Undisplaced fractures, having an intact periosteal sleeve, heal approximately twice as rapidly as displaced fractures. The

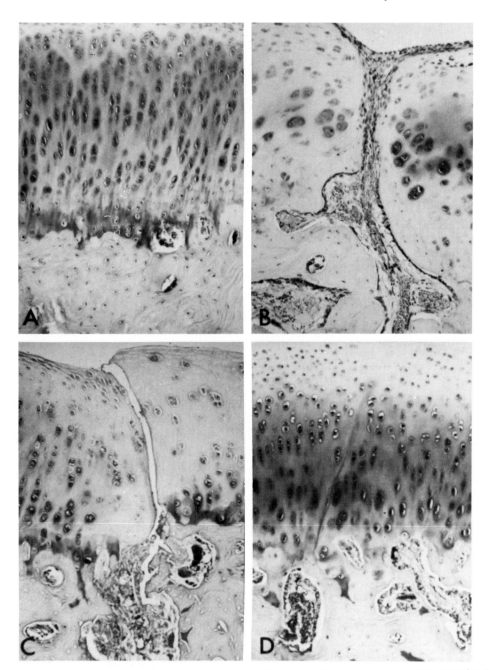

Figure 15.24. Photomicrograph of the experimental fracture site in articular cartilage (safranin O stain). *A*, normal intact articular cartilage of the femoral condyle of a rabbit. *B*, after four weeks of cast immobilization the fracture in the cartilage has healed by fibrous scar tissue. *C*, after four weeks of cage activity the fracture has failed to heal. *D*, after four weeks of continuous passive motion (CPM) the fracture in the cartilage has healed well by cartilage.

greater the initial displacement, the more extensive is the tearing of the periosteal sleeve and consequently, the more prolonged is the healing time of the fracture.

4. Blood Supply to the Fragments

If both fracture fragments have a good blood supply and are therefore alive, the fracture will heal provided there are no other complications. If, however, one fragment has lost its blood supply and is therefore dead, the living fragment must become united, or fused, to the dead fragment in the same manner as living bone in a host site becomes united, or fused to a dead bone graft; union will be slow and rigid immobilization of the fracture will be required. If both fragments are avascular, bony union cannot occur until they are revascularized, despite rigid immobilization of the fracture.

ASSESSMENT OF FRACTURE HEALING IN PATIENTS

The state of union of a fracture is assessed by both clinical and radiographic examination. The clinical examination for union consists of applying bending, twisting and compression forces to the fracture to determine the presence, or absence, of movement (Fig. 15.25). If there is considerable movement at the fracture site, both you and the patient will see it as well as feel it; if, however, there is only minimal movement, the patient alone will feel it because it is painful. Thus, if neither you nor the patient

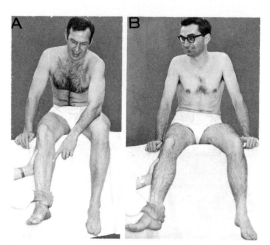

Figure 15.25. Clinical assessment of fracture healing in patients. *A*, bending and twisting forces applied to this man's leg produce only minimal movement at the fracture site but cause the patient local pain as he is indicating. His fracture is not yet clinically united. *B*, bending and twisting forces applied to this man's leg produce neither movement nor pain at the fracture site. Therefore, his fracture is clinically united.

is able to detect movement at the fracture site, the fracture is *clinically united*.

At the time of *clinical union*, radiographic examination reveals evidence of bony callus, but the fracture line is still apparent since clinical union precedes radiographic consolidation (Figs. 15.21, 22). At this stage immobilization is no longer required, but the healing bone has not regained its normal strength; consequently, it must still be protected from undue stress until *radiographic consolidation* has been achieved as evidenced by a bony callus that completely bridges the fracture and obliterates the fracture line (Figs. 15.21, 22). The re-establishment of the medullary cavity in shaft fractures and the re-establishment of trabeculae across fractures in cancellous bone are radiographic evidence of the *remodeling phase* of united fractures.

Abnormal Healing of Fractures

The healing of a given fracture may be *abnormal* in one of three different ways:

1. The fracture may heal in the normally expected time but in an unsatisfactory position with residual bony deformity (*mal-union*).

2. The fracture may heal eventually but it takes considerably longer than the normally expected time to do so (*delayed union*).

3. The fracture may fail completely to heal by bone (*non-union*) with resultant formation of either a *fibrous union* or a false joint (*pseudarthrosis*).

Mal-union, delayed union and non-union are discussed further in this chapter in the section that deals with the recognition and treatment of the complications of fractures.

Complications of Fractures

Fortunately the majority of fractures are uncomplicated either by any serious associated injury or by any serious reaction to injury. Consequently, with reasonable treatment the injured patient may be expected to make a full recovery from his fracture without any significant disability. By contrast, however, some fractures are either accompanied or followed by *complications*, some of which have serious local consequences, others of which endanger not only limb but even life itself.

Before proceeding to a discussion of the general principles of fracture treatment, you should be aware of the possible complications of fractures lest you make the error of focusing all your attention on the fractured bone alone and thereby of overlooking an associated complication. A fracture in a given patient may be complicated *initially* by an associated injury, or it may become complicated subsequently, either *early* or *late*. The complication may be *local* at the fracture site, or it may be *remote* in other organs. Furthermore, the complication may be caused by the original injury or it may be *iatrogenic* in that it is caused by the treatment of the injury.

Those complications of fractures that are the result of the injury itself are classified below; those that are the result of treatment and are therefore iatrogenic are classified separately following a discussion of fracture treatment. The recognition and treatment of *all* complications of fractures are discussed together in a subsequent section of this chapter.

CLASSIFICATION OF THE COMPLICATIONS OF THE ORIGINAL INJURY

I. Initial (Immediate) Complications
   A. Local Complications (Associated Injuries)
      1. Skin Injuries
         a) From without
            Abrasions, laceration, puncture wound, penetrating missile wound, avulsion, loss of skin
         b) From within
            Penetration of the skin by a fracture fragment
      2. Vascular Injuries
         a) Injury to a major artery
            Division, contusion, arterial spasm
         b) Injury to a major vein
            Division, contusion
         c) Local hemorrhage
            External
            Internal
               Into soft tissues— hematoma
               Into body cavities—
                  intracranial hemorrhage, hemothorax, hemoperitoneum, hemarthrosis
      3. Neurological Injuries
         a) Brain
         b) Spinal cord
         c) Peripheral nerves
      4. Muscular Injuries
         Division (usually incomplete)
      5. Visceral Injuries
         a) Thoracic—heart and great vessels, trachea, bronchi and lungs
         b) Intra-abdominal—gastrointestinal tract, liver, spleen, urinary tract
   B. Remote Complications
      1. Multiple Injuries
         Simultaneous injuries to other parts of the body (unrelated to a fracture)
      2. Hemorrhagic shock
II. Early Complications
   A. Local Complications
      1. Sequelae of immediate complications
         Skin necrosis, gangrene, Volkmann's ischemia, gas gangrene, venous thrombosis, visceral complications
      2. Joint Complications
         Infection (septic arthritis)—from an open injury
      3. Bony Complications
         Infection (osteomyelitis) at fracture site—from an open injury
         Avascular necrosis of bone— usually of one fragment
   B. Remote Complications
      1. Fat Embolism
      2. Pulmonary Embolism
      3. Pneumonia
      4. Tetanus
      5. Delirium Tremens
III. Late Complications

A. Local Complications
1. Joint Complications
   a) Persistent joint stiffness
   b) Post-traumatic degenerative joint disease
2. Bony Complications
   a) Abnormal fracture healing Mal-union, delayed union, non-union
   b) Growth disturbance—from epiphyseal plate injury
   c) Persistent infection (chronic osteomyelitis)
   d) Post-traumatic osteoporosis
   e) Sudeck's post-traumatic painful osteoporosis
   f) Refracture
3. Muscular Complications
   a) Post-traumatic myositis ossificans
   b) Late rupture of tendons
4. Neurological Complications
   Tardy nerve palsy
B. Remote Complications
1. Renal calculi
2. Accident neurosis

The General Principles of Fracture Treatment

The six general principles of treatment for all musculoskeletal conditions discussed in Chapter 6 are just as applicable to *traumatic* musculoskeletal conditions (such as fractures, dislocations and associated soft tissue injuries) as they are to *non-traumatic* musculoskeletal disorders. A review of these general principles is in order before you proceed to learn about their application to the treatment of fractures and associated injuries.

1. FIRSTLY DO NO HARM

While some of the problems and complications of fractures are caused by the *original injury*, others are caused by the *treatment* of the injury and are therefore *iatrogenic*. The increasing frequency of lawsuits that are initiated by dissatisfied patients against their physicians or surgeons attests to the incidence and significance of such iatrogenic complications. To a large extent iatrogenic complications are *preventable* and hence their prevention is one of the important general principles of fracture treatment. The recognition, prevention and treatment of such complications are discussed in a subsequent section of this chapter but a few examples are listed here: (a) Further damage to important soft tissues by careless first aid treatment and reckless transportation of the patient to the hospital as well as within it. (b) Damage to soft tissues such as skin, blood vessels and nerves by incorrectly applied plaster casts as well as by excessive traction. (c) Opening the path to infection of the fracture site by the careless and injudicious application of open reduction with internal skeletal fixation.

2. BASE TREATMENT ON AN ACCURATE DIAGNOSIS AND PROGNOSIS

The necessity for accurate clinical and radiographic diagnosis of fractures and associated injuries has already been stressed. In addition to *diagnosing* a fracture, as well as any associated soft tissue injury, you must gather the information necessary to make a reasonable estimate of the *prognosis* of the injury because your choice of the specific method of treatment for a given fracture in a given patient must be based on its prognosis.

The following factors are of particular importance in relation to the healing of uncomplicated fractures: age of the patient, site and configuration of the fracture, amount of initial displacement, and the blood supply to the fracture fragments. The significance of these factors has already been discussed in a previous section of this chapter. In general, when good external (periosteal) callus can be expected, as in a shaft fracture without excessive periosteal disruption, or when a combination of good external (periosteal) and internal (endosteal) callus can be expected, as in an impacted metaphyseal fracture, perfect reduction and rigid fixation (rigid immobilization) are not essential. By contrast, when healing can be expected to occur from internal (endosteal) callus *alone*, as in a fracture of the neck of the femur where the periosteum is exceedingly thin, or in an intra-articular fracture of a small bone, such as the carpal scaphoid, perfect reduction and rigid fixation are essential.

Your first decision is whether or not the fracture requires reduction and if so, what type of reduction—closed or open. Your second decision concerns the type of immobilization required—external or internal.

3. SELECT TREATMENT WITH SPECIFIC AIMS

The *specific aims* of fracture treatment are: (a) to relieve pain, (b) to obtain and maintain satisfactory position of the fracture fragments; (c) to allow, and if necessary to encourage bony union; (d) to restore optimum function not only in the fractured limb or spine but also in the patient as a person.

(a) *To relieve pain.* Since bone is relatively insensitive, the pain from a fracture arises from the associated injury to the soft tissues, including periosteum and endosteum. The pain is aggravated by movement of the fracture fragments, associated muscle spasm and progressive swelling in a closed space. Thus, the pain from a fracture can usually be relieved by immobilizing the fracture site and by avoiding an unduly tight encircling bandage or cast. During the first few days after a fracture, however, analgesics may also be required.

(b) *To obtain and maintain satisfactory position of the fracture fragments.* Some fractures are either undisplaced, or displaced so little that *no* reduction is indicated. Reduction of a fracture to obtain a satisfactory position is indicated only when you anticipate that reduction will be necessary to obtain good *function*, to prevent subsequent degenerative joint disease or to obtain an acceptable clinical appearance of the injured part, but not necessarily a perfect radiographic appearance of the bone since you must always remember that you are treating a patient and his fracture rather than a radiograph. The maintenance of satisfactory position of the fracture fragments usually requires some degree of immobilization

which may be achieved by a variety of methods such as continuous traction, a plaster-of-Paris cast, and internal skeletal fixation depending upon the degree of stability or instability of the reduction.

(c) *To allow and, if necessary, to encourage bony union.* In most fractures union will occur provided it is given a chance, or allowed to occur by not disturbing the natural healing processes. In certain fractures, however, such as those with severe tearing of the periosteum and surrounding soft tissues or those with avascular necrosis of one or both fragments, union must be encouraged by the judicious use of autogenous bone grafts, either early or late in the healing process.

(d) *To restore optimum function.* During the period of immobilization of the healing fracture, disuse atrophy of regional muscles must be prevented by active static (isometric) exercises of those muscles that control the immobilized joints and active dynamic (isotonic) exercises of all other muscles in the limb or trunk. The preservation of good muscle power and tone throughout this period improves local circulation and greatly facilitates subsequent restoration of normal joint motion and optimum function not only in the fractured limb or spine but also in the patient as a person. After the period of immobilization, active exercises should be continued even more vigorously. Rehabilitation of the whole person, as discussed in Chapter 6, is always important but usually presents problems only when the fracture has involved a particularly long period of treatment or is associated with serious complications.

4. COOPERATE WITH THE "LAWS OF NATURE"

The musculoskeletal tissues react to a fracture in accordance with "laws of nature" as described in a previous section of this chapter dealing with the normal healing of uncomplicated fractures. Your treatment must respect and cooperate with these natural laws of tissue behavior lest you delay, or even prevent normal healing. For example, inadequate protection and immobilization, excessive traction with resultant distraction at the fracture site, operative destruction of blood supply to fragments, and postoperative infection, all delay fracture healing and may even prevent it. Your treatment of a fracture should be planned to create the ideal setting and circumstances in which the natural restorative powers of your patient and his tissues can reach their full potential. In addition, a knowledge of the natural laws of late remodeling of a healed fracture at various sites and at various ages is important in determining how much deformity at the site of a fracture can be accepted.

5. BE REALISTIC AND PRACTICAL IN YOUR TREATMENT

When considering a specific method of treatment for a given patient with a given fracture, common sense and sound judgement will lead you to ask yourself three important questions concerning the proposed method.

(a) *Precisely what am I aiming to accomplish by this method of treatment; what is its specific aim or goal?* The specific aims of fracture treatment have been discussed above.

(b) *Am I, in fact, likely to accomplish this aim or goal by this method of treatment?* You can answer this question in part as a result of your knowledge of the previously discussed factors in the prognosis of fractures. In addition, as you will learn later, certain fractures, such as displaced fractures of the lateral condyle of the humerus in children and displaced fractures of the neck of the femur in adults, cannot be adequately treated by means of external immobilization alone; they require accurate reduction and internal fixation.

(c) *Will the anticipated end result justify the means or method; will it be worth it to your patient in terms of what he will have to endure—the risks, the discomfort, the period away from his home, work, or school?* This question is of particular importance in fracture treatment. For example, intertrochanteric fractures of the femur in the elderly will nearly always unite whether treated by continuous traction and prolonged immobilization of the patient as well as of the limb (bed rest), or by operative reduction with internal skeletal fixation and early mobilization of the patient as well as of the limb. For an elderly patient, however, the risk of prolonged bed rest is too great in that it may initiate a series of pathological events that lead to his progressive deterioration and even to his death. Under such circumstances operative treatment is preferable since it carries less risk for the elderly person than prolonged bed rest.

6. SELECT TREATMENT FOR YOUR PATIENT AS AN INDIVIDUAL

A given fracture may present an entirely different problem for one individual than it does for another, particularly in relation to age, sex, occupation and any coexistent disease. For example, residual deformity of a healed fracture (mal-union) of the clavicle presents little problem for a young child (because it will remodel over the growing years) or for a laboring man (because he is not concerned about its appearance), but it may be quite distressing for a female model or an actress. Likewise, mal-union of a finger fracture may not interfere significantly with hand function for a taxi driver but it may be catastrophic for a concert pianist. Therefore, your choice of the specific method of fracture treatment must be tailored to fit the particular needs of your particular patient.

Preliminary Care For Patients With Fractures

During the interval between the time an individual is injured and the time he receives definitive treatment, an interval that may vary from less than an hour to several hours or even longer (and always *seems* longer to the unfortunate victim and his relatives), much can be done to deal with life-threatening complications, to prevent further injury and to make the victim more comfortable. This preliminary care for patients with fractures is best considered in three phases: (1) immediate care outside a hospital (first aid); (2) care during transportation to hospital; (3) emergency care in a hospital.

1. IMMEDIATE CARE OUTSIDE A HOSPITAL (FIRST AID)

When you happen upon the scene of an accident you, as a medical doctor, should always accept your moral obligation to stop and render help to the injured. The summoning of emergency services—police, firemen, ambulance—can usually be delegated to someone else while you create order out of disorder, make a rapid assessment of the situation and initiate immediate care of the injured on the basis of the following priorities which are discussed in order of their urgency.

(a) Obstructed Airway

If the injured person is unconscious (from fainting, shock or head injury), his airway may become obstructed by his tongue having dropped back into his pharynx or by aspiration of mucus, blood, vomitus or a foreign body. This life-threatening complication can usually be relieved by gently rolling the person into the prone position, pulling the jaw and tongue forward and clearing his pharynx with your finger.

(b) External Hemorrhage

The most effective method of controlling external hemorrhage is firm manual pressure applied to the open wound through a temporary dressing improvised from the cleanest material available. Local pressure on an extremity wound is not only more effective than a tourniquet but also much safer; a tourniquet that is applied too loosely occludes only the venous return and thereby increases the bleeding, whereas a tourniquet that is applied too tightly or left on too long causes permanent damage to blood vessels, nerves and other soft tissues.

(c) Shock

At the scene of an accident you can at least help to prevent shock, or to prevent an increase in severity of existing shock, by controlling hemorrhage and by minimizing pain. Pallor combined with cold, moist skin and a weak, rapid pulse are the most obvious manifestations of shock. Careless and rough handling of an injured person aggravates both pain and shock and therefore must be avoided. Neither food nor fluids should be given by mouth during the preliminary treatment of an injured person who may require a general anesthetic shortly after his admission to hospital.

(d) Fractures and Dislocations

Obvious fractures and dislocations of the limbs should be *splinted* before the person is moved, not only to minimize pain but also to prevent further injury to the soft tissues. Traction applied slowly and steadily is the most effective and least painful way of straightening a gross deformity and of holding an injured limb while it is being splinted. An injured upper limb is best splinted by being bound to the person's trunk and an injured lower limb can be bound to the opposite lower limb. Temporary limb splints can also be improvised from many available objects (Fig. 15.26). Spinal injury may be less obvious but its presence or absence should be determined by testing for local tenderness along the spine before the injured person is moved, since movement, particularly flexion, of an injured spinal column endangers the spinal cord and nerve roots.

Pertinent information concerning the circumstances of the accident, injuries sustained and their emergency treatment should be transmitted to ambulance attendants so that it will be available to hospital attendants.

2. TRANSPORTATION

Persons with major injuries deserve gentle care while being placed in an ambulance or other suitable vehicle; unless there is no alternative they should not be squeezed into the narrow confines of a car seat. A person who has sustained a spinal injury requires extremely careful handling; he should be lifted onto a stretcher or some suitable alternative such as a door by at least two, and preferably four individuals in such a way that his spine is kept straight while he is lifted as "an immobilized unit." When possible a short spinal board should be strapped to the victim's back before he is moved (Fig. 15.27).

During the trip to hospital in an ambu-

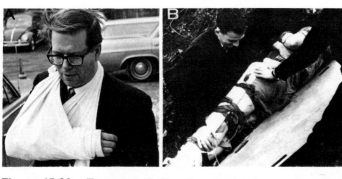
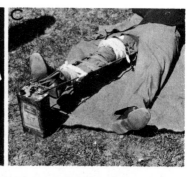

Figure 15.26. Temporary limb splints at the scene of an accident. *A*, upper limb splint. A short board has been bandaged to this man's fractured forearm before the sling was applied. For an injury above the elbow a second sling or bandage can be used to bind the upper limb to the trunk. *B*, lower limb splint. A long board has been bandaged to this man's injured lower limb and then the two lower limbs have been bound together. He was also thought to have a spinal injury and consequently is being gently rolled onto a long spinal board. *C*, temporary Thomas splint that has been applied by an ambulance attendant for a man with an open fracture of the femur. The pressure dressing over the open wound and the splint have been applied before the accident victim is transported to hospital.

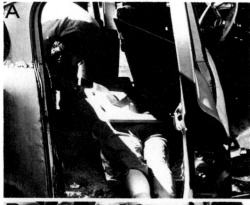

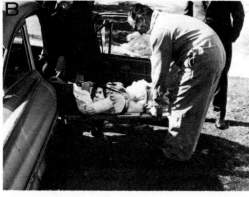

Figure 15.27. Moving an accident victim who has a suspected spinal injury. *A*, a short spinal board is being strapped to the victim's back even before he is extracted from the wrecked automobile. *B*, the victim is then extracted as an immobilized unit.

lance, good care and comfort are much more important to the injured person than careless speed; there is seldom justification for an ambulance driver to break local traffic laws and furthermore, a jolting, swinging ride is painful and dangerous for the injured person as well as dangerous to others. The modern well-equipped ambulance should be in effect a mobile minor emergency room complete with suction and an oxygen inhalator (Fig. 15.28). The use of helicopters as air ambulances will undoubtedly become more frequent in the future, particularly in situations where ground travel is impractical or unsatisfactory, such as rough terrain or dense highway traffic. Ambulance attendants in particular merit and appreciate commendation when they have effectively carried out their part of the preliminary care of the injured.

3. EMERGENCY CARE IN A HOSPITAL

In the emergency or accident room of a hospital you will have the facilities necessary to provide continuation of preliminary care for the injured patient at a more sophisticated level (Fig. 15.29). Pertinent data concerning the nature of the accident and the patient's subsequent condition, including some indication of the amount of blood loss, should be obtained from those who have

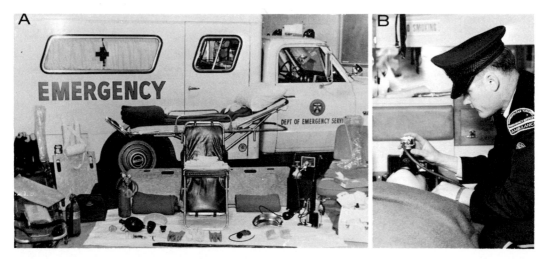

Figure 15.28.   A modern, well-equipped ambulance. The displayed equipment on the left includes stretchers, spinal boards, air splints, oxygen tanks, positive pressure face mask, suction apparatus, gloves and simple surgical instruments. On the right an accident victim receiving oxygen from an inhalator in the ambulance.

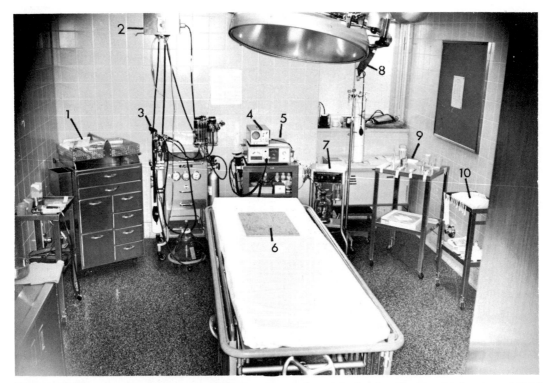

Figure 15.29.   An emergency or accident room equipped to treat patients who have sustained critical injuries. The equipment shown includes the following: *1*, anesthetic instruments to provide an airway (pharyngeal airways, laryngoscopes, endotracheal tubes). *2*, ceiling source of oxygen, nitrous oxide and suction. *3*, anesthetic machine. *4*, electrocardiograph with oscilloscope. *5*, defibrillator. *6*, board on stretcher (to provide firm surface under the patient's thorax in the event that closed cardiac massage is required). *7*, auxiliary suction machine. *8*, blood pump for rapid transfusion. *9*, drugs for cardiac arrest—ready for immediate injection. *10*, cut-down tray for cannulation of a vein.

brought him to hospital. Emergency treatment is based on the same priorities as first aid care.

(a) Obstructed Airway

Persistent obstruction of the patient's airway may be relieved by suction and the insertion of a pharyngeal airway but may require tracheal intubation or even an emergency tracheostomy. Supportive oxygen therapy is frequently necessary.

(b) External Hemorrhage

If local pressure has not arrested external hemorrhage from an open wound, it may be necessary to clamp one or more vessels after which the wound is covered with a temporary sterile dressing. Internal hemorrhage secondary to closed fractures is usually underestimated; for example, an adult with a closed fracture of the femoral shaft may lose from 1000 to 2000 ml of blood into his tissues and with a fracture of the pelvis he may lose even more.

(c) Shock

Prevention of shock and urgent treatment of either impending or established shock are imperative before definitive treatment of any fracture is instituted. Vital signs including pulse rate, respiratory rate, blood pressure and level of consciousness are monitored and recorded. Blood is obtained for typing and cross-matching and at the same time an intravenous infusion is started; in severe shock, the central venous pressure should also be monitored via a catheter inserted into a peripheral vein and passed proximally into the vena cava. While waiting for compatible whole blood, intravenous administration of fluids such as glucose and water, plasma or plasma expanders or lactated Ringer's solution help to control shock temporarily but, of course, hemorrhagic shock is best treated by transfusion of whole blood. Provided there is no head injury or significant abdominal inury, severe pain should be relieved by morphine or a comparable narcotic which may have to be given intravenously if the peripheral circulation is inadequate.

(d) Fractures and Dislocations

Once treatment for the first three priorities has been initiated, a rapid but systematic physical examination is conducted. Vascular impairment and nerve injury should be assessed and their presence or absence recorded before definitive fracture treatment is initiated; otherwise there may be doubt whether such a lesion when discovered subsequently has been caused by treatment or by the original injury.

After a rapid assessment of the patient's obvious injury or injuries, the whole patient

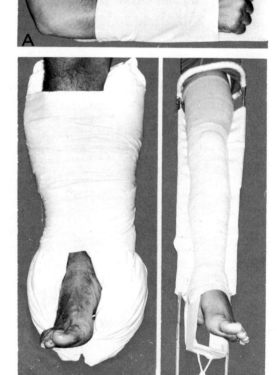

Figure 15.30. Temporary splints for fractured limbs prior to radiographic examination. *A*, arm splint for a forearm fracture, a simple covered board and bandages. *B*, pillow splint for a fractured leg or ankle. There is less risk of circulatory disturbance and skin maceration with this type of splint than with an air splint. *C*, Thomas splint for a fractured femur.

(including all body systems) must be carefully examined for other fractures as well as for soft tissue injuries and visceral lesions. More injuries escape early detection because of an inadequate physical examination in the emergency assessment of the patient and consequent failure to proceed with further investigation than from incorrect interpretation of radiographs.

Before a patient's fractured extremity is subjected to radiographic examination, it should be *splinted* not only to minimize pain but also to protect the related soft tissues from further injury (Fig. 15.30). For the same reasons the patient and his injured part should be moved as little as possible during the radiographic examination; it is most important to shift the tube and film of the radiographic equipment in order to obtain various projections rather than to shift the patient or his fractured extremity (Fig. 15.31). The projections and extent of the radiographic examination required for accurate diagnosis are discussed in an earlier section of this chapter.

Throughout the emergency treatment for an injured patient, compassionate care for the patient and considerate care of his injured tissues as well as kindly communication with his relatives are essential, deserved and appreciated. As much information as possible should be obtained about the patient, particularly concerning any pre-existing disorder and its treatment, before definitive treatment of the fracture is undertaken.

Specific Methods of Definitive Fracture Treatment

Having learned the broad *general principles* of treatment as applied to fractures, you will now wish to learn the various *specific methods* of definitive fracture treatment. In the subsequent two chapters these specific methods of treatment are discussed in relation to specific fractures in children and in adults. In this chapter, however, all of these methods are discussed as a group so that you may consider them in perspective and also in order that discussion of treat-

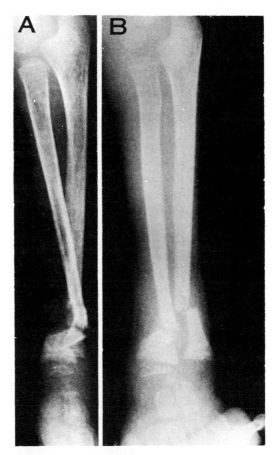

Figure 15.31. This child had an unstable fracture of the distal end of his radius and ulna. Radiographs requested: anteroposterior and lateral projections (the child's forearm should have been splinted prior to radiographic examination). *A*, a lateral projection of both proximal and distal fracture fragments. *B*, a lateral projection of the proximal fragments and an anteroposterior projection of both distal fragments. Obviously, between the two exposures the child's forearm has been rotated through the unstable fracture sites by the technician. The child would have complained of much pain at this time and might even have sustained further injury to the related soft tissues.

ment for specific fractures in the subsequent two chapters may be more meaningful to you.

For each specific method of fracture treatment there are favorable circumstances in which the method *should* be used (*indications*) as well as unfavorable circumstances in which it should *not* be used (*contraindications*). A knowledge of the indications and contraindications is of great importance in selecting a specific method, or combination of methods of treatment, for your particular patient with his particular fracture. There is not always unanimity of opinion, even among "fracture experts," about indications and contraindications in relation to the treatment of various fractures. Opinions are based not only on general principles but also on individual experience and preference, as well as on our present state of knowledge. With continuing advances in knowledge and improvement in methods and techniques, indications and contraindications become modified. You will appreciate, moreover, that there may be more than one pathway by which to reach a desired goal in fracture treatment, but some pathways are smoother, easier and safer for your patient than others.*

The specific methods of treatment are discussed together with their indications and risks. Contraindications for the various methods of treatment can be considered in a more general way now. The absence of an indication for a specific method represents a contraindication in itself. In addition there are three main situations which represent a contraindication for a specific method of treatment: (1) the fracture is not sufficiently serious to require the method; (2) the fracture cannot be adequately treated by the method; (3) either the patient or the fracture is likely to be made worse by the method.

While studying the specific methods of fracture treatment outlined below, you should bear in mind the four basic goals or aims of all fracture treatment: (1) to relieve pain; (2) to obtain and maintain satisfactory position of the fracture fragments; (3) to allow, and if necessary encourage, bony union; (4) to restore optimum function, not only in the fractured limb or spine but also

in the patient as a person. The fourth goal is discussed further in a subsequent section in relation to after-care and rehabilitation for patients with fractures.

In the broad spectrum of fracture treatment, two completely divergent schools of thought have emerged and both have gained much support—on the one hand, the Swiss AO/ASIF system of precise open reduction and rigid internal fixation, and on the other hand, the American functional fracture-bracing system (each of which is described in a subsequent section of this chapter). Although seemingly, on the surface, the exact antithesis of one another, these two relatively new methods of fracture management have one important common denominator, namely the preservation of function in the injured limb and, in particular, the prevention of iatrogenic joint stiffness ("fracture disease").

SPECIFIC METHODS OF TREATMENT FOR CLOSED FRACTURES

1. Protection Alone (Without Reduction or Immobilization)

Protection of a fracture from the usual forces applied to the particular bone as well as from further injury can be accomplished in the upper limb by means of a simple sling and in the lower limb by relief of weight bearing with crutches, at least for older children and adults (Fig. 15.32).

Indications. (Fig. 15.33). Protection alone is indicated for undisplaced or relatively undisplaced, stable fractures of the ribs, phalanges, metacarpals—and in children—of the clavicle. A second indication is that group of fractures, such as mild compression fractures of the spine and impacted fractures of the upper end of the humerus, in which the total result will be better without either reduction or immobilization. Protection alone is also indicated after clinical union has been obtained by other means, but before complete radiological consolidation has been established.

Risks. The protection provided may not be adequate for the particular patient (especially a child or an uncooperative adult) in

---

* This paragraph is paraphrased from a comparable paragraph in Chapter 6 for the sake of both clarity and emphasis.

which case the fracture may become displaced; hence, the need for radiographic examinations of the fracture site at regular intervals during the healing process.

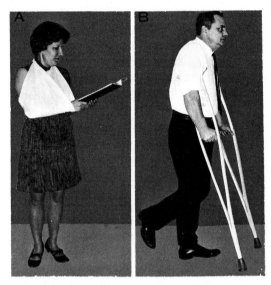

Figure 15.32. Protection alone (without reduction or immobilization). Simple sling for an upper limb injury and crutches with non-weightbearing on an injured lower limb.

2. Immobilization By External Splinting (Without Reduction)

Immobilization of a fracture by external splinting is only *relative* immobilization, as opposed to rigid fixation, since some motion can still occur inside the limb or trunk at the fracture site during the early phases of healing. Relative immobilization is usually achieved by the use of plaster-of-Paris casts of varying design and occasionally by metallic or plastic splints (Fig. 15.34).

Indications. (Fig. 15.35). Immobilization by external splinting without reduction is indicated for fractures that are relatively undisplaced and yet unstable. Such fractures merely require maintenance of the existing position of the fracture fragments during the healing process. A fracture of a long bone in which there is only sideways shift of the fragments in relation to one another but with good contact and no significant angulation or rotation does not require reduction; it does, however, require relative immobilization. The immobilizing splint or cast must be carefully applied and molded to prevent further displacement.

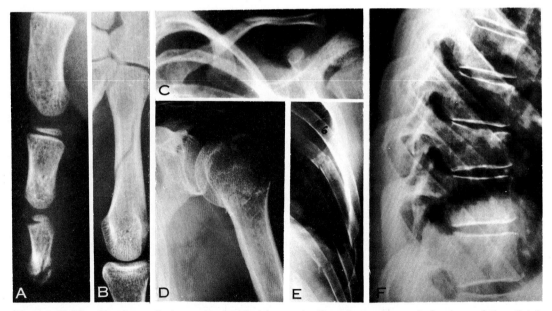

Figure 15.33. Fractures that can be treated by protection alone. *A,* crush fracture of the distal phalanx. *B,* undisplaced fracture of a metacarpal. *C,* green-stick fracture of the clavicle in a young child. *D,* impacted compression fracture of the surgical neck of the humerus in an elderly adult. *E,* undisplaced fractures of ribs (7th, 8th and 9th). *F,* mild compression fracture of the thoracic spine.

Risks. Despite the fact that the fracture is relatively undisplaced at the time it is immobilized by a cast or splint, subsequent muscle pull and gravitational forces may

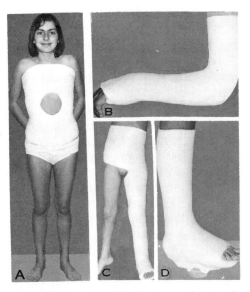

Figure 15.34. Immobilization by external splinting (without reduction)—plaster-of-Paris casts of varying design. *A*, body cast; *B*, above elbow cast; *C*, hip spica cast; *D*, below knee walking cast.

cause further displacement such as angulation, rotation or overriding which is unacceptable; hence the need for repeated radiographic examinations. Improperly applied casts or splints may cause local pressure sores over bony prominences or constriction of a limb with resultant impairment of venous or arterial circulation—or both.

3. Closed Reduction By Manipulation Followed By Immobilization

Closed reduction of a fracture, a form of surgical manipulation, is by far the commonest method of treatment for the majority of displaced fractures in both children and adults. Immobilization of the fracture by means of a plaster-of-Paris cast is the commonest method of *maintaining* the reduction.

The precise technique of manipulative reduction, which is usually performed under anesthesia (general, regional, or local), varies with each fracture but in general it involves placing the fracture fragments where they were at the time of maximal displacement and then reversing the path of displacement. This requires some knowledge of the likely mechanism of the fracture as

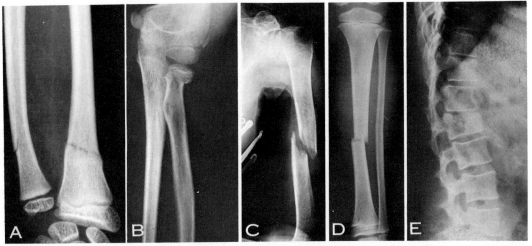

Figure 15.35. Fractures that can be treated by external splinting (without reduction). *A*, undisplaced fracture of the radius and ulna of a child. *B*, undisplaced fracture of the neck of the radius in a child. *C*, oblique fracture of the shaft of the humerus in an elderly lady. You probably noticed the metallic corset stays, but did you detect the second fracture? There is a coexistent impacted compression fracture of the surgical neck of the humerus. *D*, stable transverse fracture of the tibial shaft. *E*, compression fracture of the second lumbar vertebra; the lumbar spine is more mobile and hence less stable than the thoracic spine.

well as a three-dimensional appreciation of the relationship of the fragments to one another and to the surrounding soft tissues. The forces involved in reduction are the opposite of those that produced the fracture (Fig. 15.36). The "feel" of stability of a reduced fracture comes only with clinical experience. The completeness of reduction is assessed by radiographs taken at right angles to each other—without moving the limb. The various techniques of closed reduction of fractures by manipulation depend on many factors and must be seen to be appreciated. These you will learn by "live demonstrations" from your surgical teachers in your own hospitals.

Plaster casts for immobilization of the fracture and maintenance of the reduction must be carefully and thoughtfully applied and molded lest the reduction be subsequently lost within the cast. Indeed, the cast should hold the fracture fragments in the same manner as the surgeon's hands were holding them in their most stable position at the completion of the reduction.

Indications. (Fig. 15.37). Closed reduction by manipulation followed by immobilization is indicated for displaced fractures that require reduction and when it is predicted that sufficiently accurate reduction can be not only *obtained* but also *maintained* by closed means.

Risks. Closed reduction that is ineptly and inaptly applied with more force than skill may cause further damage to soft tissues including blood vessels, nerves and even the periosteum. Excessive traction in the longitudinal axis of the limb during reduction may even produce arterial spasm, particularly at the elbow and knee, with resultant Volkmann's ischemia (which is discussed in a subsequent section of this chapter). Likewise, progressive swelling of a limb within the confines of a tight and rigid cast may also seriously impair circulation. Pressure sores over bony prominences and pressure injuries to peripheral nerves over bony prominences (especially the lateral popliteal nerve where it crosses the neck of the fibula) may also occur as a result of incorrectly applied casts.

Fractures in which the reduction is not sufficiently stable, particularly oblique, spiral and comminuted fractures, may become displaced subsequently within the cast and, hence, repeated radiographic assessments of the position of the fragments are essential. These risks, however, are minimal when the appropriate technique of manipulative reduction is applied to an appropriate type

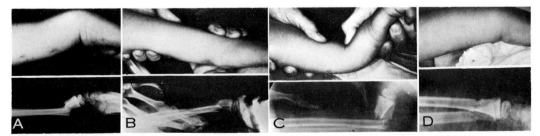

Figure 15.36.   Closed reduction of a fracture by manipulation. *A*, fractures of the distal end of radius and ulna with angulation and overriding in a child. *B*, longitudinal traction corrects the angulation but does not reduce the fractures because the intact periosteal hinge will not allow the fracture fragments to be distracted sufficiently to obtain reduction. (These radiographs were taken for teaching purposes; normally, the surgeon's hands would not be exposed to radiation.) *C*, the fracture deformity must first be increased (to the extent that it was with the "follow through" immediately after the fracture). Then the distal fragment can be moved distally so that the fracture surfaces can be engaged. Only after this manipulation to correct the overriding is angulation corrected. The intact periosteal hinge on the concave side of the angulation then prevents over-correction of the fracture deformity. (The role of the intact periosteal hinge is depicted by line drawings in Fig. 15.11.) *D*, the reduced fracture is ready to be immobilized in a well molded plaster cast that will maintain the reduction.

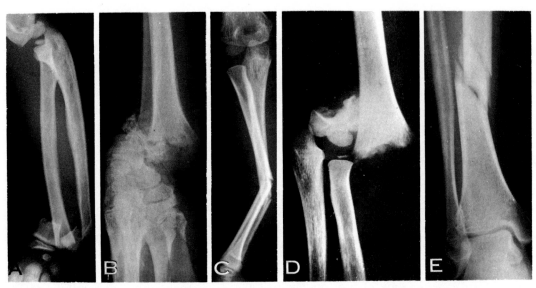

Figure 15.37. Fractures that can be treated by closed reduction followed by immobilization. *A*, displaced fractures of the distal end of the radius and ulna of a child. *B*, Colles' fracture of the distal end of the radius of an adult. *C*, green-stick fracture of the shaft of the radius and ulna of a child. *D*, displaced supracondylar fracture of the humerus in a child. *E*, angulated spiral fracture of the tibial shaft in an adult.

of fracture by an appropriately experienced surgeon and the signs of circulatory impairment and pressure are appreciated following reduction.

4. Closed Reduction by Continuous Traction Followed by Immobilization

Closed reduction of a fracture by means of continuous traction can be achieved in a variety of ways. For fractures in young children continuous traction can be applied through the skin by means of extension tape (*skin traction*) (Fig. 15.38). For older children and adults in whom greater traction force is required, it is best applied through bone by means of a transverse rigid wire or pin (*skeletal traction*) (Fig. 15.39). Furthermore, the traction device may be fixed to the end of the bed (*fixed traction*) or it may be balanced by cords with pulleys and weights (*balanced traction*).

Traction in the long axis of the limb is effective in re-aligning fracture fragments only because the remaining intact soft tissues surrounding the fracture are put on the stretch and thereby guide the fragments into alignment. Continuous traction on the distal fragment is designed to overcome the previously mentioned effects of muscle pull and gravity on the fracture fragments and should be arranged so as to bring the distal fragment in line with the proximal fragment. For example, in a subtrochanteric fracture of the femur, the proximal fragment is pulled into flexion, abduction and external rotation by the muscles attached to the lesser and greater trochanters; thus, traction should be applied to the distal fragment in flexion, abduction and external rotation in order to align it with the proximal fragment. Under certain circumstances, however, manipulative reduction is required to reduce the fracture and continuous traction is employed to maintain the reduction. When the fracture has healed to the point that traction is no longer required to prevent re-displacement, continuous traction can be replaced by immobilization of the limb or trunk in an appropriate cast, after which the patient may be able to return home while awaiting clinical union of the fracture.

Indications. (Fig. 15.40). Closed reduction by continuous traction is indicated for unstable oblique, spiral or comminuted frac-

tures of major long bones, and unstable spinal fractures. Skeletal traction is also applicable to the treatment of fractures complicated by vascular injuries, excessive

swelling or skin loss in which an encircling bandage or cast would be dangerous.

Risks. Excessive longitudinal traction, particularly if applied several hours or longer after the fracture occurred, may produce arterial spasm with resultant Volkmann's ischemia. Ineptly applied skin traction, excessive traction or both may result in superficial skin loss, whereas skeletal traction may become complicated by pin track infection which reaches the bone. Furthermore, continuous traction, if inaccurately applied and monitored, may fail to achieve and maintain adequate reduction of the fracture. Excessive traction may also distract the fracture fragments with resultant delayed union or even nonunion; osteoblasts can creep but cannot leap. These risks, however, like those of closed reduction, are largely preventable, but their prevention requires clinical vigilance by an experienced surgeon.

5. Closed Reduction Followed by Functional Fracture-Bracing

In 1961 Dehne advocated the early use of weight-bearing plaster casts in the treatment of fractures of the tibia. Two years later, Sarmiento expanded upon this concept by conceiving the principle of early function combined with allowing motion at the joints above and below the fractured bone. This specific method of fracture treatment is variously known as "closed functional treatment," "cast-bracing" or "functional fracture-bracing." Adapting the principles involved in fitting prostheses to amputation

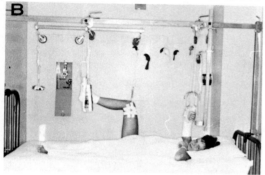

Figure 15.38. Continuous skin traction. *A*, continuous fixed skin traction combined with a Thomas splint for a boy with an unstable fracture of the femur. *B*, continuous balanced skin traction on the arm for a boy with an unstable fracture of the humerus. Note also the skeletal traction on the femur for an unstable subtrochanteric fracture of the femur in the same boy.

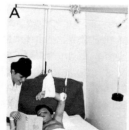
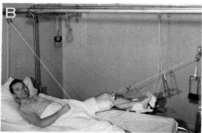
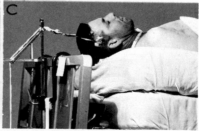

Figure 15.39. Continuous skeletal traction. *A*, continuous skeletal traction through the olecranon for an unstable supracondylar fracture of the humerus in a child. *B*, continuous balanced skeletal traction through the upper end of the tibia for an unstable fracture of the femur in an adult. *C*, continuous skeletal traction through tongs in the outer table of the skull for an unstable fracture-dislocation of the cervical spine.

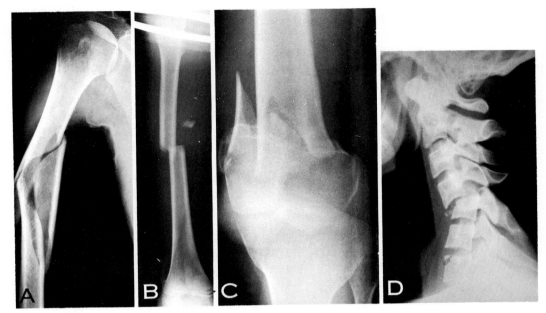

Figure 15.40.   Fractures that can be treated by continuous traction. *A*, unstable comminuted fracture of the shaft of the humerus. *B*, unstable fracture of the shaft of the femur. *C*, unstable comminuted supracondylar fracture of the femur. *D*, unstable fracture-dislocation of the cervical spine.

stumps (e.g. patella tendon-bearing for below knee prostheses), Sarmiento first used plaster casts and more recently plastic (Orthoplast) splints, both of which are hinged at the level of joints.

The principle of functional fracture-bracing is based on the following concepts: (1) that rigid immobilization of fracture fragments is not only unnecessary but also undesirable for fracture healing; (2) that function and the resultant motion at the fracture site actually stimulate healing through abundant callus formation; (3) that such function prevents iatrogenic joint stiffness; (4) that somewhat less than perfect (anatomical) reduction of a fracture of the shaft of a long bone does not create significant problems concerning either function or appearance (cosmesis). A beneficial socioeconomic "spin-off" of this method of fracture treatment is the combination of a shorter period of hospitalization, no risk of infection and a more rapid return to normal activities, including work.

The initial treatment consists of closed reduction of the fracture followed by immobilization in a plaster cast for a period of three to four weeks (i.e. until the acute pain and swelling have subsided and the soft tissues have begun to heal). At the end of this preliminary period the hinged cast-brace, or plastic brace is applied to splint the fracture and yet allow motion in the joints above and below the fractured bone. (Figs. 15.41 and 15.42). The encircling external splint combined with the viscoelastic nature of the soft tissues creates a "hydraulic effect" that prevents any initial shortening of the limb from increasing. In large series of patients with fractures of long bones treated by this method, the incidence of non-union has been only 1%.

Indications. Closed reduction followed by functional fracture-bracing is indicated for fractures of the shaft of the tibia, the distal third of the femur, the humerus and the ulna in adults. The method is *contraindicated*, however, for fractures that can be more effectively treated by open reduction and internal skeletal fixation, including intertrochanteric fractures of the femur, subtrochanteric and mid-shaft fractures of the femur, shaft of the radius and intra-articular fractures.

Risks. Although functional fracture-brac-

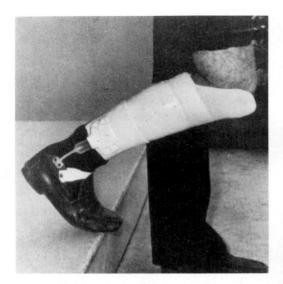

Figure 15.41. Functional fracture-brace for a fracture of the shaft of the tibia in an adult. Note that the well molded and close fitting plastic (Orthoplast) brace allows full motion of both the ankle and the knee and in this sense is much more "functional" than a plaster cast that immobilizes both joints.

ing is relatively risk-free there is a possibility that the method will fail to maintain an acceptable position of the fracture fragments in which case alternative methods such as open reduction and internal fixation may still be applied.

6. Closed Reduction by Manipulation followed by External Skeletal Fixation

External skeletal fixation of fractures, first devised by Stader, a veterinary surgeon, for the purpose of avoiding the use of plaster casts in animals, was modified for humans over three decades ago by Roger Anderson. After a long period of relatively little utilization, external skeletal fixation is currently creating a rebirth of clinical interest and application.

In its simplest form, two or three metal pins are inserted percutaneously through the bone above and below the fracture site and held rigidly together by external bars to provide firm (but not rigid) fixation of the fracture "at a distance" (Fig. 15.43). In recent years devices such as the Hoffman type of external fixation have become increas-

ingly sophisticated to provide more rigid fixation in three dimensions (Fig. 15.44).

Indications. (Fig. 15.45). Closed reduction by manipulation followed by external skeletal fixation is primarily indicated for se-

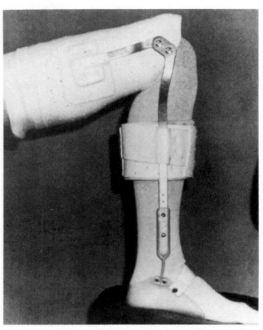

Figure 15.42. Functional fracture-brace for a fracture of the distal third of the femur in an adult. Note that the brace, which has a metal hinge at the knee and a plastic hinge at the ankle allows motion at the hip, knee and ankle.

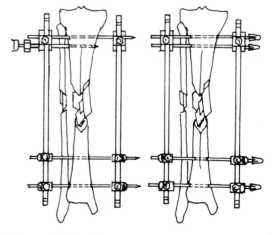

Figure 15.43. Simplest form of external skeletal fixation to provide fixation of a comminuted fracture of the tibia "at a distance."

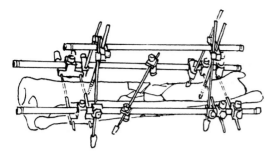

Figure 15.44. More sophisticated form of external skeletal fixation to provide more rigid fixation in three dimensions.

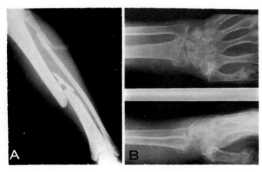

Figure 15.45. Fractures that can be treated by closed reduction and external skeletal fixation. *A*, unstable comminuted fracture of the tibia in an adult. *B*, unstable comminuted Colles' fracture of the distal end of the radius in an adult.

verely comminuted (and hence unstable) fractures of the shaft of the tibia or femur—especially Type 3 open fractures with extensive injuries to soft tissues including arteries and nerves the repair of which necessitates immobilization of the fracture site. For such fractures this method offers the distinct advantage of allowing changes of the wound dressing as well as the application of skin grafts. External skeletal fixation may also be indicated for unstable fractures of the pelvis, humerus, radius and even metacarpals.

Risks. The main risk of external skeletal fixation is pin track infection with, or without, osteomyelitis. If the pins are inserted by means of a high-speed power drill the surrounding bone may be "burnt to death" by the heat of friction, in which case superimposed infection will produce a ring sequestrum (Fig. 15.68).

7. Closed Reduction by Manipulation followed by Internal Skeletal Fixation

After accurate manipulative reduction of an unstable fracture, the reduction can be maintained by the percutaneous insertion of metallic nails or intramedullary rods across the fracture site for the purpose of providing *internal skeletal fixation* of the fracture (Fig. 15.46). Both the closed manipulative reduction of the fracture and the "blind" insertion of the internal skeletal fixation are performed using radiographic control, either by means of repeated single radiographs or short periods of fluoroscopy with an image intensifier. Fractures should never be reduced under ordinary fluoroscopy because of the radiation hazard to the patient as well as to the surgeon.

Indications. (Fig. 15.47). Manipulative reduction followed by internal skeletal fixation is indicated for certain fractures in which accurate reduction can be obtained by closed means but cannot or should not be maintained by external immobilization. The

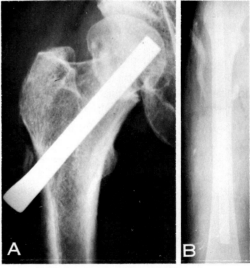

Figure 15.46. Closed reduction followed by internal skeletal fixation. *A*, Smith-Petersen nail that has been inserted percutaneously across a fracture of the neck of the femur after closed reduction. This so-called "blind" nailing of a fracture is not really blind; it is performed under radiographic control. *B*, intra-medullary rod that has been inserted percutaneously across a fracture of the shaft of the femur after closed reduction.

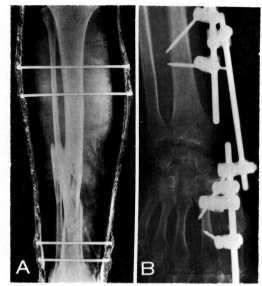

Figure 15.47. Fractures that can be treated by closed reduction and internal skeletal fixation. *A*, fracture of the neck of the right femur in an adult. *B*, fracture of the neck of the left femur in a child.

commonest indication for *internal* skeletal fixation is the unstable fracture of the neck of the femur; after accurate reduction a tri-flange nail is driven across the fracture site through a small skin incision using radiographic control. Certain fractures in the mid-shaft of the long bones that can be accurately reduced by closed means also lend themselves to "blind" intramedullary nailing under radiographic control.

Risks. The closed manipulative reduction may fail to obtain a satisfactory position of the fracture fragments and the skeletal fixation may fail to achieve sufficiently rigid fixation of the fracture. Since with internal skeletal fixation the skin is traversed, the risk of infection is ever present.

8. Open Reduction Followed By Internal Skeletal Fixation

Open reduction has an important place in the treatment of uncomplicated closed fractures but should never be undertaken lightly; when the results are good they are very good, but when they are bad they are horrid—and may even be catastrophic! The fracture site is exposed surgically so that the fracture fragments may be reduced perfectly *under direct vision*. A fracture that is open to inspection, however, is also open to infection. Indeed, the operative reduction of fractures should be performed (or at least supervised) only by an experienced surgeon and only in a favorable setting such as an operating theater that has a consistently low infection rate and is properly equipped with adequate instruments. To convert a closed fracture to an infected fracture is a terrible tragedy.

Once the fracture has been reduced at open operation, the reduction must be maintained by *rigid internal fixation* which is achieved by using some type of metallic device, a technique that is sometimes referred to as *osteosynthesis*. Surgical skill is required to avoid unnecessary further damage to the surrounding soft tissues and in particular to the blood supply of the fracture fragments. The surgeon must constantly think as a biologist with reverence for living tissues rather than merely as a carpenter of cortical bone, even though the technical application of internal fixation must of course be structurally sound.

A wide variety of mechanical devices have been developed to provide rigid internal fixation of fractures. These metallic devices, each of which has its special uses and advantages, include various types of transfixion screws, onlay plates held by screws, intramedullary nails and rods, smooth and threaded pins, encircling bands and wire sutures (Fig. 15.48).

The AO/ASIF System of Internal Fixation. In 1958 a small group of Swiss surgeons including Müller, Allgower and Willeneger, who were dissatisfied with the existing systems and techniques of internal fixation of fractures, formed a study group called AO (Arbeitsgemeinshaft für Osteosynthesefragen or Association for Osteosynthesis) which was subsequently called ASIF (Association for the Study of Internal Fixation). These innovative surgeons and their research colleagues, who are primarily concerned with biomechanical improvements of the internal fixation for fractures, have de-

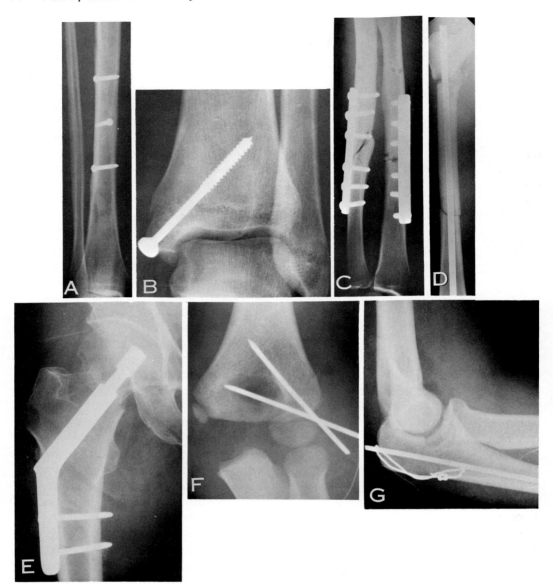

Figure 15.48.   Metallic devices used for internal fixation of fractures. *A*, transfixion screws for a long oblique fracture of the tibia. *B*, lag screw (compression screw) for an avulsion fracture of the medial malleolus. *C*, heavy onlay compression plate and screws (AO compression device), for fractures of the radius and ulna. (One screw in the ulna is incorrectly placed in that it traverses a fracture line.) *D*, intramedullary rod for a segmented fracture of the femur. *E*, nail-plate combination for a fracture of the neck of the femur. *F*, Kirschner wires for a fracture of the lateral condyle of the humerus in a child. *G*, intramedullary Kirschner wire and a "tension relieving" figure-eight wire loop (AO device) for a fracture of the olecranon.

veloped the best system, techniques and equipment available for this purpose.

The principle of the AO/ASIF system is the achievement of sufficiently rigid internal fixation of fracture fragments that external immobilization is not necessary and full, active function of muscles and joints is possible very soon after operation. The underlying reason for this system is the avoidance of what this group refers to as "*fracture disease*," i.e. the iatrogenic sequelae of prolonged immobilization of extremities—joint stiffness, muscle atrophy, disuse osteoporosis and chronic edema. In essence, the aim of the AO/ASIF system is the rapid recovery of function in the injured limb. As mentioned in an earlier section of this chapter, fracture healing in the presence of rigid, stable internal fixation (applied under compression) is of the "direct" or "primary" type.

The surgeon who treats fractures must be skilled in all methods of fracture treatment and not just in a system of internal fixation lest he exemplify the phenomenon stated by Abraham Maslow, namely that "if the only tool you have is a hammer, you tend to see every problem as a nail."

Indications. (Fig. 15.49). Open reduction and internal skeletal fixation of a closed fracture should be undertaken only for definite and justifiable indications which may be either absolute (a matter of necessity) or relative (a matter of judgment). Open operation is indicated *to obtain* reduction when closed reduction by manipulation would clearly be impossible, or has already been proven to be so. Examples are displaced avulsion fractures, intra-articular fractures in which reduction of the joint surface must be perfect, displaced fractures in children that cross the epiphyseal plate, and fractures in which soft tissues have become interposed and trapped between the fragments. With grossly unstable fractures it may be possible to *obtain* reduction by closed means, but impossible to *maintain* the reduction and hence for these fractures operative treatment is indicated, not so much for the reduction of the fracture as for the maintenance of reduction by *internal fixation*. Examples are intertrochanteric fractures of the femur, fractures of both bones of the forearm in adults, and displaced fractures of phalanges.

Open reduction and internal fixation of a fracture are also indicated where there is a coexistent vascular injury that requires exploration and repair. Operative treatment of a fracture may be indicated to *facilitate nursing care* of the patient and thereby prevent serious complications as with unstable intertrochanteric fractures of the femur in the elderly, extremity fractures associated with severe head injury and fracture-dislocations

of the spine complicated by paraplegia. Under certain circumstances a *pathological fracture* through a metastatic neoplasm merits internal fixation (with or without methylmethacrylate) to relieve pain and thereby make the remaining months of the patient's life more bearable.

In general, combined open reduction and internal fixation is *contraindicated* in fractures of the shaft of the tibia and the shaft of the humerus (both of which can usually be adequately managed by functional fracture bracing).

Risks. The most serious risk of open operative reduction of fractures is *infection*. Even in the best of operating rooms every operative wound becomes *contaminated* by bacteria from the air and the longer the wound is open, the more bacteria enter it; furthermore, the torn and bruised muscles, as well as the fracture hematoma itself, serve as an ideal culture medium for bacteria. The fact that *contamination* does not invariably lead to *infection* attests to the local and general resistance of the host; nevertheless, the risk is real and an infected fracture is a catastrophe. Operative reduction of a fracture also carries the risk of further *damage to the blood supply* of the fracture fragments which, in turn, may lead to delayed union and even non-union. Unless the device used for internal fixation does in fact provide rigid immobilization of the fracture fragments in a suitable position of reduction, there is a possibility of continued movement at the fracture site and hence a risk of *metal failure* and of delayed union or non-union. In addition, *postoperative adhesions* between muscle groups may lead to persistent restriction of joint motion.

The controversial concept of using less rigid or semi-flexible plates to diminish the "stress protection" of bone offers some theoretical advantages but is still in the investigative stage, both experimentally and clinically.

9. Excision of a Fracture Fragment and Replacement by an Endoprosthesis

For certain fractures of the hip and elbow the results of internal fixation are relatively

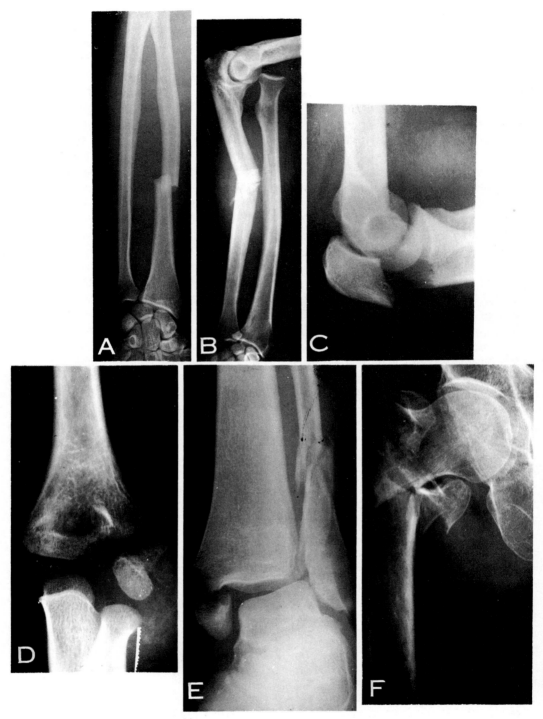

Figure 15.49.   Fractures that are best treated by open reduction and internal fixation. *A*, fracture of the shaft of the radius and subluxation of the inferior radioulnar joint in an adult. *B*, fracture of the shaft of the ulna and anterior dislocation of the proximal end of the radius (Monteggia fracture-dislocation) in an adult. *C*, widely separated intra-articular fracture of the olecranon. *D*, displaced fracture of the lateral condyle of the humerus in a child. *E*, fracture-subluxation of the ankle with an avulsion fracture of the medial malleolus and a comminuted fracture of the shaft of the fibula. *F*, comminuted intertrochanteric fracture of the femur.

unsatisfactory because of the high incidence of avascular necrosis of the articular fragment, non-union of the fracture and post-traumatic degenerative joint disease. Under these circumstances, the articular fragment may be excised and replaced by a suitable endoprosthesis to provide a prosthetic joint replacement (Fig. 15.50).

Indications. (Fig. 15.51). Because of the

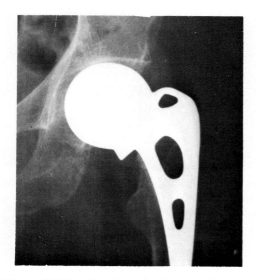

Figure 15.50. Excision of a fracture fragment and replacement by a prosthesis. In this elderly patient who had a femoral neck fracture, the proximal fragment (femoral head and neck) has been excised and replaced by an endoprosthesis, the stem of which penetrates the distal fragment.

high incidence of avascular necrosis of the femoral head and non-union of the fracture, displaced intracapsular fractures of the neck of the femur in the elderly cannot always be managed satisfactorily by internal fixation. Excision of the proximal fragment (femoral head) combined with replacement with an endoprosthesis overcomes both of these problems and permits earlier mobilization of the patient as well as of the hip. Comminuted fractures of the radial head in adults are not amenable to internal fixation and, since residual incongruity of the joint leads to post-traumatic degenerative joint disease, it is preferable to excise the radial head. If the elbow joint is grossly unstable as a result of coexistent ligamentous injury, the radial head may be replaced by an endoprosthesis. If, however, the elbow joint is not unstable, no endoprosthesis is required and the patient is left with an excision arthroplasty. Excision of the radial head is, of course, contraindicated in children because of the resultant loss of the epiphyseal growth at this site. Severely comminuted fractures of the patella are best treated by excision of the entire patella and reconstruction of the quadriceps mechanism.

Risks. As with other methods of operative treatment of fractures, the most serious risk is *infection*, a complication that is particularly serious in the presence of an endoprosthesis. Indeed, severe infection may even

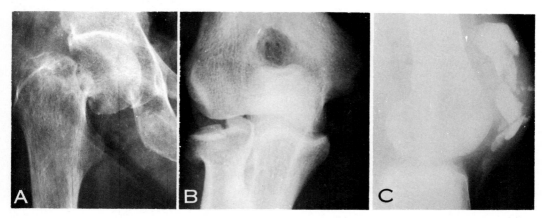

Figure 15.51. Fractures that may require excision of a fragment. *A*, fracture of the femoral neck in an elderly adult. The fragment should be replaced by an endoprosthesis. *B*, comminuted, intra-articular fracture of the radial head in an adult. *C*, severely comminuted (shattered) patella.

necessitate removal of the endoprosthesis with a resultant false joint (excision arthroplasty). There is also a risk, particularly in the elderly hip, that the endoprosthesis will gradually migrate through osteoporotic bone of the pelvis or femur.

TREATMENT FOR OPEN FRACTURES

Since open (compound) fractures have communicated with the external environment through the skin and have therefore already been complicated by *bacterial contamination*, they carry the serious risk of becoming further complicated by *infection*. Thus, they merit special consideration with particular emphasis on the *prevention of infection*.

The extent of the skin wound of an open fracture varies considerably. It may be a small *puncture wound* caused by penetration of the skin from within by a sharp, jagged spike of bone, or by penetration of the skin from without by a missile such as a bullet (Fig. 15.10). The wound may be a sizeable *tear* in the skin through which bare bone is still protruding (Fig. 15.52). Alternatively, the wound may consist of extensive *lacerations* from without (Fig. 15.53) or even *avulsion* of a large area of skin and subcutaneous fat (Fig. 15.54). The soft tissue injury associated with an open fracture is usually even more extensive than is immediately apparent; the external blood loss through the open wound prior to hospital admission is also frequently underestimated.

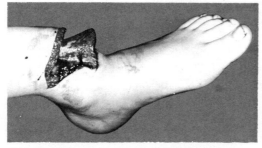

Figure 15.52. Open fracture of the distal end of the tibia. The protruding tibial fragment has penetrated the skin from within and the skin has been further torn by severe displacement at the moment of injury.

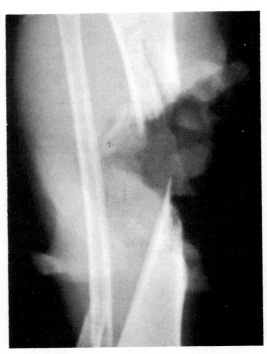

Figure 15.53. Open fracture of the shaft of the tibia. The blades of a power lawn mower penetrated the skin from without and fractured the tibia. There is extensive soft tissue loss as well as loss of a large segment of bone. Did you also notice the associated closed fracture of the fibula?

Classification of Open Fractures

From the extensive experience of over 1000 open fractures of long bones, Gustilo and Anderson were able to distinguish three distinct categories of such injuries and hence to develop the following classification based on the severity of the soft tissue injury: Type 1—a clean wound less than 1 cm in length (usually from within); Type 2—a laceration more than 1 cm in length but without extensive soft tissue damage, skin flaps or avulsions; Type 3—extensive soft tissue damage such as skin flaps, avulsions, muscle and nerve injuries and major arterial injury. A special category of Type 3 open fractures includes those caused by either gunshots or farm accidents.

They recommended primary closure of the skin in Types 1 and 2 open fractures (this is controversial) but delayed primary closure in Type 3 open fractures. Using antibiotics

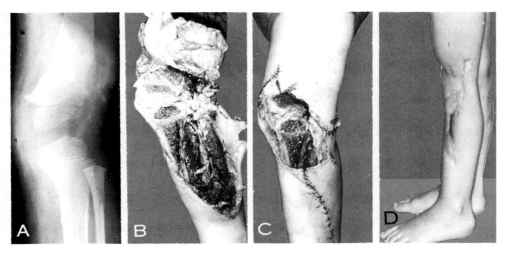

Figure 15.54.   *A*, an open fracture of the distal end of femur and proximal end of tibia in a child. A power saw has lacerated and avulsed skin and has cut out a portion of femur and tibia. *B*, clinical appearance of the limb showing the extensive skin lacerations, avulsion of skin, extensive damage to underlying soft tissues and bones. *C*, after debridement and partial closure of the wound. The residual skin deficit was covered later by a split thickness skin graft. *D*, one year later there is extensive scarring but good function. Nevertheless, further reconstructive surgery will be required because of a growth disturbance in the injured epiphyseal plates.

(usually one of the cephalosporins) before, during and after operation, the over-all infection rate was 2.4% while the infection rate for Type 3 injuries alone was 10%.

Open fractures represent a surgical emergency; they require expert treatment based on well established guidelines in order to minimize the risk of infection. The following aspects of treatment for open fractures are particularly important.

1. Cleansing of the Wound. Gross dirt, bits of clothing and other foreign material should be literally washed away by extensive irrigation as well as by mechanical cleansing with large amounts of sterile water or saline (rather than merely camouflaged by strong antiseptics which cause further tissue damage). Residual material should be carefully picked out of the wound. The wound may even have to be opened further in order to allow adequate assessment of the degree of contamination.

2. Excision of Devitalized Tissue (Debridement). Since tissues that have lost their blood supply not only prevent primary wound healing but also enhance infection, the surgical excision of all devitalized tissue,

such as skin, subcutaneous fat, fascia, muscle and loose fragments of bone, is essential. Foreign material such as bits of clothing and dirt should also be removed; in addition it is wise to obtain a culture of the wound at the time of operation.

3. Treatment of the Fracture. When the open wound is small, such as a puncture wound from within, the fracture can usually be treated by closed means, after the wound has been cleansed, debrided and closed. When the wound is extensive, however, the fracture may require either skeletal traction or open reduction with skeletal fixation. External skeletal fixation "at a distance" above and below the fracture is often of value. In general, internal fixation should be avoided since its mere insertion tends to traumatize and devitalize more tissue and thereby tends to increase the risk of infection. Under certain circumstances, however, such as excessive instability of the fracture, or an associated vascular injury, internal fixation is justified since the risks of its application are less serious than the risks of alternative methods.

4. Closure of the Wound. Even when the

open fracture is treated within "the golden period" of the first six or seven hours and contamination is not extensive, *immediate primary closure* of the wound is contraindicated, in keeping with the aphorism "Leave open fractures open." After the first week, provided no infection has developed, *delayed primary closure* of the wound is indicated. Loss of skin may necessitate the delayed application of split thickness skin grafts. Suction drainage should be used to prevent accumulation of blood and serum in the depths of the wound. Delayed primary closure is particularly applicable in grossly contaminated open fractures sustained on the battlefield or in major disasters.

5. Antibacterial Drugs. In order to be effective in the prevention of infection, antibacterial drugs must be administered in large doses before and during treatment of the wound as well as after such treatment. Even so, antibacterial treatment is no guarantee against infection because many bacteria are resistant to the various drugs; furthermore, antibacterial drugs cannot reach any tissue in the wound that has lost its blood supply. The aforementioned surgical care of the wound is of much greater importance than antibacterial therapy.

6. Prevention of Tetanus. All patients with open fractures require preventive measures against the uncommon but serious complication of tetanus. If the patient has been previously immunized by tetanus toxoid, a booster dose of toxoid should be given. If there has been no previous immunization, or if there is inadequate information available, immediate passive immunity can be achieved by the use of 250 units of tetanus immune globulin (human). Active immunity with tetanus toxoid is initiated at the same time.

Anesthesia for Patients With Fractures

During the first hour or so after a fracture has occurred, the patient's tissues are somewhat "numb" and it may be possible to reduce certain fractures without anesthesia. Even under these circumstances,

however, reduction should be performed without anesthesia only if the physician or surgeon is confident that he can accomplish this with one deft manipulation and if the patient is not unduly tense and nervous. There is no justification for the use of "vocal" anesthesia, a combination of the physician's or surgeon's futile vocal reassurances and the patient's anguished vocal complaints.

Certain fractures, such as the Colles' fracture at the lower end of the radius in adults, are amenable to reduction after *infiltration* of a local anesthetic agent in and around the fracture site. Other fractures in the limbs can be reduced under regional anesthesia such as is provided by a brachial plexus block for the upper limb and by a spinal anesthetic for the lower limb.

In general, the majority of fractures requiring reduction are best treated under *general* anesthesia which provides not only for complete comfort but also the muscle relaxation so helpful in reducing a fracture. The risk of aspiration of stomach contents during the induction of general anesthesia as well as during the recovery period merits special mention in relation to patients with fractures. After a significant injury, such as a fracture, gastric motility virtually ceases for many hours and consequently, if the patient has ingested food or drink shortly before or after the injury, his stomach retains a mixture of undigested food and gastric acid—either of which can cause death if aspirated into the trachea or lungs. Under these circumstances therefore (unless there is a serious complication such as an open fracture or a vascular injury), general anesthesia should be delayed until approximately six hours after the ingestion of food or drink; even after this period, special precautions (such as removal of gastric contents through a tube) are necessary to prevent the serious complication of aspiration. The welfare of the patient must always take precedence over the convenience of his physician or surgeon. Temporary splints should not be removed nor should the fractured part be moved during the preliminary stages of anesthesia lest the painful stimulus initiate either cardiac arrest or laryngeal spasm.

After-Care and Rehabilitation for Patients With Fractures

You will recall that the four aims of all fracture treatment are: (1) to relive pain; (2) to obtain and maintain satisfactory position of the fracture fragments; (3) to allow and if necessary to encourage bony union; (4) to restore optimum function. The greatest of these is *restoration of function*, for what does it profit a man if he gains union of his fracture in a satisfactory position but fails to regain useful function of the injured part?

The more function that can be *preserved* during the treatment of the patient's fracture, the less function will have to be *restored*. Thus, rehabilitation of a patient begins with the immediate care of his injury, continues through the emergency treatment, the definitive treatment and beyond until the patient is restored to normal or as near normal as the injury permits.

Excessive and persistent *edema* in soft tissues produces glue-like adhesions with resultant joint stiffness and therefore should be prevented or minimized by appropriate elevation of the fractured limb during the early phase of fracture healing, as well as by improvement of venous return through active exercises of all regional muscles. Muscles that are not used soon exhibit *disuse atrophy*, which can be prevented by active static (isometric) exercises of those muscles that control the immobilized joints, and active dynamic (isotonic) exercises of all other muscles of the limb or trunk. Supervised *physiotherapy* is particularly important in the after care of *adults* with fractures; the patient must be helped to help himself. All joints that are not immobilized by the fracture treatment should be put through a full range of motion daily—by the patient (Fig. 15.55).

In addition to preservation of function in the muscles and joints after a fracture, you must think of preserving healthy function in the *patient's mind*, since the patient's attitude of mind toward his injury determines to a considerable extent the rate at which he

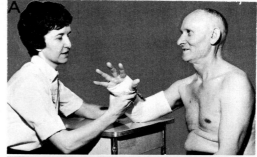
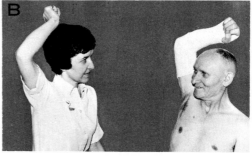

Figure 15.55. Supervised physiotherapy. The physiotherapist is teaching and encouraging the patient (who has a fracture of radius and ulna) to actively move all joints in the fractured limb that are not immobilized.

will recover from it. Indeed, *psychological considerations* added to good care of the patient's fracture can usually prevent unnecessary despondency, depression and undue concern about the future. Many patients regain function readily, some need help and others who are more timid and self-centered need constant encouragement in their efforts.

After the period of external immobilization of the fracture, active exercises should be continued even more vigorously until normal muscle power and joint motion have been regained. If necessary, the patient should be re-trained in the activities of daily living and occupation, usually through supervised *occupational therapy* (Fig. 15.56). In addition, after a period away from work the patient's *general* condition has often deteriorated and he may need to embark upon a program of general physical fitness before returning to work; this is often best accomplished in a rehabilitation center.

Rehabilitation of the whole person, as dis-

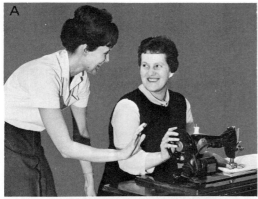

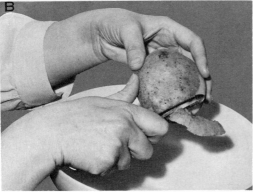

Figure 15.56. Supervised occupational therapy. The occupational therapist is re-training and encouraging this patient (who is recovering from a Colles' fracture of the distal end of her radius) in activities of daily living appropriate for her occupation as a homemaker.

cussed in Chapter 6, is always important and is especially so when the fracture has necessitated a particularly long period of treatment or has been associated with serious complications.

Complications of Fracture Treatment

Complications that are *iatrogenic* in that they are caused by the *treatment* of the fracture are classified below. These complications are to a large extent *preventable*; as you will see, they are related to three main factors: excessive local pressure, excessive traction and infection.

CLASSIFICATION OF COMPLICATIONS OF FRACTURE TREATMENT

1. Skin Complications
   Pressure lesions (pressure sores)
   Bed sores (decubitus ulcers)
   Cast sores (cast ulcers)

2. Vascular Complications
   Traction and pressure lesions
   Volkmann's ischemia
   Gangrene
3. Neurological Complications
   Traction and pressure lesions
4. Joint Complications
   Infection (septic arthritis) complicating open operative treatment of a closed injury
5. Bony Complications
   Infection (osteomyelitis) complicating open operative treatment of a closed injury

Recognition and Treatment of Complications

Some of the complications discussed below are caused by the *initial injury* that produced the fracture, whereas others are iatrogenic in that they are caused by the *treatment of the fracture*. Both groups of complications have been classified previously.

Your total care of the injured must include constant diligence and vigilance lest in your preoccupation with the fracture itself you overlook either the initial presence or the subsequent development of a significant complication. The detection of complications requires that you attend to every complaint of the patient, examine him clinically at frequent intervals, assess any positive clinical findings and when necessary, proceed with special investigations.

INITIAL AND EARLY COMPLICATIONS

A. Local Complications

Skin Complications. The skin may have sustained an abrasion (friction burn) with particles of dirt having been ground into the dermis. Such abrasions must be thoroughly cleansed under anesthesia in order to prevent the late unsightly tattoo effect of residual pigmentation from dirt under the re-epithelialized surface (Fig. 15.57).

The management of associated lacerations, puncture wounds, penetrating missile wounds, avulsion of skin and skin loss have been discussed in relation to the treatment of open fractures.

Gross swelling within a fractured limb may stretch the overlying skin and compromise

particularly vulnerable to injury in association with certain specific fractures and dislocations (Fig. 15.61).

Arterial Division. A major artery may be completely or incompletely divided either by the sudden displacement of a sharp fracture fragment from within or by an object or

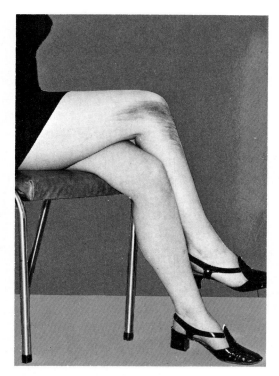

Figure 15.57. Tattoo effect from residual pigmented dirt that should have been removed from the abrasion and which is now covered by epithelium. This unsightly blemish is preventable.

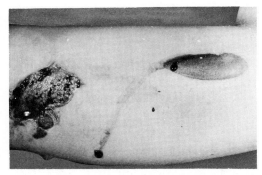

Figure 15.58. Blisters, or blebs, in the skin of the forearm in association with a fracture of the radius and ulna. One bleb has ruptured and the other is seeping serum.

the circulation to its superficial layers with resultant *blister* or *bleb* formation (Fig. 15.58).

During fracture treatment, an area of skin may be constantly compressed between a firm surface on the outside and an underlying bony prominence. Thus, a patient who is not turned regularly or is insensitive to pain may develop a *bed sore* (decubitus ulcer), particularly over the sacrum and heels (Fig. 15.59). Furthermore, excessive local pressure from an incorrectly applied plaster-of-Paris cast may produce a *pressure sore* (cast sore) (Fig. 15.60). These iatrogenic complications, which are preventable, may necessitate extensive skin grafting.

Vascular Complications. *Arterial Complications (Injury to a Major Artery).* Small blood vessels are torn at the time of all fractures but injury to a major artery is uncommon. Nevertheless, such a complicating injury is serious because of the sequelae of persistant arterial occlusion. Major arteries are

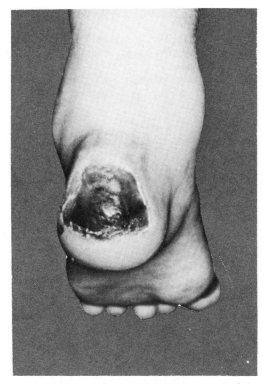

Figure 15.59. Bed sore (decubitus ulcer) of the heel in an elderly comatose patient. This lesion is preventable.

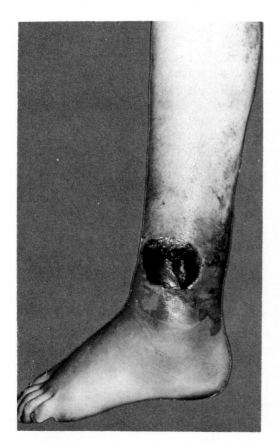

Figure 15.60. Pressure sore (cast sore) over the lateral aspect of the leg from excessive local pressure of an ineptly molded plaster cast. This iatrogenic complication, which is preventable, required a skin graft.

missile that has penetrated the deep tissues from without. A completely torn artery usually retracts and stops bleeding spontaneously, whereas one that is incompletely torn tends to continue bleeding; in either instance there is a residual hematoma locally and ischemia distally. In addition, incomplete division of an artery may lead to the development of a pulsating hematoma (false aneurysm).

Arterial Spasm. When a major artery is subjected to sudden and severe traction, either at the time of fracture or during treatment of the fracture, it may react by *persistent spasm* of its muscular coat with resultant occlusion. Although the artery has not been

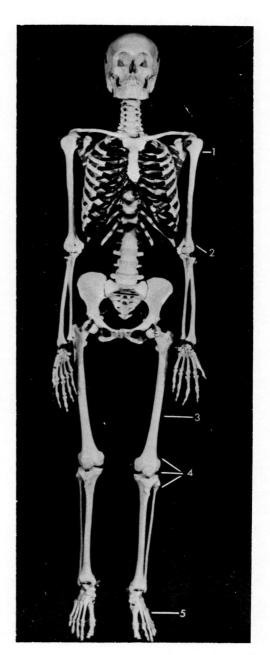

Figure 15.61. Sites of vascular complications in relation to fractures. *1*, axillary artery—fracture-dislocations and dislocations of the shoulder. *2*, brachial artery—supracondylar fractures of the humerus. *3*, femoral artery—fractures of the shaft of the femur. *4*, popliteal artery—fractures distal end of femur and proximal end of tibia, dislocation of the knee. *5*, dorsalis pedis artery—fractures in the forefoot.

divided, there is usually a tear in the intima which leads to thrombosis. Secondary arterial spasm may spread both proximally and distally to include collateral arteries in which case the resultant ischemia distally becomes even more extensive.

Arterial Compression. Occasionally a major artery becomes trapped and compressed between two fracture fragments. Compression of an artery can also be iatrogenic due to the combination of an excessively tight encircling plaster-of-Paris cast or bandage externally, and progressive swelling within a closed space internally.

Arterial Thrombosis. After any arterial injury that results in persistent occlusion, thrombosis is a potential sequel. As you might expect, the presence of pre-existing arteriosclerosis increases the risk of post-traumatic arterial thrombosis.

Recognition of Arterial Complications. External hemorrhage from a divided artery is obvious, whereas internal hemorrhage is evidenced only by a progressively enlarging local swelling. Complete arterial occlusion in a limb is associated with initial pallor of the skin distally, loss of arterial pulse, coolness of the skin and later, mottled, dark discoloration which heralds gangrene (Fig. 15.62). If the presence of a peripheral pulse is questionable, it is probably absent. A surface Doppler probe is of considerable help in detecting a peripheral pulse that is too weak to be palpable. Arteriography is helpful in localizing the precise site of arterial occlusion (Fig. 15.63).

Compartment Syndromes. When the increased pressure of progressive edema within a rigid osteofascial compartment of either the forearm or the leg threatens the circulation to the enclosed (intracompartmental) muscles and nerves, the phenomenon is called a "compartment syndrome." Formerly known as *Volkmann's ischemia*, compartment syndromes most frequently involve the flexor compartment of the forearm and the anterior tibial compartment of the leg (although any osteofascial compartment may be affected). Since tissues outside the

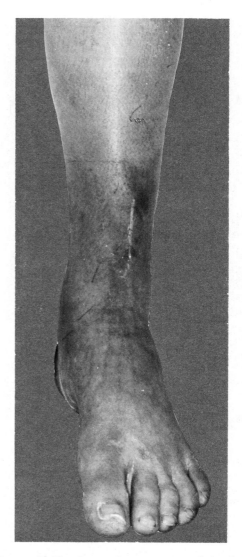

Figure 15.62. Impending gangrene of the foot and distal part of the leg in a 15-year-old boy who had sustained a closed fracture of the proximal end of the tibia. No pulse could be detected below the knee and the skin was cool with mottled dark discoloration.

compartment are spared, the skin and the distal part of the limb, although transiently affected, survive and hence, the disorder is quite different from that of gangrene.

The progressive intracompartmental pressure from edema initially compromises capillary blood flow to muscle which, in turn, produces more edema and consequently a

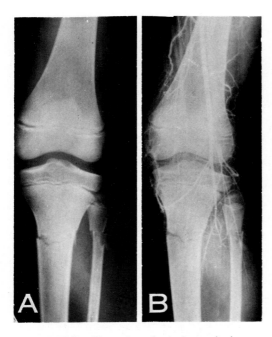

Figure 15.63. The value of arteriography in vascular occlusion. *A*, the knee region of a 15-year-old boy with a relatively undisplaced fracture of the proximal end of the tibia and fibula. The fracture, which was said to have been angulated, had been reduced 8 hours previously; the foot immediately became white and pulseless. The appearance of the boy's foot on admission is shown in Figure 15.62. *B*, an arteriogram immediately after admission reveals the exact site of vascular occlusion just distal to the bifurcation of the popliteal artery. Exploration of the arteries was performed forthwith; the arteries were decompressed after which blood flow was restored. The boy's foot did not become gangrenous but because of the 8-hour delay before arterial exploration he did develop Volkmann's ischemia of the leg muscles and a subsequent Volkmann's contracture.

vicious cycle is established. Peripheral nerves within the compartment can withstand only two to four hours of ischemia but they do have some potential for regeneration. By contrast, muscle can survive up to six hours of ischemia but cannot regenerate. Indeed, in due course, necrotic muscle is replaced by dense fibrous scar tissue that gradually shortens to produce a *"compartmental contracture"* or *Volkmann's contracture.*

A compartment syndrome may be secondary to one of two quite different phenomena: (1) proximal (extracompartmental) occlusion of the main artery supplying the compartment; (2) intracompartmental injury to either bone or soft tissue (or both). In both types, the intracompartmental pressure rises rapidly to dangerous levels, and unless this pressure is relieved expeditiously by a complete surgical fasciotomy, ischemic *necrosis* and consequent ischemic *contracture* are inevitable.

The injuries that are most frequently complicated by a compartment syndrome are: (1) displaced supracondylar fractures of the humerus with damage to the brachial artery in children; (2) excessive longitudinal traction in the treatment of fractures of the femoral shaft in children with resultant arterial spasm; (3) fractures (as well as surgical osteotomies) of the proximal third of the tibia; (4) drug-induced coma with resultant pressure on major arteries from lying on a hard surface in an awkward position for a prolonged period.

The *clinical picture* of a compartment syndrome with impending compartmental ischemia, or Volkmann's ischemia, is characterized by severe pain (from muscle ischemia), transient decrease in peripheral circulation with resultant relative pallor and coolness of the skin as well as puffy swelling of the hand or foot and, subsequently, ischemic disturbance of the involved peripheral nerve function as evidenced by paresthesia, hypoesthesia and paralysis. Thus the clinical warnings of impending intracompartmental ischemia are pain, pallor, puffiness, paresthesia and paralysis. If the underlying cause is extracompartmental the peripheral pulse is likely to be absent but if the cause is intracompartmental the peripheral pulse may be palpable. Furthermore, if the extracompartmental injury also involves serious damage to major peripheral nerves supplying sensation to the compartment, pain may not be a feature; this can be dangerously misleading. When the peripheral nerves are intact, passive extension of the fingers and wrist (or toes and ankle) aggravates the pain.

The injudicious use of analgesics for severe and persistent pain may well mask the compartmental ischemia and should be avoided.

In recent years it has become possible to measure intracompartmental interstitial fluid pressure by means of the transcutaneous insertion of a catheter of various types, e.g. the slit catheter (Rorabeck) or the wick catheter (Mubarak). The normal resting intracompartmental pressure is from 0 to 8 mm Hg. Pressures over 30 mm Hg represent an absolute indication for immediate decompression of the compartment by complete surgical fasciotomy throughout the complete length of the compartment. The fascia, of course, must be left wide open and the skin may have to be left open also— at least until the swelling subsides in a few days at which time delayed primary closure can be performed.

Treatment of Vascular Complications. Occlusion of a major artery represents a surgical emergency since within a few hours of its onset the results of the associated ischemia become irreversible. Indeed, treatment of the vascular complication takes precedence over treatment of the associated fracture itself. A series of therapeutic measures must be instituted immediately in the following order: (1) any constricting cast or bandage must be *completely* removed (and not just cut); (2) any distortion of the fractured limb or extreme position of a nearby joint should be lessened; (3) if the fracture is being treated by continuous traction, the amount of traction should be decreased; (4) if these measures fail to restore adequate peripheral circulation, an emergency arteriogram is indicated; and if there is no improvement within half an hour, the artery should be explored surgically. Sympathetic denervation by anesthetic block is of doubtful value.

At operation, if the artery has been divided, it should be repaired by direct suture; if this is not possible, continuity can be achieved either by means of an autogenous vein graft or a plastic arterial prosthesis. Associated division of a major vein should also be repaired. If the artery is merely compressed it can be released, and provided there is no associated arterial spasm, flow will be re-established. An arterial thrombus should be removed and if the artery is severely contused or if there has been an intimal tear, it may be necessary to resect the damaged portion of the vessel and restore its continuity by direct suture, vein graft or prosthesis. Persistent arterial spasm may be more difficult to relieve; if the local application of warm papaverine does not relieve the spasm, the constricted portion of the artery can sometimes be permanently dilated by means of intra-arterial injection of saline beginning proximally and dilating the vessel a segment at a time as described by Mustard. As a last resort, division of the artery and ligature of the cut ends may break the spasm in the artery and its collateral vessels and thereby re-establish distal circulation, at least in young children.

Even after re-establishment of the arterial blood flow there is likely to be a residual compartment syndrome; consequently the compartment(s) supplied by that artery may need to be decompressed by surgical fasciotomy as described above.

After operative treatment for a vascular complication, internal fixation of the fracture is indicated to prevent further movement at the site of the arterial injury.

Sequelae of Arterial Complications. 1. *Gangrene.* Persistent total ischemia distal to an arterial lesion results in necrosis of all tissues including skin (*gangrene*). The ischemic tissues become mummified and the skin eventually comes to resemble dark leather. This irreversible complication necessitates amputation through viable tissues.

2. *Compartment Syndrome (Volkmann's Ischemic Contracture).* Persistent occlusion of deep arteries for approximately six hours or longer produces ischemia of muscles and nerves with resultant necrosis. Necrotic muscle is subsequently replaced by fibrous

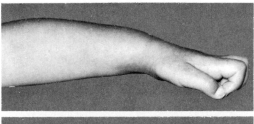
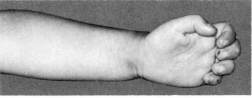

Figure 15.64. Volkmann's ischemic contracture of muscles of the forearm in a 6-year-old child. After reduction of a supracondylar fracture of the humerus the child had complained of severe pain in the forearm. Regrettably, his surgeon prescribed large doses of analgesics which relieved the pain somewhat; in the meantime he developed severe Volkmann's ischemia of nerves and muscles in the forearm. In these photographs taken 6 months later, you can see that he has severe deformities and serious disability as a result of progressive contracture of the necrotic muscles which have been replaced by fibrous tissue. This tragic outcome could have been prevented.

scar tissue which causes the involved muscle to become permanently short (contracture) (Fig. 15.64). After the establishment of persistent Volkmann's ischemia of muscle, but before the development of muscle contracture, surgical resection of the infarcted area of muscle decompresses the nerves and may prevent contracture. Established Volkmann's ischemic contracture, however, necessitates major reconstructive operations including muscle release, nerve grafts and tendon transfers to minimize the severe disability. The most important aspect of Volkmann's ischemia is its *prevention*. Furthermore, impending Volkmann's ischemia, if recognized and treated very early, can be reversed.

3. *Intermittent Claudication.* When an arterial lesion has not been sufficiently severe or persistent to produce either gangrene or Volkmann's ischemic contracture, but has not been completely repaired, the sequelae

of the persistent *relative* ischemia include pain, which is initiated by muscle activity and relieved by rest (*intermittent claudication*). In addition, there may be persistent muscle weakness, numbness and coldness in the limb.

4. *Gas Gangrene.* The uncommon but serious complication of fulminating infection by an anaerobic bacteria, *Clostridium welchii*, produces rapidly progressive edema and gas formation in the local tissues; the blood supply is soon occluded with the resultant development of *gas gangrene.*

After an incubation period of 24 to 48 hours, the patient experiences severe and constant local pain and becomes acutely ill. There is a characteristic foul, fetid odor associated with gas gangrene. Physical examination may reveal local soft tissue crepitus indicating the presence of gas; the gas can also be detected radiographically as discussed in Chapter 5 (Fig. 5.16).

The local wound should be re-opened and debrided immediately. The patient should be given systemic antibacterial therapy, usually penicillin and one of the tetracyclines. Treatment in a hyperbaric oxygen chamber for several two-hour periods usually results in dramatic improvement in the clinical picture both locally and systemically.

Venous Complications. Division of a Major Vein. A major vein may be completely or incompletely divided either by the displacement of a fracture fragment from within or by an object or missile that has penetrated the deep tissues from without. Injuries to major veins should be repaired surgically in order to prevent the late sequelae of persistent venous congestion distally.

Venous Thrombosis and Pulmonary Embolism. The veins of the lower limbs and pelvis are more susceptible to thrombosis after a fracture than those of the upper limbs. Adults are more susceptible to thrombosis than children. The main factor that precipitates thrombosis is *venous stasis*, which can be caused by local pressure on a vein from prolonged bed rest or from a tight encircling plaster-of-Paris cast or bandage. Venous stasis is aggravated by inactivity of muscles which normally have a pumping action on venous return from the limb. After a fracture the venous lesion is usually a phlebothrombosis as opposed to an inflammatory thrombosis (thrombophlebitis). The thrombus is only loosely adherent to the wall of the vein and may therefore come loose and pass to the lungs to produce *pulmonary embolism.* Approximately one half of pulmonary emboli, however, arise from a previously undetected thrombosis ("silent thrombosis").

Diagnosis. When the venous thrombosis is in the calf, the patient complains of local pain and there is tenderness in the midline posteriorly as well as distal swelling due to congestion. Passive dorsiflexion of the ankle aggravates the pain (Homan's sign). When the thrombosis is in the thigh, the entire lower limb becomes swollen. A venogram is often helpful in localizing the site of thrombosis.

The complication of pulmonary embolism varies in severity. A small pulmonary embolus may go undetected or may cause only mild chest pain. An embolus of moderate size is manifest by the sudden onset of chest pain, dyspnea and sometimes hemoptysis; a friction rub may be heard and subsequently, radiographic examination reveals a triangular shaped area of increased density in the lung, representing the infarcted segment (Fig. 15.65).

A massive pulmonary embolus, however, produces a dramatic onset of severe chest pain. The patient immediately blanches and literally drops dead.

Prevention of Venous Thrombosis. The key to prevention of venous thrombosis is the underlying venous stasis which can be prevented to a large extent by avoiding constant local pressure on veins and by encouraging the patient to actively contract all muscles in the injured limb as well as to move about as much as possible within the limits imposed by the treatment of his fracture. For adults confined to bed, the use of the elastic stocking seems to be of value in the prevention of deep venous thrombosis.

Treatment of Venous Thrombosis. As soon

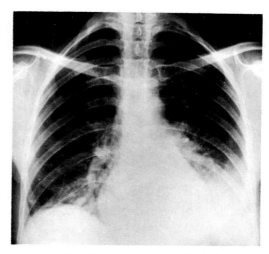

Figure 15.65. Pulmonary infarct in the left lower lobe of the lung due to pulmonary embolism in a 35-year-old woman. Five days after closed reduction of a fractured tibia, the patient experienced the sudden onset of severe pain in the left side of the chest as well as left shoulder-tip pain (referred from the left diaphragm). This radiograph reveals a triangular area of density representing the infarcted segment as well as evidence of a pleural effusion.

as this complication is recognized, the patient should be treated with appropriate anticoagulant drugs. Recent thrombosis in the femoral vein is best treated by surgical thrombectomy, not only to decrease the risk of pulmonary embolism but also to prevent the late sequelae of persistent venous obstruction in the lower limb.

Neurological Complications. Complicating injuries to brain, spinal cord or peripheral nerves in association with a fracture may be caused either by the original injury or, less commonly, by inept treatment of the fracture itself. Neurological complications are relatively common in association with specific fractures and dislocations (Fig. 15.66). The etiology, diagnosis and treatment of these injuries are discussed in Chapter 12.

Visceral Complications. Thoracoabdominal viscera may be injured at the time of an accident independent of any fractures; they may also be injured, however, by penetration of a sharp fracture fragment of a nearby bone. Thus, displaced fractures of the ribs may damage the heart and produce a hem-

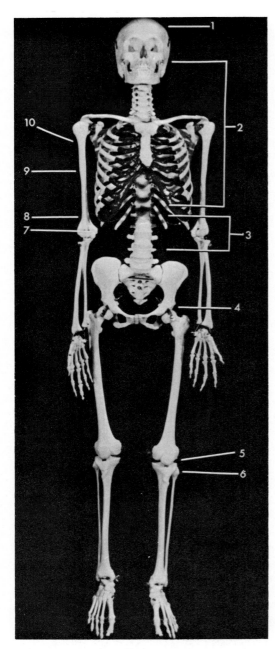

Figure 15.66. Sites of neurological complications in relation to fractures. *1*, brain—skull fractures. *2*, spinal cord—cervical and thoracic spine fractures and dislocations. *3*, cauda equina—lumbar spine fractures and dislocations. *4*, sciatic nerve—posterior dislocations and fracture-dislocations of the hip. *5*, medial and lateral popliteal nerves—dislocations of the knee. *6*, lateral popliteal nerve—vulnerable to external pressure from bandages and casts. *7*, ulnar nerve—avulsion fracture-separation of the medial epicondyle. *8*,

opericardium or may perforate the pleura to produce a hemothorax; they may even perforate the lung, to produce a hemopneumothorax. Displaced fractures of the lower ribs may perforate the liver, spleen or kidneys, Fractures of the thoracic and lumbar spine may result in paralytic ileus and gastric dilatation. Displaced fractures of the pelvis may rupture the bladder or urethra and less commonly, the colon or rectum.

Joint Complications. *Infection of a Joint (Septic Arthritis).* After an open intra-articular fracture, and less commonly after open operation on a closed intra-articular fracture, the serious complication of *septic arthritis* may ensue. Unless treated early and effectively, septic arthritis leads inevitably to destruction of articular cartilage with the resultant development of degenerative joint disease.

The diagnosis and treatment of septic arthritis are discussed in Chapter 10.

Bony Complications. *Infection of Bone (Osteomyelitis).* Open fractures are particularly susceptible to *infection*, which involves all layers of the soft tissues as well as bone at the fracture site. The treatment of open fractures is discussed in an earlier section of this chapter; it is aimed at minimizing the risk of acute osteomyelitis and its sequelae—chronic osteomyelitis, delayed union and even non-union.

A closed fracture may become infected after open operation—a terrible tragedy (Fig. 15.67). Furthermore, bone may become infected locally along the track of a metal pin used either for continuous skeletal traction or external skeletal fixation (*pin track osteomyelitis*). Indeed, a ring of bone surrounding the pin track may not only become infected, but may also become necrotic and form a *ring sequestrum* (Fig. 15.68).

Avascular Necrosis of Bone. Post-trau-

median nerve—supracondylar fractures of the humerus. *9*, radial nerve—fractures of the shaft of the humerus. *10*, circumflex nerve—dislocations and fracture-dislocations of the shoulder.

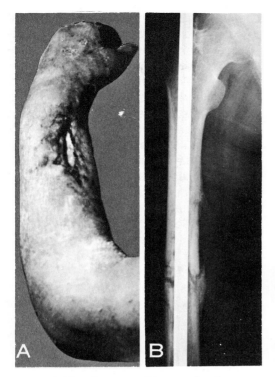

Figure 15.67.   Osteomyelitis complicating open reduction of fractures. *A*, severe osteomyelitis of the radius complicating open reduction of a closed fracture in a young man. The wound has broken open and necrotic infected bone is exposed in its depths. The patient's disability will be greatly increased and prolonged as a result of this serious complication. *B*, severe osteomyelitis of the shaft of the femur complicating open reduction and intramedullary rod fixation of a closed fracture in a young woman. Subperiosteal new bone can be seen at each end of a necrotic, infected fragment (sequestrum). This infection will be exceedingly difficult to control; the sequestrum will have to be excised and the entire area irrigated continuously with a combination of antibiotic and a detergent such as alevaire. The intramedullary nail will have to be removed as soon as there is sufficient new bone formation to provide stability at the fracture site.

matic avascular necrosis of bone is usually caused by disruption of the nutrient vessels at the time of the original injury but may also be iatrogenic as a result of excessive dissection during open reduction of fractures and dislocations. It is a serious complication since it leads not only to delayed union but

also to subsequent joint incongruity and degenerative joint disease (Fig. 15.69). The complication of avascular necrosis occurs most commonly after certain specific fractures and dislocations because of the precarious blood supply to bone at these sites (Fig. 15.70).

Post-traumatic avascular necrosis of bone is also discussed in Chapter 13.

B. Remote Complications

Fat Embolism Syndrome. Fat globules can be found in the circulation of most adults after a major fracture of the long bone. For-

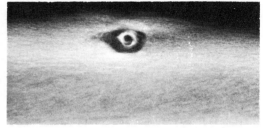

Figure 15.68.   A typical ring sequestrum in the anterior cortex of the tibia due to the complication of a pin track infection at the site of a pin that had been used for continuous skeletal traction. The radioopaque ring-shaped sequestrum is surrounded by a radiolucent area of osteolytic resorption of bone. The infection subsided after removal of the sequestrum.

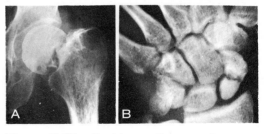

Figure 15.69.   Post-traumatic avascular necrosis of bone. *A*, avascular necrosis of the femoral head complicating a fracture of the femoral neck in a 40-year-old woman. Note also that there is non-union of the fracture. *B*, avascular necrosis of the proximal half of the scaphoid complicating a fracture in a 22-year-old man. The fracture has failed to unite one year after injury and will require bone grafting.

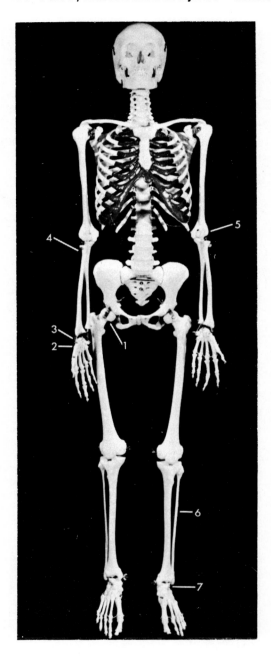

Figure 15.70. Sites of avascular necrosis of bone in relation to fractures. *1*, femoral head—fractures of the femoral neck, dislocations of the hip. *2*, lunate—dislocations of the lunate. *3*, scaphoid—fractures of the scaphoid. *4*, radial head—fractures of the neck of the radius. *5*, lateral condyle (capitellum)—fractures of the lateral condyle. *6*, middle segment of a comminuted fracture. *7*, body of the talus—fractures of the neck of the talus.

tunately, however, only a small percentage of such patients develop detectable systemic fat embolization and a significant respiratory distress syndrome with severe arterial hypoxia, the combination of which constitutes the *fat embolism syndrome.* It is probably relatively common in mild, and hence clinically undetected (sub-clinical) forms, since small fat emboli are frequently discovered as an unsuspected finding at postmortem examination of adult accident victims who may have died *with* fat emboli but not necessarily *because of* fat emboli. Most susceptible to the serious complication of clinical fat embolism syndrome are previously healthy young adults who have sustained severe fractures, especially when associated with other injuries ("multiple injuries," or "polytrauma"). Elderly persons who sustain fractures of the upper end of the femur are also susceptible. This syndrome, although rare in previously normal children, may complicate fractures in those who have some type of pre-existing systemic collagen disease with or without corticosteroid therapy.

Etiology and Pathogenesis. Although fat embolization from bone marrow has been proven to occur, the precise pathogenesis of fat embolism syndrome is both conjectural and controversial. However, it would seem that stress-induced changes in lipid metabolism as well as in blood coagulation (as may result from severe trauma) may cause coalescence of chylomicrons to form macroglobules of fat that produce fat embolization and resultant arterial hypoxia with metabolic and respiratory acidosis. Indeed, there may well be several mutually compatible explanations.

Clinical Features. Detectable fat embolism usually develops after a latent period of two or three days although in very severe cases it may become manifest within a few hours of injury. Since the symptoms and signs are manifestations of emboli in various organs they might be anticipated. Pulmonary emboli cause respiratory distress with dyspnea, hemoptysis, tachypnea and cyanosis; cerebral emboli are manifest by headache and irritability followed by delirium, stupor and even coma; cardiac emboli cause tachycardia and a drop in blood pressure. Transient skin lesions become apparent as multiple petechial hemorrhages (which may be due to a transient thrombocytopenia rather than to emboli), particularly in the skin of the upper chest and axillae as well as in the conjunctivae (Fig. 15.71). The patient also develops a fever. The prognosis in patients who exhibit pulmonary insufficiency and coma is grave in that the mortality rate is approximately 20%, a fatal outcome usually being related to a combination of pulmonary and cerebral lesions. Furthermore, fat embolism syndrome has been estimated to be the major cause of death in 20% of fatalities associated with fractures.

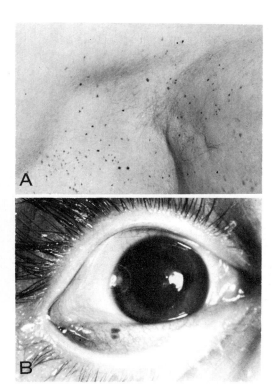

Figure 15.71. Petechial hemorrhages associated with fat embolism: *A*, over the lateral chest wall and axilla and *B*, in the conjunctiva of the lower lid. Two days previously the patient had sustained fractures of both femora in an automobile accident.

Radiographic Features. In well established fat embolism, radiographic examination of the lungs reveals multiple areas of consolidation—a "snow storm" appearance.

Laboratory Features. Since there is no pathognomonic laboratory test for fat embolism syndrome, the diagnosis is primarily clinical. In approximately half the patients with clinically recognizable fat embolism, the serum fatty acids are elevated and there is free fat in the sputum and urine. The hemoglobin usually drops sharply very early in the process. The partial pressure of oxygen in the blood (PO_2) is reduced well below the normal level of 100 mm—sometimes as low as 60 mm. Thrombocytopenia is often present.

Prevention of Fat Embolism. Since fat embolism is related at least in part to disturbed metabolism, efforts should be made to prevent metabolic and respiratory acidosis by good general care of the injured patient, including high carbohydrate intake plus constant maintenance of fluid and electrolyte balance. Such care of all adults who have sustained two or more fractures definitely decreases the incidence of fat embolism (Hillman).

Treatment of Established Fat Embolism. Once fat embolism is established, the use of heparin increases the rate of hydrolysis and removal of emboli; and corticosteroids may decrease the tissue injury in the lungs. Blood volume and electrolytes should be restored. Intravenous alcohol is of doubtful value and may even mask the cerebral symptoms. Low molecular weight dextran infusion may help to improve the microcirculation in the involved organs. In the presence of respiratory distress, endotracheal intubation or, if necessary, a tracheostomy followed by mechanically assisted respiration with oxygen, improves the patient's clinical condition by decreasing cerebral anoxia. Constant monitoring of PO_2, PCO_2 and arterial pH provides the best appraisal of the patient's metabolic status and serves as a guide to corrective therapy.

Pulmonary Embolism. This complication

has been discussed in a previous section of this chapter dealing with venous thrombosis.

Pneumonia. When treatment of a patient's fracture involves complete and prolonged bed rest, the convalescent period may become complicated by *hypostatic pneumonia.* The elderly are particularly susceptible. Likewise, painful fractures of the ribs with associated limitation of respiratory excursion may lead to the development of pneumonia. Treatment includes appropriate antibiotic therapy as well as deep breathing exercises, frequent turning of the bedfast patient and, if necessary, bronchoscopic suction.

Tetanus. Tetanus, which is caused by *Clostridium tetani*, is a preventable complication of open wounds. Nevertheless, at least 300 persons still die each year in North America as a result of this tragic complication, which even with treatment has a mortality rate of 50%.

Etiology and Pathogenesis. The *Clostridium tetani*, being an anaerobic organism, thrives in devitalized or dead tissue where it produces a powerful neurotoxin; the neurotoxin is carried by the lymphatics and bloodstream to the central nervous system where it soon becomes fixed in anterior horn cells after which it can no longer be neutralized by antitoxins. The site of entry may vary from an apparently insignificant puncture wound to a severe open fracture wound. Although the incubation period may vary considerably it is usually between 10 and 14 days.

Clinical Features. The effect of the powerful neurotoxin is to initiate tonic, and later clonic, contractions of skeletal muscles (*tetanic spasms*). Spasms of the neck and trunk muscles produce the characteristic arched back posture ("*opisthotonus*"), spasms of the jaw muscles produce trismus ("*lock jaw*"), while spasms in the fascial muscles account for the sardonic grin (*risus sardonicus*) (Fig. 15.72). Eventually involvement of intercostal muscles and diaphragm leads to fatal asphyxia.

Prevention. The prevention of tetanus has been described in the preceding section of

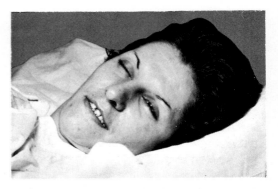

Figure 15.72. Risus sardonicus of severe tetanus in a 35-year-old woman. The sardonic grin is caused by tetanic spasms of her facial muscles; she was acutely ill and at this stage was semicomatose.

this chapter in relation to the treatment of open fractures.

Treatment. Established tetanus requires the intravenous administration of large doses of tetanus immune globulin (human), heavy sedation and, in the presence of severe muscle spasms and respiratory involvement, endotracheal intubation and mechanically assisted respiration. Antibacterial therapy is of little value in the treatment of established tetanus but may be helpful in preventing or controlling associated infections.

Delirium Tremens. When a chronic alcoholic sustains a major injury and is admitted to hospital, his source of alcohol is abruptly withdrawn. During the ensuing few days he may exhibit dramatic and even alarming *withdrawal symptoms* which are characterized by disorientation, anxiety, agitation and disturbing visual hallucinations. Understandably the development of delirum tremens (the "D.T.'s") interferes with treatment of the patient's injuries and may also mimic such complications as head injury and fat embolism.

LATE COMPLICATIONS

A. Local Complications

Late Joint Complications. *Joint Stiffness.* Transient stiffness is an anticipated sequel in any joint that has been immobilized during the period of a fracture; it can be minimized during the period of immobilization by active contraction of all muscle groups controlling the joint and can usually be successfully treated by active movement of the joint after the immobilization has been discontinued. This transient type of joint stiffness is not considered a complication.

Persistent joint stiffness, by contrast, is a significant complication since it retards restoration of normal function in the injured limb. Such joint stiffness is most likely to complicate fractures that are close to a joint or those that actually involve a joint surface. Rare in childhood, the incidence of persistent joint stiffness rises with advancing years and is particularly common in joints which have had pre-existing degenerative changes.

The commonest causes are peri-articular adhesions, intra-articular adhesions, adhesions between the muscles and bone and post-traumatic myositis ossificans (post-traumatic ossification in muscle).

Peri-articular Adhesions. After a fracture near a joint, adhesions may develop between the fibrous capsule and ligaments as well as between these structures and nearby muscles and tendons. Such adhesions impair the normal gliding between these structures. Forceful passive movement at this stage may actually cause more adhesions. After a period of extensive physiotherapy (involving active movements only), however, when no further improvement in joint motion is being obtained, a gentle manipulation of the joint under general anesthesia frequently yields a considerable increase in joint movement which, of course, must be retained by further physiotherapy. Under these circumstances, continuous passive motion (CPM) may prove to be of value.

Intra-articular Adhesions. Intra-articular fractures, dislocations and fracture-dislocations are invariably associated with a hemarthrosis and subsequent fibrinous deposits on the synovium and articular cartilage which lead to firm adhesions within the joint between folds of synovium and between the synovium and the cartilage. After a period of extensive physiotherapy, any persistent joint stiffness in large joints such as the knee and shoulder usually responds to gentle manipulation under anesthesia. Such manipulation however, is contra-indicated in small joints such as those of the hand.

As with peri-articular adhesions, so also with intra-articular adhesions, CPM may prove helpful in both prevention and treatment.

Adhesions Between Muscles and Between Muscles and Bone. Severely displaced fractures are always associated with extensive tearing of surrounding muscles. Likewise, during open reduction of fractures the surrounding muscles may be damaged. Subsequent formation of fibrous scar tissue binds muscles to each other as well as to the underlying bone. This phenomenon is particularly common after fractures of the lower end of the femur where the adhesions involving the quadriceps muscle result in persistent limitation of knee flexion. Physiotherapy is helpful in restoring joint motion but manipulation is contraindicated because of the risk of producing additional muscle tears and consequently additional adhesions. Surgical release of the adhesions sometimes becomes necessary for this type of persistent joint stiffness. We have already used CPM immediately after such operations with benefit.

Post-traumatic Degenerative Joint Disease. Any residual incongruity of joint surfaces following an intra-articular fracture, dislocation or fracture-dislocation, particularly in weight-bearing joints, leads inevitably to the gradual development of degenerative joint disease with subsequent use of the joint as discussed in Chapter 11 (Fig. 15.73). This complication emphasizes the necessity for perfect restoration of joint surfaces after injury. An additional cause of post-traumatic degenerative joint disease in the weight-bearing joints is malunion, particularly malalignment, of fractures with residual excessive stresses being applied to one area of the joint (Fig. 15.74).

The treatment of degenerative disease of various joints is discussed in Chapter 11.

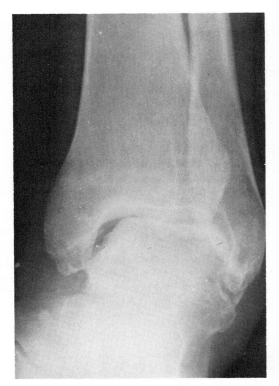

Figure 15.73. Post-traumatic degenerative joint disease in the ankle of a 57-year-old man who had injured his ankle 25 years previously.

Bony Complications. *Abnormal Healing of Fractures.* The healing of a fracture may be abnormal in one of three ways: (1) union may occur in the usual time but in an abnormal position (*mal-union*); (2) union may be delayed beyond a reasonable time (*delayed union*); (3) union may fail to occur (*non-union*).

Mal-union. As the term *mal-union* implies, union has occurred but badly, in the sense that the fracture has united in an unsatisfactory position of significant deformity. Minor degrees of residual deformity (angulation, rotation, shortening, lengthening) are common but do not present significant problems either in relation to appearance or function. Major degrees of residual deformity, however, particularly angulatory deformity, are significant in relation to both appearance and function as well as to the late complication of degenerative joint disease (Fig. 15.75). Mal-union frequently necessitates a correc-

tive osteotomy; in most instances, however, mal-union is preventable.

Delayed Union. Under certain circumstances, healing of a given fracture is much slower than the estimated rate of healing for that particular fracture. This slow type of fracture healing is referred to as *delayed union.* Successive clinical and radiographic examinations reveal evidence of slow but steady progression toward union with no radiographic sclerosis of the bone ends; patience is required by both the patient and his surgeon (Fig. 15.76). Occasionally, however, the surgeon must encourage union by means of an autogenous bone graft.

Non-union. Complete failure of a fracture to unite by bone after a much longer period than normal is referred to as *non-union*, of which there are two types. In one type of

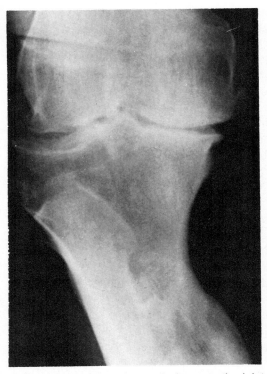

Figure 15.74. Post-traumatic degenerative joint disease in the knee of a 60-year-old man. The degenerative joint disease is secondary to excessive wear on the medial side of the knee joint which in turn has resulted from the long-standing varus malalignment of a mal-united tibia. The deformity had been present for 20 years.

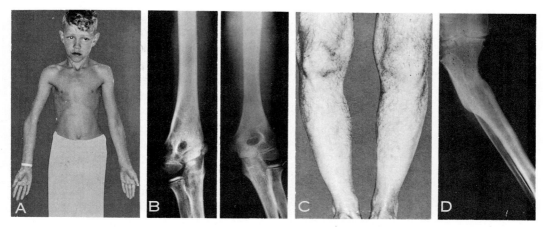

Figure 15.75.   Mal-union of fractures. *A*, cubitus varus ("gun stock deformity") of the right elbow of a boy due to mal-union of a supracondylar fracture of the humerus. Did you also notice that he has a congenital cataract of his right eye? *B*, cubitus varus of the right elbow. The loss of carrying angle of the right elbow is apparent when compared with the normal carrying angle of the left elbow. *C*, genu varum ("bow leg") of the right leg in a 60-year-old man due to mal-union of a fractured tibia 20 years previously. *D*, marked varus deformity of a mal-united tibia. Note the degenerative joint disease of the knee, especially in the medial compartment.

non-union the fracture has healed by fibrous tissue only (*fibrous non-union*) but it may have some potential for bony union provided it is rigidly immobilized internally for a sufficiently long period of time and provided any local deterrent to fracture healing, such as infection, is eradicated (Fig. 15.77). Once radiographic examination reveals that the bone ends have become sclerosed, the surgeon should encourage union by autogenous bone graft.

In the second type of non-union, however, continued movement at the fracture site stimulates the formation of a false joint (*pseudarthrosis*) complete with a synovial-like capsule, synovial cavity and synovial fluid (Fig. 15.78). An established non-union cannot possibly unite even with prolonged immobilization and therefore requires bone grafting. Autogenous cancellous bone grafts are much more effective than large cortical grafts.

Electrical Stimulation of Fracture Healing. During the past two decades one facet of biophysics that has become particularly relevant to fracture healing has been the electrical stimulation of osteogenesis as an alternative to bone grafting in the treatment of delayed union and non-union of fractures (as discussed in Chapter 6). When bone is stressed by bending forces, *stress-generated electrical potentials* develop—electronegative on the concave (compression) side and electropositive on the convex (tension) side. Furthermore, *biolectrical potentials* which are dependent on cellular viability arise in living unstressed bone—electronegative in sites of bone growth and repair, and electropositive in other sites. It has also been shown that the application of relatively small amounts of electrical currents to bone stimulates osteogenesis around the negative electrode (cathode).

On the basis of these biophysical data the following three systems of electrical stimulation have been developed for the treatment of delayed union and non-union of fractures in humans: (1) constant direct current through percutaneous wire cathodes (semi-invasive) (Brighton); (2) constant direct current through implanted electrodes and an implanted power pack (invasive) (Dwyer and Paterson); (3) inductive coupling through electromagnetic coils (non-invasive) (Bassett and deHaas).

Although each of these systems has its

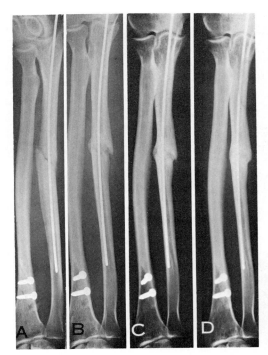

Figure 15.76. Delayed union of an oblique fracture of the shaft of the ulna in a 35-year-old woman. The fracture had been treated by open reduction and intramedullary nailing; a coexistent fracture of the distal end of the radius had been treated by open reduction and screw fixation. *A*, two months after injury the fracture line in the ulna is clearly visible and there is little callus. *B*, four months after injury, union in the ulna is delayed but still progressing; the fracture of the radius has united. *C*, nine months after injury the ulna is still not united but union is progressing slowly. *D*, one year after injury union, though delayed, has finally occurred.

advantages and disadvantages, all three have been proven to be effective in that, for properly selected patients, they all provide an over-all success rate of approximately 80%. All three systems are effective in the treatment of delayed unions and of fibrous non-unions but are ineffective when there is an established false joint (pseudarthrosis).

The factors that favor delayed union and non-union include the following: (1) severe disruption of the periosteal sleeve at the time of the original fracture, or subsequently at the time of open operation; (2) loss of blood supply to one or both fracture fragments; (3) inadequate immobilization of the fracture;

shearing forces are particularly harmful; (4) an inadequate period of immobilization; (5) distraction of fracture fragments by excessive traction; (6) persistent interposition of soft tissues in the fracture site; (7) infection at the fracture site from an open fracture (or from an open operation); (8) a local and progressive disease of bone (certain types of pathological fractures).

Persistent Infection of Bone. If osteomyelitis that has complicated an open fracture or open reduction of a closed fracture is not completely eradicated, it persists and be-

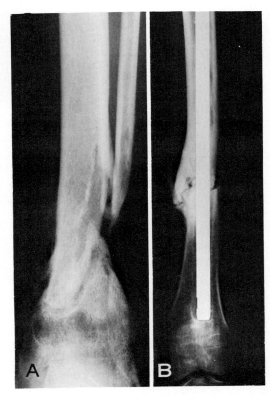

Figure 15.77. Non-union of fractures. *A*, non-union of a comminuted fracture of the tibia in a 24-year-old woman despite 18 months of immobilization. Note the sclerosis of the bone ends. This is a fibrous non-union which requires bone grafting. *B*, infected non-union of the closed femoral shaft fracture that had been treated one year previously by open reduction and intramedullary nailing in a 30-year-old man. The fracture line is still apparent, the bone ends are sclerosed and there is evidence of persistent movement around the nail in the distal fragment. This fracture will not unite until the infection has been eradicated.

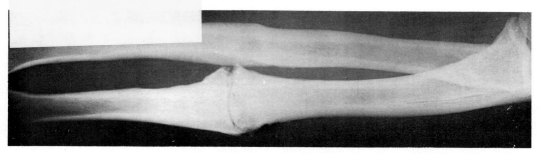

Figure 15.78.   Non-union of the ulna with formation of a pseudarthrosis in a 60-year-old man whose fracture had occurred 20 years previously. The patient still complained of pain and local tenderness; this type of non-union requires bone grafting and internal fixation.

comes chronic osteomyelitis which may be extremely resistant to treatment, as discussed in Chapter 10. Furthermore, local chronic osteomyelitis frequently leads to delayed union or even non-union (*infected non-union*) and the fracture cannot heal until the infection is completely controlled (Fig. 15.77*B*).

Post-Traumatic Osteoporosis. During the period of immobilization of a fractured limb, particularly if the patient has failed to maintain good tone in muscles controlling immobilized joints, the bones atrophy (*disuse atrophy*, *disuse osteoporosis*), since bone resorption exceeds bone deposition (Fig. 15.79). Minor degrees of disuse osteoporosis are common, but if the osteoporosis is severe and persistent it retards restoration of normal function of the limb. Intensive physiotherapy and gradual increase in the stresses applied to the osteoporotic bones tend to reverse the process.

Sudeck's Post-Traumatic Painful Osteoporosis (Reflex Sympathetic Dystrophy). Certain individuals, particularly those who are somewhat fearful and inhibited, seem predisposed to develop the troublesome complication of Sudeck's post-traumatic painful osteoporosis. The initial injury, which is usually in the distal part of a limb, may or may not include a fracture and may even be trivial.

This complication is usually detected by the unexpected failure of the patient to regain normal function in the hand or foot a few months after the injury at a time when most patients would have recovered fully.

The patient complains of severe pain in the hand or foot and is disinclined to use it. The joints become stiff, the soft tissues are edematous and the skin is moist, mottled, smooth and shiny. Radiographic examination reveals an exaggerated degree of disuse osteoporosis (Fig. 15.80).

Sudeck's post-traumatic painful osteoporosis is a prolonged complication that is difficult to treat. Local warmth and active exercises are helpful. Occasionally repeated sympathetic blocks are required to relieve the symptoms. Recovery is slow and may take many months, but is relatively sure.

Refracture. The bone at the site of a completely healed fracture that has become remodeled is just as strong as it was before the fracture. Nevertheless, during the relatively long period between clinical union and complete consolidation, the fracture is still relatively susceptible to *refracture*. This complication is uncommon in adults but occasionally occurs in children who, with few inhibitions and little fear, return to vigorous activity including sports at the earliest possible opportunity (Fig. 15.81).

A different type of re-fracture, which is seen both in children and adults, occurs not at the exact site of the original fracture but at the site of a screw, a site that is always weaker than normal bone (Fig. 15.82).

Metal Failure. A metallic device that is used to obtain internal fixation of a fracture serves only as a temporary internal splint to maintain reduction of the fracture fragments during the early weeks or months of healing. When fracture healing proceeds normally,

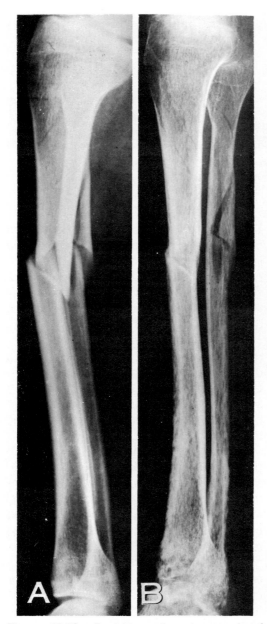

Figure 15.79. Post-traumatic osteoporosis of the tibia and fibula after a period of immobilization. A, spiral fracture of the tibia and fibula in a young adult. B, three months later the fractures are uniting but note the marked osteoporosis, particularly in the distal fragments.

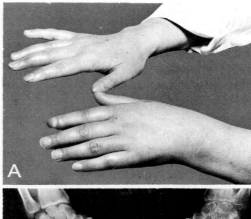

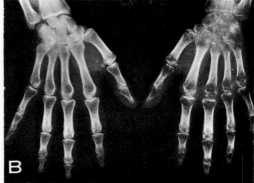

Figure 15.80. Sudeck's painful post-traumatic osteoporosis (reflex sympathetic dystrophy) in the left hand of a 30-year-old woman three months after a fracture of the radius. A, note that the left hand is swollen and the skin is smooth and shiny. B, an exaggerated degree of osteoporosis in the left hand most striking in the areas of cancellous bone.

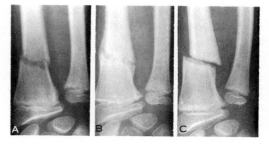

Figure 15.81. Refracture. A, fracture of the distal end of the radius in a 13-year-old boy. B, six weeks after injury the fracture has become clinically united but not yet radiographically consolidated. C, three months after the initial injury and before the fracture had become consolidated, the boy sustained a second injury and consequently a refracture through the still relatively weak area of the original fracture. Note the amount of epiphyseal growth (a few millimeters) that has taken place since the original fracture.

the metal is subjected to diminishing stress until the fracture is completely united after which the metal is no longer stressed. By contrast, however, with delayed union and non-union there is persistent movement and

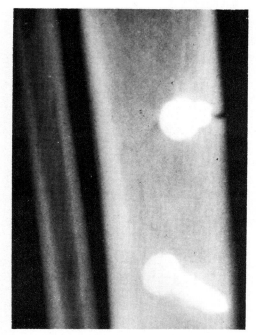

Figure 15.82. Refracture of the tibia that has occurred, 5 years after the original injury, not through the site of the original fracture but through the weakened site of a screw.

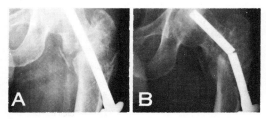

Figure 15.83. Metal failure. *A*, non-union of a fracture of the femoral neck in an elderly adult. The metal nail is unable to withstand the repeated stresses of continual movement at the fracture site and is beginning to bend. *B*, two months later the metal has fatigued, has failed completely and has broken.

hence repeated stress on the metal at the fracture site over a period of many months or even years. Under these circumstances, the metal may "fatigue" as a result of local rearrangement of its molecular structure; a crack develops and eventually the metallic device fails completely and breaks (Fig. 15.83).

Muscular Complications. *Traumatic*

Myositis Ossificans (*Post-traumatic Ossification*). Occasionally, after a fracture, a dislocation or even an isolated muscle injury, particularly in the region of the elbow and thigh of children and young adults, a rapidly enlarging painful tender mass develops in the injured tissues. This mass, which is in part a hematoma is initially radiolucent but soon radiographic examination reveals evidence of extensive ossification (Fig. 15.84). This new bone formation in an abnormal site is referred to as *heterotopic ossification* and develops between (rather than within) the torn muscle fibers. Patients with severe

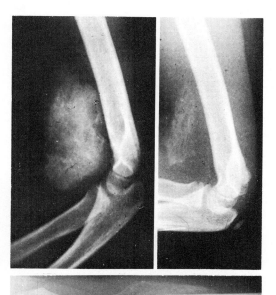

Figure 15.84. Post-traumatic myositis ossificans. *Left*, three weeks after a posterior dislocation of the elbow that had been reduced but not immobilized, radiographic examination of the child's elbow reveals evidence of extensive ossification in the soft tissues. At this stage there was marked limitation of elbow motion. *Right*, six months later, after no treatment other than active exercises, the area of myositis ossificans has been to a large extent resorbed. The range of elbow motion was almost normal. *Bottom*, post-traumatic myositis ossificans in the anterior aspect of the thigh of a 20-year-old football player 4 weeks after he had sustained a direct blow to this area. This type of post-traumatic ossification also tends to be resorbed spontaneously.

head injuries or paraplegia are particularly prone to develop this complication. Understandably, this painful lesion is accompanied by considerable limitation of motion in the related joint.

The treatment for post-traumatic myositis ossificans consists of local rest by splinting during the active stage. Passive stretching or manipulation of the related joint is contraindicated since it tears more muscle fibers and aggravates the entire process. The same is true of attempts to excise the lesion in the early stages; furthermore, the microscopic appearance of the lesion at this stage is dangerously similar to that of osteosarcoma for which it could be tragically mistaken. Left completely alone, the heterotopic new bone is to a large extent resorbed spontaneously over the ensuing months; the residual lesion is no longer painful and joint motion improves.

Late Rupture of Tendons. In the region of the wrist and ankle, tendons glide along smooth bony grooves but after a metaphyseal fracture that heals with an irregularity in the cortex, these grooves are no longer smooth. Consequently, over a period of months a tendon may gradually become frayed from the friction and finally rupture. This complication of a fracture is not common, but it occasionally occurs in the extensor pollicis longus tendon after a Colles' fracture of the distal end of the radius.

Neurological Complications. *Tardy Nerve Palsy.* A residual valgus deformity of the elbow after either mal-union or non-union of a fracture results in excessive stretching of the ulnar nerve as well as friction between the nerve and the distal end of the humerus during flexion and extension of the elbow. Gradually, over a period of years, from 10 to 20, the nerve becomes thickened by intraneural fibrosis; symptoms and signs of an ulnar nerve lesion become apparent (Fig. 15.85). The only effective treatment for this late complication is surgical transposition (relocation) of the ulnar nerve to the anterior aspect of the elbow.

B. Remote Complications

Renal Calculi. Patients, particularly adults, who are confined to bed for many

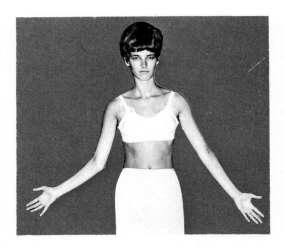

Figure 15.85. Tardy ulnar palsy. This 20-year-old girl had residual cubitus valgus secondary to malunion of a fractured lateral condyle 15 years previously. She had just recently developed symptoms and signs of an incomplete tardy ulnar nerve palsy.

weeks or months as a result of multiple complicated fractures, have a tendency to develop radio-opaque renal calculi of the calcium type. The combined underlying factors responsible for this complication are inadequate drainage of urine from the dependent calyces and the hypercalcemia associated with generalized disuse osteoporosis. Renal calculi can be prevented to a large extent by an increased fluid intake (at least 4,000 ml per day) and frequent turning of the patient. As soon as it is feasible the patient should be allowed out of bed, not only to facilitate renal drainage but also to minimize disuse osteoporosis.

Accident Neurosis. When a patient's fracture or dislocation has resulted from an accident for which he is entitled to industrial compensation, accident insurance or liability insurance, he may either wittingly or unwittingly develop patterns of neurotic behavior. Such a patient, although not necessarily a malingerer, consistently denies that he is able to return to his former occupation. Even extensive rehabilitation may fail to accelerate the patient's recovery and occasionally psychiatric examination is required. In some instances, recovery becomes possible only after legal settlement of the patient's claim.

SPECIAL TYPES OF FRACTURES

Four types of fractures merit separate consideration. These fractures, which are "special" in that they are markedly different from ordinary fractures, include *stress fractures*, *pathological fractures*, *birth fractures*, and *fractures that involve the epiphyseal plate*. The latter two types of fractures are discussed in Chapter 16.

Stress Fractures (Fatigue Fractures)

Just as metal may fatigue as a result of repeated stresses and consequently develop a small crack or fatigue fracture, so also may bone, particularly if it is subjected to unaccustomed stresses for which it has not had time to become "conditioned" by the normal process of work hypertrophy. Thus, when an individual who is "out of condition" or "out of training" begins to participate in activities such as long marches, track and field activities or ballet dancing, one of the weight-bearing bones may fatigue as a result of the repeated stresses and develop a small crack (*stress fracture* or *fatigue fracture*). Unlike metal however, living bone can react to fatigue by healing and therefore, the crack does not proceed to a displaced fracture.

The more common clinical examples of stress or fatigue fractures are: the second, third or fourth metatarsals in military recruits (march fracture) (Fig. 15.86), the lower end of the fibula in runners; the upper third of the tibia in jumpers and ballet dancers.

Clinically, when the fatigue fracture first develops, the patient experiences the insidious onset of local pain that is aggravated by activity and relieved by rest; local deep tenderness can be readily detected. The tiny crack may not become readily apparent radiographically until subperiosteal and endosteal new bone appears during the healing process (Fig. 15.87).

Treatment consists of desisting from the responsible activity until the crack has healed. Subsequently, gradual resumption of activity results in sufficient work hypertrophy of the bone to increase its strength and thereby gradually "condition" it for the stresses of the particular activity involved.

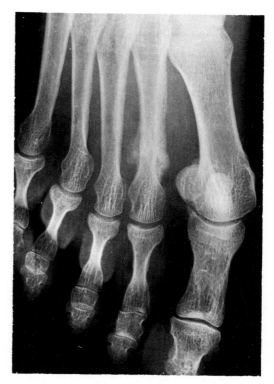

Figure 15.86. Stress fracture, or fatigue fracture, of the neck of the second metatarsal in a 45-year-old woman who had recently undertaken an exercise program including long walks. She had complained of pain for 3 weeks prior to this radiograph which reveals abundant callus surrounding the stress fracture. In the metatarsals, such fractures are usually referred to as "march fractures."

Pathological Fractures

Whereas an ordinary fracture occurs through ordinary or normal bone, a *pathological fracture* is one that occurs through abnormal bone, bone that is pathological, weaker and hence more susceptible to fracture than normal bone. The pathological bone may be so weak that it is fractured by a trivial injury, or even by normal use; nevertheless, even if the pathological bone breaks as a result of a major injury it is still a pathological fracture.

On the basis of your knowledge gained from the preceding chapters, you will appreciate that pathological fractures can occur in a wide variety of disorders, some localized, some disseminated and others generalized. The following is a classification of

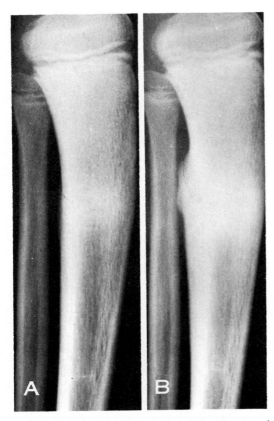

Figure 15.87. Stress fracture of the upper end of the tibia in a 10-year-old boy who had recently become involved in strenuous track and field activities. *A*, the initial radiograph, taken after the boy had been complaining of local pain for only one week, reveals only a tiny crack and slight sclerosis. *B*, five weeks later radiographic examination reveals the stress fracture more clearly as well as the subperiosteal and endosteal new bone of the healing process.

disorders in which pathological fractures are most likely to occur:

CLASSIFICATION OF DISORDERS THAT PREDISPOSE BONE TO PATHOLOGICAL FRACTURE

   I. Congenital Abnormalities (Chapter 8)
      Localized
      Congenital defect of tibia (leading to pseudarthrosis)
      Disseminated
      Enchondromatosis
      Generalized
      Osteogenesis imperfecta (fragile bones)
      Osteopetrosis (chalk bones)

  II. Metabolic Bone Disease (Chapter 9)
      Rickets
      Osteomalacia
      Scurvy
      Osteoporosis
      Hyperparathyroidism
 III. Disseminated Bone Disorders of Unknown Etiology (Chapter 9)
      Polyostotic fibrous dysplasia
      Skeletal reticuloses
         Hand-Schüller-Christian disease, eosinophilic granuloma Gaucher's disease
  IV. Inflammatory Disorders (Chapter 10)
      Hematogenous osteomyelitis
      Osteomyelitis secondary to wounds
      Tuberculous osteomyelitis
      Rheumatoid arthritis
   V. Neuromuscular Disorders (with Disuse Osteoporosis) (Chapter 12)
      Paralytic disorders
         Poliomyelitis, paraplegia (spina bifida and acquired paraplegia)
      Disorders of muscle
      Muscular dystrophy
  VI. Avascular Necrosis of Bone (Chapter 13)
      Post-traumatic avascular necrosis
      Post-irradiation necrosis
 VII. Neoplasms of Bone (Chapter 14)
      Primary neoplasms and neoplasm-like lesions
         Non-osteogenic fibroma
         Monostotic fibrous dysplasia
         Simple bone cyst
         Enchondroma
         Angioma
         Aneurysmal bone cyst
      True primary neoplasms of bone
      A. Osteogenic neoplasms
         Osteosarcoma
      B. Chondrogenic neoplasms
         Benign chondroblastoma
         Chondromyxoid fibroma
         Chondosarcoma
      C. Collagenic neoplasms
         Fibrosarcoma
      D. Myelogenic neoplasms
         Plasma cell myeloma
         Ewing's tumor
         Reticulum cell sarcoma

Hodgkin's disease
Acute leukemia
Osteoclastoma (giant cell tumor)
Metatastatic neoplasms in bone
Metastatic carcinoma
Metastatic neuroblastoma

CLINICAL FEATURES AND DIAGNOSIS

Occasionally a pathological fracture is the first manifestation of an abnormality of bone in which case further investigation is required to establish the precise nature of the underlying disorder. The clinical features, in addition to those of the fracture, are those of the underlying condition and have been described in preceding chapters indicated in the classification.

PROGNOSIS OF PATHOLOGICAL FRACTURES

Most pathological fractures will unite since the rate of bone deposition in fracture healing is usually more rapid than the rate of bone resorption of the underlying pathological process (Fig. 15.88). A pathological fracture through an area of osteomyelitis, however, will not usually unite until the infection has been controlled. In certain highly malignant primary neoplasms such as osteosarcoma, the rate of bone destruction and resorption may be almost as great as that of bone deposition; under these circumstances, union will be markedly delayed and amputation is indicated (Fig. 15.89). Pathological fractures through metastatic neoplasms in the limbs usually merit internal fixation combined with irradiation and, if indicated, hormone therapy; the fracture thus treated will usually unite and in the meantime, the patient, who is already doomed by his disease, will be spared much misery, pain and disability during the remaining months of his life (Fig. 15.90).

DISLOCATIONS AND ASSOCIATED INJURIES

Much of what you have learned about fractures from the preceding section of this chapter is equally applicable to dislocations and associated injuries. Certain special features of joint injuries, however, merit special consideration.

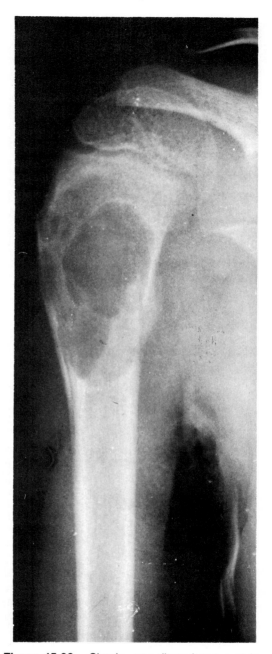

Figure 15.88. Simple, or solitary bone cyst in the metaphyseal region of the upper end of the humerus in a 10-year-old boy. Note the healing pathological fracture through the weakened cortex on the medial side. The boy had sustained a minor injury 3 weeks previously.

Normal Joint Stability

Synovial joints are designed to permit smooth movement through a normal range that is specific for each joint. Three struc-

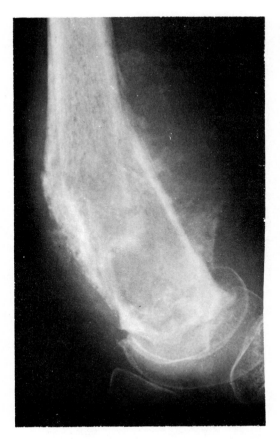

Figure 15.89. Pathological fracture through an osteosarcoma in the lower end of the femur in a 9-year-old girl. The angulated femur is beginning to unite by subperiosteal callus despite the presence of the rapidly growing neoplasm; nevertheless, since union will be delayed and refracture is likely, amputation is indicated.

tural factors are responsible for preventing an abnormal range of motion and thereby for providing *joint stability*: (1) the reciprocal contours of the opposing joint surfaces; (2) the integrity of the fibrous capsule and ligaments; (3) the protective power of muscles that move the joint. Thus, a defect in any one or any combination of these structures may result in loss of joint stability.

The relative importance of these stabilizing factors varies with each type of joint. In a ball and socket joint, such as the hip, the joint contours are the most important factor; in a hinge joint such as the knee, ligaments are the most important factor; in a freely mobile joint such as the shoulder, however,

joint stability depends mostly on the integrity of the fibrous capsule and the protective power of surrounding muscles.

Physical Factors in the Production of Joint Injuries

Whereas a fracture of a bone is a break in its continuity, dislocation of a joint is a *structural loss of its stability*. The physical factors that suddenly force a joint beyond its normal range of motion cause a *tension failure* either in the bony components of the joint or in the fibrous capsule and ligaments. These structures are particularly vulnerable to tension failure when the muscles controlling the joint are either weak or are "caught off guard" at the moment of injury. The causative force of tension failure is usually an indirect injury in which the initial force is transmitted through the bones to the involved joint.

Descriptive Terms Pertaining to Joint Injuries

A direct blow to a joint usually produces a *contusion* of the joint but, if sufficiently

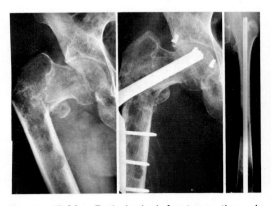

Figure 15.90. Pathological fractures through metastatic neoplasms. *Left,* pathological intertrochanteric fracture of the femur through a metastasis from carcinoma of the breast in a 55-year-old woman. *Middle,* the same pathological fracture after open reduction and internal fixation with a nail and plate. The patient was thereby relieved of pain. *Right,* pathological fracture of the femoral shaft through a metastasis from carcinoma of the lung in a 60-year-old man. The fracture had not become displaced and the intramedullary nail had been driven down the femur from above (under radiographic control) without exposing the fracture site. The patient's pain was relieved.

severe, may produce an *intra-articular fracture*. An indirect injury produces sudden tension on a ligament which may result in severe stretching of the ligament with minor tears and some hemorrhage (*ligamentous sprain*) without loss of joint stability. A more severe injury produces a major *ligamentous tear* that may be either partial or complete with resultant loss of joint stability. If the ligament itself does not tear, it may avulse a fragment of its bony attachment at either end (*ligamentous avulsion*).

The term *ligamentous strain*, by contrast, refers to the gradual elongation of a ligament that results from repeated mild stretching over a prolonged period of time.

There are three degrees of joint instability: (1) *occult joint instability* (which is apparent only when the joint is stressed) (Fig. 15.91); (2) *subluxation* (less than a luxation) in which the joint surfaces have lost their normal re-

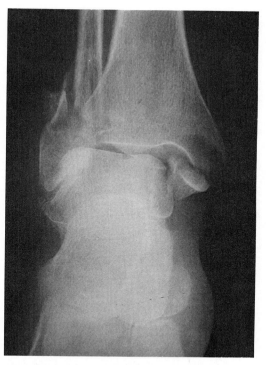

Figure 15.92. Traumatic subluxation of the ankle joint associated with a fracture of the medial malleolus and the distal end of the fibula—a fracture-subluxation. The joint surfaces have lost their normal relationship but still retain considerable contact.

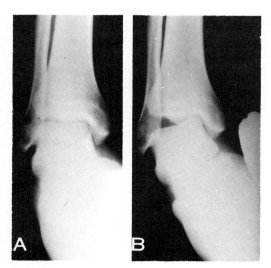

Figure 15.91. Occult joint instability. *A,* anteroposterior radiograph of the ankle of a football player who, after an inversion injury of his ankle had pain, swelling and local tenderness over the lateral aspect of the joint. The radiograph is normal but this does not exclude occult joint instability. *B,* anteroposterior radiograph of the same ankle while it is being stressed (stress radiograph) with the patient under general anesthesia. Note the marked opening up of the ankle joint (talar tilt) on the lateral side indicating joint instability associated with a complete tear of the lateral ligament of the ankle. The stress simulates the original injury.

lationship but still retain considerable contact (Fig. 15.92); (3) *dislocation* (luxation) in which the joint surfaces have completely lost contact (Fig. 15.93).

Either a dislocation or a subluxation may have occurred only momentarily at the time of injury and may have reduced spontaneously leaving no radiographic evidence of the seriousness of the injury unless the joint is stressed. When the dislocation is accompanied by fracture, either intra-articular or extra-articular, it is referred to as a *fracture-dislocation* (Fig. 15.94). As with fractures, a joint injury may be *closed* (simple) or *open* (compound) either from within or from without (Fig. 15.93).

The joints most susceptible to traumatic dislocation are the shoulder, elbow, enterphalangeal joints, hip and ankle. Internal derangements of the knee joint due to a torn meniscus are discussed in Chapter 17.

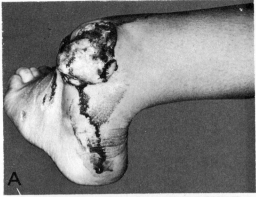
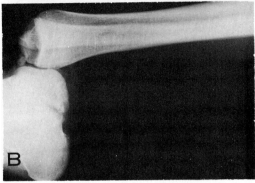

Figure 15.93. Open traumatic dislocation (luxation) of the ankle joint. *A*, the distal ends of the fibula and tibia have burst through the skin from within at the time of the dislocation. *B*, the radiograph (taken in the same projection as the photograph) reveals that the joint surfaces of the ankle joint have completely lost contact.

Associated Injury to the Fibrous Capsule

The fibrous capsule and contiguous periosteum may be stripped up from the bony margin of the joint and stretched by the causative injury resulting in an *intracapsular dislocation.* More often, however, the fibrous capsule is torn and one bone end perforates the rent in the capsule to produce an *extracapsular dislocation.* Occasionally the bone end becomes trapped in the dislocated position by the relatively small rent in the capsule, and this phenomenon is referred to as a *buttonhole dislocation,* which may be impossible to reduce by closed methods. Occasionally, at the time of closed reduction of a dislocation, a flap of torn capsule becomes trapped between the joint

surfaces, and by preventing perfect reduction, results in residual subluxation of the joint.

The Diagnosis of Joint Injuries

Many of the clinical features of traumatic dislocation and subluxation are comparable to those already discussed in a previous section of this chapter in relation to the clinical features of fractures. Because of normal proprioceptive sensation in joints, however, the patient is usually aware that a given joint has "gone out of place." The associated joint instability and stretching of the injured structures cause pain and muscle spasm; in addition, there is decreased function of the involved part.

Physical examination in the presence of a complete dislocation usually reveals *swelling* (unless the dislocated joint is deep, as in the hip), *deformity* (angulation, rotation, loss of normal contour, shortening) and *abnormal movement* (occurring through the unstable joint) (Fig. 15.95). There is *local tenderness*

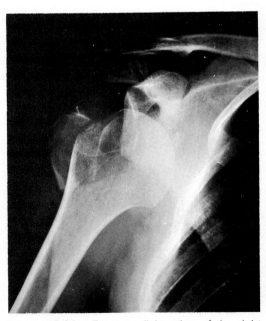

Figure 15.94. Fracture-dislocation of the right shoulder in an adult. Note the fracture of the greater tuberosity of the humerus and the dislocation of the humeral head in relation to the glenoid cavity.

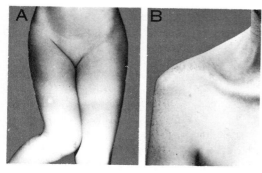

Figure 15.95. Clinical deformity associated with traumatic dislocations. *A*, the typical clinical deformity of traumatic posterior dislocation of the right hip—flexion, adduction, internal rotation and apparent shortening. *B*, the typical clinical deformity of traumatic inferomedial dislocation of the right shoulder; the normal round contour of the shoulder has been lost and the shoulder looks square.

over a sprained or torn ligament. Dislocations and subluxations may go unrecognized because of inadequate physical examination and consequent failure to obtain the appropriate radiographic examination. Physical examination must also include a diligent search for any associated injuries to spinal cord, peripheral nerves or major vessels.

Radiographic examination reveals the typical features of a subluxation (Fig. 15.92) or of a dislocation (Fig 15.93). At least two projections at right angles to each other (anterioposterior and lateral) are essential for accurate diagnosis (Fig. 15.96). In the absence of radiographic evidence of a dislocation or subluxation, despite clinical evidence of significant ligamentous injury, additional radiographs taken while the joint is being stressed (under local or general anesthesia) are helpful in the diagnosis of occult joint instability (Fig. 15.91).

The Normal Healing of Ligaments

Unlike bone, which heals without a scar, torn ligaments heal by fibrous scar tissue which is not as strong as the normal ligament. Partial tears in a ligament heal reasonably well provided the tendon is protected during the healing process. With complete tears of ligaments, however, there is usually

a considerable gap between the shredded ends of the ligament—a gap that can heal only with fibrous scar tissue. Under these circumstances, even if the torn ligament heals, it is both elongated and relatively weak.

The time required for normal healing of a torn ligament varies directly with its size and the forces to which it is normally subjected. Thus, the ligaments of the finger joints may be healed in three weeks, whereas the major ligaments of the knee may require three months. The healing time for torn ligaments is somewhat shorter in children than in adults but the influence of age is much less marked in ligamentous healing than it is in fracture healing.

Complications of Dislocations and Associated Injuries

The complications of the original injury that produced the dislocation or subluxation are much the same as those of fractures which have been classified and discussed in an earlier section of this Chapter. The immediate local complications include associated injury to skin, blood vessels, peripheral nerves and spinal cord as well as multiple

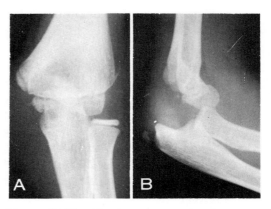

Figure 15.96. The importance of at least two radiographic projections at right angles to each other (anteroposterior and lateral). *A*, the anteroposterior projection reveals some evidence of disturbance in this child's elbow (the radial head is not in correct relationship with the capitellum) but it is not striking. *B*, the lateral projection clearly reveals a posterior dislocation of the elbow.

injuries. The early local complications include infection (septic arthritis) after an open joint injury and avascular necrosis of one of the articulating bone ends (especially the head of the femur). Late complications of dislocations, subluxations and occult joint instability include persistent joint stiffness, persistent joint instability and recurrent dislocation, post-traumatic degenerative joint disease, post-traumatic osteoporosis, reflex sympathetic dystrophy and post-traumatic myositis ossificans.

General Principles of Treatment for Joint Injuries

The six general principles of fracture treatment discussed in an earlier section of this chapter are equally applicable to the treatment of dislocations and associated injuries. Dislocations and subluxations must be reduced perfectly in order to restore normal congruity of the joint surfaces.

Specific Types of Joint Injuries

CONTUSION

When a joint receives a direct blow, the synovial membrane reacts to the injury by producing an effusion; synovial vessels may even rupture with a resultant hemarthrosis. Radiographic examination is necessary to exclude the possibility of an associated intra-articular fracture.

LIGAMENTOUS SPRAIN

An acute sprain, or strain, of a ligament is caused by a sudden stretching of the ligament with minor (incomplete) tears and resultant local hemorrhage. The sprain is manifest by local swelling, tenderness and pain that is aggravated by those movements of the joint that put the sprained ligament on the stretch. Since the ligament has not been unduly elongated, however, there is no joint instability.

Radiographic examination is required to exclude a dislocation, subluxation or a fracture; additional radiographs taken while the joint is being stressed are essential to exclude occult joint instability (Fig. 15.91).

Treatment of a simple ligamentous sprain is aimed at protecting the injured ligament from further stretching during the healing process. Complete immobilization is seldom necessary, except for severe pain, but appropriately applied adhesive strapping can serve as a temporary (external) ligament that relieves pain by restricting undesired motion while permitting other movements of the joint (Fig. 15.97). Active exercises are important not only to maintain joint motion but also to increase the protective power of the muscles that control the joint.

DISLOCATIONS AND SUBLUXATIONS

In order to restore normal congruity to the joint surfaces, perfect reduction of dislocations and subluxations must be achieved, either by closed manipulation or, when nec-

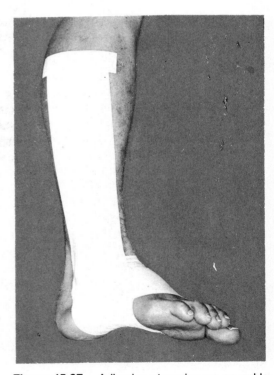

Figure 15.97. Adhesive strapping on an ankle in the treatment of a lateral ligamentous strain. Each strip of adhesive begins on the lateral aspect of the ankle, encircles the foot and extends up the lateral aspect of the leg while the foot is held in eversion (to relieve tension on the strained ligament). The adhesive strapping, which serves as a temporary external ligament, restricts inversion at the subtalar joint but permits dorsiflexion and plantar flexion at the ankle joint.

essary, by open reduction. After reduction of the dislocation or subluxation, consideration must then be given to the torn ligaments in order to prevent the complication of residual joint instability and resultant recurrent dislocation of the joint.

Torn Ligaments. A complete tear of certain

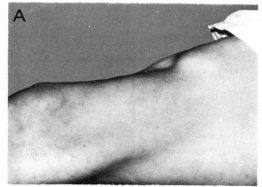

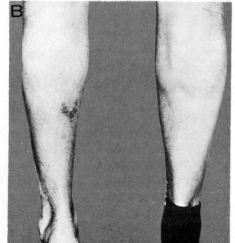

Figure 15.98. Rupture of muscles. *A*, rupture of the musculotendinous junction of the left quadriceps muscle in the suprapatellar region of a hockey player (as seen from the lateral aspect). Note the retracted muscle belly proximally and the gap distally. This injury required surgical repair. *B*, rupture of the musculotendinous junction of the medial head of the left gastrocnemius of a tennis player. Note the ecchymosis and loss of normal contour of the calf. Since only one head of the gastrocnemius muscle has ruptured, it retracts relatively little. Elevation of the heel of the shoe reduces the tension on the calf muscles and hence relieves pain on walking during the healing process.

major ligaments, such as the collateral ligament of the knee, should be repaired surgically as soon as possible after the injury since the results of delayed or late repair are less satisfactory than those of immediate repair. For many other ligaments however, such as the lateral ligament of the ankle or the collateral ligaments of the fingers, the reduced joint need only be immobilized to protect the injured ligaments and capsule from further stretching during the healing process. Immobilization of a joint after reduction of a dislocation is necessary to obtain stability. In the elbow and hip, immobilization is also helpful in preventing the complication of post-traumatic myositis ossificans.

MUSCLE INJURIES

When severe tension is suddenly applied to an already contracted muscle, some of the muscle bundles may rupture and thereby produce the painful local lesion well known to athletes and trainers as a "charley horse." Occasionally a more extensive rupture occurs at the musculotendinous junction of a major muscle such as the quadriceps femoris or the gastrocnemius (Fig. 15.98).

TENDON INJURIES
Closed Tendon Injuries

A normal tendon seldom ruptures even with strenuous activity but, if it has become frayed by friction or has degenerated, it may rupture with even normal activity. In either case reconstructive operations are required to either repair or replace the abnormal part of the ruptured tendon. Sudden tension on a normal tendon may avulse a fragment of its bony insertion; the commonest example of this injury is the mallet finger (baseball finger, cricket finger) (Fig. 15.99).

Open Tendon Injuries

Clean open division of tendons in most sites can be treated by immediate surgical repair. The complex and intricate arrangement of flexor tendons in the hand, however,

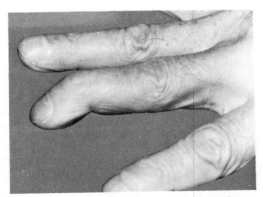

Figure 15.99. Mallet finger (baseball finger, cricket finger). The distal interphalangeal joint of this man's right middle finger was suddenly forced into acute flexion as he miscaught a ball. A small fragment of the insertion of the long extensor tendon into the base of the distal phalanx was avulsed so that he lost active extension of the joint. Alternatively, the thin extensor tendon may rupture proximal to insertion. The resultant deformity bears some resemblance to a mallet. Treatment is discussed in Chapter 17.

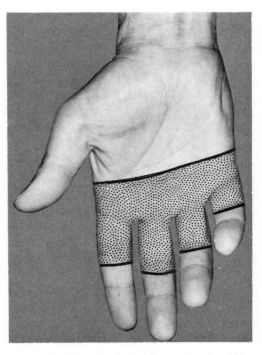

Figure 15.100. The critical area for flexor tendon injuries in the hand ("no man's land"). In this area both the profundus and sublimus tendons for each finger pass through an unyielding fibrous tunnel; consequently adhesions between repaired tendons and the fibrous tunnel are almost inevitable in this area.

presents special problems since adhesions between injured tendons interfere significantly with hand function. When both the profundus and sublimis tendons are divided at the wrist or in the proximal part of the palm, only the profundus tendon should be repaired. When both tendons are divided in the *critical area* ("no man's land") between the distal palmar crease and the proximal interphalangeal joint, neither should be repaired primarily; late repair by tendon graft is necessary (Fig. 15.100). Distal to this area the lacerated profundus tendon can be either repaired or the proximal end advanced and sutured to bone; if, however, the proximal end has retracted into the palm, the distal end can be sutured to the middle phalanx, thereby crossing the distal interphalangeal joint as a tenodesis and providing stability of the joint in slight flexion.

MULTIPLE CRITICAL INJURIES

Victims of major accidents have usually sustained multiple critical injuries to more than one organ system, since accidents respect neither anatomical nor physiological barriers.

Priorities

In the emergency care of the critically injured, the saving of time means the saving of life. Total care must proceed expeditiously and effectively on the basis of the following priorities:

1. Airway and aeration of lungs.
2. Hemorrhage—external and internal.
3. Shock—hemorrhagic (hypovolemic, oligemic) shock.

These three priorities are of particular importance because they demand emergency care in all patients with multiple injuries.

The following list of priorities in order of decreasing urgency refer to injuries involving specific organ systems:

4. Respiratory injuries—bronchi, lungs, chest wall.
5. Neurological injuries—brain, spinal cord.

6. Gastrointestinal injuries—bowel, liver (and also spleen).

7. Urological injuries—kidney, bladder.

8. Musculoskeletal injuries—Fractures, dislocations, and associated soft tissue injuries.

The state of respiration and of circulation merit top priority since if they can be restored to normal, all other organ systems will be able to function—unless they have been directly injured. If either the respiratory or circulatory system fails to respond to emergency care, however, the victim succumbs to his injuries.

Throughout the phase of emergency care, the critically injured patient should be moved as little as possible. He should not be transported to the radiology department; instead, radiographic equipment should be brought to the emergency resuscitation room for urgent examination. The emergency care of patients with fractures has been outlined in a previous section of this chapter; the total care of the patient with *multiple* injuries presents additional problems about which you will learn from your textbooks on trauma in general.

Responsibility for the Care of the Critically Injured

Although several physicians and surgeons representing various specialties may be involved as a treatment team in the total care of the patient who has sustained multiple critical injuries, one surgeon must serve as the team captain. He must assume the role of leadership and accept the coexistent responsibility for the total welfare of the patient. He should, of course, seek the help of professional colleagues as necessary and coordinate the efforts of all, but a critically injured patient is in dangerous jeopardy when the final responsibility for his lifesaving care is divided.

SUGGESTED ADDITIONAL READING

Akeson, W. H., Coutts, R. D. and Woo, S. L.-Y.: Principles of less rigid internal fixation with plates. Can. J. Surg. 23:235–239, 1980.

Alho, A.: Fat embolism syndrome. Etiology, pathogenesis and treatment. Acta Chirurg. Scand. (Suppl.) 499: 75–85, 1980.

Allbrook, D. M.: Muscle breakdown and repair. In *Scientific Foundations of Orthopaedics and Traumatology*, edited by Owen, R., Goodfellow, J. and Bullough, P. London, William Heinemann Medical Books, 1980.

Allgower, M. and Spiegel, P. G.: Internal fixation of fractures. Evolution of concepts. Clin. Orthop. 138: 26–29, 1979.

Apley, A. G. and Solomon, L.: *Apley's System of Orthopaedics and Fractures*, 6th ed. London, Butterworth, 1982.

Bassett, C. A. L., Mitchell, S. N. and Gaston, S. R.: Treatment of ununited tibial diaphyseal fractures with pulsing electromagnetic fields. J. Bone Joint Surg. 63A: 511–523, 1981.

Bassett, C. A. L., Valdes, M. G. and Hernandez, E.: Modification of fracture repair with pulsing electromagnetic fields. J. Bone Joint Surg. 64A: 888–895, 1982.

Becker, R. O.: The significance of electrically stimulated osteogenesis. Clin. Orthop. 141: 266–274, 1979.

Bentley, G.: Repair of articular cartilage. In *Scientific Foundations of Orthopaedics and Traumatology*. edited by Owen, R., Goodfellow, J. and Bullough, P. London, William Heinemann Medical Books, 1980.

Brand, R. A.: Fracture healing. In *The Scientific Basis of Orthopaedics*, edited by Albright, J. A. and Brand, R. A. New York, Appleton-Century-Crofts, 1979.

Briggs, B. T. and Chao, E. Y. S.: The mechanical performance of the standard Hoffmann-Vidal external fixation apparatus. J. Bone Joint Surg. 64A: 566–573, 1982.

Brighton, C. T.: The treatment of non-unions with electricity. Current concepts Review J. Bone Joint Surg. 63A: 847–851, 1981.

Brighton, C. T.: Present and future of electrically induced osteogenesis. In *Clinical Trends in Orthopaedics*, edited by Straub, L. R. and Wilson, P. D. Jr. New York, Thieme-Stratton, 1982.

Brooker, A. F. and Edwards, C. C.: *External Fixation—The Current State of the Art.* Baltimore, Williams & Wilkins, 1979.

Charnley, John: *The Closed Treatment of Common Fractures*, 3rd ed. Edinburgh, Churchill-Livingstone, 1961.

deHaas, W. G., Watson, J. and Morrison, D. M.: Noninvasive treatment of ununited fractures of the tibia using electrical stimulation. J. Bone Joint Surg. 62B: 465–470, 1980.

Dehne, E., Metz, C. W., Deffer, P. A. and Hall, R. M.: Nonoperative treatment of the fractured tibia by immediate weightbearing. J. Trauma 1: 514–533, 1961.

Devas, M. B.: *Stress Fractures*. Edinburgh, Churchill-Livingstone, 1975.

Dwyer, A. F. and Wickham, G. G.: Direct current stimulation in spine fusion. Med. J. Aust. 1: 73–75, 1974.

Edmondson, R. S. and Flowers, M. W.: Intensive care in tetanus: management, complications and mortality in 100 cases. Br. Med. J. 1: 1401–1404, 1979.

Friedenberg, Z. B. and Brighton, C. T.: Bioelectricity and fracture healing. Plast. Reconstr. Surg. 68: 435–443, 1981.

Genant, H. K., Wilson, J. S., Bovill, E. G., Brunelle, F. O., Murray, W. R. and Rodrigo, J. J.: Computed tomography of the musculoskeletal system. J. Bone Joint Surg. 62A: 1088–1101, 1980.

Gossling, H. R. and Donohue, T. A.: Fat embolism syndrome. J.A.M.A. 241: 2740–2742, 1979.

Gozna, E. R., Harrington, I. J. and Evans, D.C.: *Biomechanics of Musculoskeletal Injury*. Baltimore, Williams & Wilkins, 1982.

Gustilo, R. B., and Anderson, J. T.: Prevention of infection in the treatment of one thousand and twenty-five open fractures of long bones. J. Bone Joint Surg. 58A: 453–458, 1976.

Ham, A. W. and Cormack, D. H.: *Histophysiology of Cartilage, Bones and Joints*. Philadelphia, J. B. Lippincott, 1979.

Heimback, R. D.: Gas gangrene: review and update. Hyperbaric Oxygen Rev. 1: 41–61, 1980.

Heppenstall, R. B. (ed.): *Fracture Treatment and Healing*. Philadelphia, W. B. Saunders, 1980.

Holden, C. E. A.: The pathology and prevention of Volkmann's ischemic contracture. J. Bone Joint Surg. 61B: 3:296–300, 1979.

Jackson, R. W. and Waddell, J. P.: Hyperbaric oxygen in the management of clostridial myonecrosis (gas gangrene). Clin. Orthop. 96: 271, 1973.

McLeod, R. A., Stephens, D. H., Beabout, J. W., Sheedy, P. F. and Hattery, R. R.: Computed tomography of the skeletal system. Semin. Roentgenol. 13: 1978.

Mears, D. C.: *Materials and Orthopaedic Surgery*. Baltimore, Williams & Wilkins, 1979.

Mubarak, S. J., Owen, C. A., Hargens, A. R., Garetto, L. P. and Akeson, W. H.: Acute compartment syndromes: diagnosis and treatment with the aid of a wick catheter. J. Bone Joint Surg. 60A: 1091–1095, 1978.

Müller, M. E.: The role of internal and/or extraskeletal fixation: probable future refinements of techniques and their applications. In *Clinical Trends in Orthopaedics*, edited by Straub, L. R. and Wilson, P. D. Jr. New York, Thieme-Stratton, 1982.

Müller, M. E., Allgower, M., Schneider, R. and Willeneger, H.: *Manual of Internal Fixation—Techniques Recommended by the AO Group*, 2nd ed. (Translated by Schatzker, J.) Berlin, Springer-Verlag, 1979.

Mustard, W. T. and Bull, C.: A reliable method for relief of traumatic vascular spasm. Ann. Surg. 155: 339–344, 1962.

Paterson, D. C., Lewis, G. N. and Cass, C. A.: Treatment of delayed union and nonunion with an implanted direct current stimulator. Clin. Orthop. 148: 117–128, 1980.

Paul, D. F., Morrey, B. F. and Helms, C. A.: Computerized tomography in orthopaedic surgery. Clin. Orthop. 139: 142–149, 1979.

Peltier, L. F.: The diagnosis and treatment of fat embolism. J. Trauma, 11: 661–667, 1971.

Perren, S. M.: Physical and biological aspects of fracture healing with special reference to internal fixation. Clin. Orthop. 138: 175–196, 1979.

Potenza, A.D.: Tendon and ligament healing. In *Scientific Foundations of Orthopaedics and Traumatology*, edited by Owen, R., Goodfellow, J. and Bullough, P. London, William Heinemann Medical Books, 1980.

Rockwood, C. A. and Green, D. P.: *Fractures*. Philadelphia, J. B. Lippincott, 1975, vols. 1 and 2.

Rorabeck, C. H., Castle, G. S. P., Hardie, R. and Logen, J.: Compartment pressure measurements. An experimental investigation using the slit catheter. J. Trauma 21: 446, 1981.

Rorabeck, C. H. and Macnab, I.: Anterior tibial compartment syndrome complicating fractures of the shaft of the tibia. J. Bone Joint Surg. 58A: 549, 1976.

Salter, R. B. and Harris, D. J.: The healing of intra-articular fractures with continuous passive motion. In *American Academy of Orthopaedic Surgeons Instructional Course Lecture Series*. St. Louis, C. V. Mosby, 1979, vol. 28, pp. 102–117.

Sarmiento, A.: The role of functional bracing and the likely further development of its technology. In *Clinical Trends in Orthopaedics*, edited by Straub, L. R. and Wilson, P. D. Jr. New York, Thieme-Stratton, 1982.

Sarmiento, A. and Latta, L. L.: *Closed Functional Treatment of Fractures*. Berlin, Springer-Verlag, 1981.

Sarmiento, A., Mullis, D. L., Latta, L. L., Tarr, R. R. and Alvarez, R.: A quantitative comparative analysis of fracture healing under the influence of compression plating vs. closed weight bearing treatment. Clin. Orthop. 149: 232–239, 1980.

Schatzker, J. and Tile, M.: The AO(ASIF) method of fracture care. In *American Academy of Orthopaedic Surgeons Instructional Course Lectures*. St. Louis, C. V. Mosby, 1980, vol. 29, pp. 41–50.

Sevitt, S.: Healing of fractures. In *Scientific Foundations of Orthopaedics and Traumatology*, edited by Owen, R., Goodfellow, J. and Bullough, P. London, William Heinemann Medical Books, 1980.

Uhthoff, H. (ed.): *Current Concepts of External Fixation of Fractures*. Berlin, Springer-Verlag, 1982.

Weisz, G. M., Rang, M. and Salter, R. B.: Post-traumatic fat embolism in children. J. Trauma 13: 529–534, 1973.

Wilson, J. N. (ed.): *Watson-Jones' Fractures and Joint Injuries*, 5th ed. Edinburgh, Churchill-Livingstone, 1976, vols. 1 and 2.

PART 4

Musculoskeletal Injuries—Specific

CHAPTER 16

Specific Fractures and Joint Injuries in Children

Your knowledge and understanding of the *general features* of fractures, dislocations and soft tissue injuries gained from Chapter 15—combined with your own good sense—will enable you to deduce, and therefore to anticipate the appropriate methods of treatment for *specific injuries* in children.

Before considering specific injuries in children, however, you would be wise to consider some of the *special features* of fractures and dislocations in the growing years. Just as in all other clinical fields of medicine and surgery, so also in the field of fractures, children cannot be considered simply as "little adults." Indeed, as you will see, fractures in children, and the reaction of children's tissues to these fractures, differ greatly from those in adults; Blount deserves special credit for emphasizing the fact that *"fractures in children are different."*

SPECIAL FEATURES OF FRACTURES AND DISLOCATIONS IN CHILDREN

The special features of fractures and dislocations are first listed and then discussed individually. You will appreciate that these differences are most striking in the infant and young child and become progressively less striking as the child approaches adulthood. The comparative terms such as "more" and "less" refer to a comparison between fractures and dislocations in children and those in adults.

1. Fractures more common.
2. Stronger and more active periosteum.
3. More rapid fracture healing.
4. Special problems of diagnosis.
5. Spontaneous correction of certain residual deformities.
6. Differences in complications.
7. Different emphasis on methods of treatment.
8. Torn ligaments and dislocations less common.
9. Less tolerance of major blood loss.

1. Fractures More Common

The higher incidence of fractures in children is explained by the combination of their relatively slender bones and their carefree capers. Some of these injuries, such as crack, or hairline fractures, buckle fractures and green-stick fractures, are not serious; whereas others, such as intra-articular fractures and epiphyseal plate fractures, are very serious indeed.

2. Stronger and More Active Periosteum

The stronger periosteum in children is less readily torn across at the time of a fracture and consequently there is more often an intact periosteal hinge that can be utilized during closed reduction of the fracture. Furthermore, the periosteum is much more osteogenic in children than it is in adults (Fig. 16.1).

3. More Rapid Fracture Healing

As mentioned in Chapter 15, the rate of healing in bone varies much more with age than it does in any other tissue in the body,

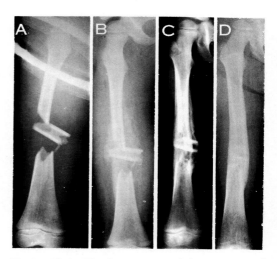

Figure 16.1 The importance of the strong and actively osteogenic periosteum in the healing process of children's fractures is demonstrated in this series of radiographs of a fractured femoral shaft in a 4-year-old child. *A*, the day of injury; a double fracture with the middle segment lying almost transversely. The strong periosteal sleeve however, would not be completely torn across. Note the metal ring of the Thomas splint. *B*, three weeks after injury abundant callus is forming from the actively osteogenic periosteum; at this stage traction was replaced by a hip spica cast. *C*, ten weeks after injury the middle segment is well incorporated in the callus and is being resorbed; the fracture was clinically united at this stage and the child was allowed to walk. *D*, six months after injury the contour of the femur is returning to normal through the process of remodeling.

particularly during childhood. This is closely related to the osteogenic activity of the periosteum and endosteum, a process that is remarkably active at birth, becomes progressively less active with each year of childhood and remains relatively constant from early adult life to old age.

Fractures of the shaft of the femur serve as an example of this phenomenon; a femoral shaft fracture occurring at birth will be united in 3 weeks; a comparable fracture at the age of 8 years will be united in 8 weeks; at the age of 12 years it will be united at 12 weeks; and from the age of 20 years to old age it will be united in approximately 20 weeks.

Non-union of children's fractures is rare, unless an unnecessary open operation has damaged the blood supply to the fracture fragments or has introduced the complication of infection.

4. Special Problems of Diagnosis

The varying radiographic appearance of a given epiphysis, both before and after the development of a secondary center of ossification, can be quite confusing; and although the various secondary centers of ossification appear at relatively constant ages, these are not easy to remember. Likewise, the radiographic appearance of the various epiphyseal plates may be puzzling to the inexperienced and may be mistaken for fracture lines. These radiographic problems of diagnosis, however, can be readily overcome in limb injuries. Just as you would naturally compare an injured limb with its normal uninjured mate during the clinical examination, so also you should compare the two limbs during the radiographic examination (Fig. 16.2).

5. Spontaneous Correction of Certain Residual Deformities

In adults the deformity of a mal-united fracture is permanent; but in children certain residual deformities tend to correct spontaneously either by extensive remodeling or by epiphyseal plate growth, and sometimes by a combination of both. Just how much spontaneous correction of the healed fracture deformity can be anticipated depends

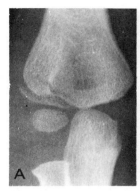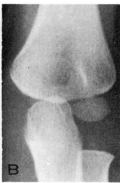

Figure 16.2 The value of a comparable radiographic examination of the opposite uninjured limb. *A*, does the radiolucent line just proximal to the capitellum of this child's right humerus represent a fracture or just part of the epiphyseal plate? *B*, comparison with the radiograph of the opposite elbow clarifies the situation; the child has a relatively undisplaced fracture of the lateral condyle of the right humerus, a potentially serious fracture as you will see in a subsequent section of this chapter.

upon the age of the child (and consequently the number of years of skeletal growth remaining) and the type of deformity (angulation, incomplete apposition, shortening, rotation). This phenomenon is therefore best considered in relation to specific deformities.

Angulation. Residual angulation near an epiphyseal plate will tend to correct spontaneously with subsequent growth *provided* that the plane of the deformity is the same as the plane of motion in the nearest joint. For example, residual anterior angulation at the site of a healed fracture in the distal end of the radius is in the same plane as the flexion and extension motion in the wrist joint; thus, in a young child it can be expected to correct to a large extent (Fig. 16.3). By contrast, residual angulation at right angles to the plane of motion of the nearest joint, for example a lateral angulation or varus deformity in the supracondylar region of the humerus which is at right angles to the flexion and extension motion of the elbow, cannot be expected to correct (Fig. 16.4). Furthermore, angulation in the middle third of a long bone, being well away from an epiphyseal plate, cannot be expected to correct spontaneously (Fig. 16.5).

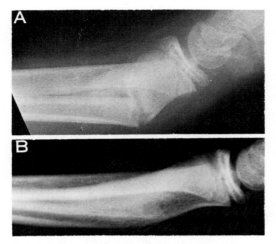

Figure 16.3 Spontaneous improvement in a residual fracture deformity with subsequent growth. *A*, lateral projection of the distal end of the radius of a 10-year-old boy 6 weeks after injury. Unfortunately the metaphyseal fracture had been allowed to unite with 35° of anterior angulation. *B*, six months later there is only 15° of anterior angulation and the corners of the angulation deformity have remodeled. Note that the epiphysis has grown away from the fracture site during these 6 months.

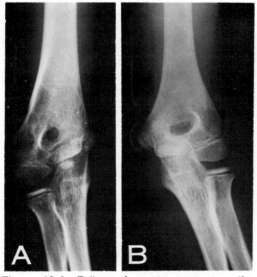

Figure 16.4 Failure of spontaneous correction of a residual fracture deformity. *A*, a supracondylar fracture of the humerus in a 9-year-old girl had been allowed to unite with 20° of lateral angulation 2 years previously. *B*, the opposite elbow has a normal carrying angle of 15°. Thus, on the injured side the normal carrying angle has not only been lost but also reversed so that there is 5° of varus. This deformity of mal-union is permanent.

Incomplete Apposition. With incomplete apposition of the fracture fragments, or even side-to-side (bayonet) apposition in children, the contour of the healed fracture improves greatly through the active process of remodeling—an example of Wolff's law (Fig. 16.6).

Shortening. After a displaced fracture of a long bone in a growing child, the associated disruption in the nutrient artery results in a compensatory increase in the blood flow at the epiphyseal ends of the bone. This phenomenon produces a temporary acceleration of longitudinal growth in the bone for as long as one year after the fracture (Fig.

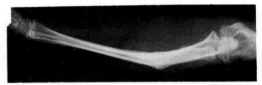

Figure 16.5 Failure of spontaneous correction of a residual fracture deformity. The fractures of the middle third of the radius and ulna of an 8-year-old girl had been allowed to unite in the unsatisfactory position of 35° of posterior angulation one year previously. This deformity of malunion is permanent.

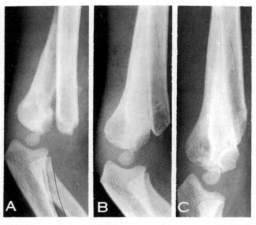

Figure 16.6 Spontaneous correction of incomplete apposition through remodeling. *A*, an unreduced supracondylar fracture of the humerus in a 4-year-old child 3 weeks after injury; note the new bone formation in the periosteal tube through which the proximal fragment is protruding. *B*, five months after injury the periosteal tube has formed a new shaft and the original shaft is becoming resorbed. *C*, one year after injury the contour of the fracture site has been markedly improved by the process of remodeling. Note that the epiphysis has grown away from the fracture site.

16.7). This is most striking after displaced femoral shaft fractures and therefore over-riding is a desirable aim in the treatment of such fractures, since the shortening will be corrected spontaneously by temporary overgrowth and the two femora will become almost the same length (Fig. 16.8).

Rotation. Residual rotational deformity at the site of a healed fracture in a long bone does not correct spontaneously regardless of the child's age or the site of the deformity.

6. Differences in Complications

Most of the complications discussed in Chapter 15 develop in both children and adults but certain differences merit consideration. Growth disturbances after epiphyseal plate injuries, of course, occur only in

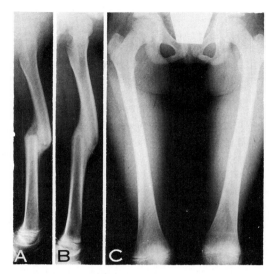

Figure 16.8 Overgrowth of the left femur after a displaced fracture of the shaft in a 9-year-old girl. *A*, lateral projection 8 weeks after injury; the fracture had been allowed to unite with 1 cm of overriding intentionally. *B*, six months after injury the united fracture is becoming remodeled. *C*, eighteen months after injury the femora are virtually equal in length as a result of overgrowth of the left femur. If the fracture had been allowed to unite end-to-end, the femur would have been 1 cm too long 18 months later and the leg length discrepancy would have been permanent.

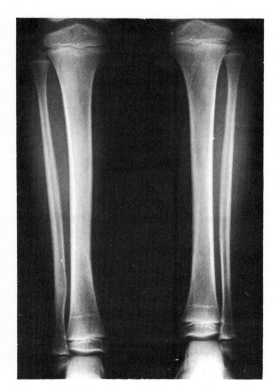

Figure 16.7 Overgrowth of a long bone after a displaced fracture. One year previously the right tibia of this 8-year-old boy had been fractured and during the ensuing year it had overgrown 1 cm. The transverse radio-opaque lines in the distal tibial metaphyses represent the site of the epiphyseal plate at the time of injury; note that there has been more growth from the epiphyseal plate of the right tibia than from that of the left. The resultant leg length discrepancy will be permanent.

children. Osteomyelitis secondary to either an open fracture or open reduction of a closed fracture tends to be more extensive in a child and, furthermore, the infection may even destroy an epiphyseal plate with resultant growth disturbance. Volkmann's ischemia of nerves and muscles is much more common in children as are post-traumatic myositis ossificans and refracture.

By contrast, persistent joint stiffness after fracture is relatively uncommon in children unless the fracture has involved the joint surface; consequently, physiotherapy and occupational therapy are seldom required in the after care of children with fractures. Likewise, fat embolism, pulmonary embolism and accident neurosis are rare in childhood.

7. Different Emphasis on Methods of Treatment

Although the *principles* of fracture treatment described in Chapter 15 are equally applicable to children and adults, there is a different emphasis on the *methods* of treatment in the two age groups. Virtually *all* fractures of the long bones in children can, and indeed should be treated by means of closed reduction, either by manipulation or by continuous traction. Of course, the emotional exuberance and physical vigor of children recovering from fractures demand that their plaster-of-Paris casts be particularly strong.

Certain fractures in children do, however, necessitate open reduction and internal skeletal fixation; for example, displaced intra-articular fractures, femoral neck fractures and certain types of epiphyseal plate injuries which are described in a subsequent section. There is no indication for excision of a fracture fragment and replacement by an endoprosthesis in children.

8. Torn Ligaments and Dislocations Less Common

Children's ligaments are strong and resilient. Furthermore, since they are stronger than the associated epiphyseal plates, sudden extension on a ligament at the time of injury results in a separation of the epiphyseal plate rather than a tear in the ligament (Fig. 16.9). This is also true, but to a lesser extent, of fibrous joint capsules; for example, the type of injury that would produce a

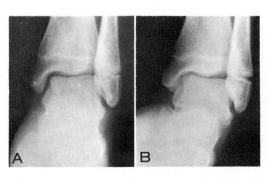

Figure 16.9. Traumatic separation of the distal fibular epiphysis in a 14-year-old boy. *A*, this radiograph appears normal because after the injury the fibular epiphysis had returned to its normal position. *B*, in this stress radiograph (taken while a varus stress is being applied to the ankle joint with the child under anesthetic) there is a tilt of the talus and the separation of the fibular epiphysis is apparent.

traumatic dislocation of the shoulder in an adult will produce a fracture-separation of the proximal humeral epiphysis in a child.

9. Less Tolerance of Major Blood Loss

The importance of percentage blood loss in relation to shock is well known. Obviously, the total blood volume is proportionately smaller in a child than in an adult; a formula for estimating the average blood volume in a child is 75 ml per kilogram of body weight. Thus, the average blood volume of a child who weighs 20 kg (44 lb) is 1500 ml. Consequently, external hemorrhage of 500 ml in such a child represents 33% of the total blood volume, whereas a similar hemorrhage in an average adult would represent only 10% of the total blood volume of 5000 ml.

SPECIAL TYPES OF FRACTURES IN CHILDREN

In addition to *stress fractures* and *pathological fractures*, which occur in both children and adults and are discussed in Chapter 15, there are two special types of fractures that are limited to childhood, namely, *fractures that involve the epiphyseal plate* and *birth fractures*.

Fractures That Involve the Epiphyseal Plate (Physis)

Epiphyseal plate fractures, or physial fractures, present special problems in relation to both diagnosis and treatment; furthermore, they carry the risk of becoming complicated by a serious disturbance of local growth and the consequent development of progressive bony deformity during the remaining years of skeletal growth.

Although the term "physis" is a relatively recent and acceptable synonym for the epiphyseal plate, the latter term is still more widely used in many countries and hence is used throughout this textbook.

ANATOMY, HISTOLOGY AND PHYSIOLOGY

The anatomy and histology of pressure and traction types of epiphyses and their epiphyseal plates have been discussed in

Chapter 2, but a few pertinent points merit emphasis. The types of epiphyses are shown in Fig. 16.10.

The weakest area of the epiphyseal plate is the zone of calcifying cartilage; and, therefore, when the epiphysis is separated by injury, the line of separation is through this zone (Fig. 16.11). Thus, the epiphyseal plate, which is radiolucent and therefore not radiographically visible, always remains attached to the epiphysis.

The blood supply of the epiphyseal plate enters from its epiphyseal surface and, therefore, if the epiphysis loses its blood supply and becomes necrotic, the plate likewise becomes necrotic and growth ceases. In most sites the blood supply to the epiphysis is not damaged at the time of injury but in the proximal femoral epiphysis and the proximal radial epiphysis the blood vessels course along the neck of the bone and cross the epiphyseal plate peripherally. Consequently in these sites epiphyseal separation frequently damages the blood supply and leads to avascular necrosis of the epiphysis as well as of the epiphyseal plate.

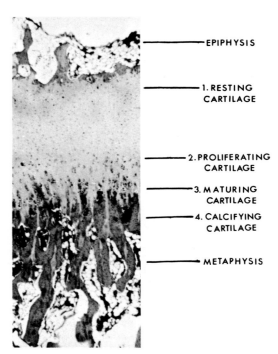

EPIPHYSIS

1. RESTING CARTILAGE

2. PROLIFERATING CARTILAGE

3. MATURING CARTILAGE

4. CALCIFYING CARTILAGE

METAPHYSIS

Figure 16.11. Low power photomicrograph of an epiphyseal plate from the proximal end of the tibia of a child.

The cartilaginous epiphyseal plate is weaker than bone and yet epiphyseal injuries account for only 15% of all fractures in childhood. The explanation for this apparent paradox is that the epiphysis is firmly attached to its metaphysis peripherally by the union of perichondrium and periosteum (Fig. 16.10). Nevertheless, as mentioned previously, epiphyseal plates are weaker than their associated ligaments and joint capsule; for this reason injuries that would result in a torn ligament or a dislocation in an adult usually produce a traumatic separation of the epiphysis in a child (Fig. 16.9).

In the lower limb more longitudinal growth takes place at the epiphyseal plates in the region of the knee than of the hip or ankle. By contrast, in the upper limb more growth takes place in the region of the shoulder and the wrist than of the elbow.

DIAGNOSIS OF EPIPHYSEAL PLATE INJURIES

You should suspect an epiphyseal plate fracture clinically in any injured child who

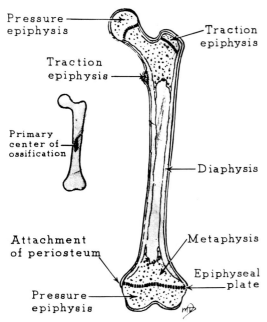

Pressure epiphysis

Traction epiphysis

Traction epiphysis

Primary center of ossification

Diaphysis

Attachment of periosteum

Metaphysis

Epiphyseal plate

Pressure epiphysis

Figure 16.10. Types of epiphyses (secondary centers of ossification) in the femur. Note the attachment of the periosteum to the epiphysis.

exhibits signs suggestive of a fracture near the end of a long bone, a dislocation or a ligamentous injury (including a sprain). Precise diagnosis, however, depends upon radiographic examination; at least two projections at right angles to each other are essential and you should also obtain comparable projections of the same region of the opposite uninjured limb (Fig. 16.2).

SALTER-HARRIS CLASSIFICATION OF EPIPHYSEAL PLATE INJURIES

The following classification is based on the mechanism of injury as well as the relationship of the fracture line to the growing cells of the epiphyseal plate; in addition, it is correlated with the method of treatment as well as the prognosis of the injury concerning growth disturbance.

Type I (Fig. 16.12)

There is complete separation of the epiphysis without any fracture through bone; the growing cells of the epiphyseal plate remain with the epiphysis. This type of injury, the result of a shearing force, is more common in newborns (from birth injury) and in young children in whom the epiphyseal plate is relatively thick.

Closed reduction is not difficult because the periosteal attachment is intact around most of its circumference. The prognosis for future growth is excellent provided the blood supply to the epiphysis is intact, which it usually is in sites other than the proximal femoral epiphysis and the proximal radial epiphysis.

Type II (Fig. 16.13)

In this, the commonest type, the line of fracture-separation extends along the epiphyseal plate to a variable distance and then out through a portion of the metaphysis thereby producing a triangular-shaped metaphyseal fragment. The growing cells of the plate remain with the epiphysis. This type of injury, the result of shearing and bending forces, usually occurs in the older child in whom the epiphyseal plate is relatively thin. The periosteum is torn on the convex side of the angulation but is intact on the concave side; thus the intact periosteal hinge is always on the side of the metaphyseal fragment.

Closed reduction is relatively easy to obtain as well as to maintain; the intact periosteal hinge and the metaphyseal fragment both prevent over-reduction. The prognosis for growth is excellent provided the blood supply to the epiphysis is intact, which it nearly always is in sites where Type II injuries occur.

Type III (Fig. 16.14)

The fracture is intra-articular, extends from the joint surface to the deep zone of the epiphyseal plate and then along the plate to its periphery. This uncommon type of injury is caused by an intra-articular shearing

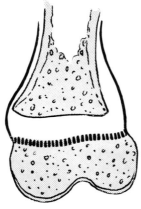

Figure 16.12. Type I epiphyseal plate injury. Separation of epiphysis.

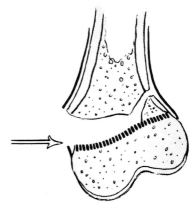

Figure 16.13. Type II epiphyseal plate injury. Fracture-separation of epiphysis.

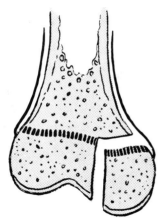

Figure 16.14. Type III epiphyseal plate injury. Fracture of part of epiphysis.

force and is usually limited to the distal tibial epiphysis.

Open reduction is usually necessary to restore a perfectly normal joint surface. The prognosis for growth is good provided the blood supply to the separated portion of the epiphysis has not been disrupted.

Type IV (Fig. 16.15)

The fracture, which is intra-articular, extends from the joint surface through the epiphysis, across the entire thickness of the epiphyseal plate and through a portion of the metaphysis. The commonest example of a Type IV injury is the fracture of the lateral condyle of the humerus.

Open reduction and internal skeletal fixation are necessary not only to restore a normal joint surface but also to obtain perfect apposition of the epiphyseal plate. Indeed, unless the fractured surfaces of the epiphyseal plate are kept perfectly reduced, fracture healing occurs across the plate and renders further longitudinal growth impossible. Thus the prognosis for growth after a Type IV injury is bad unless perfect reduction is both obtained and maintained.

Type V (Fig. 16.16)

This relatively uncommon injury results from a severe crushing force being applied through the epiphysis to one area of the epiphyseal plate. It is most likely to occur in the region of the knee and ankle.

Because the epiphysis is not usually dis-

placed, the diagnosis of a Type V injury is difficult. Weight bearing must be avoided for at least three weeks in the hope of preventing further compression of the epiphyseal plate. The prognosis of Type V injuries is decidedly poor since premature cessation of growth is almost inevitable.

To these five basic types of epiphyseal plate injuries, Rang has subsequently added a sixth type, namely the rare injury to the peripheral perichondrial ring, or zone of Ranvier, which encircles the plate. Although this type of injury can be caused by a direct blow, it is more often due to an open slicing mechanism by a sharp object such as the blade or blades of a power lawn mower. This Type VI injury carries a bad prognosis for subsequent growth because a local bony bridge tends to form across the epiphyseal plate.

Recently, Ogden has published an encyclopedic classification of epiphyseal injuries that comprises nine types and 18 subtypes.

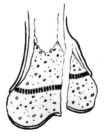 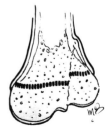

Figure 16.15. Type IV epiphyseal plate injury. *Left,* fracture of epiphysis and epiphyseal plate. *Right,* bony union will cause premature closure of the plate.

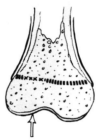 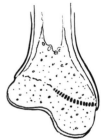

Figure 16.16. Type V epiphyseal plate injury. *Left,* crushing of epiphyseal plate. *Right,* premature closure of the plate on one side with a resultant angulatory deformity.

HEALING OF EPIPHYSEAL PLATE INJURIES

After reduction of a separated epiphysis, as in Types I, II and III injuries, endochondral ossification on the metaphyseal side of the epiphyseal plate is only temporarily disturbed. Thus, within two or three weeks of replacement of the epiphysis, endochondral ossification has resumed and has united the epiphyseal plate to the metaphysis. This special type of fracture healing accounts for the clinical observation that these three types of epiphyseal separations heal in only half the time required for union of a fracture through the metaphysis of the same bone in a child of the same age. Type IV and Type V injuries by contrast must heal in the same manner as any other fracture through cancellous bone.

PROGNOSIS CONCERNING GROWTH DISTURBANCE

The following factors will help you to estimate the prognosis of a given epiphyseal plate injury in a given child.

1. Type of Injury

The prognosis for each of the five classified types of epiphyseal plate injury has been discussed above.

2. Age of the Child

This is really an indication of the amount of growth normally expected in the particular epiphyseal plate; obviously, the younger the child at the time of injury, the more serious any growth disturbance will be.

3. Blood Supply to the Epiphysis

Disruption of the blood supply to the epiphysis is associated with a poor prognosis for reasons already discussed.

4. Method of Reduction

Unduly forceful manipulation of a displaced epiphysis may crush the epiphyseal plate and thereby increase the likelihood of growth disturbance.

5. Open or Closed Injury

Open injuries of the epiphyseal plate carry the risk of infection which, in turn, is likely to destroy the plate and result in premature cessation of growth.

POSSIBLE EFFECTS OF GROWTH DISTURBANCE

Fortunately, 85% of epiphyseal plate injuries are uncomplicated by growth disturbance. In the remaining 15%, however, the clinical problem associated with the dread complication of premature cessation of growth depends on several factors including the bone involved, the extent of the disturbance in the epiphyseal plate and the amount of growth normally expected from that particular epiphyseal plate.

If the entire epiphyseal plate ceases to grow in a single bone the result is a progressive limb length discrepancy (Fig. 16.17). If, however, the involved bone is one of a parallel pair (such as tibia and fibula, or radius and ulna) progressive length discrepancy between the two bones will in addition produce a progressive angulatory deformity in the neighbouring joint (Fig. 16.18). If growth ceases in only one part of the plate (for example on the medial side) but continues in the remainder, the result will be a progressive angulatory deformity (Fig. 16.19).

Premature cessation of growth does not necessarily occur immediately after an injury to the epiphyseal plate; indeed, growth may be only retarded for a period of six months, or even longer, before it ceases completely.

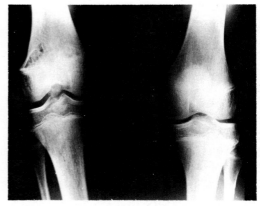

Figure 16.17. Progressive leg length discrepancy secondary to premature cessation of growth in the entire distal femoral epiphyseal plate. A Type IV epiphyseal plate injury had occurred 2 years previously in this 11-year-old boy; the discrepancy will continue to increase during the remaining years of growth.

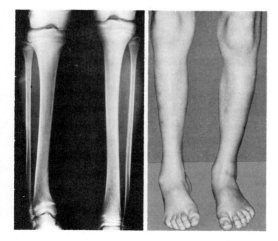

Figure 16.18. Progressive leg length discrepancy and progressive angulatory deformity in a 9-year-old girl 18 months after a Type IV epiphyseal plate injury of the right medial malleolus. Growth has ceased in the medial part of the tibial epiphyseal plate and has continued in the lateral part, as well as in the epiphyseal plate of the fibula. The result is a varus deformity of the ankle. Note also that the right tibia is shorter than the left.

Resection of Bony Bridges

On the basis of experimental investigations in animals, Langenskiold has devised the surgical procedure of resection of an established bony bridge that is tethering the epiphyseal plate and causing a growth disturbance, either peripherally or centrally. The resultant defect is then filled with an autogenous fat graft to prevent recurrence of the bridge. Provided that the bony bridge has not already extended to cover more than one-third of the surface of the epiphyseal plate (as demonstrated by tomography in the anteroposterior and lateral projections) this procedure usually enables resumption of symmetrical growth and sometimes even achieves some correction of the existing angulatory deformity. More recently, Bright has recommended filling the defect with a silicone-rubber implant with results that are comparable to those of Langenskiold.

On the orthopaedic horizon is the technical possibility through microsurgery of transplantation of an expendable autogenous epiphyseal plate (such as that of the proximal end of the fibula) to the site of a prematurely closed plate.

SPECIAL CONSIDERATIONS IN THE TREATMENT OF EPIPHYSEAL PLATE INJURIES

From the foregoing discussion you will appreciate that injuries involving the epiphyseal plate must be treated gently and as soon after injury as possible. Types I and II injuries can nearly always be treated by closed reduction. Type III injuries frequently require open reduction and Type IV injuries always require open reduction and internal fixation. The period of immobilization required for Types, I, II and III injuries is only half of that required for a metaphyseal fracture of the same bone in a child of the same age.

The parents of a child who has sustained an epiphyseal plate injury should always be given some indication of the prognosis concerning future growth without causing them undue anxiety. Furthermore, the child should

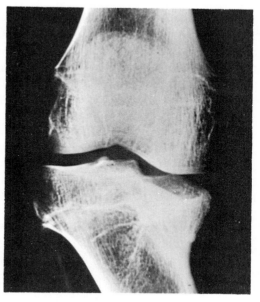

Figure 16.19. Progressive angulatory deformity of the knee in a 15-year-old boy 3 years after a Type V injury involving the medial part of the upper tibial epiphyseal plate. Growth has ceased on the medial side but has continued on the lateral side with a resultant progressive varus deformity of the knee.

be carefully examined both clinically and radiographically at regular intervals for at least one year and often longer to detect any growth disturbance.

Specific epiphyseal plate injuries are discussed on a regional basis along with specific fractures and dislocations in a subsequent section of this chapter.

AVULSION OF TRACTION EPIPHYSES

A sudden traction force applied through either a ligament or a tendon to a traction epiphysis (apophysis) may result in an avulsion of the epiphysis through its epiphyseal plate. Examples of such injuries are avulsion of the medial epicondyle of the humerus and the lesser trochanter of the femur. Since the epiphyseal plates of these traction epiphyses do not contribute to the longitudinal growth of the bone, such injuries are not complicated by a growth disturbance.

Birth Fractures

During the difficult delivery of a large baby, especially a breech presentation, when the threat of fetal anoxia may necessitate rapid extraction of the baby, one limb may be difficult to disengage from the birth canal and a bone may be inadvertently fractured or an epiphysis separated; only rarely is a previously normal joint dislocated by a birth injury. This usually unavoidable mishap is uncommon but when it does occur it is usually the proximal bones of the limbs that are injured.

Multiple birth fractures are nearly always pathological and the commonest cause is osteogenesis imperfecta (Chapter 8). Birth fracture of the tibia is rare and when it does occur it is nearly always a pathological fracture—congenital pseudarthrosis of the tibia (Chapter 8).

When either the humerus or the femur is fractured during delivery, the obstetrician feels and usually hears the bone break. When an epiphysis is separated however, it tends to slide off the metaphysis and the obstetrician may neither feel nor hear it. Thus the diagnosis of epiphyseal separations necessitates careful and repeated physical examination of the newborn.

Parents are understandably distressed when their new baby has sustained a birth fracture—and so is the obstetrician. The physician or surgeon who treats the newborn infant's injury, however, should gently inform the parents not only that such an injury is unavoidable under the circumstances but also that it is much less serious than fetal anoxia which the obstetrician had undoubtedly prevented by rapid extraction of their baby.

Specific birth injuries are discussed below in order of decreasing incidence.

SPECIFIC BIRTH FRACTURES

Clavicle

The slender newborn clavicle is the most susceptible bone to fracture during delivery, particularly in a broad-shouldered baby. The infant tends not to move the affected limb during the first week; this "pseudo paralysis" can be differentiated from the true paralysis of a brachial plexus injury by clinical examination (although, of course, the two may coexist). Radiographic examination confirms the presence of a fractured clavicle.

The fracture unites with remarkable rapidity, a strikingly large callus becoming apparent both clinically and radiographically within 10 days. Simple protection with a sling and bandage is the only treatment required.

Humerus

The humeral shaft is particularly susceptible to a birth fracture during a difficult breech delivery. The complete fracture is in the shaft and is frequently associated with a radial nerve injury; the latter, being only a neuropraxia, however, recovers completely. The newborn infant's fractured arm is obviously floppy and the diagnosis is readily confirmed radiographically (Fig. 16.20).

The infant's arm should be bandaged to the chest for a period of two weeks by which time the fracture is always clinically united. Mild residual angulatory deformities improve with subsequent growth but rotational deformities are permanent.

Rarely, the proximal humeral epiphysis is separated by a birth injury.

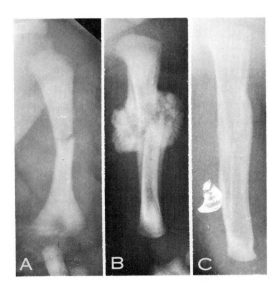

Figure 16.20. Birth fracture of the humerus. *A*, the day of birth. *B*, ten days later there is profuse callus formation; the fracture at this stage was clinically united. *C*, ten weeks later a remarkable amount of remodeling has occurred.

Femur

Birth fractures of the femur are most likely to occur during the delivery of a baby who has presented as a frank breech. The clinical deformity and floppiness of the lower limb are apparent and radiographic examination confirms the diagnosis of a fracture which is usually in the mid shaft. Overhead (Bryant's) skin traction on both lower limbs provides adequate alignment of the fracture, which is clinically united within three weeks.

Traumatic separation of the distal femoral epiphysis is more difficult to recognize clinically and may escape detection until the knee becomes enlarged by extensive new bone formation (Fig. 16.21). Overhead (Bryant's) skin traction is required for two weeks. Being a Type I epiphyseal plate injury in an epiphysis that has a good blood supply, the prognosis for subsequent growth is excellent.

Traumatic separation of the proximal femoral epiphysis is difficult to differentiate clinically from dislocation of the hip, but the latter is rare as a birth injury. Radiographi-

cally the differentiation may also be difficult since at birth the head, neck and greater trochanter are completely unossified; indeed the radiographic differentiation from a congenitally dislocated hip at birth may require an arthrogram. Within three weeks, however, radiographic examination reveals evidence of new bone formation in the metaphyseal region indicating a traumatic epiphyseal separation (Fig. 16.22). Treatment consists of immobilization of the hip in abduction and flexion in a spica cast for two weeks. The prognosis for subsequent growth is good since at birth the proximal femoral epiphysis consists of the head, neck and greater trochanter, and therefore, at this stage, separation of the entire epiphysis does not jeopardize its blood supply.

Spine

Fortunately birth injuries of the spine are rare but they are extremely serious since they may be complicated by complete paraplegia.

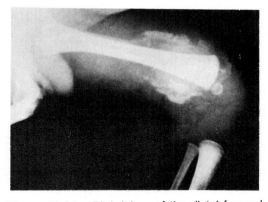

Figure 16.21. Birth injury of the distal femoral epiphysis. In this radiograph taken 10 days after birth, the center of ossification of the distal femoral epiphysis is seen to be displaced posteriorly (normally it is in line with the central axis of the femoral shaft). The marked new bone formation from the elevated periosteum would have taken approximately 10 days to develop and therefore, by deduction, this Type I epiphyseal plate injury probably occurred at birth. The injury had been unsuspected at the time of the difficult breech delivery but the radiograph was taken 10 days later because of the gross clinical swelling of the infant's knee.

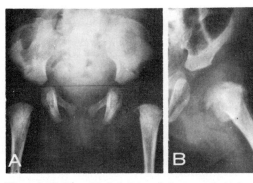

Figure 16.22. Birth injury of the proximal femoral epiphysis. *A*, six days after birth there is obvious lateral displacement of the metaphysis of the left femur in relation to the acetabulum (the normal hip serves as a helpful comparison). Clinically, the infant was thought to have congenital dislocation of the left hip. The center of ossification does not appear until approximately 6 months of age. Note the slight new bone formation, however, around the metaphysis; this differentiates an epiphyseal plate injury from a dislocation of the hip. *B*, eight weeks later there is further new bone formation and early remodeling.

SPECIFIC FRACTURES AND DISLOCATIONS

The Hand

Apart from crush injuries of the distal phalanges, fractures of the hand are much less common in children than in adults.

In children a hyperflexion injury of the distal interphalangeal joint may produce a fracture-separation through the epiphyseal plate, a *childhood type of mallet finger* which can be differentiated from avulsion of the extensor tendon by a lateral radiograph. The finger should be immobilized with the distal joint in extension for three weeks.

Phalangeal fractures must be accurately reduced to avoid a persistent angulatory deformity (Fig. 16.23). Rotational deformity in a finger, which is most likely to occur through a *separation of the proximal phalangeal epiphyseal plate*, should also be corrected since such deformity seriously impairs function of the hand (Fig. 16.24).

Displaced *intra-articular fractures of finger* joints merit open reduction and internal fixation with fine Kirschner wires to restore a perfect joint surface.

Metacarpophalangeal dislocation of the thumb is not uncommon in children as a result of a hyperextension injury (Fig. 16.25). The first metacarpal head escapes through a small tear in joint capsule which then tends to grip the narrow neck of the metacarpal and act as a button hole. For this reason, the dislocation may be frustratingly difficult to reduce by closed manipulation and frequently requires open reduction followed by

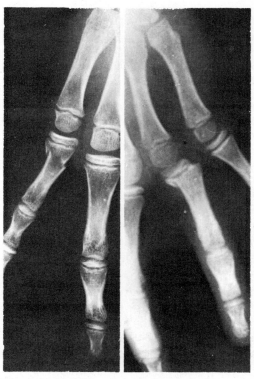

Figure 16.23 (left).   Fracture through the metaphysis of the proximal phalanx of the little finger with angulation. If this angulatory fracture deformity is not reduced, there would be a permanent deformity of the finger.

Figure 16.24 (right).   Type II fracture-separation of the epiphysis of the proximal phalanx of the ring finger. Only slight displacement is apparent in this radiograph, which was taken 3 weeks after injury. Clinical examination at this time, however, revealed a 45° rotational deformity of the finger; as a result, this finger crossed over its neighbor during flexion. Since the epiphyseal plate injury had unfortunately been allowed to heal with this deformity, a corrective osteotomy of the phalanx was required to restore normal function in the child's hand.

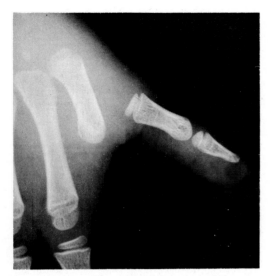

Figure 16.25. Traumatic dislocation of the metacarpophalangeal joint of the thumb of a child. In this particular child the dislocation could not be reduced by closed manipulation and consequently open reduction was required.

immobilization of the joint in the stable position of moderate flexion for three weeks.

Older boys who fight with more force than finesse may sustain a *fracture of the neck of the mobile fifth metacarpal.* This fracture responds well to closed reduction; the depressed metacarpal head can be elevated by pressure along the axis of the proximal phalanx with the metacarpophalangeal joint flexed to a right angle. The fracture should be immobilized for four weeks with the finger in moderate flexion.

Fractures of the carpal bones are rare in childhood possibly because of their relatively large cartilaginous component during the growing years. Nevertheless, *fractures of the carpal scaphoid* sometimes occur in older boys and may require the same prolonged immobilization as they do in adults.

Severe injuries of the hand, particularly tendon injuries and open fractures, should be treated by a surgeon who has a special interest and skill in surgery of the hand.

The Wrist and Forearm

Fractures in the region of the wrist and forearm are extremely common in childhood because of frequent falls in which the forces are transmitted from the hand to the radius and ulna.

DISTAL RADIAL EPIPHYSIS

Fracture-separation is by far the commonest epiphyseal plate injury in the body, accounting for approximately half of the total. This injury occurs frequently in older children and may be accompanied by a green-stick fracture of the ulna. It is a Type II injury as indicated by the separation of the entire epiphysis with a small triangular-shaped metaphyseal fragment (Fig. 16.26). Since this fracture-separation results from a forced hyperextension and supination injury, it can be reduced by a combination of flexion and pronation. The reduced fracture-separation should be immobilized in an above elbow cast with the forearm in pronation for a period of three weeks (epiphyseal separations heal twice as rapidly as fractures through the cancellous area of the same bone in the same child). Being a Type II injury, the prognosis for subsequent growth is excellent.

DISTAL THIRD OF RADIUS AND ULNA

Incomplete Fractures

In young children the most frequent fracture in this region is the *buckle type* (Fig. 16.27), which requires protection alone for three weeks.

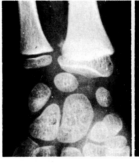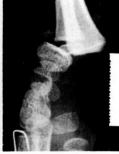

Figure 16.26. Type II fracture-separation of the distal radial epiphysis. In the anteroposterior projection the epiphyseal plate of the radius is not apparent because the epiphysis is displaced and angulated. In the lateral projection the backward displacement and angulation of the epiphysis are apparent. Note the small triangular shaped metaphyseal fragment which is attached to the epiphysis and its epiphyseal plate.

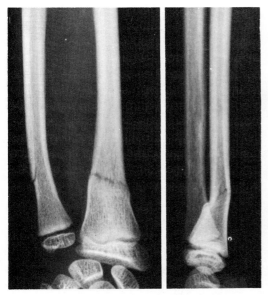

Figure 16.27. Buckle fracture of the distal metaphysis of the radius and a crack fracture of the ulna in a child. The angulation deformity with buckling, or crumpling of the thin dorsal cortex is apparent in the lateral projection. This is sometimes referred to as a "torus" fracture because of the ridge on the cortex (*L. torus*, ridge or protuberance).

may be more stable with the forearm in the neutral position. In either case a well molded, above-elbow plaster cast is required for six weeks.

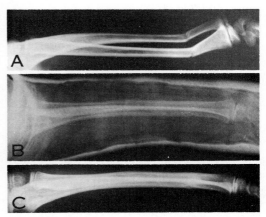

Figure 16.28. *A*, green-stick fractures of the distal third of the radius and ulna in a 7-year-old boy with anterior angulation. *B*, reduced position of the fractures in a plaster cast; the remaining intact portion of the cortex of each bone was deliberately cracked through at the time of reduction. *C*, six weeks later both fractures have united in a satisfactory position.

Green-stick fractures of the distal metaphyseal region of the radius and ulna require closed reduction by manipulation if the angulation is significant. The angulation is gradually corrected to the point when the remaining intact part of the cortex is heard and felt to crack through (Fig. 16.28). Indeed, if this is not done, the angulatory deformity will not be completely corrected and furthermore it may even recur during the period of immobilization.

Complete Fractures

Displaced fractures of the distal metaphyseal region of the radius and ulna are particularly common in childhood (Fig. 16.29). They may be difficult to reduce unless the significance of the intact periosteal hinge as discussed in Chapter 15 is appreciated (Figs. 15.11 and 15.34). When the radius alone is fractured, the injury has been one of supination; consequently the reduction is most stable in pronation. When both the radius and ulna are fractured, the reduction

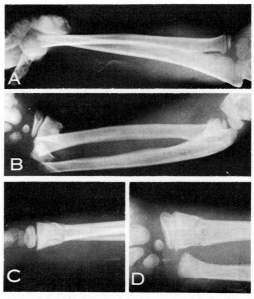

Figure 16.29. Displaced fractures of the distal metaphysis of the radius and ulna with marked overriding. *A* and *B*, before reduction. *C* and *D*, immediately after closed reduction utilizing the intact periosteal hinge (as depicted in Figs. 15.11 and 15.34).

Moderate residual angulation, either anterior or posterior, though not desirable, is acceptable since it tends to correct spontaneously with subsequent growth as already mentioned (Fig. 16.3).

MIDDLE THIRD OF RADIUS AND ULNA

Green-stick fractures of the middle third of the radius and ulna can be completely reduced by closed manipulation provided the aforementioned practice of cracking through the remaining intact part of the cortex is utilized (Fig. 16.30). Indeed, unless the angulatory deformity is well corrected, the normal rotation of the radius around the ulna during supination and pronation will be permanently restricted.

Displaced fractures of the middle third of the radius and ulna are unstable and may be difficult to reduce as well as to keep reduced. Just how much of the fracture deformity is due to angulation and how much is due to rotation is often better assessed by looking at the child's two forearms than by looking at the radiographs.

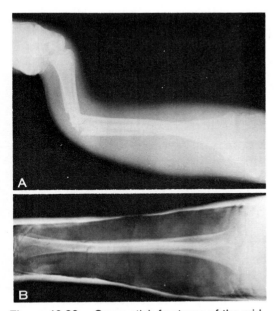

Figure 16.30. Green-stick fractures of the middle third of the radius and ulna of a 14-year-old boy. *A*, note the gross angulation. *B*, reduced position of the fractures in a plaster cast; the remaining intact portion of the cortex of each bone was deliberately cracked through at the time of reduction.

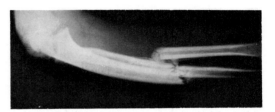

Figure 16.31. Displaced fractures of the middle third of the radius and ulna of a 15-year-old child. Six weeks after injury, the position of the fragments is obviously unsatisfactory; the ulna is out to length but there is marked overriding of the radial fracture and a rotational deformity at both fractures. At this time (after 6 weeks of healing) the fractures could not be reduced by closed manipulation and consequently open reduction and internal fixation were required. Closed reduction would have been possible at an earlier stage had the loss of position of the fragments been detected by repeated radiographic examinations during the first few weeks.

Both angulation and rotation at the fracture site must be corrected, but side-to-side (bayonet) apposition of both fractures is acceptable. Nevertheless, it is usually possible to obtain end-to-end apposition first of one fracture and then of the other, after which the most stable position of the reductions can be assessed; it is usually, but not invariably, the mid-position between supination and pronation. Immobilization in a well molded, above-elbow cast with the forearm in the most stable position should be maintained for eight weeks (healing through cortical bone is slower than through cancellous bone).

Unstable fractures of both bones of the forearm should be examined radiographically each week for at least four weeks in order to detect any deterioration in the position of the fragments (Fig. 16.31). If angulation recurs during the period of immobilization, remanipulation is best performed about two weeks after the injury at which time the fracture sites have become "sticky" and the reduction is likely to be more stable. Loss of apposition with resultant overriding should be corrected by remanipulation as soon as it is recognized.

Fractures of both bones of the forearm in children may be difficult to treat and are

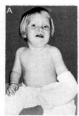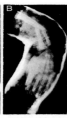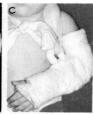

Figure 16.32. Avoidable pitfall in the treatment of fractures of both bones of the forearm in a child. *A,* this 2-year-old child has reason to cry. The incorrectly applied above-elbow cast for her fractured forearm had been gradually slipping off during the preceding 3 days. Note that the fingers have disappeared into the cast and that the elbow of the cast is no longer at the level of the child's elbow. It is on the way to becoming a "shopping bag cast," one which the mother brings back in her shopping bag. *B,* the child's fractures have become angulated since they are now at the level of the elbow of the cast. A second reduction was required. *C,* after the second reduction a well molded cast was applied and was suspended from the child's neck; these precautions prevent the cast from slipping off.

often not treated well. There is virtually no indication for open reduction of these fractures in children. Some of the avoidable pitfalls of treatment are depicted as examples in order that you too may avoid them (Figs. 16.32 and 16.33).

PROXIMAL THIRD OF RADIUS AND ULNA

Fracture of the shaft of the ulna combined with dislocation of the radiohumeral joint (Monteggia fracture-dislocation) is a serious injury not only because it is a fracture-dislocation but also because the dislocation component of the injury is so frequently unrecognized and consequently remains untreated (Fig. 16.34). Because of the firm attachment of the radius to the ulna through the fibrous interosseous membrane, a fracture of the middle or proximal third of the ulna cannot become angulated unless its attached mate, the radius, either fractures also or else dislocates at its proximal end. Thus, as was pointed out in Chapter 15, whenever you see a child with an angulated fracture of the ulna you should be certain that the radiographic examination includes the full length of the forearm (Fig. 15.15).

In children, closed reduction of a Monteggia fracture-dislocation can usually be obtained by correcting the angulation of the ulnar fracture and replacing the radial head in proper relationship with the capitellum (Fig. 16.35). Immobilization of the limb in a cast with the elbow in acute flexion is necessary for six weeks to maintain the reduction; active exercises may be required to help regain elbow motion after removal of the cast.

Neglected residual dislocation of the radiohumeral joint is difficult to treat even a few months after the injury and necessitates an extensive reconstructive operation (Fig. 16.34). If six months or more have elapsed from the time of injury, the dislocation is better left unreduced since elbow stiffness after surgical correction may be more troublesome than the joint instability associated with the residual dislocation.

The Elbow and Arm

Fractures and dislocations of the elbow in children are common injuries; they are also serious not only because of inherent difficulties in obtaining adequate reduction but also because of the high incidence of complications.

One very common but minor injury, "pulled elbow," also merits discussion in this section.

PULLED ELBOW

Children of pre-school age are particularly vulnerable to a sudden pull or jerk on their arms and frequently sustain the common minor injury well known to family physicians and pediatricians as *"pulled elbow."*

Clinical Features

The history is characteristic; a parent, nursemaid or older sibling, while lifting the small child up a step by the hand or pulling him away from potential danger, exerts a strong pull on the extended elbow. The resulting injury of "pulled elbow" is sometimes referred to as "nursemaid's elbow"; although the nursemaid may cause the injury, it is the child who suffers it (Fig. 16.36).

The child begins to cry and refuses to use the arm, which he protects by holding it with the elbow flexed and the forearm pronated.

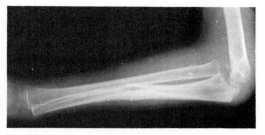

Figure 16.34. Healed fracture of the shaft of the ulna combined with dislocation of the radial head (Monteggia fracture-dislocation). The radial head should always be opposite the capitellum. The child had been treated for the fractured ulna 3 months previously but the dislocated radial head had not been recognized. Unfortunately, at this stage reconstructive surgery on the ulna and radiohumeral joint is required.

Understandably, the parent fears that "something must be broken" and seeks medical attention.

Diagnosis

Physical examination reveals a crying or fretting child but the only significant local finding is painful limitation of forearm supination. Radiographic examination is consistently negative.

Pathological Anatomy

Pulled elbow is essentially a *transient subluxation of the radial head.* For years it was assumed that in children under the age of five years, the diameter of the cartilaginous radial head was no larger than that of the radial neck and that consequently, in this age group the radial head could easily be pulled through the annular ligament. This

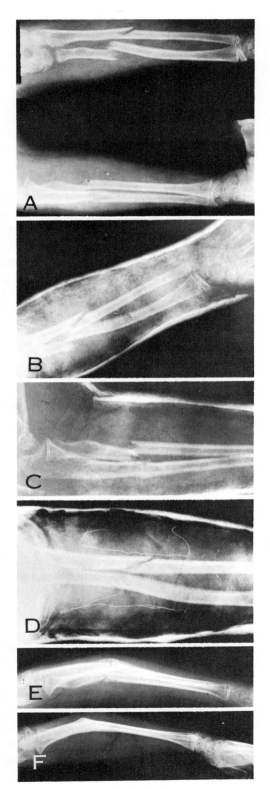

Figure 16.33. Avoidable pitfalls in the treatment of unstable fractures of both bones of the forearm

in an 8-year-old girl. *A,* initial radiographs. *B* and *C,* the position obtained by closed reduction was unsatisfactory. The surgeon did not appreciate the rotational deformity at the fracture sites. *D,* the surgeon then performed an open reduction of both fractures but failed to secure the reduction by means of internal fixation. *E,* six weeks after injury the fractures have united with an unacceptable amount of angulation (mal-union). The surgeon apparently felt this would correct spontaneously with subsequent growth. *F,* one year later the angulation remains unchanged. In addition to an ugly clinical deformity, there was gross restriction of pronation and supination of the forearm.

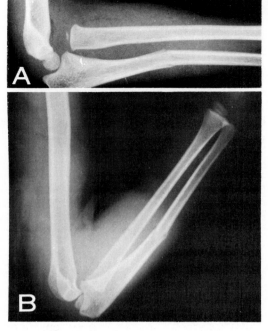

Figure 16.35. Fresh fracture of the shaft of the ulna combined with dislocation of the radial head. *A*, before reduction. *B*, after closed reduction of the angulated ulna and the dislocated radial head.

also reveal that with the elbow flexed, sudden supination of the forearm frees the incarcerated part of the annular ligament which then resumes its normal position.

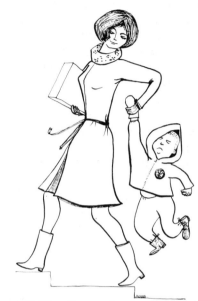

Figure 16.36. The mechanism of injury that produces a "pulled elbow" in a young child.

assumption, however, is incorrect. Anatomical studies in the postmortem room reveal that in children of all ages the diameter of the radial head is always larger than that of the neck. In young children, however, the distal attachment of the annular ligament to the radial neck is thin and weak.

In postmortem studies that we have conducted with the elbow joint exposed, we demonstrated that in young children a sudden pull on the extended elbow while the forearm is pronated produces a tear in the distal attachment of the annular ligament to the radial neck. The radial head penetrates part way through this tear as it is distracted from the capitellum and then the proximal part of the annular ligament slips into the radiohumeral joint where it becomes trapped between the joint surfaces when the pull is released (Fig. 16.37). The subluxation, therefore, is transient and this explains the normal radiographic appearance of the elbow. The source of pain is the pinched annular ligament. The postmortem studies

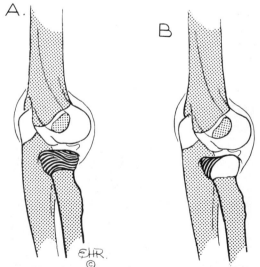

Figure 16.37. Schematic representation of the pathological anatomy of a "pulled elbow." *A*, normal arrangement of the annular ligament. *B*, in the "pulled elbow" there is a tear in the distal attachment of the annular ligament through which the radial head has protruded slightly; the proximal portion of the annular ligament has slipped into the radiohumeral joint where it has become trapped.

Treatment

On the basis of the foregoing explanation of the pathological anatomy of pulled elbow, its treatment is rational and simply consists of a deft supination of the child's forearm while the elbow is flexed. A slight "click" can usually be felt over the anterolateral aspect of the radial head as the annular ligament is freed from the joint. Within moments the child's pain is relieved and he begins to use his arm again.

If the child has been sent to the radiology department prior to treatment, the radiographic technician frequently, and unwittingly, "treats" the pulled elbow while the forearm is being passively supinated to obtain the anteroposterior projection.

After-treatment consists of a sling for two weeks to allow the tear in the attachment of the annular ligament to heal. In addition, the parents are advised about the harmful effects of pulling or lifting their small child by the hand.

PROXIMAL RADIAL EPIPHYSIS

Fracture-separation of the proximal radial epiphysis is produced by a fall that exerts a compression and abduction force on the elbow joint. It is a Type II epiphyseal plate injury with a characteristic metaphyseal fragment and the radial head becomes tilted on the neck (Fig. 16.38).

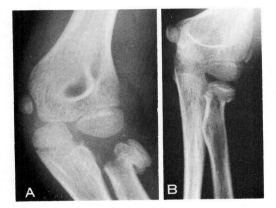

Figure 16.38. Type II fracture-separation of the proximal radial epiphysis in a child. *A*, note the valgus deformity of the elbow, the angulation at the fracture site and the loss of contact of the radiohumeral joint surfaces. *B*, the position of the fragments after closed reduction is satisfactory.

Treatment

Satisfactory closed reduction can usually be obtained by pressing upwards and medially on the tilted radial head while an assistant holds the arm with the elbow extended and adducted. Residual angulation of less than 40° is compatible with acceptable function. Occasionally, open reduction is necessary to restore congruity between the joint surface of the radial head and that of the capitellum. Internal fixation is not necessary. Even if it has lost all soft tissue attachments, the radial head should *never* be excised during childhood. Indeed, removal of the radial epiphysis also includes its epiphyseal plate from the proximal end of the radius; as you might anticipate, this produces a progressive discrepancy in length between the radius and ulna due to relatively less growth in the radius and consequently the hand becomes progressively deviated toward the radial side. After reduction, either closed or open, the child's elbow should be immobilized for three weeks at a right angle with the forearm supinated since this is the most stable position.

Complications

Since the blood supply to the intra-articular radial head is precarious, displaced fracture-separations through the epiphyseal plate may be complicated by avascular necrosis of the epiphysis. The small volume of the radial epiphysis, however, permits fairly rapid revascularization and regeneration. Little deformity of the replaced radial head ensues, but necrosis of the epiphyseal plate results in premature cessation of growth at this site and a length discrepancy between the radius and ulna. Nevertheless, this result is far superior to the results of removing the radial head in children.

DISLOCATION OF THE ELBOW

Posterior dislocation of the elbow joint occurs relatively frequently in young children as a result of a fall on the hand with the elbow flexed. The distal end of the humerus is driven through the anterior capsule as the radius and ulna dislocate posteriorly (Fig. 16.39).

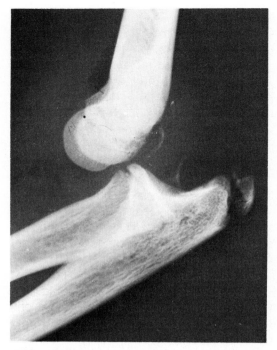

Figure 16.39. Posterior dislocation of the elbow joint in a child. The apparently separated fragment of bone at the proximal end of the ulna is a traction epiphysis rather than a fracture fragment.

through the attached medial ligament in association with two types of injuries. In one type the medial epicondyle is avulsed at the time of a posterior dislocation of the elbow and is therefore carried posteriorly; as the dislocation is reduced so also is the separation of the medial epicondyle.

More frequently, however, the injury that avulses the medial epicondyle is severe abduction of the extended elbow with or without a transient lateral dislocation of the joint; the medial epicondyle is carried distally. There is marked local swelling and tenderness. In the absence of a permanent lateral dislocation of the elbow, however, radiographic examination reveals only moderate separation of the medial epicondyle from the distal end of the humerus (Fig. 16.40). If there is doubt about the diagnosis, comparable radiographic projections of the opposite elbow are helpful.

Treatment

Stability of the elbow joint is the most important aspect of this second type of avul-

Treatment

Closed reduction is readily accomplished by reversing the mechanism of injury; traction is applied to the flexed elbow through the forearm which is then brought forward. The reduced elbow should be maintained in the stable position of flexion above a right angle in a plaster cast for a period of three weeks after which gentle active exercises are begun.

Fracture-dislocations of the elbow are discussed in relation to the specific fractures of the medial epicondyle and lateral condyle of the humerus.

Complications

The complication of *post traumatic myositis ossificans* which may develop after dislocation of the elbow is discussed in Chapter 15 (Fig. 15.79).

MEDIAL EPICONDYLE

Avulsion of the medial epicondyle (attraction epiphysis) results from sudden traction

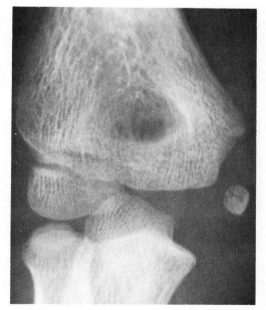

Figure 16.40. Avulsion of the medial epicondyle (a traction epiphysis) from the distal end of the humerus in a 6-year-old child. The medial epicondyle has shifted distally approximately 1 cm to reach the level of the joint line of the elbow.

sion injury and should always be assessed under general anesthesia to determine the optimum form of treatment. If the elbow is stable when subjected to an abduction force, the relatively slight separation of the medial epicondyle requires only immobilization with the elbow in flexion for three weeks; under these circumstances, even if the epicondyle heals by fibrous union, there is no growth disturbance and the long term result will be satisfactory. If, however, the elbow is grossly unstable when subjected to an abduction force, open reduction and internal fixation are indicated to restore stability of the joint (Fig. 16.41).

Complications

A traction injury of the ulnar nerve is a frequent complication of the abduction type of avulsion of the medial epicondyle; the prognosis for recovery of the nerve lesion is excellent and the presence of such a lesion in itself is not an indication for open reduction.

Occasionally, at the moment of spontaneous reduction of a lateral dislocation, the avulsed medial epicondyle is trapped in the elbow joint. Under these circumstances the medial epicondyle can be freed from the joint by closed manipulation but since open reduction and internal fixation are indicated to restore stability to the elbow, the trapped

medial epicondyle is best freed at the time of operation.

LATERAL CONDYLE

Fractures of the lateral condyle of the humerus in children are relatively common, frequently complicated and regrettably often inadequately treated. The fracture line begins at the joint surface, passes through the cartilaginous portion of the epiphysis medial to the capitellum, crosses the epiphyseal plate and extends into the metaphysis. Thus, a fracture of the lateral condyle represents a Type IV epiphyseal plate injury, the serious significance of which is discussed in an earlier section of this chapter (Fig. 16.15).

These fractures are inherently unstable since they are predominantly intra-articular; the only periosteal covering therefore is on the metaphyseal fragment and this is frequently completely disrupted. Consequently, even when the fracture appears undisplaced initially, it has a tendency to become displaced subsequently with serious sequelae.

Radiographically, an undisplaced fracture of the lateral condyle may escape detection unless comparable projections of the opposite elbow are obtained (Fig. 16.2). The lateral condyle (which includes the capitellum and the lateral portion of the metaphysis) may be relatively undisplaced, moderately angulated or even completely distracted and rotated (Fig. 16.42). With severe injuries there even may be an associated dislocation of the elbow and, hence, a fracture-dislocation.

Treatment

Even undisplaced fractures of the lateral condyle are potentially serious because of their instability. They may be treated initially by immobilization of the arm in a plaster cast with the elbow at a right angle; during the first two weeks, however, repeated radiographic examinations are essential since even during immobilization the fracture may become displaced in which case immediate open reduction and internal fixation are indicated.

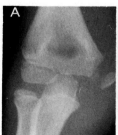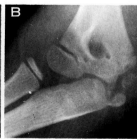

Figure 16.41. Instability of the right elbow joint of a 7-year-old boy in association with avulsion of the medial epicondyle. *A,* anteroposterior projection of the elbow showing moderate separation of the medial epicondyle. *B,* this stress radiograph taken with the boy under anesthetic and with an abduction force being applied to the elbow reveals gross instability of the joint; the medial epicondyle has been pulled further distally.

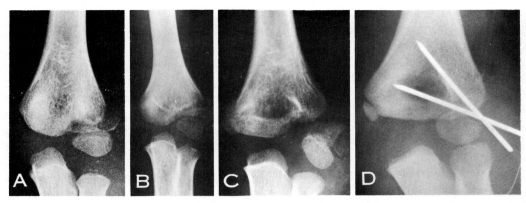

Figure 16.42. Fractures of the lateral condyle of the humerus in children, a Type IV epiphyseal plate injury. *A*, relatively undisplaced. *B*, moderately angulated. *C*, completely distracted and rotated. *D*, after open reduction and internal fixation of the fracture with Kirschner wires.

Displaced fractures of the lateral condyle represent one of the relatively few absolute indications for open reduction and internal fixation in children. Since these fractures are Type IV epiphyseal plate injuries, even relatively minor displacement must be perfectly reduced and the reduction must be constantly maintained by internal fixation in order to avoid an otherwise inevitable growth disturbance (Fig. 16.42*D*). After operation, the arm should be immobilized in a plaster cast with the elbow at a right angle for three weeks. The metallic internal fixation (usually Kirschner wires) should then be removed and gentle active exercises should be started.

Complications

If union is delayed because of inadequate fixation, the associated hyperemia may cause an overgrowth on the lateral side of the elbow with resultant cubitus varus (loss of carrying angle) (Fig. 16.43*A*). Failure to obtain and maintain perfect reduction of a fractured lateral condyle of the humerus leads to serious growth disturbance at the epiphyseal plate (Fig. 16.43*B*). If the fracture is complicated by avascular necrosis of the capitellum, there is not only a growth disturbance and deformity but also a marked secondary enlargement of the radial head (Fig. 16.44). Inadequate treatment of a fractured lateral condyle may even result in a complete non-union, one of the few exam-

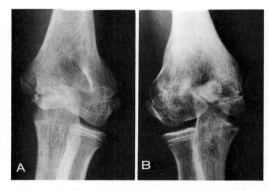

Figure 16.43. Growth disturbances complicating fractures of the lateral condyle of the humerus. *A*, cubitus varus 1 year after a fracture of the lateral condyle due to overgrowth of the lateral part of the epiphyseal plate. *B*, notch in the distal end of the humerus 2 years after a fracture of the lateral condyle (due to premature cessation of local epiphyseal plate growth).

ples of this complication of fractures in childhood (Fig. 16.45). The resultant cubitus valgus (increased carrying angle) is eventually further complicated by the gradual development of a tardy ulnar palsy as discussed in Chapter 15 (Fig. 15.80).

SUPRACONDYLAR FRACTURE OF THE HUMERUS

Of the significant injuries about the elbow, displaced supracondylar fractures of the humerus are the most common and certainly the most serious. Not only are they associated with a high incidence of mal-union with

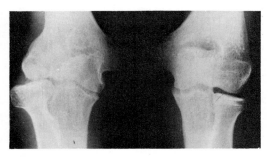

Figure 16.44. The late effects of avascular necrosis of the right capitellum which occurred 5 years previously as a complication of a fracture of the lateral condyle of the humerus. Note the growth disturbance of the distal end of the humerus, the deformity of the capitellum and the secondary enlargement of the radial head.

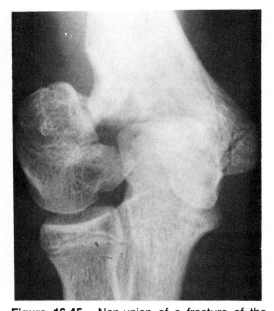

Figure 16.45. Non-union of a fracture of the lateral condyle in a 12-year-old boy 6 years after an injury that had been thought to be a "sprained elbow." The boy's elbow was deformed and unstable but had a reasonable range of motion. Reconstructive surgery at this stage would be unlikely to improve the unfortunate situation.

residual deformity but also with the serious risk of Volkmann's ischemia of nerves and muscles of the forearm with resultant contracture.

The following discussion refers to the extension type of supracondylar fracture which comprises 99% of the total.

Pathological Anatomy

The flared but flat distal metaphysis of the humerus is indented posteriorly (the olecranon fossa) and also anteriorly (the coronoid fossa); consequently, it is a relatively weak site in the upper limb. As a result of either a hyperextension injury or a fall on the hand with the elbow flexed, the forces of injury are transmitted through the elbow joint which grips the distal end of the humerus like a right-angled wrench. Thus, the resultant fracture is consistently immediately proximal to the elbow joint. When the injury is severe there is considerable "follow-through" of the fragments at the moment of fracture. The jagged end of the proximal fragment is driven through the anterior periosteum and the overlying brachialis muscle into the plane of the brachial artery and median nerve and comes to rest in the subcutaneous fat of the antecubital fossa; it may even penetrate the skin from within thereby creating an open fracture (Fig. 16.46).

Diagnosis

Clinically there is an obvious deformity in the elbow region which soon becomes grossly swollen and tense as a result of extensive internal hemorrhage. The state of the peripheral circulation and the function of the peripheral nerves should be assessed immediately; impairment of the circulation demands urgent reduction of the fracture. Radiographic examination provides striking evidence of the displacement of the fragments but little evidence of the severe soft tissue damage (Fig. 16.47). The distal fragment lies posteriorly and hence there is an

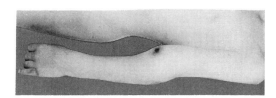

Figure 16.46. Clinical appearance of a child's arm with an open supracondylar fracture of the humerus. Note the wound in the antecubital fossa (the fracture was open from within), the gross swelling and the striking extension deformity just proximal to the elbow joint.

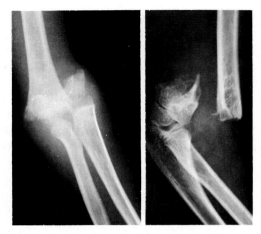

Figure 16.47.   Displaced supracondylar fracture of the right humerus in a 7-year-old girl. *Left*, in the anteroposterior projection the distal fragment of the humerus is displaced medially and proximally. *Right*, in the lateral projection the distal fragment is displaced posteriorly and proximally. The jagged end of the proximal fragment is lying in the soft tissues of the antecubital fossa.

intact posterior hinge of periosteum. In addition, the distal fragment is displaced either medially or laterally, more often the former. When it is displaced medially there is an intact medial hinge of periosteum, whereas when it is displaced laterally there is an intact lateral hinge; these facts are important in relation to treatment, as you will see.

Treatment

Undisplaced supracondylar fractures require only immobilization of the arm with the elbow flexed for three weeks. Most displaced supracondylar fractures of the humerus can be treated by closed reduction which is made possible by utilizing the intact periosteal hinge. Thus, gentle traction on the forearm (with the elbow slightly flexed to avoid traction on the brachial artery) brings the fragments into general alignment after which any rotational deformity and any medial or lateral displacement are corrected. At this stage—and not before—the elbow is flexed beyond a right angle. This maneuver tightens the posterior hinge of periosteum and helps to maintain the reduction. If the distal fragment was originally displaced medially, the forearm is then pronated since

this tightens the medial hinge and closes the fracture line on the lateral side thereby preventing any varus deformity at the fracture site. If, however, the distal fragment had been displaced laterally, the forearm is supinated since this tightens the lateral hinge and closes the fracture on the medial side thereby preventing any valgus deformity at the fracture site.

After reduction of the fracture, anteroposterior and lateral radiographs are obtained by rotating the tube of the X-ray machine (rather than by rotating the child's arm) in order that the reduction is not lost (Fig. 16.48). The peripheral circulation is again assessed and, if it is inadequate, the elbow must be allowed to extend slightly. The child's arm is then immobilized in a special type of cast which does not constrict the area of maximal swelling (Fig. 16.49).

Children who require closed reduction of a supracondylar fracture of the humerus should be admitted to the hospital for at least a few days for observation with particular reference to peripheral circulation in the limb. A well reduced fracture is stable and hence comfortable; persistent pain therefore may be a warning signal of ischemia and

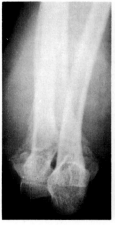
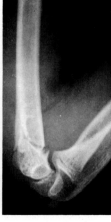

Figure 16.48.   After closed reduction of the supracondylar fracture shown in Figure 16.47, the position of the fragments is satisfactory. *Left*, the anteroposterior projection is taken with the elbow flexed. *Right*, the position of the arm has not been altered for the lateral projection. Flexion of the elbow helps to maintain the reduction.

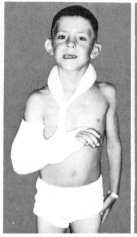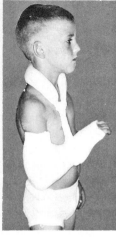

Figure 16.49.   Above-elbow cast with neck sling attached for immobilization of a reduced supracondylar fracture of the humerus. The cast maintains the elbow in flexion and the forearm in pronation. Note that it does not extend into the antecubital fossa and therefore does not constrict the soft tissues in the region of the elbow.

should not be masked by sedation. Repeated radiographic examinations are required during the first 10 days to assess the position of the fracture fragments within the cast.

Healing of supracondylar fractures is rapid and consequently, the cast should always be removed after only three weeks. Immobilization for a more prolonged period is nearly always followed by prolonged elbow joint stiffness even in children because of the extensive soft tissue damage.

After removal of the cast in three weeks, the child's elbow always lacks extension. Active exercises are the only safe way of regaining joint motion and may have to be carried out for several months or even longer before a full range of motion is regained. Passive stretching of the joint is decidedly deleterious and should always be avoided.

Supracondylar fractures in which the reduction is grossly unstable as well as those with excessive soft tissue swelling or impairment of circulation are best treated by continuous skeletal traction through either a transverse pin or a vertical screw in the olecranon (Fig. 16.50).

For an unstable supracondylar fracture of

the humerus, an acceptable alternative to skeletal traction is closed reduction followed by the transcutaneous insertion of two Kirschner wires across the fracture side (under image intensification).

The rare flexion type of supracondylar fracture in which the distal fragment is displaced anteriorly is not serious. It requires closed reduction and immobilization of the elbow in extension.

Complications

1. *Volkmann's Ischemia (Flexor Compartment Syndrome).* The most serious complication of displaced supracondylar fractures of the humerus in children is Volkmann's ischemia of nerves and muscles of the forearm—a form of compartment syndrome due to proximal extracompartmental occlusion of the brachial artery. The brachial artery may be caught and thus kinked in the fracture site, a complication that can be relieved only by reduction of the fracture. Moreover, the brachial artery, often contused at the

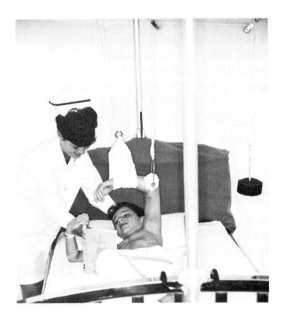

Figure   16.50.   Continuous   skeletal   traction through a pin in the olecranon for a grossly unstable supracondylar fracture of the humerus. The position of the fragments must be monitored every few days by radiographic examination during the first 2 weeks in order that the line and amount of traction may be adjusted as necessary to prevent mal-union.

moment of fracture, is prone to develop severe arterial spasm, particularly if the subsequent manipulation of the fracture has been forceful or if there is rapidly progressive swelling within the unyielding fascial compartment of the arm. Excessive flexion of the elbow aggravates the tightness of the deep fascia in the antecubital fossa and may compress the brachial artery; a tight encircling cast may have the same effect.

The dread complication of Volkmann's ischemia, its recognition and urgent treatment, as well as subsequent Volkmann's contracture, are fully discussed in Chapter 15 under the heading of "Compartment Syndromes," along with other arterial complications. It should be reviewed in Chapter 15 at this time since it is particularly pertinent to supracondylar fractures of the humerus in children (Fig. 15.59).

2. *Peripheral Nerve Injury.* Although the median nerve and less commonly the radial and ulnar nerve may be injured at the moment of fracture, they are not divided and consequently the prognosis for recovery is excellent.

3. *Mal-union.* A common complication of displaced supracondylar fractures of the humerus is mal-union, particularly residual *cubitus varus* (Fig. 16.51). Once thought to be the result of an epiphyseal growth disturbance, this unsightly deformity is now known to be the result of fracture healing in an unsatisfactory position (mal-union). It can and should be *prevented* by accurate reduction of the fracture.

Mal-union, if sufficiently severe, necessitates a supracondylar osteotomy of the humerus after the child has regained a full range of elbow motion.

SHAFT OF THE HUMERUS

Fractures of the humeral shaft are not common in childhood and when they do occur, they are the result of a fairly severe injury. The fracture is usually in the midshaft, less commonly in the proximal metaphysis, and tends to be unstable (Fig. 16.52).

Relatively undisplaced stable fractures of the humeral shaft or proximal metaphysis

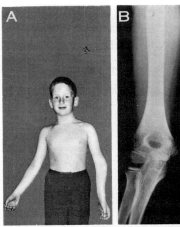
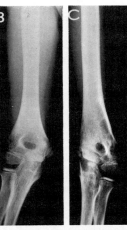
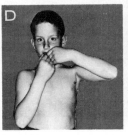
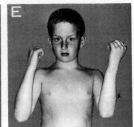

Figure 16.51. Cubitus varus (reversal of the carrying angle) of the left elbow of a 9-year-old boy due to mal-union of a supracondylar fracture of the humerus 1 year previously. *A*, note the unsightly deformity (sometimes referred to as a "gun stock" deformity). *B* and *C*, radiographs of this boy's upper limbs. Unfortunately the supracondylar fracture of the left humerus had been allowed to unite in a position of varus. *D*, because of the altered plane of the elbow joint the boy cannot put the left hand to his mouth without abducting his shoulder. *E*, for the same reason his hand and forearm are deviated laterally when he keeps his elbow to his side (this could create problems for a dinner partner seated on his left side). The appearance and function of this boy's arm can be improved by a supracondylar osteotomy of the humerus.

can be adequately treated by a sling and a thoracobrachial bandage which binds the arm to the chest. Most displaced fractures can be managed by closed reduction followed by a shoulder spica cast for six weeks (Fig. 16.53). Markedly unstable fractures, particularly those in older children, may require continuous skeletal traction (as shown in Fig. 16.50) for a few weeks to maintain alignment and correct rotation after which the fracture is sufficiently "sticky" that the

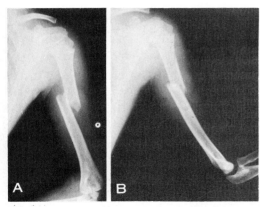

Figure 16.52. Unstable fracture of the mid-shaft of the left humerus in a 7-year-old boy. Prior to the radiographic examination, this boy's arm should have been splinted so that his arm could not be moved through the fracture site. *A*, an anteroposterior projection of both the proximal and the distal fragments. *B*, this is a lateral projection of the distal fragment but almost an anteroposterior projection of the proximal fragment. Obviously, between the two exposures the child's arm has been rotated approximately 90° through the unstable fracture site by the technician. The child would have experienced much pain at this time and might even have sustained further injury to the related soft tissues.

traction can be replaced by a shoulder spica cast. An above-elbow cast suspended by a loop around the neck (a "hanging cast") is an inefficient method of providing traction during the first few weeks, especially during sleep, and is uncomfortable for a child.

The commonest complication of a fracture of the mid-shaft of the humerus is an associated injury of the radial nerve which winds around the humerus at this level; the prognosis for spontaneous recovery, however, is good.

The Shoulder
PROXIMAL HUMERAL EPIPHYSIS

The type of injury that in an adult would produce a dislocation of the shoulder produces a Type II *fracture-separation of the proximal humeral epiphysis* in a child since the joint capsule is stronger than the epiphyseal plate (Fig. 16.54).

If the displacement is only slight, closed reduction can usually be obtained after which a sling and thoracobrachial bandage

are used to immobilize the shoulder for three weeks.

If the displacement is marked, closed reduction can be difficult unless the intact periosteal hinge is utilized; this necessitates applying traction to the arm while it is held directly over the child's head in line with the trunk, a maneuver that pulls the distal fragment into line with the epiphysis. The reduction is frequently most stable in this position,

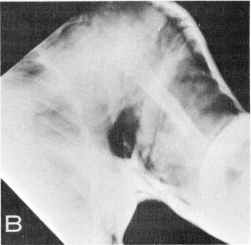
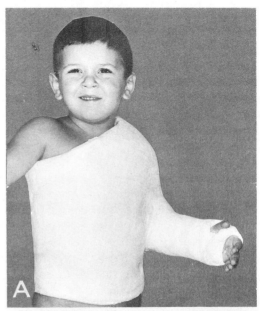

Figure 16.53. *A*, shoulder spica cast for immobilization of an unstable fracture of the mid-shaft of the humerus in a 5-year-old boy. *B*, anteroposterior projection through the cast showing the satisfactory position of the fragments.

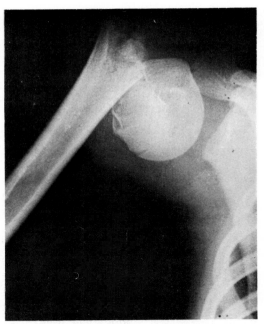

Figure 16.54. Type II fracture-separation of the right humeral epiphysis in a 14-year-old boy. Note the large metaphyseal fragment and the marked displacement of the fracture. The humeral head has retained its normal relationship with the glenoid cavity of the scapula.

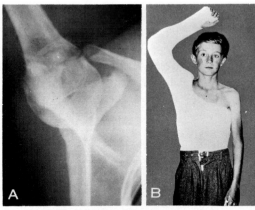

Figure 16.55. *A*, reduced Type II fracture-separation of the right proximal humeral epiphysis in the boy whose initial radiograph is shown in Figure 16.54. Note that the arm is in the overhead position. *B*, shoulder spica cast for immobilization of this boy's arm in the overhead position.

in which case the shoulder is immobilized in the overhead position in a shoulder spica cast for a period of two weeks, after which the spica can be replaced by a sling for an additional week (Fig. 16.55).

Even with imperfect reduction of the separated epiphysis, union occurs through the intact portion of the periosteal tube; moreover, spontaneous correction of deformity and remodeling of the proximal end of the humerus usually produce a satisfactory result. There is virtually no indication for open reduction of these Type II epiphyseal injuries.

CLAVICLE

Fractures of the clavicle are the most common but the least serious of all childhood fractures. Preschool children in particular tumble almost daily and when they land on their hands, elbows or shoulders, their slender clavicles are subjected to indirect forces which may produce a fracture. These common fractures are not serious, however, since they virtually all unite rapidly and there are almost no permanent sequelae (Fig. 16.56).

Green-stick fractures of the clavicle require only a sling to provide protection from further injury for three weeks. Displaced fractures of the clavicle in young children (under the age of 10 years) usually do not require reduction; they are best treated by means of a snug figure-eight bandage, not so much to hold the fragments in perfect position as to hold them relatively still and thereby to make the child comfortable (Fig. 16.57). The parents are instructed to tighten

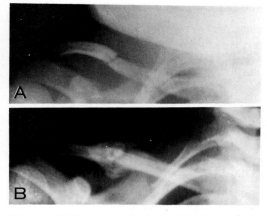

Figure 16.56. *A*, undisplaced fracture of the right clavicle in a 2-year-old boy. *B*, three weeks after injury there is abundant callus formation; the fracture callus was both visible and palpable as a lump.

The Ankle and Leg

During childhood all significant fractures about the ankle involve an epiphyseal plate and therefore should be considered in relation to the particular type of epiphyseal plate injury as classified in an earlier section of this chapter.

TYPE I INJURY OF THE DISTAL FIBULAR EPIPHYSIS

Avulsion of the distal fibular epiphysis may be caused by a sudden inversion injury of the ankle. If the epiphysis returns immediately to its normal position, the child may seem to have merely sprained his ankle since radiographic examination will be negative. Marked local tenderness at the site of the epiphyseal plate is an indication to obtain stress radiographs, which may reveal evidence of occult joint instability due to separation of the epiphysis as previously described (Fig. 16.9).

Treatment consists of a below-knee walking cast for three weeks. The prognosis for subsequent growth is excellent.

TYPE II INJURY OF THE DISTAL TIBIAL EPIPHYSIS

Even severely displaced Type II epiphyseal plate injuries around the ankle can be readily reduced by closed means. Furthermore, the reduction can be well maintained

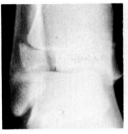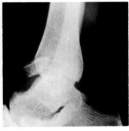

Figure 16.66. Type III injury of the distal tibial epiphysis in a 14-year-old boy. Note that the displacement of the anterolateral corner of the epiphysis is more obvious in the lateral projection than in the anteroposterior projection.

provided there is appropriate molding of the plaster cast (Fig. 16.65). Healing is usually complete within three weeks and the prognosis for subsequent growth is excellent.

TYPE III INJURY OF THE DISTAL TIBIAL EPIPHYSIS

In older children who are almost fully grown, a severe ankle injury may fracture the anterolateral corner of the distal tibial epiphysis—the last part of the epiphysis to become fused to the metaphysis.

This injury is more readily detected in the lateral radiographic projection than in the anteroposterior projection (Fig. 16.66). Since the fracture is intra-articular, open reduction is indicated to obtain perfect restoration of the joint surfaces.

TYPE IV INJURY OF THE DISTAL TIBIAL EPIPHYSIS

A severe inversion injury of the ankle may produce a Type IV fracture through the medial portion of the distal tibial epiphyseal plate. The fracture line, which begins at the ankle joint surface, crosses the epiphyseal plate and extends into the metaphysis. As with Type IV injuries elsewhere, the fracture is unstable.

This is a treacherous injury, which requires open reduction and internal fixation to obtain and maintain perfect apposition of the fracture fragments. Indeed, even a slight residual disparity at the level of the fractured surfaces of the epiphyseal plate leads inevitably to a serious growth disturbance (Fig. 16.67).

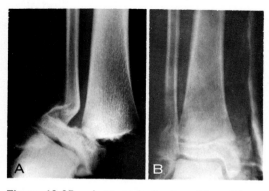

Figure 16.65. *A*, severely displaced Type II fracture-separation of the distal tibial epiphysis combined with a green-stick fracture of the distal third of the fibula in a 13-year-old boy. The intact periosteal hinge is on the lateral aspect of the tibia. *B*, after closed reduction the fragments are in satisfactory position and the reduction is maintained by a well molded plaster cast.

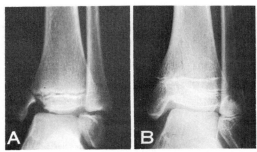

Figure 16.67. Type IV injury of the distal tibial epiphysis. *A*, note that the fracture line begins at the joint surface, crosses the epiphyseal plate and extends into the metaphysis. The entire medial malleolus is shifted medially and proximally. This fracture should have been treated by open reduction and internal fixation. Did you also notice the Type I injury of the distal fibular epiphysis? *B*, one year after injury a growth disturbance is apparent; the medial part of the distal tibial epiphysis has ceased growing while the lateral part has continued to grow. The varus deformity of the ankle will be progressive.

TYPE V INJURY OF THE DISTAL TIBIAL EPIPHYSIS

When a child gets one foot caught, for example between the pickets of a fence, and then falls, the severe angulation of the ankle produces a tremendous compression force on the distal tibial epiphysis and epiphyseal plate. The result may be a Type V epiphyseal plate injury.

Despite the paucity of clinical and radiographic evidence of the injury, the prognosis concerning subsequent growth is very poor indeed (Fig. 16.68). When a Type V injury is suspected, the child should be kept from bearing weight on the ankle for at least three weeks in an attempt to prevent further compression of the epiphyseal plate. Regardless of treatment, however, subsequent growth disturbance is almost inevitable.

FRACTURE OF THE TIBIA

The majority of tibial shaft fractures in children are relatively undisplaced and this may be explained in part by the strong periosteal sleeve which is not readily torn across. Consequently, such fractures are relatively stable and can be adequately treated by closed reduction; widely displaced open fractures of the tibia and fibula,

however, can result from major trauma such as an automobile accident (Fig. 16.69).

Closed reduction of a fractured tibial shaft must correct both angulatory and rotational deformities; the reduction is best maintained by the application of a long-leg cast with the knee flexed to a right angle not only to control rotation but also to prevent the child from bearing weight. After four weeks in such a cast the fracture is usually sufficiently healed that a long-leg walking cast can be applied and retained for an additional four weeks. There is virtually no indication for open reduction of an uncomplicated fracture of the tibial shaft in children.

Correction of alignment is particularly important when the fracture is in the proximal metaphysis of the tibia since neither valgus nor varus deformities can be expected to correct spontaneously with subsequent growth (Fig. 16.70). Furthermore, in this particular site a flap of interposed pes anserinus and periosteum in the fracture site may prevent accurate reduction, in which case the

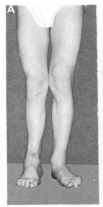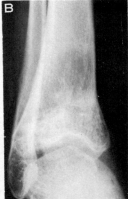

Figure 16.68. Type V injury of the distal tibial epiphysis. *A*, clinical varus deformity of the ankle in a 9-year-old boy 5 years after a fall from a considerable height. He landed on his right foot and was thought to have sustained "only a sprained ankle." One year later he began to develop a progressive deformity of his ankle. Note also the shortening of the right leg. *B*, a radiograph of the ankle reveals a growth disturbance of the distal tibial epiphysis. Growth had ceased in the medial part of the epiphyseal plate due to a Type V crushing injury but had continued in the lateral part and also in the fibular epiphysis with a resultant varus deformity and shortening.

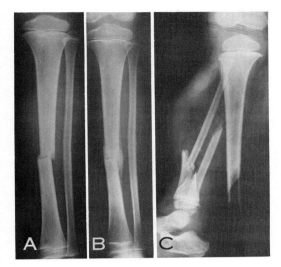

Figure 16.69. Fractures of the tibial shaft. *A*, relatively undisplaced and stable fracture of the tibial shaft in a 6-year-old girl. No reduction was required. *B*, six weeks later the fracture is clinically united. *C*, widely displaced open fracture of the tibia and fibula of a 5-year-old boy who was run over by a truck. The skin was split open from the ankle to the knee and there was extensive soft tissue damage. Note the marked overriding and external rotation at the fracture site. After thorough debridement the fractures were reduced and the soft tissues were repaired. Both bones and soft tissues healed without infection.

flap should be surgically released to prevent the combination of malunion and progressive growth disturbance. Fractures of the proximal third of the tibia and fibula are potentially serious because of the risk of injury to the anterior and posterior tibial arteries at the upper border of the interosseous membrane as previously described in Chapter 15 (Fig. 15.58).

The Knee and Thigh

The most significant injuries about the knee in children involve the epiphyseal plate of either the proximal tibial epiphysis or the distal femoral epiphysis.

TYPE II INJURY OF THE PROXIMAL TIBIAL EPIPHYSIS

The attachment of the proximal tibial epiphysis to the metaphysis is particularly strong because of its irregular contour; consequently, a severe injury is required to separate it. A severe hyperextension injury of the knee may produce a Type II fracture-separation of the proximal tibial epiphysis which, though not common, is serious because of the risk of injury to the popliteal artery (Fig. 16.71).

TYPE II INJURY OF THE DISTAL FEMORAL EPIPHYSIS

The distal femoral epiphysis is more often separated from its metaphysis than is the proximal tibial epiphysis. A hyperextension injury may produce a Type II fracture-separation of the epiphysis; the metaphysis of the femur tears the posterior periosteum and is driven posteriorly into the soft tissues of the popliteal fossa, where it may injure the popliteal artery as well as the medial or lateral popliteal nerves.

Clinical examination reveals a grossly swollen knee because of the associated hemarthrosis; radiographic examination reveals a striking displacement of the epiphysis (Fig. 16.72).

This fracture-separation may be difficult to reduce unless the child is lying face-down. Reduction then becomes comparable to that

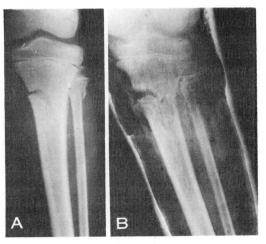

Figure 16.70. *A*, slightly angulated fracture in the metaphyseal region of the upper end of the left tibia of a 9-year-old boy. Even this slight angulation should be corrected by manipulation and no weight bearing should be allowed in the early stages of healing. Regrettably, the boy was treated with a long-leg walking cast. *B*, with weight bearing the angulation increased over the ensuing 6 weeks. This angulatory deformity cannot be expected to correct spontaneously.

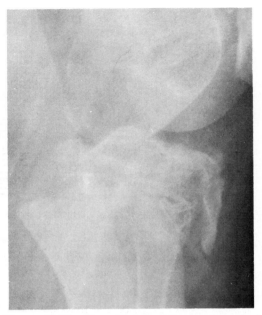

Figure 16.71. Type II injury of the proximal tibial epiphysis in a 14-year-old boy who was hit on the anterior aspect of the tibia by an automobile. This injury was complicated by severe damage to the popliteal artery, which necessitated local resection of the damaged portion of the artery and replacement by a vein graft.

duction is maintained by completely flexing the knee since this tightens the intact anterior hinge of periosteum. The lower limb is immobilized in a cast in this position for only three weeks after which active exercises are begun. Since this is a Type II injury, the prognosis concerning subsequent growth is excellent.

TYPE IV INJURY OF THE DISTAL FEMORAL EPIPHYSIS

Fortunately, this serious type of epiphyseal plate injury is uncommon at the knee. Being a Type IV fracture that traverses the joint surface as well as the epiphyseal plate, the prognosis concerning subsequent growth is very poor unless the reduction is perfect (Fig. 16.73).

This type of injury is extremely important to recognize because with accurate open reduction and secure internal fixation, the otherwise inevitable growth disturbance can be prevented.

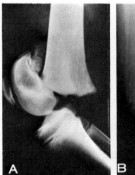 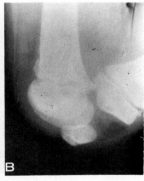

Figure 16.72. *A*, type II injury of the distal femoral epiphysis in a 13-year-old boy as the result of a hyperextension injury of the knee. Note the large triangular-shaped fragment anteriorly, the side of the intact periosteal hinge. *B*, after reduction the epiphysis is in good position and the reduction is maintained by the flexed position of the knee.

for a supracondylar fracture of the humerus; traction is applied to the leg with the knee slightly flexed after which the epiphysis can be pushed into its normal position. The re-

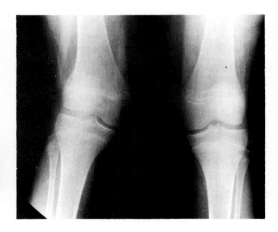

Figure 16.73. Type IV injury of the right distal femoral epiphysis of a 12-year-old boy 1 year after injury. The fracture began at the joint surface of the lateral femoral condyle, crossed the epiphyseal plate and extended into the metaphysis. The lateral condyle was displaced proximally and should have been treated by open reduction and internal fixation but unfortunately it was not. One year after injury growth has ceased in the lateral part of the epiphyseal plate but has continued in the medial part with a resultant progressive valgus deformity.

TRAUMATIC DISLOCATION OF THE PATELLA

Older children and adolescents, particularly girls who have some degree of genu valgum and generalized ligamentous laxity, may sustain a lateral dislocation of the patella due to an abduction, external rotation injury to the knee. The patient experiences sharp pain, her knee gives way completely and she falls.

Diagnosis

Physical examination reveals a grossly swollen knee due to a gross hemarthrosis. The patella can be felt lying on the lateral aspect of the knee; sometimes, however, the patella has already slid back into its normal position spontaneously before the patient is seen. Radiographic examination must include a tangential superoinferior (skyline) projection to detect the presence of an associated osteochondral fracture of either the medial edge of the patella or the lateral lip of the patellar groove, the site of impact as the patella dislocates laterally.

Treatment

If there is no osteochondral fracture, the dislocated patella can be reduced by closed manipulation with the knee in the extended position. The knee is then immobilized in a cylinder cast (ankle to groin) in extension for a period of six weeks. The presence of an osteochondral fracture is an indication for open operation with removal of the fragment and repair of the torn soft tissues. During and after the period of immobilization, quadriceps exercises are important in attempting to prevent recurrence of the dislocation.

Complications

Recurring dislocation of the patella is a troublesome complication of this injury (Fig. 16.74). Moreover, with each dislocation, the articular cartilage of the patella is injured and this leads to the development of chondromalacia of the patella and eventually to degenerative joint disease of the knee. Thus, recurring dislocation of the patella is an indication for a reconstructive operation which involves the release of tight structures on the lateral side of the joint, repair of the

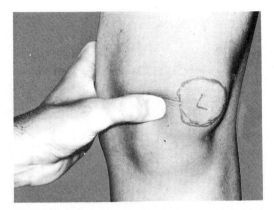

Figure 16.74. Recurring dislocation of the left patella in a 14-year-old girl who exhibited generalized ligamentous laxity. The patella could almost be dislocated by simply pushing it laterally with the thumb.

fibrous joint capsule on the medial side and redirection of the line of pull of the patellar tendon by means of a tenodesis (using the semitendinosus tendon). In a growing child this type of operation is safer than that in which the tibial tubercle is transplanted since interference with the tibial tubercle (which includes part of the proximal tibial epiphyseal plate) may cause a serious growth disturbance.

INTERNAL DERANGEMENTS OF THE KNEE

The semilunar cartilages (menisci) of the knee in children are resilient and relatively resistant to disruption. For this reason torn menisci are uncommon in young children. Nevertheless, they may occur in older children and adolescents as a result of injuries incurred in such sports as skiing, football and hockey. Meniscal injuries and their treatment are discussed in Chapter 17.

FRACTURES OF THE FEMORAL SHAFT

Displaced fractures of the femoral shaft are common in childhood and merit special consideration. Usually involving the middle third of the femur, the fracture may be transverse, oblique, spiral or even comminuted depending on the mechanism of injury. Even with marked displacement of the fragments, however, at least part of the strong periosteal sleeve remains intact, a point of consid-

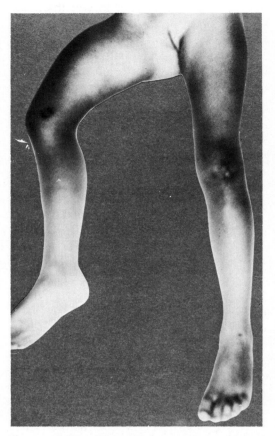

Figure 16.75. Clinical deformity in the thigh of a child with a displaced fracture of the right femoral shaft. Note the angulation, external rotation and shortening.

is immobilized in a hip spica cast until it is clinically united. There is virtually no indication for open reduction of an uncomplicated femoral shaft fracture in a child. The type and duration of traction depends on the age of the child.

Children under two years of age and 30 lb weight can be treated by overhead (Bryant's) skin traction which is applied to both lower limbs (Fig. 16.76). In children over the age of two years, however, overhead traction is potentially dangerous because of the risk of femoral arterial spasm and consequent Volkmann's ischemia of nerves and muscles (a compartment syndrome comparable to that seen in the upper limb as a complication of supracondylar fractures of the humerus).

Thus in children over the age of two years, fractures of the femoral shaft are best treated by continuous traction of the fixed type in a Thomas splint which is slightly bent at the knee, the child lying on an inclined frame (Fig. 16.77).

Reduction of femoral shaft fractures in children is achieved gradually by the traction apparatus rather than by manipulation. Angulatory and rotational deformities must be erable importance in relation to treatment as well as to healing of the fracture.

Diagnosis

The diagnosis is obvious from clinical examination alone because of the typical deformity (Fig. 16.75). Since these fractures are extremely unstable it is essential to apply a temporary splint before radiographic examination is undertaken, not only to spare the child unnecessary pain but also to prevent further injury to the femoral artery.

Treatment

The basis of treatment for unstable fractures of the femoral shaft in children is continuous traction until the fracture is "sticky" (partially healed and hence relatively stable and painless), after which the healing femur

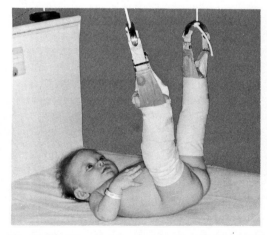

Figure 16.76. Continuous overhead (Bryant's) skin traction in the treatment of a fracture of the shaft of the left femur in a 6-month-old baby girl. Note that both lower limbs are included in the traction and that the baby's buttocks are just clear of the bed.

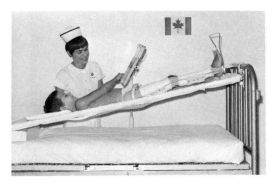

Figure 16.77. Continuous skin traction combined with a Thomas splint slightly bent at the knee for the treatment of an unstable fracture of the mid shaft of the right femur in an 8-year-old boy.

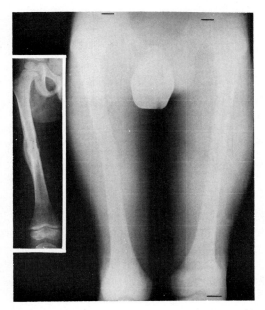

Figure 16.78. Overgrowth of the right femur after a perfectly reduced fracture of the mid-shaft at age 5 years (*inset*). Eight years later the right femur is 1.2 cm longer than the left.

completely corrected since these deformities do not correct spontaneously. For reasons discussed at the beginning of this chapter, temporary overgrowth always occurs after displaced fractures of the femoral shaft. The average amount of overgrowth is 1 cm and any residual discrepancy in length one year after the fracture is permanent (Fig.

16.78). It will be obvious to you therefore that the ideal position in which to allow the fragments to unite is side-to-side (bayonet) apposition with approximately 1 cm of over-riding. This intentional shortening is compensated within one year by the overgrowth as discussed in an earlier section of this chapter (Fig. 16.8).

Remodeling of the healed femoral shaft fracture is remarkable during the growing years; although residual angulation and rotation at the fracture site do not correct spontaneously, side-to-side apposition is beautifully remodeled over a period of years (Fig. 16.79). In adolescents—particularly those with a severe brain injury, or multiple injuries, it may be preferable to deal with the femoral shaft fracture by means of an intramedullary rod.

Complications

The most serious complication of femoral shaft fractures in children is Volkmann's ischemia (compartment syndrome) of nerves and muscles due to femoral arterial spasm; the spasm, which in turn may be secondary to a tear of the intima, is further aggravated by excessive traction on the fractured limb. The clinical manifestations of impending Volkmann's ischemia in the lower limb are the same as those in the upper limb—pain, pallor, puffiness, pulselessness, paresthesia

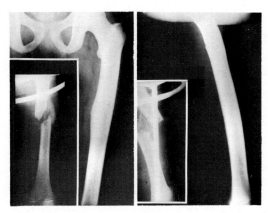

Figure 16.79. Remodeling after a displaced fracture of the femoral shaft at age 6 years (*insets*). Seven years later the fracture deformity has been beautifully remodeled.

and paralysis. Thus, children being treated for a fracture of the femoral shaft should not be given analgesics. A well controlled fracture should not be a source of pain and therefore if the child has severe and constant pain—especially pain in the calf—the most likely cause is impending ischemia; analgesics may mask this important warning signal and for this reason are contraindicated.

The moment impending Volkmann's ischemia is suspected all encircling bandages should be removed immediately; the skin traction should be replaced by skeletal traction through the distal metaphysis of the

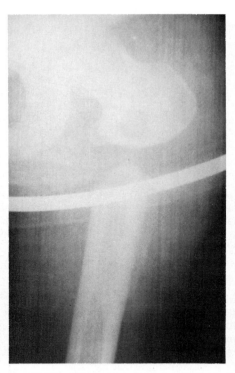

Figure 16.81. Subtrochanteric fracture of the left femur of a 14-year-old girl. Note the ring of the Thomas splint. In this anteroposterior projection the proximal fragment is flexed to 90°; you are looking into its medullary cavity which is represented by the round radiolucent area.

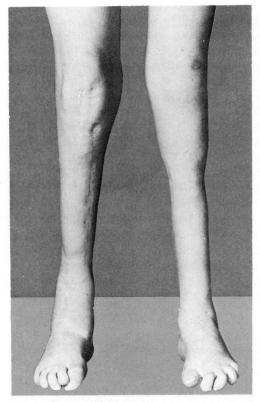

Figure 16.80. Residual Volkmann's ischemic contracture of both lower limbs in a 7-year-old boy who had been treated in overhead (Bryant's) traction for bilateral fractured femora at age 5 years, much beyond the age when overhead traction is safe. During the first 2 days of traction the boy had complained of severe pain in both legs. The ill-advised use of analgesics relieved the pain somewhat and this masked the relentless development of severe Volkmann's ischemia until the nerve and muscle damage was irreversible. This is a preventable tragedy!

femur with the hip and knee flexed. If the peripheral circulation has not been re-established within half an hour, exploration of the artery is indicated as described in Chapter 15 in relation to Volkmann's ischemia. The permanent effects of Volkmann's ischemia and subsequent Volkmann's ischemic contracture are tragic (Fig. 16.80).

FRACTURES OF THE SUBTROCHANTERIC REGION OF THE FEMUR

When the femoral fracture is just distal to the trochanters, the muscles inserted into the proximal fragment, particularly the iliopsoas and the glutei, pull it into a position of acute flexion, external rotation and abduction (Fig. 16.81). Therefore, in order to obtain correct alignment of the fracture fragments, continuous traction must be so arranged as to bring the distal fragment up to and in line

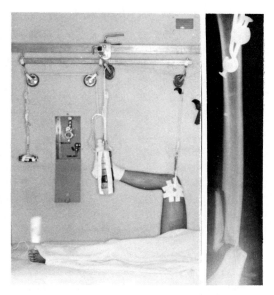

Figure 16.82 (left).   Continuous skeletal traction through a pin in the distal metaphysis for treatment of a subtrochanteric fracture of the femur. The distal fragment is thereby brought into line with the flexed proximal fragment.

Figure 16.83 (right).   Lateral projection of the same fractured femur as shown in Figure 16.81 (inverted). Note the metal pin and stirrup in the region of the distal end of the femur. The distal fragment has been brought into line with the flexed proximal fragment. The comminution was not apparent in the anteroposterior projection.

with the proximal fragment. This is best accomplished by continuous skeletal traction through the distal metaphysis of the femur with the thigh flexed, externally rotated and abducted (Figs. 16.82 and 16.83). The remainder of the treatment is comparable to that for a fracture of the mid-shaft of the femur in a child of the same age.

The Hip and Pelvis

FRACTURES OF THE FEMORAL NECK

The femoral neck in the child, unlike that in the elderly adult, is extremely strong and consequently a severe injury is required to fracture it. Fractures of the femoral neck, therefore, are not common but they are serious; the combination of the severe injury and the precarious blood supply to the femoral head lead, as you might expect, to a high incidence of post-traumatic avascular necrosis. Moreover, as with femoral neck

fractures in adults, they are extremely unstable and cannot be adequately treated either by closed reduction and external immobilization or by continuous traction.

Treatment

Displaced femoral neck fractures in children, therefore, represent an absolute indication for internal skeletal fixation (Fig. 16.84). Since a child cannot be expected to refrain from weight bearing during the healing phase of the fracture, it is necessary to supplement the internal fixation with a hip spica until the fracture is clinically united; this usually requires three months.

Complications

If internal skeletal fixation has not been used, or if it has been inadequate, fractures of the femoral neck in children are likely to be complicated by *non-union* and a progressive coxa vara deformity (Fig. 16.85).

When the femoral head has lost its blood supply by disruption of its vessels at the time of a fracture, the result is *post-traumatic avascular necrosis*, a complication that occurs in approximately 30% of children with this injury. There is little radiographic evidence of this complication until several months have elapsed. The ossific nucleus stops growing for at least six months after the injury and at first appears *relatively* ra-

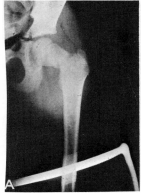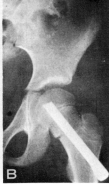

Figure 16.84.   *A*, fractured neck of femur in a 10-year-old boy. Note the ring of the Thomas splint. *B*, after closed reduction and percutaneous nailing, the fragments are in satisfactory position. Three threaded pins would have been equally satisfactory for internal fixation of this fracture.

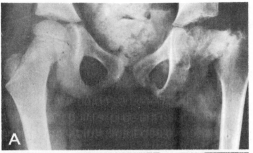

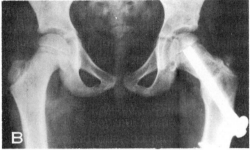

Figure 16.85. *A,* non-union of a fracture of the left femoral neck in a 9-year-old boy. Note the sclerosis at the fracture site and the coxa vara deformity with resultant shortening of the limb. This fracture should have been treated by internal skeletal fixation. *B,* correction of the deformity and union of the fracture were obtained by means of an operation which included bone grafting and the use of a nail and plate.

dio-opaque (relative to the post-traumatic osteoporosis of the living bone in the acetabulum and femoral shaft). Later, when the ossific nucleus is being revascularized and re-ossified, it appears *absolutely* radio-opaque as new bone is laid down on dead trabeculae. Subsequently, the femoral head may become deformed as described in the section on Legg-Perthes' disease in Chapter 13. The treatment of the complication of post-traumatic avascular necrosis of the femoral head in children is the same as that previously described for Legg-Perthes' disease.

TYPE I INJURY OF THE PROXIMAL FEMORAL EPIPHYSIS

This uncommon but serious injury carries the same risk of avascular necrosis of the femoral head and resultant premature closure of the underlying epiphyseal plate as do fractures of the femoral neck and for the

same reasons (Fig. 16.86). Like the femoral neck fracture, a Type I injury of the proximal femoral epiphysis should be treated by internal skeletal fixation, usually with two or more threaded wires; after the injury has healed the threaded wires should be removed to avoid a growth disturbance.

TRAUMATIC DISLOCATION OF THE HIP

The normal hip joint is most vulnerable to dislocation when it is in a position of flexion and adduction. In this position, a force transmitted along the shaft of the femur (as may occur from a dashboard injury or a fall on the flexed knee) may drive the femoral head

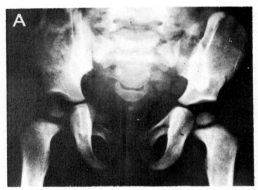

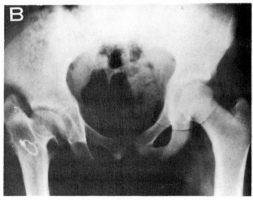

Figure 16.86. Type I injury of the proximal femoral epiphysis in a 1-year-old child who had been struck by a truck. *A,* note the obvious fractures of the pelvis. Less obvious is the increased distance between the proximal femoral epiphysis and metaphysis on the right side indicating a Type I epiphyseal separation. *B,* ten years later there is deformity of the femoral head (coxa plana), marked shortening of the femoral neck and coxa vara. (The wire loop is at the site of a previous osteotomy of the femur.)

posteriorly over the labrum, or lip, of the acetabulum to produce a posterior dislocation. Less force is required to dislocate the hip in a child than in an adult. Since the femoral head escapes through a rent in the capsule, it is an extracapsular type of dislocation.

Diagnosis

The clinical deformity of a posterior dislocation of the hip—flexion, adduction and internal rotation—is characteristic (Fig. 16.87). Traumatic anterior dislocation of the hip is rare in childhood but when it does occur, the hip is held in the opposite position—extension, abduction and external rotation. Posterior dislocation is obvious radiographically (Fig. 16.88).

Treatment

As long as the hip is dislocated, the torn capsule and surrounding structures constrict the femoral neck vessels and thereby jeopardize the blood supply to the femoral head. For this reason traumatic dislocation

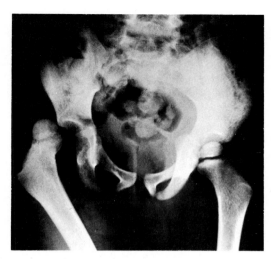

Figure 16.88. Traumatic posterior dislocation of the right hip suffered by the same patient shown in Figure 16.87.

of the hip represents an emergency; the dislocation should be reduced as soon as possible in an attempt to prevent the serious complication of avascular necrosis of the femoral head. Indeed, in children whose hips are reduced within eight hours from the time of injury, the incidence of avascular necrosis is low, whereas in those whose hips have remained unreduced for longer than eight hours, the incidence of this complication is high (approximately 40%).

Closed reduction is accomplished by applying upward traction on the flexed thigh and by forward pressure on the femoral head from behind. After reduction, which must be perfect both clinically and radiographically, a hip spica cast is applied with the hip in its most stable position—extension, abduction and external rotation. Immobilization of the reduced hip is maintained for eight weeks to allow strong healing of the torn capsule.

Complications

The acetabular margin, being largely cartilaginous in children, is seldom fractured and the sciatic nerve is seldom injured. The complication of post-traumatic avascular necrosis of the femoral head has been described above in relation to fractures of the femoral neck.

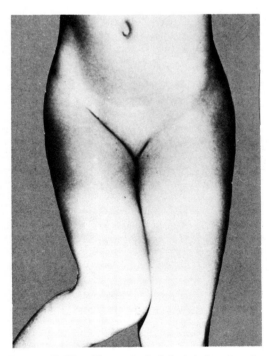

Figure 16.87. The typical clinical deformity of a child with traumatic posterior dislocation of the right hip--flexion, adduction, internal rotation and apparent shortening.

The longer the hip remains dislocated, especially after 12 hours, the higher is the incidence of this complication.

Soft tissue interposition of capsule or labrum in the joint prevents perfect reduction; the residual subluxation leads to degenerative arthritis and consequently, such soft tissue interposition (which is often best detected by computed tomography) should be removed surgically.

Pelvis

The pelvis of a child is more flexible and hence more yielding than that of an adult because of the cartilaginous components at the sacroiliac joints, triradiate cartilages and symphysis pubis. Consequently, serious fractures of the pelvis are not common in childhood although they do occur as the result of a severe injury such as an automobile accident.

The most important aspects of fractures of the pelvis in children are not the fractures themselves but rather the associated complications, extensive internal hemorrhage from torn vessels and extravasation of urine from rupture of the bladder or urethra.

Diagnosis

Physical examination reveals local swelling and tenderness; and in unstable fractures there may also be deformity of the hips as well as instability of the pelvic ring. Special radiographic projections are required to assess the precise nature of a pelvic fracture since the anteroposterior projection provides only a two-dimensional concept of the injury and the lateral projection, which would normally provide the third dimension, is unsatisfactory because of overlap of the two innominate bones. Thus, in order to obtain a three-dimensional concept of the disturbed anatomy of the injury, it is necessary to obtain: (1) an anteroposterior projection; (2) a tangential projection in the plane of the pelvic ring (with the tube directed upward 50°); (3) an inlet projection looking down into the pelvic ring with the tube directed downwards 60°. Computed tomography has proven to be useful in obtaining a three-dimensional appreciation of the precise sites of the fractures and the position of the fragments in the pelvis, including the acetabulum.

Treatment

The *emergency care* of a child with a fractured pelvis centers on the two major complications.

The pelvis is a particularly vascular area and consequently displaced fractures of the pelvis may tear vessels (such as the large superior gluteal artery) with resultant major hemorrhage. Thus a child may lose as much as 60% of his circulating blood volume into the peripelvic and retroperitoneal tissues and hence develop severe hemorrhagic shock. The recognition and treatment of shock have been discussed in Chapter 15.

While the child's shock is being treated, a catheter should be inserted into the bladder to investigate the possibility of associated injury to the bladder or urethra. If there is blood in the urethra and a catheter cannot be passed, the urethra is almost certainly torn. Hence a suprapubic cystotomy must be performed pending surgical repair of the urethra. If the catheter can be passed into the bladder and the urine contains blood, a cystogram should be carried out immediately to determine if the bladder has been ruptured, in which case it should be repaired as soon as possible.

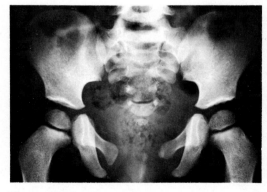

Figure 16.89. Traumatic separation of the symphysis pubis in a 2-year-old child. Both sacroiliac joints have been spread open also. The separation was reduced by internal rotation of both hips and the reduction was maintained in a hip spica cast.

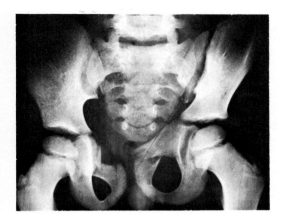

Figure 16.90. "Bucket-handle" type of unstable fracture of the pelvis of a 9-year-old boy who was run over by a truck. Note the vertical fracture just lateral to the left sacroiliac joint and the fractures of the superior pubic rami. The left half of this child's pelvis has been displaced forward and inward. The displacement was reduced by external rotation of the left hip and the reduction was maintained in a hip spica cast.

Since the bone of the pelvis is principally of the cancellous type, and since its blood supply is abundant, fractures of the pelvis unite rapidly. Treatment of the various types of fractures is aimed at correcting significant fracture deformities in order to prevent malunion and resultant disturbance of function.

STABLE FRACTURES OF THE PELVIS

Fractures that do not transgress the pelvic ring do not interfere with stability of the pelvis in relation to weight bearing and hence do not require reduction.

In children, particularly in athletic boys, a sudden violent pull on the hamstring muscles may avulse their origin, the ischial apophysis. This injury usually heals well but may result in a fibrous union.

Isolated fractures of the ilium are of little significance and require only protection from weight bearing until pain subsides within a few weeks.

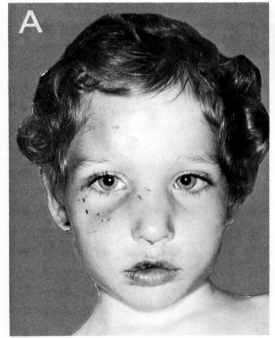
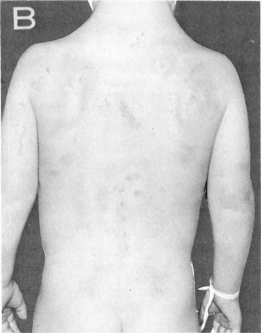

Figure 16.91.   Child abuse. This sad-looking 5-year-old girl was brought to hospital with a history of having "fallen in the garden." Note the bruising and abrasions over the right side of her face. Further examination revealed multiple bruises in various stages of resolution over the girl's trunk and limbs. These physical findings suggest repeated assaults.

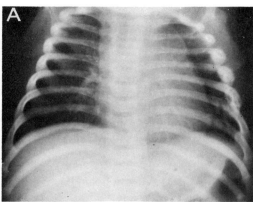

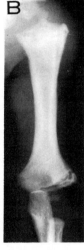
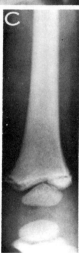

Figure 16.92. Child abuse. A 1-year-old child suspected of being the victim of child abuse. *A*, note the multiple rib fractures on the left side of the chest, some of which are fresh and others of which are partially healed. *B*, note the callus formation in the region of the proximal metaphysis of the humerus as well as the partially healed fracture of the lateral condyle. *C*, a healing epiphyseal plate injury is apparent in the child's femur. These multiple radiographic findings are typical of child abuse.

A "straddle" injury of the pelvis (which may occur as a child loses his footing while walking along the top of a fence) may cause one or more fractures of the inferior pubic rami, but more important is likely to produce a tear of the urethra.

UNSTABLE FRACTURES OF THE PELVIS

Complete separation of the symphysis pubis and opening out of the pelvic ring is best reduced by internally rotating both hips;

the reduction is maintained in a well molded hip spica cast (Fig. 16.89).

Lateral compression of the pelvis may produce a "bucket handle" fracture in which the fractured half of the pelvis rolls forward and inward (Fig. 16.90). In children this type of fracture can usually be managed by externally rotating the lower limb and the reduction can be maintained by the application of a well molded hip spica cast.

Unstable fractures in which one-half of the pelvis is driven proximally by an upward thrust require continuous skeletal traction through the femur to obtain and maintain reduction.

CHILD ABUSE

Distasteful and difficult to understand as it may be, the tragic truth remains that some infants and small children are, in fact, physically abused within their own homes by a disturbed parent or even an older brother or sister. Such *child abuse* tends to be repeated and often results in multiple musculoskeletal injuries, frequently referred to by the sickening synonym "battered baby syndrome," a repulsive, yet realistic term.

Fractures in children under the age of three years are not very common but it has been estimated that 25% of fractures in this age group are caused by child abuse.

Diagnosis

The victim of such pathological behavior may not be brought for medical attention immediately. When the child is brought, the history of injury given by the parents is often evasively vague and may even be deliberately misleading. There is usually something mysterious about the mishap and this should arouse your suspicion.

Physical examination may reveal multiple bruises, often in varying stages of resolution which suggests multiple assaults over a period of time. The child usually has a sad countenance—and for good reason (Fig. 16.91).

Radiographic examination under such circumstances needs to be extensive and should include the skull, chest and all four limbs. Skull fractures, multiple rib fractures and epiphyseal separations in the limbs are the most characteristic skeletal injuries. These multiple injuries may also be in varying stages of healing, an observation that usually indicates repeated assaults (Fig. 16.92).

Treatment

Infants and children suspected of having been physically abused should be admitted to hospital for complete investigation (as well as photographic documentation). The physician or surgeon who suspects child abuse has a moral, and indeed a legal, obligation to report the *suspicion* of such abuse to the local authorities who then proceed with the necessary investigation and action. Records of previous attendance at the hospital should be studied. Indeed, if a central registry of physically abused children is kept in the community, this should also be consulted since the parents may not consistently bring their child to the same hospital, particularly in a large community.

Regrettably, if these protective and preventive steps are not taken, a significant percentage of these helpless and hapless little victims will eventually succumb to multiple injuries—particularly cerebral injuries—that are wittingly and willfully being inflicted upon them.

Suggested Additional Reading

Apley, A. G. and Solomon, L.: *Apley's System of Orthopaedics and Fractures*, 6th ed. London, Butterworth, 1982.

Arino, V. L., Lluck, E. E., Ramirez, A. M., Ferrer, J., Rodriguez, L. and Baixauli, F.: Percutaneous fixation of supracondylar fractures of the humerus in children. J. Bone Joint Surg. 59A: 914–916, 1977.

Baker, R. H., Carroll, N., Dewar, F. P., and Hall, J. E.: The semitendinosus tenodesis for recurrent dislocation of the patella. J. Bone Joint Surg. 54B: 103–109, 1972.

Bassett, C. A. L., Mitchell, S. N. and Gaston, S. R.: Treatment of ununited tibial diaphyseal fractures with pulsing electromagnetic fields. J. Bone Joint Surg. 63A: 511–523, 1981.

Bassett, C. A. L., Valdes, M. G. and Hernandez, E.: Modification of fracture repair with pulsing electromagnetic fields. J. Bone Joint Surg. 64A: 888–895, 1982.

Blount, W. P.: *Fractures in Children*. Baltimore, Williams & Wilkins, 1955.

Briggs, B. T. and Chao, E. Y. S.: The mechanical performance of the standard Hoffmann-Vidal external fixation apparatus. J. Bone Joint Surg. 64A: 566–573, 1982.

Bright, R. W.: Operative correction of partial epiphyseal plate closure by osseous-bridge resection and silicone-rubber implant. An experimental study in dogs. J. Bone Joint Surg. 56A: 655–664, 1974.

Brighton, C. T.: The treatment of non-unions with electricity. Current concepts review. J. Bone Joint Surg. 63A: 847–851, 1981.

Brighton, C. T.: Present and future of electrically induced osteogenesis. In *Clinical Trends in Orthopaedics*, edited by Straub, L. R. and Wilson, P. D. Jr. New York, Thieme-Stratton, 1982.

Brooker, A. F., and Edwards, C. C.: *External Fixation— The Current State of the Art*. Baltimore, Williams & Wilkins, 1979.

Canale, S. T. and Bourland, W. L.: Fracture of the neck and intertrochanteric region of the femur in children. J. Bone Joint Surg. 59A: 431–443, 1977.

Charnley, John: *The Closed Treatment of Common Fractures*, 3rd ed. Edinburgh, Churchill-Livingstone, 1961.

deHaas, W. G., Watson, J. and Morrison, D. M.: Non-invasive treatment of ununited fractures of the tibia using electrical stimulation. J. Bone Joint Surg. 62B: 465–470, 1980.

Edmondson, R. S. and Flowers, M. W.: Intensive care in tetanus: management, complications and mortality in 100 cases. Br. Med. J. 1: 1401–1404, 1979.

Friedenberg, Z. B. and Brighton, C. T.: Bioelectricity and fracture healing. Plast. Reconstr. Surg. 68: 435–443, 1981.

Genant, H. K., Wilson, J. S., Bovill, E. G., Brunelle, F. O., Murray, W. R., and Rodrigo, J. J.: Computed tomography of the musculoskeletal system. J. Bone Joint Surg. 62A: 1088–1101, 1980.

Gossling, H. R. and Donohue, T. A.: Fat embolism syndrome. J.A.M.A. 241: 2740–2742, 1979.

Gozna, E. R., Harrington, I. J. and Evans, D. C.: *Biomechanics of Musculoskeletal Injury*. Baltimore, Williams & Wilkins, 1982.

Gustilo, R. B., and Anderson, J. T.: Prevention of infection in the treatment of one thousand and twenty-five open fractures of long bones. J. Bone Joint Surg. 58A: 453–458, 1976.

Hall, J. E., Micheli, L. J. and McNanama, G. B. Jr.: Semitendinosus tenodesis for recurrent subluxation or dislocation of the patella. Clin. Orthop. 144: 31–35, 1979.

Ham, A. W. and Cormack, D. H.: *Histophysiology of Cartilage, Bones and Joints*. Philadelphia, J. B. Lippincott, 1979.

Harder, J. A., Bobechko, W. P., Sullivan, R. and Daneman, A.: Computerized axial tomography to demonstrate occult fractures of the acetabulum in children. Can. J. Surg. 24: 409–411, 1981.

Helfer, R. E., Hempe, C. H. (Eds.): *The Battered Child*, 2nd ed. Chicago, University of Chicago Press, 1974.

Heppenstall, R. B. (ed.): *Fracture Treatment and Healing*. Philadelphia, W. B. Saunders, 1980.

Holden, C. E. A.: The pathology and prevention of Volkmann's ischemia contracture. J. Bone Joint Surg. 61B: 3: 296–300, 1979.

Jackson, A. D. M.: Wednesday's children: a review of child abuse. J. R. Soc. Med. 75: 83–88, 1982.

Jackson, R. W. and Waddell, J. P.: Hyperbaric oxygen in the management of clostridial myonecrosis (gas gangrene). Clin. Orthop. 96: 271, 1973.

Jacobs, J.: Child abuse (editorial). Can. Med. Assoc. J. 124: 1423–1425, 1981.

Kennedy, J. C. (ed.): *The Injured Adolescent Knee.* Baltimore, Williams & Wilkins, 1979.

Kettlekamp, D. B.: Management of patellar malalignment. Current concepts review. J. Bone Joint Surg. 63A: 1344–1347, 1981.

Kirby, R. M., Winquist, R. A. and Hansen, S. T. Jr.: Femoral Shaft fractures in adolescents: a comparison between traction plus cast treatment and closed intramedullary nailing. J. Pediatr. Orthop. 1: 193–197, 1981.

Langenskiold, A.: Surgical treatment of partial closure of the growth plate. J. Pediatr. Orthop. 1: 3–11, 1981.

Matsen, F. A. III and Veith, R. G.: Compartmental syndromes in children. J. Pediatr. Orthop. 1: 33–41, 1981.

McDonald, G. A.: Pelvic disruptions in children. Clin. Orthop. 151: 13–134, 1980.

Mubarak, S. J. and Carroll, N. C.: Volkmann's contracture in children. J. Bone Joint Surg. 61B: 285–293, 1979.

Mubarak, S. J., Owen, C. A., Hargens, A. R., Garetto, L. P. and Akeson, W. H.: Acute compartment syndromes: diagnosis and treatment with the aid of a wick catheter. J. Bone Joint Surg. 60A: 1091–1095, 1978.

Mustard, W. T. and Bull, C.: A reliable method for relief of traumatic vascular spasm. Ann. Surg. 155: 339–344, 1962.

Offierski, C. M.: Traumatic dislocation of the hip in children. J. Bone Joint Surg. 63B: 194–197, 1981.

Ogden, J. A.: *Skeletal Injury in the Child.* Philadelphia, Lea & Febiger, 1982.

Palmer, E. E., Niemann, K. M. W., Vesley, D. and Armstrong, J. H.: Supracondylar fracture of the humerus in children. J. Bone Joint Surg. 60A: 653–656, 1978.

Paterson, D. C., Lewis, G. N. and Cass, C. A.: Treatment of delayed union and nonunion with an implanted direct current stimulator. Clin. Orthop. 148: 117–128, 1980.

Paul, D. F., Morrey, B. F. and Helms, C. A.: Computerized tomography in orthopaedic surgery. Clin. Orthop. 139: 142–149, 1979.

Peterson, H. A.: Operative correction of post fracture arrest of the epiphyseal plate: Case report with ten-year follow-up. J. Bone Joint Surg. 62A: 1018–1020, 1980.

Rang, M.: *The Growth Plate and Its Disorders.* Edinburgh, E. & S. Livingstone, 1969.

Rang, M.: *Children's Fractures.* 2nd ed. Philadelphia, J. B. Lippincott, 1983.

Ratliff, A. H. C.: Traumatic separation of the upper femoral epiphysis in young children. J. Bone Joint Surg. 50B: 757–770, 1968.

Rorabeck, C. H., Castle, G. S. P., Hardie, R. and Logan, J.: Compartment pressure measurements. An experimental investigation using the slit catheter. J. Trauma 21: 446, 1981.

Rorabeck, C. H. and Macnab, I.: Anterior tibial compartment syndrome complicating fractures of the shaft of the tibia. J. Bone Joint Surg. 58A: 549, 1976.

Salter, R. B. and Best, T.: The pathogenesis and prevention of valgus deformity following fractures of the proximal metaphyseal region of the tibia in children. J. Bone Joint Surg. 55A: 1324, 1973.

Salter, R. B. and Harris, D. J.: The healing of intra-articular fractures with continuous passive motion. In *American Academy of Orthopaedic Surgeons Instructional Course Lectures.* St. Louis, C. V. Mosby, 1979, vol. 28, pp. 102–117.

Salter, R. B. and Harris, W. R.: Injuries involving the epiphyseal plate. J. Bone Joint Surg. 45A: 587–622, 1963.

Salter, R. B. and Zaltz, C.: Anatomic investigations of the mechanism of injury and pathological anatomy of "pulled elbow" in young children. Clin. Orthop. 77: 134–143, 1971.

Sharrard, W. J. W.: *Pediatric Orthopaedics and Fractures*, 2nd ed. Oxford, Blackwell Scientific Publications, 1979.

Siffert, R. S.: Injuries to the growth plate and to the epiphysis. In *American Academy of Orthopaedic Surgeons Instructional Course Lectures.* St. Louis, C. V. Mosby, 1980, vol. 29, pp. 62–78.

Silverman, F. N.: *Problems in pediatric fractures. Semin. Roentgenol. 13: 167–176, 1978.*

Taylor, L. and Newberger, E. H.: Special article: Child abuse in the international year of the child. N. Engl. J. Med. 301: 1205–1212, 1979.

Weber, B. G.: Fibrous interposition causing valgus deformity after fracture of the upper tibial metaphysis in children. J. Bone Joint Surg. 59B: 290–292, 1977.

Weisz, G. M., Rang, M. and Salter, R. B.: Post-traumatic fat embolism in children. J. Trauma 13: 529–534, 1973.

Wilson, J. N. (ed.): *Watson-Jones' Fractures and Joint Injuries*, 5th ed. Edinburgh, Churchill-Livingstone, 1976, vols. 1 and 2.

CHAPTER 17

Specific Fractures and Joint Injuries in Adults

The Care of Athletes
The Care of the Elderly and Their Fractures

Your knowledge and understanding of the *general features* of fractures, dislocations and soft tissue injuries gained from Chapter 15—combined with your own good sense—will enable you to deduce, and therefore anticipate, the appropriate methods of treatment for *specific injuries* in adults.

From Chapter 16 you will have learned about the special features of fractures and dislocations in *children* in comparison with such injuries in adults. The differences between fractures in children and in adults are sufficiently important in your understanding of fracture treatment that they merit further emphasis.

SPECIAL FEATURES OF FRACTURES AND DISLOCATIONS IN ADULTS

The special features of fractures and dislocations in adults are first listed and then discussed individually. These features are relatively constant in both young and middle-aged adults; special problems associated with fractures in the elderly are discussed in a separate section at the end of this chapter.

In the present section the comparative terms such as "more" and "less" refer to a comparison between fractures and dislocations in adults and in children; the following features pertain to adults.

1. Fractures less common but more serious.
2. Weaker and less active periosteum.
3. Less rapid fracture healing.
4. Fewer problems of diagnosis.
5. No spontaneous correction of residual fracture deformities.
6. Differences in complications.
7. Different emphasis on methods of treatment.
8. Torn ligaments and dislocations more common.
9. Better tolerance of major blood loss.

1. Fractures Less Common But More Serious

Buckle fractures and green-stick fractures—which are so common in children—do not occur in adults, and crack, or hairline fractures are relatively uncommon. More force is required to break a bone in the adult and consequently when a fracture does occur it tends to be significantly displaced; furthermore, it is more likely to be complicated. Added to these features are the slower rate of fracture healing and the greater socioeconomic loss due to time away from work and other responsibilities of adulthood.

2. Weaker and Less Active Periosteum

In adults the periosteum is relatively thin and weak; consequently it is readily torn across at the time of a fracture and there is less often an intact periosteal hinge that can be utilized during closed reduction of the fracture. This is particularly true in sites where the bone lies subcutaneously (such as the shaft of the ulna and of the tibia) or where a portion of the bone (such as the neck of the femur) lies within a synovial joint. Furthermore, the periosteum is much less osteogenic in adults than in children and this important biological factor accounts largely for the less rapid fracture healing in adults.

3. Less Rapid Fracture Healing

Throughout adult life the rate of normal fracture healing in a given bone is relatively constant—but always considerably slower than during childhood. Fractures of the shaft of the femur serve as an example; a femoral shaft fracture occurring at birth will be united in 3 weeks; a comparable fracture at the age of 8 years will be united in 8 weeks; at the age of 12 years it will be united in 12 weeks; and from the age of 20 years to old age it will be united in approximately 20 weeks.

Related to the slower rate of union of fractures in adults is the higher incidence of delayed union and non-union. Thus, in adults, fracture healing is not only slower than in children, it is also less certain.

4. Fewer Problems of Diagnosis

Since in adults there are no separate centers of ossification and all epiphyseal plates have closed, there are fewer problems of radiographic diagnosis of fractures than in children. Nevertheless, at least two radiographic projections at right angles to each other are just as important in the diagnosis of fractures in adults as in children.

5. No Spontaneous Correction of Residual Fracture Deformities

In adults, the deformity of a mal-united fracture is permanent since residual angulation, shortening or rotation at the site of a healed fracture cannot correct spontaneously. The process of remodeling in the shaft of a long bone can still occur in the adult, albeit more slowly and less completely than in the child. Consequently, the sharp corners of an incompletely reduced shaft fracture gradually become smooth through the process of remodeling—an example of Wolff's law. Nevertheless, residual angulation, shortening and rotation persist; therefore, in adults, these deformities must be adequately corrected during the initial treatment of the fracture.

6. Differences in Complications

Most of the complications discussed in Chapter 15 can develop in both children and adults but certain differences merit consideration. Open fractures are more common in adults as are major arterial injuries, gangrene, venous thrombosis, pulmonary embolism, fat embolism, pneumonia and renal calculi. Delirium tremens and accident neurosis are virtually confined to adult life. Persistent joint stiffness after fracture is a much more common complication in adults than in children and its prevention requires vigorous measures throughout the period of fracture treatment and after care. [We are currently conducting prospective investigations concerning the clinical application of the new concept of *continuous passive motion* (CPM) to the immediate post-operative care of patients following open reduction and internal fixation of intra-articular fractures and also following ligament reconstruction.] As mentioned above, delayed union and non-union are also more common in adults than in children. The complication of growth disturbance, of course, does not occur during adult life.

7. Different Emphasis on Methods of Treatment

Although the *principles* of fracture treatment described in Chapter 15 are equally applicable to children and adults, there is a different emphasis on the *methods* of treatment in the two age groups. Adults tend to be more reliably cooperative during treatment and consequently their undisplaced and impacted fractures can be more reasonably treated by protection alone than can such fractures in children. By contrast, displaced and unstable fractures (particularly of the forearm bones and femur) in adults frequently require open reduction and internal fixation, whereas virtually all such long bone fractures in children can and should be treated by closed means. In an elderly person who has sustained a severely displaced fracture of the neck of the femur with disruption of blood supply to the femoral head, the most reasonable initial method of treatment may be excision of the femoral head and neck fragment and replacement by an endoprosthesis; this method of treatment, of course, would not be indicated for any type of fracture in a child.

In recent years there has been increasing use of three specific methods of fracture treatment in adults, namely functional fracture-bracing, external skeletal fixation and the AO/ASIF, or AO, system of rigid internal fixation. Before proceeding further in this chapter you may wish to review the discussions of these three methods in Chapter 15.

8. Torn Ligaments and Dislocations More Common

Ligaments and fibrous joint capsules are less resilient in adults than in children; consequently they are more often either completely torn across or avulsed with a small fragment of attached bone. Moreover, the type of injury that produces a separation of an epiphysis through its epiphyseal plate in a child is likely to produce a dislocation, or even a fracture-dislocation, in an adult. These observations account for the increased incidence of major ligamentous tears and dislocations in adults.

9. Better Tolerance of Major Blood Loss

Hemorrhage of 500 ml in a child who weighs 20 kg (44 lb) represents 33% of the total blood volume, whereas a similar hemorrhage in an average adult would represent only 10% of the total blood volume. It must be remembered, however, that the elderly do not tolerate major blood loss as well as young and middle-aged adults.

SPECIFIC FRACTURES AND DISLOCATIONS
The Hand
GENERAL FEATURES

Fractures and dislocations in the hand are not only common in adults but also poten-tially serious. Such injuries are often considered to be minor and consequently are treated with indifference; these important injuries, however, should always be treated with deference rather than with indifference in order to prevent permanent disability.

Hand function is closely related to anatomical form—especially in the fingers and thumb—and because of the close relationship of gliding tendons to bones, fractures involving the phalanges in particular must be accurately reduced; there is but a small margin of tolerable imperfection in the treatment of hand injuries.

The injured hand is prone to become grossly swollen and, since the damaging effects of persistent edema are particularly disabling in the fingers and thumb, the injured hand must always be kept elevated to prevent this complication. Fractured digits should be immobilized for as short a time as possible and almost never more than three weeks lest adhesions produce a permanent loss of joint motion. In general, fingers should be immobilized in the flexed position of function—and *never* in an extended position as on a straight splint. After the period of immobilization the patient should actively exercise his fingers—if necessary under supervision. Fingers should *never* be passively manipulated since manipulation of such small joints usually produces an excessive reaction and leads to permanent stiffness of the injured finger.

PHALANGES
Distal Phalanx

Crush injuries of the distal phalanx are common, particularly in industry; they are also frequently caused by the finger tip being caught in a closing door. Since the finger tips have such highly developed sensation, crush injuries are particularly painful. The fracture of the distal phalanx is usually comminuted and the soft tissues are infiltrated by an enlarging hematoma in a relatively closed space. Indeed, a tense subungual hematoma may require decompression through a small drill hole in the nail for relief of pain. Treatment of the fracture is of secondary importance to treatment of the injured soft tissues. A simple aluminum splint serves to protect the crushed finger tip from further injury during the healing phase.

Mallet Finger ("Baseball Finger," "Cricket Finger")

Sudden, unexpected passive flexion of the distal interphalangeal joint with the extensor tendon under tension may avulse a fragment of bone from the base of the distal phalanx into which the tendon is inserted. Alternatively, the extensor tendon may rupture just proximal to its insertion. In either case, the distal interphalangeal joint remains flexed and can no longer be actively extended—the typical mallet finger deformity (Fig. 17.1). Treatment of the acute injury consists of splinting the finger in a molded plaster cast with the distal interphalangeal joint extended and the proximal interphalangeal joint flexed (the position in which there is least tension on the extensor tendon). Immobilization is continued for three weeks. Since healed bone is stronger than healed tendon, the results are more satisfactory when a fragment of bone has been avulsed than when the tendon ruptures. If the bony fragment is sufficiently large that it includes a significant part of the joint surface, open reduction and fine wire fixation of the avulsion fracture are indicated.

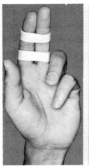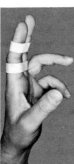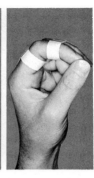

Figure 17.2. Adhesive strapping for an undisplaced fracture of the proximal phalanx of the index finger. The adjacent uninjured finger serves as a splint and the two fingers are free to move together as a unit.

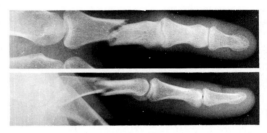

Figure 17.3. Displaced and unstable fracture of the proximal phalanx of the index finger of a working man. The alignment is satisfactory.

Middle and Proximal Phalanges

Most fractures of the middle and proximal phalanges are the result of either crushing or hyperextension injuries. Because of the close relationship of the fracture to the flexor tendons, accurate skeletal alignment is essential.

Undisplaced phalangeal fractures are usually stable because of the relatively intact periosteal tube. They are best treated by strapping the injured finger to an adjacent finger—the "buddy system"—which protects the fractured phalanx and yet allows movement of the finger joints (Fig. 17.2).

Displaced phalangeal fractures tend to be unstable (Fig. 17.3). There is frequently anterior angulation at the fracture site. After closed manipulation (using the principle of the intact periosteal hinge) the reduction can usually be maintained by means of a padded malleable aluminum splint that extends

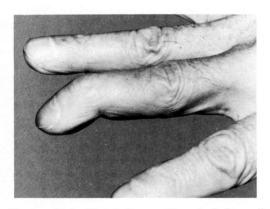

Figure 17.1 Mallet finger ("baseball finger," "cricket finger"). The distal interphalangeal joint of this man's right middle finger was suddenly forced into acute flexion as he miscaught a ball. A small fragment of the insertion of the long extensor tendon into the base of the distal phalanx was avulsed so that he lost active extension of the joint. The resultant deformity bears some resemblance to a mallet.

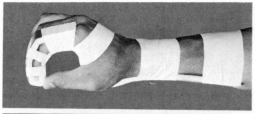

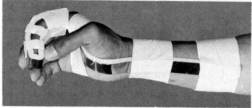

Figure 17.4. Padded malleable aluminum splint taped to the injured finger and forearm. The splint immobilizes the wrist as well as the finger in the position of function and thereby reduces tension on the long flexor and extensor tendons.

above the wrist (Fig. 17.4). Unstable oblique fractures that tend to slip with simple immobilization require either continuous traction through the finger tip (with the finger held in flexion by a cast) or, preferably, open reduction of the fracture and internal fixation with fine Kirschner wires.

Intra-articular phalangeal fractures involve the joint surface and, if displaced, should be treated by open reduction and internal fixation either fine Kirschner wires or tiny AO screws.

SPRAINS AND DISLOCATIONS OF THE INTERPHALANGEAL JOINTS

A sudden abduction or adduction injury to a finger may either partially or completely tear a collateral ligament. If the ligamentous tear is *incomplete*, the finger is painful and swollen but the injured joint is stable. The sprained finger should be immobilized in flexion by means of a malleable aluminum splint for three weeks.

Lateral or medial dislocation of the interphalangeal joint indicates a *complete* tear of the collateral ligament. The dislocation is readily reduced by traction and indeed this is often performed either by the patient or another person immediately after the injury. It is likely that some so-called sprains of interphalangeal joints have been associated

with a momentary subluxation or dislocation in which case there has been a complete tear of a collateral ligament. After reduction of a dislocated interphalangeal joint, the finger should be immobilized in the flexed position for three weeks.

Recovery of a full range of painless motion is notoriously slow after dislocation of an interphalangeal joint and may take as long as six months or even a year. With persistent active exercises, however, full function is eventually regained; in the meantime the patient requires reassurance and encouragement.

DISLOCATION OF THE METACARPOPHALANGEAL JOINTS

A metacarpophalangeal joint is usually dislocated by a severe hyperextension injury. The metacarpal head is driven through a rent in the anterior capsule of the joint and comes to lie immediately under the skin of the palmar surface (Fig. 17.5). Closed reduc-

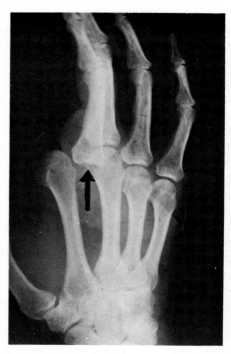

Figure 17.5. Posterior dislocation of the metacarpophalangeal joint of the right index finger. The head of the metacarpal was easily palpable immediately under the skin of the palmar surface. Closed reduction was possible in this particular patient.

tion may be possible by a combination of hyperextension of the joint followed by traction. Sometimes, however, closed reduction is impossible because of the "button hole" effect of a relatively small tear in the capsule, the edges of which grip the metacarpal neck tightly and do not permit the metacarpal head to be reduced. Under these circumstances open reduction becomes necessary. After reduction the metacarpophalangeal joint is immobilized in a position of flexion for three weeks.

METACARPALS

The metacarpal bones (with the exception of the first metacarpal) are closely bound to one another and consequently, isolated fractures of the metacarpals tend to be stable. Furthermore, since the metacarpals are covered to a large extent by muscle, they have a good blood supply and consequently, metacarpal fractures usually heal rapidly. Undisplaced fractures of a metacarpal require only protection from further injury for a period of three weeks (Fig. 17.6).

Fracture of the Neck of the Fifth Metacarpal

Sometimes referred to as a "boxer's fracture," this injury is more appropriately considered a "street fighter's fracture" since it results from an unskillful blow with the clenched fist (a boxer punches with the second and third metacarpals rather than with the more mobile fifth metacarpal). There is characteristic depression of the metacarpal head and posterior angulation at the fracture site (Fig. 17.7). Reduction can be accomplished by flexing the metacarpophalangeal joint and the proximal interphalangeal joint to a right angle and then pushing the metacarpal head back into position by means of pressure along the long axis of the proximal phalanx. The reduced fracture should be

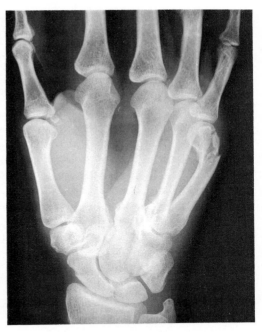

Figure 17.7. Angulated fracture of the neck of the right fifth metacarpal ("street-fighter's fracture") in a man who had become engaged in a brawl with more vigor than skill.

immobilized with the finger in this position in a padded plaster cast but never for longer than two weeks for fear of a flexion contracture of the finger. If the fracture is unstable, the distal fragment can be transfixed by a transverse percutaneous Kirschner wire to the fourth and third metacarpals, the protruding portion of the wire being incorporated in a below-elbow cast.

Fracture of Multiple Metacarpals

Severe crushing injuries of the hand may produce multiple metacarpal fractures with resultant instability. Such fractures are best stabilized by means of longitudinal intramedullary Kirschner wires.

FRACTURE-DISLOCATION OF THE FIRST CARPOMETACARPAL JOINT (BENNETT'S FRACTURE)

In adults a longitudinal force along the axis of the first metacarpal with the thumb flexed may produce a serious intra-articular fracture-dislocation of the carpometacarpal joint. A small triangular-shaped fragment of the base of the metacarpal remains in proper

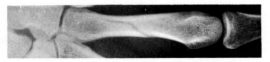

Figure 17.6. Undisplaced fracture of a metacarpal. No immobilization was required.

relationship with the trapezium but the remainder of the metacarpal, which carries with it the major portion of the joint surface, is dislocated and assumes a position of flexion (Fig. 17.8). Clinically, there is marked local swelling, tenderness and reluctance to use the thumb.

Closed reduction, though not easy, is usually possible, provided the first metacarpal is extended and the below-elbow cast is carefully molded to press the base of the metacarpal inward and the head of the metacarpal outward. If the reduction cannot be maintained in a cast, continuous tape traction on the thumb may have to be added, the traction being attached to an outrigger

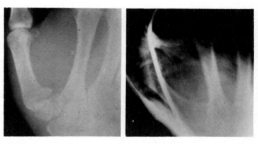

Figure 17.9. Fracture-dislocation of the first carpometacarpal joint (Bennett's fracture). *Left*, initial radiograph. *Right*, post-reduction radiograph. The first metacarpal has been extended at the carpometacarpal joint. The wire seen in this radiograph is part of an outrigger to which traction was applied. Careful molding of the cast, however, is more important than traction.

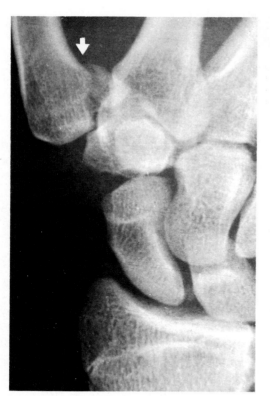

Figure 17.8. Fracture-dislocation of the first carpometacarpal joint (Bennett's fracture) in the hand of a young man who fell on his hand with the thumb flexed. Note the oblique intra-articular fracture line (*arrow*), the small triangular fragment which has remained in its normal relationship with the joint, and the dislocation of the main portion of the first metacarpal which is in a position of flexion.

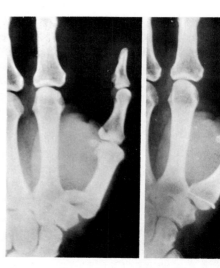

Figure 17.10. Fracture-dislocation of the first carpometacarpal joint (Bennett's fracture). *Left*, initial radiograph showing considerable displacement of the first metacarpal. The small triangular-shaped fragment has remained in proper relationship with the joint. *Right*, after open reduction and internal fixation with a wire loop.

loop which is incorporated into the cast (Fig. 17.9). Occasionally the fracture-dislocation is so unstable that open reduction and internal fixation with either a Kirschner wire or a wire loop are indicated (Fig. 17.10). Residual incongruity of the first carpometacarpal joint may lead to post-traumatic degenerative joint disease but this complication is seldom disabling.

FRACTURES OF THE SCAPHOID

Fractures of the carpal scaphoid are relatively common in young adults, particularly in males. The responsible injury is usually a fall on the open hand with the wrist dorsiflexed and radially deviated. The scaphoid, which spans the joint line between the proximal and distal rows of carpals, bears the brunt of injury at this level.

No other fracture in adults is more frequently overlooked at the time of injury than a fracture of the scaphoid. Sometimes the patient dismisses the injury as a "sprain"—an uncommon injury at the wrist—and does not seek medical attention. Occasionally the physician or surgeon makes the same error but more often radiographs are obtained and the error lies in the interpretation of the radiographs. Fractures of the scaphoid are potentially serious in that they have a high incidence of complications and hence, accurate diagnosis is most important.

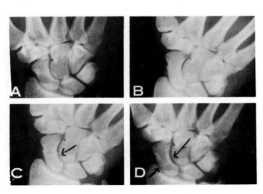

Figure 17.11. Undisplaced fracture of the scaphoid in a young man who thought he had "sprained" his wrist. *A*, two days after injury. There is no radiographic evidence of fracture. *B*, eight days after injury there is still no evidence of fracture. *C*, twelve days after injury a small crack fracture is visible through the waist of the scaphoid (*arrow*). *D*, ten weeks after injury the fracture has healed as indicated by the thin line of increased radiographic density (*arrows*). This series of radiographs emphasizes the importance of obtaining radiographs one week and, if necessary, two weeks after a wrist injury if there is clinical suspicion of a fractured scaphoid. The hairline fracture becomes more apparent after a week or so, partly because of slight resorption of bone at the fracture site and partly because of slight separation of the fragments.

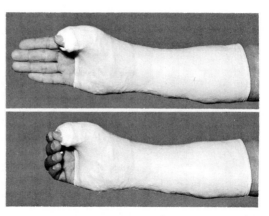

Figure 17.12. Plaster cast for treatment of a fractured scaphoid. The cast immobilizes all joints of the thumb but in a functional position so that it can be opposed by the index and middle fingers. The cast should be close-fitting and well molded.

Clinical Features

The patient experiences pain on the radial side of the wrist, particularly on dorsiflexion and radial deviation. There is usually only slight swelling but marked local tenderness in the region of the anatomical "snuff box."

Radiographic Features

The scaphoid is not clearly outlined in anteroposterior projections of the wrist and requires special oblique projections. An undisplaced fracture of the scaphoid may not be apparent in the initial radiographs but becomes apparent after a week or more (Fig. 17.11).

Treatment

Since isolated fractures of the scaphoid are relatively undisplaced, no reduction is required; but the fragments should be immobilized in a below-elbow cast that incorporates all joints of the thumb (Fig. 17.12). Such treatment should be initiated on the basis of a clinical diagnosis even in the absence of initial radiographic confirmation of a fracture. The scaphoid has no muscle attachments and is covered to a large extent by articular cartilage. Consequently, its blood supply is precarious and fracture union may be seriously impaired. Furthermore, the relative absence of periosteum places the burden of fracture healing on endosteal callus formation. For these reasons, healing of a fractured scaphoid is characteristically slow, requiring at least three months and often much longer.

Complications

For reasons already mentioned, fractures of the scaphoid are prone to become complicated by *avascular necrosis*, *delayed union*, *non-union* and *post-traumatic degenerative joint disease*.

Avascular necrosis of the proximal pole of the scaphoid complicates approximately one-third of transverse fractures. The avascular fragment exhibits a relative radiographic density between two and three months after injury since it does not share in the disuse osteoporosis of the surrounding vascular bones (Fig. 17.13). This complication may also lead to non-union. Since revascularization of the proximal pole is exceedingly slow in adults and almost invariably results in degenerative joint disease of the wrist, painful established avascular necrosis may be treated by excision of the necrotic fragment, or, if necessary, by arthrodesis of the wrist.

Delayed union can be assumed if the fracture has not united within four months; it is an indication for an inlay bone graft.

Non-union is a relatively common complication. Indeed, some patients seek medical attention after a recent injury (but many

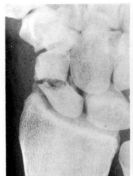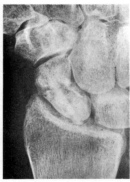

Figure 17.14. Non-union of a fractured scaphoid. *Left*, nine months after the initial injury. Note the sclerosis at the fracture line and also the cyst formation in the proximal fragment. *Right*, the same man's scaphoid three months after bone grafting. The fracture has united and the bone graft is well incorporated.

months after a previously undiagnosed injury) and are found to have an established non-union that was merely aggravated by the recent injury. Thus, the symptoms of a non-union of the scaphoid may be minimal. Radiographically, the unhealed fracture line is obvious and in addition there may be cyst formation at the fracture site and sclerosis of the fracture surfaces (Fig. 17.14A). If the non-union is causing symptoms and is not of more than a year's duration, inlay bone grafting is indicated with or without excision of the adjacent radial styloid (Fig. 17.14B).

Degenerative joint disease usually supervenes one year or more after either avascular necrosis of the proximal pole or non-union of the fracture. The arthritic changes involve not only the radiocarpal joint but also the intercarpal joints and thus, if the associated pain is disabling, arthrodesis of the wrist is justified.

DISLOCATION OF THE LUNATE

Anterior dislocation of the lunate is an uncommon but serious injury that may escape detection. Occurring as the result of a fall on the completely dorsiflexed wrist, the lunate is squeezed out of place toward the palmar surface where it comes to lie—rotated through 90°—in the floor of the carpal tunnel.

Clinically, the wrist is swollen and the

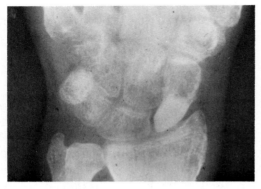

Figure 17.13. Avascular necrosis of the proximal pole of the scaphoid three months after a fracture. The proximal pole is radiographically dense in relation to the surrounding bone because being avascular it has not shared the disuse osteoporosis of immobilization.

patient experiences pain on attempting to extend the fingers. There may be evidence of a median nerve lesion from compression within the carpal tunnel. Radiographic examination of the wrist requires two projections; the diagnosis is much more obvious in the lateral projection (Fig. 17.15).

Treatment of a recent anterior dislocation consists of strong traction on the hand and direct pressure over the lunate; occasionally,

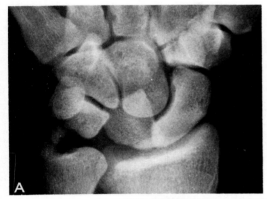
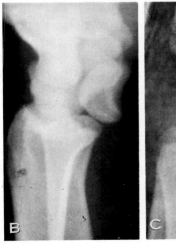
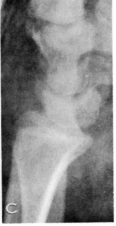

Figure 17.15. Anterior dislocation of the lunate. *A*, the anteroposterior radiograph reveals that the joint surfaces of the lunate are not congruous with those of the adjacent carpal bones and this always indicates a dislocation. The displacement, however, is not striking. *B*, in the lateral radiograph, dislocation of the lunate is obvious. The lunate has been rotated forward through 90°. *C*, post-reduction radiograph revealing that the lunate has been restored to its normal relationship to the distal end of the radius as well as to the carpal bones.

open reduction is required to replace the lunate to its normal position in the carpus. For late unrecognized dislocations, excision of the lunate may be required.

Complications include *median nerve compression* (which usually recovers completely after reduction of the lunate) and *avascular necrosis* of the lunate (similar to Kienbock's disease, which is discussed in Chapter 13). *Degenerative joint disease* of the wrist is a common sequel to avascular necrosis of the lunate and may even necessitate arthrodesis of the wrist.

Other less common injuries of the wrist include *perilunar dislocation of the carpus* in which the lunate remains in its normal relationship with the distal end of the radius but the rest of the carpus is dislocated posteriorly in relation to the lunate. A variant of this injury, *transcaphoid perilunar dislocation*, is associated with a transverse fracture of the scaphoid.

The Wrist and Forearm

DISTAL END OF THE RADIUS (COLLES' FRACTURE)

A fracture through the flared-out distal metaphysis of the radius—the Colles' fracture—is the commonest fracture in adults over the age of 50 years and occurs more frequently in women than in men. Thus, this fracture has the same age and sex incidence as fractures of the neck of the femur and for the same reason; both fractures occur through bone that has become markedly weakened by a combination of senile and post-menopausal osteoporosis.

The incidence of Colles' fracture is particularly high when walking conditions are slippery since the typical mechanism of injury is as follows: the patient either slips or trips, and in an attempt to break her fall, lands on her open hand with the forearm pronated and breaks her wrist. The forces that fracture the distal end of the radius therefore, involve not only dorsiflexion and radial deviation but also supination, all of which accounts for the typical fracture deformity.

The fracture pattern is relatively constant,

the main fracture line being transverse within the distal 2 cm of the radius. There may be only two major fragments but comminution of the thin cortex is common—especially in the osteoporotic bone of the elderly. The ulnar styloid is frequently avulsed. The distal end of an intact radius extends beyond the distal end of the ulna and the joint surface is angulated 15° toward the anterior (palmar) aspect of the wrist. After a Colles' fracture these relationships are reversed and there is always some degree of subluxation of the distal radioulnar joint.

Clinical Features

The clinical deformity—frequently referred to as a "dinner fork deformity"—is typical; in addition to swelling there is an obvious jog just proximal to the wrist due to the posterior displacement and posterior tilt of the distal radial fragment (Fig. 17.16). The

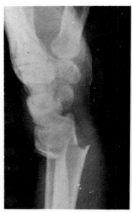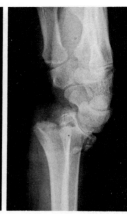

Figure 17.17. (*left*).   Lateral radiograph of a *stable* type of Colles' fracture. There is little comminution.

Figure 17.18. (*right*).   Lateral radiograph of an *unstable* type of Colles' fracture. There is gross comminution, particularly of the dorsal cortex, and also marked crushing of the cancellous bone.

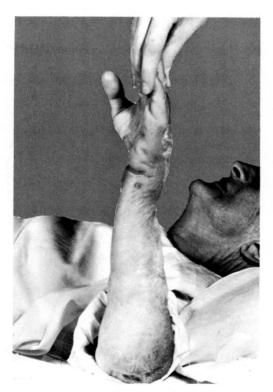

Figure 17.16.   Typical clinical deformity ("dinner fork deformity") of a displaced fracture of the distal end of the radius (Colles' fracture) in an elderly woman. Note the jog just proximal to the wrist.

hand tends to be radially deviated and though often less obvious clinically, the wrist appears supinated in relation to the forearm.

Radiographic Features

Two main types of Colles' fracture can be differentiated radiographically. In the *stable type* there is one main transverse fracture line with little cortical comminution (Fig. 17.17). In the *unstable type* there is gross comminution, particularly of the dorsal cortex, and also marked crushing of the cancellous bone (Fig. 17.18). The intact periosteal hinge is on the dorsal aspect of the fracture in both types.

Treatment

Undisplaced Colles' fractures (which are uncommon) require only immobilization in a below elbow cast for four weeks. *Displaced* fractures can usually be well reduced by closed manipulation, but the major problem is maintenance of reduction—particularly in the unstable type of Colles' fracture. In this type, with comminution of the dorsal cortex and crushing of the cancellous bone, the reduced fracture tends to slip back toward the pre-reduction position of deformity. The blood supply to bone at the distal end of the radius is excellent and consequently, bony union is assured; the main problem is not union but *mal-union*.

Satisfactory analgesia for reduction of a Colles' fracture can be obtained by infiltration of the fracture hematoma with a local anesthetic agent since muscle relaxation is not required. General anesthesia is preferred by some surgeons but carries a somewhat higher risk, especially for the elderly patient.

Closed reduction is obtained by utilizing the principle of the intact periosteal hinge described in Chapter 15 (Fig. 15.36). The fracture deformity is first increased to disimpact the fragments and to slacken the intact periosteal hinge on the dorsal surface, after which the distal fragment is moved distally to engage the proximal fragment; at this point—and not before—the dorsal displacement is corrected by pushing the distal fragment forward, the angulation is straightened, the radial deviation is corrected by placing the hand in marked ulnar deviation and the supination deformity is corrected by placing the forearm in full pronation. These maneuvers bring the distal radius out to length, tighten the intact periosteal hinge and thereby help to maintain the reduction.

The plaster cast that is then applied must hold the reduced position of the fracture, just as the surgeon's hands do at the end of the reduction (Figs. 17.19 and 17.20). Thus, the cast—whether it be of the fully encircling type or of the three-quarters slab type held by bandages—must be carefully molded (rather than tight and constricting) to maintain the reduction. The thumb and fingers must be left free to move. Usually the cast extends only to the elbow, but if the fracture is very unstable, the elbow should be included in the cast—at least for the first three weeks—to maintain the forearm in complete pronation. Repeat radiographs are obtained one and two weeks after reduction since it is during this period that the fracture may slip into an unsatisfactory position; moreover, up to the end of two weeks the fracture is sufficiently mobile that the position can still be improved, if necessary, by remanipulation. Immobilization is continued for a total of six weeks.

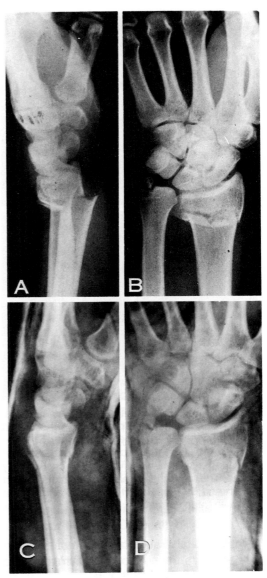

Figure 17.19. Stable type of Colles' fracture. *A* and *B*, initial radiographs. There is little comminution. *C* and *D*, post-reduction radiographs. Note that the radius is out to length and that the tilt of the distal fragment has been corrected. Did you also notice the fracture through the styloid process of the ulna?

Sarmiento recommends immobilizing the reduced Colles' fracture in supination and the subsequent use of functional fracture-bracing.

For extremely comminuted and hence extremely unstable Colles' fractures, particularly in persons under 60 years of age, ex-

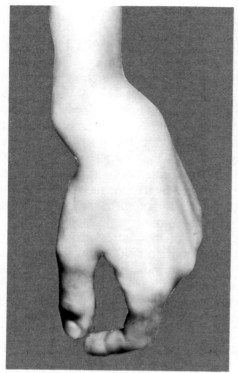

Figure 17.22. Typical clinical deformity of a severe fracture of the shaft of the radius and dislocation of the distal radioulnar joint (Galeazzi fracture-dislocation) in a 35-year-old man. The deformity is more proximal with this injury than it is with a Colles' fracture.

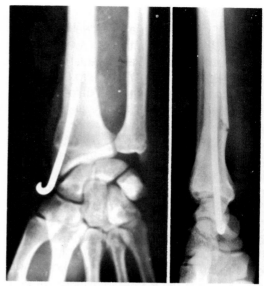

Figure 17.24. Post-reduction radiographs of the same patient illustrated in Figures 17.22 and 17.23. The radial fracture has been completely reduced and has been immobilized with a Rush intramedullary nail. A compression-type plate and screws are just as satisfactory in the treatment of this fracture and are sometimes easier to apply from a technical point of view. Note that the dislocation of the inferior radioulnar joint has also been reduced.

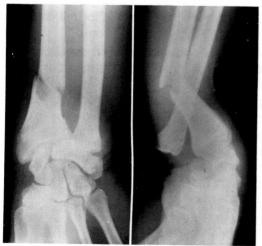

Figure 17.23. Fracture of the shaft of the radius and dislocation of the distal radioulnar joint (Galeazzi fracture-dislocation) in the patient whose clinical deformity is shown in Figure 17.22. Note that the nature of the injury is much more obvious in the lateral projection than in the anteroposterior projection.

dislocation of the distal radioulnar joint (Fig. 17.24).

Isolated Fractures of the Proximal Two-Thirds of the Radial Shaft

When the radial shaft is fractured in its upper two-thirds, the fragments tend to override and rotate. As a result of the shortening of the radius there is, of course, some degree of subluxation at the distal radioulnar joint. Isolated fractures of the radial shaft are difficult to reduce by closed means and reduction, if obtained, is difficult to maintain.

The most suitable form of treatment is open reduction of the radius and internal fixation with either an AO compression plate and screws or an intermedullary nail (Fig. 17.25).

Complications include *delayed union* and even *non-union*. *Mal-union* is a significant complication and usually involves a rotational deformity at the fracture site. If, for example, there is a 40° external rotational deformity (supination deformity) at the fracture site at the time of healing, the patient will have at least 40° loss of pronation of the forearm (Fig. 17.26).

Fractures of the Radius and Ulna

For reasons already mentioned, fractures of both bones of the forearm in adults are more difficult to treat than comparable fractures in children. Usually the result of a severe injury, these fractures are most commonly sustained by young and middle-aged adults. A direct injury usually produces transverse fractures at the same level (most frequently in the middle third) whereas an indirect injury, which almost always involves rotation, tends to produce oblique or spiral fractures at different levels. Because of the relationship between the paired radius and ulna during supination and pronation, both fractures must be perfectly reduced in relation to alignment and rotation.

Closed reduction of both fractures *may* be possible using traction and varying degrees of pronation or supination depending on the deformity. In general, fractures of the distal third are most stable in pronation, those in the middle third are most stable in the mid-position and those in the proximal third are most stable in supination. The explanation for this generalization lies in the level of the fracture of the radius in relation to the insertion of the various muscles that normally pronate or supinate it. Even if ac-

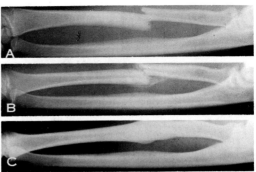

Figure 17.26. Fracture of the shaft of the radius in an adolescent boy. *A*, initial radiographs reveal that the distal fragment at the fracture site is broader than the proximal fragment and this indicates a rotation deformity. There is also loss of the normal bowing of the radial shaft. This fracture was left unreduced and was immobilized in an above-elbow plaster. *B*, six weeks later the radiograph reveals adequate callus formation. It was reported at the time of this radiograph that the fracture was clinically united. *C*, six months later the radiograph reveal consolidation of the fracture. Nevertheless, the rotational deformity has persisted and at this stage the patient was unable to pronate his forearm beyond the mid-position. Supination was only slightly limited. This patient would have been better treated by open reduction and internal fixation of the fracture in order to prevent mal-union.

curate closed reduction can be obtained, however, fractures of both bones of the forearm are unstable and tend to redisplace despite a carefully molded above-elbow cast.

Nevertheless, Sarmiento recommends treating fractures of both bones of the forearm by functional fracture-bracing (after 3 to 6 weeks in an above-elbow cast) and has found that the position of supination is satisfactory regardless of the level of the fractures.

Open reduction is usually required for fractures of both bones of the forearm in adults, either as primary treatment or as secondary treatment after failure of closed reduction. The radius and ulna should be approached through separate incisions to minimize the risk of *cross-union* between the two bones. The most effective form of internal fixation for these fractures is an AO compression plate and screws (Fig. 17.27). The radius usually heals more rapidly than

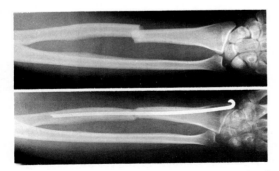

Figure 17.25. Isolated fracture of the shaft of the radius in a 25-year-old man. *Top*, initial radiograph revealing a transverse fracture with overriding of the fragments and consequent shortening of the radius. *Bottom*, the same patient's forearm four months after open reduction and intramedullary nailing with a Rush nail. The fracture has united satisfactorily.

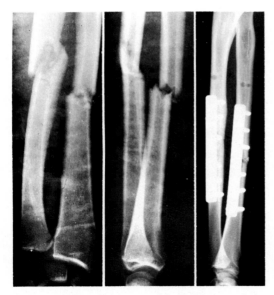

Figure 17.27. Fracture of both bones of the forearm in a 20-year-old man. *Left* and *center*, initial radiographs revealing displacement. *Right*, postoperative radiograph. Both fractures were dealt with by open reduction and the application of AO compression plates and screws. Rigid fixation of the fractures was obtained at the time of operation and union progressed satisfactorily.

the ulna but both fractures must be immobilized for at least three months.

Complications include *delayed union* and even *non-union* (especially in the ulna). In either case, autogenous cancellous bone grafting is indicated. Any residual deformity of angulation or rotation should be corrected at the same time, and under these circumstances a cortical onlay bone graft and screws may also be required. If *cross-union* develops between the radius and ulna (due to communication between the two fracture hematomata) there is a complete bony block to supination and pronation. Surgical treatment of this complication seldom yields satisfactory results.

Fracture of the Shaft of the Ulna and Dislocation of the Proximal Radioulnar Joint (Monteggia Fracture-Dislocation)

For reasons already mentioned, an angulated fracture of the proximal half of the ulna is invariably accompanied by a dislocation of the proximal radioulnar joint. Thus, radiographic examination for fractures in the forearm should always include both the wrist and elbow joints lest a fracture-dislocation be overlooked.

In the common type of Monteggia fracture-dislocation, a hyperextension and pronation injury produces a fracture of the proximal half of the ulna with anterior angulation and anterior dislocation of the proximal radioulnar joint (Fig. 17.28). This injury can also be produced by a direct blow over the ulnar border of the forearm.

Monteggia fracture-dislocations in adults are best treated by open reduction of the ulna in order that its length and alignment may be perfectly restored. Internal fixation of the fracture should be obtained by means of either a compression plate and screws or an intramedullary nail. In addition it is usually necessary in adults to perform an open reduction of the dislocated proximal radioulnar joint and to repair the ruptured annular ligament. The limb should be immobilized in an above-elbow cast with the forearm in supination for approximately three months.

A rare variation of Monteggia fracture-dislocation is the flexion type which is caused by a flexion injury and which is characterized by posterior angulation of the fractured ulna and posterior dislocation of the proximal radioulnar joint. This type of injury is treated using the same principles as for the extension type of Monteggia fracture-dislocation.

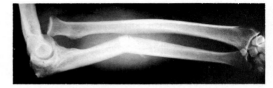

Figure 17.28. Fracture of the shaft of the ulna and dislocation of the proximal radioulnar joint (Monteggia fracture-dislocation). Note the over-riding and anterior angulation at the fracture site in the ulna and the associated anterior and upward dislocation of the radial head. Unless the radiographic examination includes the elbow region, the dislocation of the radial head may escape detection.

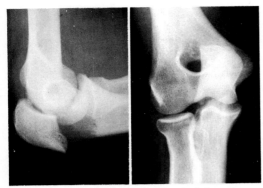

Figure 17.29. Avulsion fracture of the olecranon in a 21-year-old woman. The true nature of the injury is much more apparent in the lateral projection than in the anteroposterior projection and this emphasizes the importance of always obtaining at least two projections at right angles to one another. Note also that in the anteroposterior projection, which was taken with the elbow extended, the fracture of the olecranon is only slightly displaced whereas in the lateral projection, which was taken with the elbow flexed, the gap at the fracture site has widened. This patient's arm should have been immobilized in a temporary splint before the radiographic examination was carried out.

The Elbow and Arm
FRACTURE OF THE OLECRANON

The commonest type of olecranon fracture is due to a fall with sudden passive flexion of the elbow combined with a sudden powerful contraction of the triceps muscle. The olecranon is literally pulled apart over the fulcrum of the trochlea; thus, it is an *avulsion* type of fracture and in many ways is comparable to an avulsion fracture of the patella.

The fracture fragments are usually pulled far apart and the patient is no longer able to actively extend the elbow against gravity. Even when there is considerable swelling, a gap can be palpated at the fracture site. Radiographic examination reveals the widely separated fracture fragments (Fig. 17.29).

Closed treatment of avulsion fractures of the olecranon is only occasionally possible; when the elbow is passively extended, the olecranon may fall back into normal position. Under these rare circumstances the elbow should be immobilized in complete extension

in a plaster cast for six weeks—an awkward position and one not well tolerated, particularly by the elderly.

The usual form of treatment is open reduction of the fracture and internal fixation using the AO principle of compression (Fig. 17.30). Unless the fixation is completely rigid, the elbow should be immobilized at a right angle for at least three weeks, after which active exercises are begun. This form of treatment is suitable even in the elderly and is more satisfactory than excision of the olecranon and suture of the triceps to the ulna.

Complications of avulsion fractures of the olecranon include *non-union* with resultant pain and weakness of extension and occasionally *degenerative joint disease* of the elbow secondary to the joint incongruity. Late operation to obtain union by bone grafting seldom provides a smooth joint surface and this emphasizes the importance of perfect reduction and rigid internal fixation in the primary treatment.

FRACTURES OF THE RADIAL HEAD

This relatively common injury in young adults is caused by a severe valgus abduction) force applied to the extended elbow, usually at the time of a fall. The concave surface of the radial head is crushed against the convex surface of the capitellum and tends to split. The cartilage of both joint

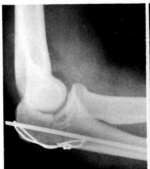
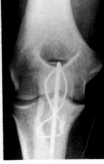

Figure 17.30. Postoperative radiograph of the same elbow shown in Figure 17.29. The combination of an intramedullary pin and a figure-eight wire loop (tension band) maintained the reduction and compressed the fragments together in accordance with the AO principle.

surfaces is damaged but it is always the radial head that fractures. The medial ligament of the elbow is stretched and, if the valgus force is sufficient, the ligament may even be torn with a resultant momentary lateral dislocation of the elbow.

The patient experiences progressive pain in the elbow as a hemarthrosis develops. Supination and pronation are limited by pain and there is local tenderness over the radial head.

Radiographic examination usually reveals the fracture but, if the fracture is completely undisplaced, several radiographs taken with the radius in varying degrees of supination and pronation may be required for its detection.

Treatment depends upon the severity of the damage to the radial head. It must be remembered, however, that the actual damage to the joint surface, as well as to the underlying bone, is always more extensive than one would imagine from the appearance of the radiographs.

Undisplaced fractures without loss of joint congruity require only protection in a sling for two weeks during which time active exercises (pronation and supination) are encouraged (Fig. 17.31).

Depressed and comminuted fractures of

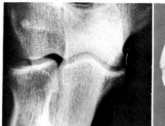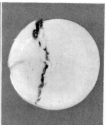

Figure 17.32. Depressed and comminuted fracture of the radial head in a young man. *Left*, initial radiograph. Note the gap in the joint surface of the radial head. The depression is not obvious in this radiograph. *Right*, The excised radial head of the same patient reveals that the fracture is more comminuted and is more extensive than one might think from the appearance of the radiographs.

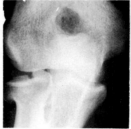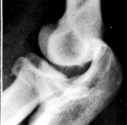

Figure 17.33. Markedly depressed and comminuted fracture of the radial head in a 40-year-old man. This type of fracture is an indication for excision of the entire head and neck of the radius.

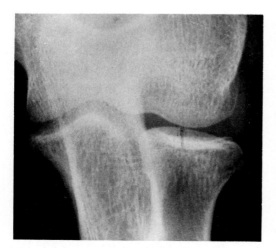

Figure 17.31. Undisplaced crack fracture of the radial head in a young woman who had a painful hemarthrosis and limitation of supination and pronation after a fall on the hand.

the radial head are best treated by excision of the entire head and neck (and not just the depressed portion) (Figs. 17.32 and 17.33). At the time of operation the elbow joint should be carefully explored in order to remove any small fragments of bone or cartilage. If the medial ligament of the elbow has been completely torn, the elbow will lack lateral stability after excision of the head and neck of the radius. Under these circumstances it may be reasonable to replace the radial head with an endoprosthesis to provide stability, but this is seldom necessary.

Complications

The most significant complication of fractures of the radial head is *post-traumatic degenerative joint disease* of the elbow—a complication of leaving a displaced fracture *in situ.* Once degenerative joint disease has developed, the pain and limitation of motion can be improved by excision of the head and neck of the radius, but the results are not as satisfactory after late excision as after immediate excision.

POSTERIOR DISLOCATION OF THE ELBOW

There are two possible mechanisms of this fairly common injury in adults: a fall on the hand with the elbow slightly flexed or, alternatively, a severe hyperextension injury of the elbow.

The distal end of the humerus is driven forward through the anterior capsule as the radius and ulna dislocate posteriorly. Thus, there is always extensive soft tissue injury to the capsule and brachialis muscle (which may be torn from its insertion into the coronoid process). The brachial artery and median nerve may also be struck by the distal end of the humerus as it is driven forward. Occasionally associated with posterior dislocation of the elbow is a minor fracture of the coronoid process, capitellum or radial head.

Clinically, the grossly swollen elbow is held in a position of semi-flexion; the olecranon is readily palpable posteriorly. Radiographic examination is essential, however, not only to confirm the clinical diagnosis but also to detect any associated fractures (Fig. 17.34a).

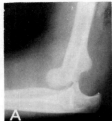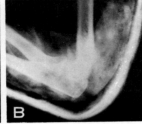

Figure 17.34. Posterior dislocation of the elbow joint in a young man. *A*, initial radiograph revealing the posterior displacement of the radius and ulna in relation to the distal end of the humerus. *B*, the post-reduction radiograph revealing that the normal relationship between the distal end of the humerus and olecranon has been restored. The patient's elbow is immobilized in flexion in a plaster cast.

Reduction of the dislocation is readily accomplished by applying traction to the flexed elbow through the forearm, which is then brought forward. The reduced elbow is then flexed above a right angle to reduce tension on the torn anterior soft tissues and is immobilized in a cast in this position for three weeks (Fig. 17.34*B*).

Complications

After dislocation of the elbow in adults, *elbow stiffness* may persist for many months. The stiffness must be treated by active exercises only, since passive stretching of the soft tissues may aggravate the soft tissue injury and actually perpetuate the stiffness. *Median nerve injury* in association with dislocation of the elbow invariably recovers. The complication of *myositis ossificans* may occur after posterior dislocation of the elbow in adults—particularly if reduction is delayed or if the elbow has been repeatedly manipulated—but it is less common in adults than in children. This complication has been discussed in Chapter 15. Major *injury to the brachial artery* is not uncommon.

FRACTURE-DISLOCATIONS OF THE ELBOW

An extremely severe fracture-dislocation of the elbow occurs when a driver or passenger has his elbow out the open window of a car at the moment the car is struck from the side by another vehicle. The elbow is dislocated and there are multiple comminuted fractures of the humerus, radius and ulna—the "sideswipe injury" of the elbow (Fig. 17.35).

Treatment of this serious injury is understandably difficult. Under anesthesia the elbow joint is reduced after which the fragments are aligned as well as possible. Open reduction and internal fixation of the multiple fractures is best delayed for a few days until the soft tissue reaction to the massive injury has subsided.

INTERCONDYLAR FRACTURES OF THE HUMERUS

The intercondylar type of fracture of the distal end of the humerus in adults results

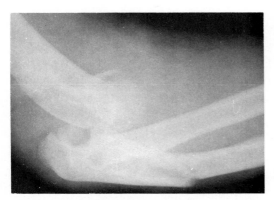

Figure 17.35. A severe fracture-dislocation of the elbow ("sideswipe injury"). Note that there are fractures of the ulna, radial head and the distal end of the humerus. Note also the posterior dislocation of the elbow joint.

from a severe fall on the point of the flexed elbow. In cross-section the articular surface of the olecranon appears wedge-shaped and, hence, it is not surprising that with such a fall the olecranon is driven like a wedge between the two condyles of the humerus and splits one or both from the shaft. Thus, the vertical component of the fracture is always intra-articular. Proximally there may be a transverse component in which case the comminuted fracture lines are T-shaped.

Clinically, the elbow region is grossly swollen and there is usually evidence of abrasions or bruises on the undersurface of the elbow indicating the mechanism of injury. Radiographic examination may require several projections to reveal the true extent of the injury. Indeed, the comminution may be extreme.

Treatment

The form of treatment depends primarily on the degree of comminution of the fracture. Of course the most important fracture to be completely reduced is the vertical fracture which extends into the elbow joint. *Single fractures* which have split off only one condyle are best treated by open reduction and internal fixation with screws to restore the joint line (Fig. 17.36). *Double fractures* with a T-shaped component may also be treated by open reduction and internal fixation of the vertical component; then the

transverse fracture can be treated by continuous skeletal traction through a pin in the olecranon. This method is preferable to prolonged operations in which an attempt is made to secure all the fragments since such surgical treatment usually leads to a permanent loss of elbow joint motion.

Severely comminuted fractures in the intercondylar region defy internal fixation and are best treated by continuous skeletal traction through a pin in the olecranon. The fragments usually become reasonably aligned and since some elbow motion is possible in the traction device, the elbow is less likely to become permanently stiff. The complication of prolonged joint stiffness is particularly common when intercondylar fractures of the humerus have been immobilized in a plaster cast for longer than three weeks.

FRACTURES OF THE SHAFT OF THE HUMERUS

Adults sustain fractures of the shaft of the humerus more readily than children. The common mechanism of injury is a direct

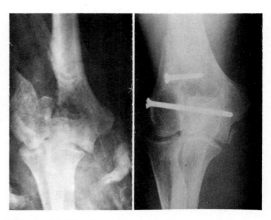

Figure 17.36. Intercondylar fracture of the humerus in a 45-year-old man. *Left*, initial radiographs (the elbow is immobilized in a temporary plaster splint). The lateral condyle has been split off from the distal end of the humerus and is not only displaced laterally but is also tilted. (The radio-opaque areas seen medially and laterally distal to the elbow are in the plaster splint and not in the patient). *Right*, post-reduction radiograph showing the lateral condyle reduced and held in position with two screws. Note that the joint line has been completely restored.

blow, in which case the fracture tends to be transverse and somewhat comminuted. Indirect injury, as is sustained from a fall on the hand, is more likely to produce a spiral fracture. It must be remembered that the humeral shaft is a common site for metastases in the adult—particularly in the elderly.

The humerus, like the femur, being surrounded by muscle, has a fairly thick periosteum, and consequently fractures of the humerus usually unite well and rapidly unless the fracture has been overdistracted (as it may be in a heavy "hanging cast"). The proximity of the radial nerve as it winds around the mid-shaft of the humerus accounts for the high incidence of radial nerve injury associated with fractures at this level.

Clinical examination reveals a flail arm which the patient tries to support with the opposite hand. A radial nerve lesion should always be sought and its presence or absence recorded at the time of the initial examination. The arm should be splinted before radiographic examination is carried out and the anteroposterior and lateral projections should be obtained by moving the radiographic tube rather than by moving the patient's fractured arm.

Treatment

Fractures of the shaft of the humerus respond well to closed treatment, the aim of which is to obtain and maintain reasonable alignment without rotational deformity. The reduction does not need to be perfect and even side-to-side (bayonet) apposition with slight shortening is acceptable. Thus, nearly all fractures of the shaft of the humerus in adults can be adequately treated by closed means. One indication for open reduction and internal fixation of the fracture is a coexistent injury to the brachial artery which necessitates arterial repair.

Transverse fractures of the humeral shaft should be reduced under anesthesia to get the fracture ends in contact and thereby provide some stability. When the alignment and rotation have been corrected, a U-shaped plaster slab (sometimes referred to as a "sugar tong splint") is applied and bandaged to the arm; a collar and wrist cuff sling are applied and for added comfort—particularly if the fracture is unstable—the upper limb can be bandaged to the chest (Fig. 17.37). Clinical union is usually achieved within six weeks, after which guarded movement of the elbow may be initiated. This form of treatment is preferable to a heavy "hanging cast" which hangs only when the patient is upright and which may distract the fracture fragments and thereby lead to delayed union; furthermore, since the "hanging cast" does not immobilize the fracture fragments, the patient experiences much discomfort during the early weeks of treatment.

Spiral and comminuted fractures of the humeral shaft do not require reduction or anesthesia; with the patient sitting upright, gravity alone is adequate to provide alignment of the fracture fragments, after which the above-mentioned U-shaped plaster splint with collar and cuff may be applied. Even slight residual angulation does not produce a clinically significant deformity at this level (Fig. 17.38).

Fractures of the shaft of the humerus are also amenable to functional fracture-bracing after an initial period of two weeks' immobilization in a plaster cast.

Complications

For reasons already mentioned, *radial nerve injury* is frequent at the time of fracture. The nerve, however, is seldom divided (neurotmesis) and since the lesion is one in

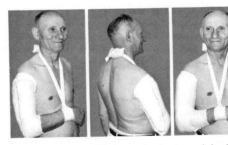

Figure 17.37. U-shaped plaster slab ("sugar tong splint") with a collar and wrist cuff sling for a fracture of the shaft of the humerus. One bandage separates the plaster from the skin and a second bandage holds the plaster slab firmly in place. If the fracture is particularly unstable, the arm can then be bandaged to the trunk as well.

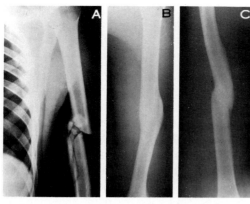

Figure 17.38. Spiral and comminuted fracture of the humeral shaft in a 44-year-old man. *A*, initial radiograph taken with the patient sitting upright. The alignment is satisfactory. The fracture was treated with a U-shaped plaster with a collar and cuff sling. *B* and *C*, one year later the fracture is consolidated; the slight varus deformity was not apparent clinically.

continuity (either neuropraxia or axonotmesis) recovery may be anticipated; therefore a radial nerve injury does not constitute an indication for open reduction. If, however, there has been no recovery of muscles innervated by the radial nerve within approximately three months (the estimated time required for regenerating nerve fibers to reach the first muscle after an axonotemesis), the nerve should be explored. Should the nerve be found to be irreparably damaged, function in the hand can be greatly improved by appropriate tendon transfers. *Delayed union* or even *non-union* may complicate a fracture of the humeral shaft, especially if the fracture has been operated upon or has been overdistracted by a "hanging cast." While fresh fractures of the humerus usually unite rapidly and well, non-union can be exceedingly difficult to treat and may need intramedullary nailing, autogenous cancellous bone grafting and a complete shoulder spica.

FRACTURES OF THE NECK OF THE HUMERUS

In elderly persons—especially women with a combination of senile and postmenopausal osteoporosis—impacted fractures of the neck of the humerus are relatively common. Resulting usually from a minor fall on the hand with forces being transmitted up the extended arm, the fracture line is transverse and the distal fragment is driven into, or *impacted*, in the proximal fragment.

Clinical examination may reveal relatively little evidence of the fracture, since it is sufficiently stable that the patient is able to move the arm reasonably well. There is local tenderness in the axilla but the arm can usually be moved passively with little pain.

Radiographic examination reveals the extent of impaction of the fracture (Fig. 17.39).

Treatment

Since *impacted* fractures of the neck of the humerus are stable, the fracture need not be immobilized and requires only protection from further injury by means of a sling during the six weeks required for union. After one week, however, the patient should remove the sling daily for a period of "pendulum" exercises to prevent shoulder stiffness; while bending forward, the patient gently swings the dependent limb back and forth and also in a circle. As soon as the

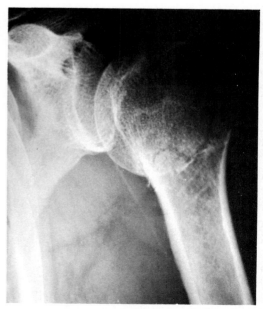

Figure 17.39. Impacted fracture of the neck of the humerus in an elderly woman. The impaction is easily seen on the medial side.

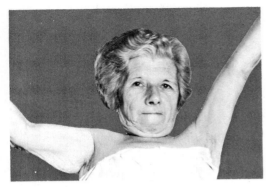

Figure 17.40. This elderly woman is abducting her shoulders four weeks after sustaining an impacted fracture of the neck of her right humerus. She will regain a useful, but not necessarily normal, range of shoulder motion.

patient no longer feels pain at the fracture site, she should be encouraged to abduct the arm against gravity (Fig. 17.40).

Fractures that are *not impacted* require more active treatment. Occurring more often in younger adults, these fractures may be markedly displaced. The short proximal fragment is usually abducted by the muscles inserted into the rotator cuff and, under these circumstances, it is necessary during closed reduction of the fracture to abduct the distal fragment and then to immobilize the patient's entire upper limb in an abduction type of shoulder spica cast for six weeks.

Complications

In the elderly the most common complication of impacted fractures of the neck of the humerus is *persistent shoulder stiffness*, a complication that is more easily prevented than treated. Prolonged physiotherapy is necessary to overcome such shoulder stiffness and occasionally after several months of therapy a gentle manipulation under anesthesia is required to regain shoulder motion. In younger adults with displaced fractures there may be coexistent *injury to the circumflex (axillary) nerve* which is manifest by deltoid muscle paralysis and a small area of diminished skin sensation over the outer aspect of the shoulder region. The prognosis for recovery of nerve function is good.

FRACTURES OF THE GREATER TUBEROSITY OF THE HUMERUS

In middle-aged and elderly adults a relatively common injury is an undisplaced fracture of the greater tuberosity of the humerus resulting from a fall directly on the point of the shoulder (Fig. 17.41). Treatment is identical to that described above for impacted fractures of the neck of the humerus.

In younger adults the greater tuberosity is more often *avulsed* by an indirect injury such as a fall on the hand with the arm adducted. Under these circumstances the greater tuberosity is usually retracted and abducted; reduction therefore necessitates abduction of the humerus and immobilization of the upper limb and trunk in a shoulder spica cast or abduction splint for six weeks.

The Shoulder
DISLOCATIONS OF THE SHOULDER

The shoulder joint is dependent for its stability on the joint capsule and surrounding muscles; the glenoid cavity, being small in relation to the head of the humerus, provides little bony stability. For this reason the shoulder joint is more often dislocated than any other joint in adults. The dislocation may be produced by either direct or indirect injury; in addition, dislocation of a shoulder may

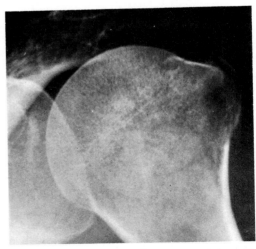

Figure 17.41. Fracture of the greater tuberosity of the humerus of a 50-year-old woman who fell directly on the outer aspect of her shoulder.

occur during the violent uncoordinated muscle contractions of a grand mal type of epileptic convulsion.

At the time of the initial shoulder dislocation the joint capsule is usually avulsed from the glenoid cavity and, since there is little bony stability of the joint, a common sequel to the initial injury is recurrent dislocation. The dislocation may be anterior and medial (subcoracoid) or less commonly, posterior; a rare injury is the inferior type of dislocation in which the head of the humerus becomes caught under the glenoid cavity and the patient cannot bring his arm down to the side (luxatio erecta).

Anterior Dislocation of the Shoulder

An injury predominantly of young adults (particularly athletes), anterior dislocation of the shoulder is usually caused by forced external rotation and extension of the shoulder; the humeral head is driven forward and frequently avulses the cartilaginous glenoid labrum and capsule from the anterior aspect of the glenoid cavity (the Bankart lesion). Less commonly, anterior dislocation is

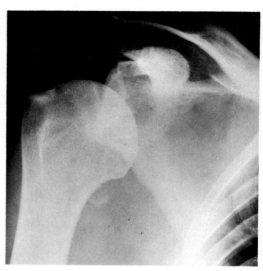

Figure 17.43. Radiographic appearance of an acute anterior dislocation of the right shoulder; note that the humeral head is no longer articulating with the glenoid cavity and is lying in the subcoracoid position.

caused by a fall on the hand or a fall directly on the posterolateral aspect of the shoulder.

The patient is immediately aware that something has "given way" or "gone out of place" and is unable to use his arm which he tends to support with his opposite hand. On physical examination the shoulder appears strikingly square due to the anterior and medial displacement of the humeral head into a subcoracoid location (Fig. 17.42). Circumflex (axillary) nerve function should always be assessed during the initial examination because it may have been injured.

Radiographic examination confirms the diagnosis; the humeral head has lost contact with the glenoid cavity and is lying in the subcoracoid position (Fig. 17.43).

Treatment. The dislocation should be reduced as soon as possible, and this can usually be accomplished by any one of three available methods. The simplest of these methods requires no anesthesia and is therefore worth a trial unless the patient is unduly nervous; the patient merely lies face down on a table with the injured arm (to which a weight is attached) hanging over the padded table edge. As the shoulder

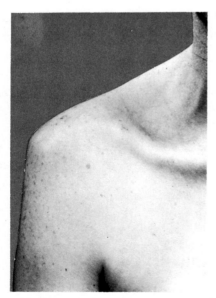

Figure 17.42. The typical clinical deformity of anterior (inferomedial) dislocation of the right shoulder in a young athlete; the normal round contour of the shoulder has been lost and the shoulder looks square. The humeral head was palpable in the subcoracoid region.

muscles relax over a period of several minutes, the humeral head frequently slips back to its normal position. If this method has not resulted in a reduction of the dislocation within ten minutes, a general anesthetic is usually indicated in order that one of the following methods may be performed. With an assistant applying constant traction to the upper limb with the shoulder in abduction, the surgeon can apply lateral and backward pressure on the dislocated humeral head with his hands and thereby reduce it. A time-honored variant of this method—dignified eponymously by the name Hippocratic method—involves the same forces but the surgeon applies the traction with his hands and the local pressure with his unshod foot in the patient's axilla (like a one-man band). The name is more dignified than the method—especially if the patient is conscious. It is perhaps appropriate to point out that the word "surgery" refers to hand work rather than to foot work. The Kocher method, which is equally effective, involves a series of four maneuvers: (1) steady traction is applied to the arm with the elbow flexed; (2) the arm is externally rotated; (3) the externally rotated arm is then adducted and flexed at the shoulder so that the elbow approaches the midline of the trunk; (4) the arm is then internally rotated until the forearm lies against the chest on the opposite side. Complete reduction should be confirmed radiographically.

After reduction of the dislocation has been obtained—by any of these methods—the patient's upper limb should be supported in a sling and bandaged to the chest to keep the shoulder adducted and internally rotated for three weeks; the avulsed capsule is thereby given a chance to heal and the risk of recurrent anterior dislocation is probably lessened, particularly in the young adult. For the elderly, three weeks' immobilization of the reduced shoulder is neither necessary nor desirable; a simple sling is adequate.

Complications. In addition to *recurrent anterior dislocation* (which is discussed in the next section of this chapter), a relatively common complication of the initial disloca-

tion is a *traction injury of the circumflex (axillary) nerve.* The patient is unable to abduct the shoulder because of deltoid paralysis and there is a small patch of diminished skin sensation over the outer aspect of the shoulder; the prognosis for recovery is good. Occasionally a coexistent *tear of the musculotendinous cuff* of the shoulder complicates a dislocation in which case the reduced shoulder should be immobilized for three weeks in an abducted position. Rarely, *interposition of the tendon of the long head of biceps* necessitates open reduction of the dislocation.

Recurrent Anterior Dislocation of the Shoulder

Since the stability of the shoulder depends to a large extent on the integrity of the joint capsule and since the capsule and anterior labrum are nearly always avulsed or stripped off the glenoid and neck of the scapula at the time of the initial dislocation of the shoulder, it is not surprising that, in some persons, especially athletes, the dislocation may recur more and more often with less and less violence. In addition to the unhealed soft tissue rent, which leaves an anterior pocket into which the humeral head may slip, there is often a residual "dent" in the posterior aspect of the head as the result of a compression fracture sustained during the initial dislocation. Such a dent allows the externally rotated humeral head to slip over the anterior margin of the glenoid cavity quite readily. Understandably, this dent cannot be detected radiographically in an anteroposterior projection but is easily seen in a special projection with the humerus internally rotated 60° (Fig. 17.44).

Treatment. In young persons recurrent anterior dislocation can be both irritating and disabling; the patient is constantly aware that if his arm is abducted and externally rotated his shoulder is likely to redislocate. Under these circumstances, surgical repair of the soft tissues is indicated. Of the large number and variety of operations designed to render such a shoulder stable, the two most commonly performed are the Bankart

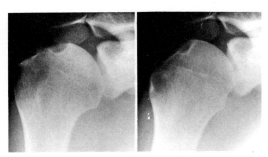

Figure 17.44. Residual dent in the posterior aspect of the humeral head after an acute anterior dislocation of the shoulder. *Left*, in this antero-posterior projection, the dent is not apparent. *Right*, in this projection (with the humerus internally rotated 60°) the dent is obvious. It is rather like a dent in a ping-pong ball.

operation, in which the labrum and capsule are reattached to the anterior margin of the glenoid cavity; and the Putti-Platt operation, in which the capsule as well as the subscapularis muscle are divided and then reefed (overlapped), thereby limiting external rotation. After operation the patient's arm should be supported in a sling and bandaged to the trunk with the shoulder internally rotated for six weeks. A successful repair enables the patient to return to full activities including athletics.

Fracture-Dislocation of the Shoulder

The greater tuberosity of the humerus is sometimes avulsed at the time of an anterior dislocation of the shoulder (Fig. 17.45). Such a fracture-dislocation can usually be treated by closed reduction of the dislocation (as described above) which brings the humeral head back into reasonable relationship with the greater tuberosity. As with an associated tear of the musculotendinous cuff, fracture-dislocations of this type require immobilization of the reduced shoulder in a position of abduction.

An uncommon but serious type of fracture-dislocation is one in which a completely displaced fracture through the neck of the humerus is associated with complete dislocation of the humeral head. For this complex injury, open reduction of the dislocation is frequently necessary; the associated frac-

ture can then be treated by closed means as previously described.

Posterior Dislocation of the Shoulder

Though much less common than anterior dislocation, posterior dislocation can occur from a fall on the front of the shoulder or on the hand with the shoulder adducted and internally rotated; it may also occur during an epileptic convulsion.

Clinically, the patient's arm seems locked in a position of adduction and internal rotation. Radiographically, the posterior dislocation is not readily detected in an anteroposterior projection since the humeral head slides only posteriorly and not medially. A special superoinferior (axillary) projection with the shoulder abducted is necessary to confirm that the humeral head is in fact lying posteriorly.

Treatment. Under anesthesia the posterior dislocation can be reduced by externally rotating the shoulder and applying forward pressure on the dislocated humeral head. Reduction should be confirmed in both the anteroposterior and superoinferior (axillary)

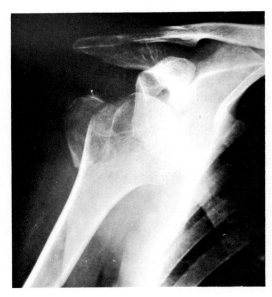

Figure 17.45. Fracture-dislocation of the right shoulder. Note the displaced fracture of the greater tuberosity of the humerus and the dislocation of the humeral head in relation to the glenoid cavity.

projections. The shoulder is then supported in a sling for three weeks.

Recurrent and Habitual Posterior Dislocation of the Shoulder

When a shoulder previously dislocated posteriorly re-dislocates as a result of another injury, the second and subsequent dislocations are referred to as *recurrent* dislocations. Surgical repair of the posterior soft tissue is indicated. When, however, the patient is able to dislocate the shoulder posteriorly at will—and likewise reduce it—the condition is one of *habitual* dislocation, and is usually associated with generalized congenital laxity of ligaments. Such a patient should be discouraged from dislocating and reducing the dislocation as a "parlor trick." Should the shoulder dislocate every time the patient's shoulder is flexed and adducted, however, surgical repair is justifiable.

RUPTURE OF THE MUSCULOTENDINOUS CUFF OF THE SHOULDER

This relatively common injury, which is frequently preceded by degenerative changes in the musculotendinous cuff, is described in Chapter 11.

SUBLUXATION AND DISLOCATION OF THE ACROMIOCLAVICULAR JOINT

The term "shoulder separation" refers to either a subluxation or a dislocation of the acromioclavicular joint—injuries that are caused by a severe fall on the top of the shoulder and are therefore frequently encountered in young men engaged in body contact sports such as football, rugger and hockey.

The acromion is driven downward while the clavicle is pulled upward by the action of the trapezius and sternomastoid muscles; the capsule of the acromioclavicular joint is torn. The coracoclavicular ligaments (trapezoid and conoid) bind the clavicle to the coracoid process of the scapula, and, if these are not torn by the injury, the acromioclavicular joint is merely *subluxated*. If, however, these ligaments are completely torn, the result is a complete *dislocation* of the acromioclavicular joint.

The patient complains of severe pain over the shoulder and there is marked local tenderness over the acromioclavicular joint. Instability of the joint may be detected clinically, especially with a complete dislocation.

Radiographic examination is best conducted with the patient standing and holding a weight in each hand. In a *subluxation* there is merely a slight depression of the acromion whereas in a *dislocation* the joint surfaces have lost contact completely (Fig. 17.46).

Treatment

Non-operative methods of strapping and plaster casts to depress the clavicle and elevate the acromion are frequently employed and may relieve the acute symptoms but are of doubtful value in restoring and maintaining the normal relationship of the clavicle to the acromion. For a *subluxation*, support of the arm in a sling for a few weeks—with or without strapping—is adequate in the realization that some degree of residual subluxation of the acromioclavicular joint is almost inevitable but also acceptable.

For a complete *dislocation*, however, non-operative methods are ineffectual although the Kenny-Howard sling halter would seem to be an exception as reported by Allman.

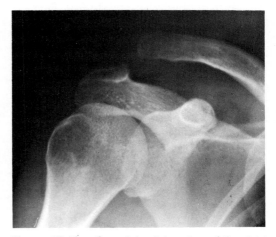

Figure 17.46. Complete dislocation of the right acromioclavicular joint in a football player. Note the marked depression of the acromion in relation to the outer end of the clavicle; the coracoclavicular ligaments (trapezoid and conoid) must be completely torn to permit this degree of displacement.

When such a halter fails the most satisfactory form of treatment is open reduction, capsular repair and the insertion of a threaded wire through the acromion, across the acromioclavicular joint and well into the clavicle. The wire is removed after six weeks. Other methods of treatment include screw fixation of the clavicle to the coracoid process and transfer of the tip of the coracoid and attached pectoralis minor muscle to the clavicle (Dewar).

Untreated or inadequately treated dislocation of the acromioclavicular joint leaves a permanent deformity as well as permanent weakness of the shoulder (Fig. 17.47).

DISLOCATION OF THE STERNOCLAVICULAR JOINT

A severe blow or fall on the front of the shoulder, which drives the outer end of the clavicle backward and the inner end forward, may produce an anterior dislocation of the sternoclavicular joint. This uncommon injury is more readily diagnosed clinically—by local tenderness and a prominence of the medial end of the clavicle—than radiographically. The dislocation can be reduced by local pressure over the dislocated end of the clavicle and the reduction can usually be maintained by the combination of a local pressure pad, strapping to hold the shoulder forward and a sling for three weeks.

Recurrent anterior dislocation of the sternoclavicular joint may necessitate a reconstructive operation which a "living suture" of fascia lata is used to retain the medial end of the clavicle in normal relationship with the sternum.

Posterior (retrosternal) dislocation of the

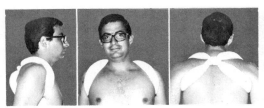

Figure 17.48. Figure-eight bandage for the treatment of a fractured clavicle in an athletic adult; the bandage, which consists of stockinette filled with cotton wool, is adjustable so that it can be tightened as necessary each day. For additional support, this bandage can be reinforced by plaster-of-Paris bandages.

sternoclavicular joint—a rare injury—may cause dangerous compression of the trachea or great vessels and may necessitate urgent open reduction.

FRACTURES OF THE CLAVICLE

The relatively strong clavicles of adults are less frequently fractured than the slender clavicles of young children. The mechanism of injury in both groups, however, is the same, namely a fall on the hand with forces being transmitted through the forearm and arm to the shoulder. The common site is the middle third of the clavicle and the lateral fragment is usually pulled inferiorly and medially by the weight of the shoulder and upper limb (Fig. 17.49A). Less commonly the fracture occurs just medial to the acromioclavicular joint.

Treatment

Since fractures of the clavicle heal well—even in adults—and perfect reduction is not essential, closed manipulation under either local or general anesthesia is usually satisfactory. Both shoulders are pulled back as far as possible and are held in this position for three weeks by means of a stout figure-eight bandage (Fig. 17.48). Although the fracture is usually clinically united in three weeks, it is not radiographically united until much later.

Complications

Mal-union of a fractured clavicle is common but is seldom a cause for concern except for young and even not-so-young women (Figs. 17-49 and 17.50). For this

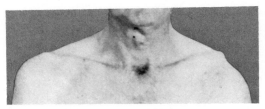

Figure 17.47. Residual deformity of an untreated dislocation of the left acromioclavicular joint. This 52-year-old working man had weakness of shoulder abduction and experienced aching in the shoulder at the end of a day's work.

group of patients the combination of careful alignment of the fracture fragments, the application of a well molded double shoulder spica cast and a few weeks' rest in bed can prevent mal-union and provides a more acceptable cosmetic result than the obvious surgical scar of an open reduction.

Delayed union may complicate a fractured clavicle that has been inadequately treated during the first few weeks (Fig. 17.49). *Non-union*, however, is very rare indeed unless the fracture has been complicated by infection after an open reduction.

The Spine
GENERAL FEATURES

Fractures, dislocations and fracture-dislocations of the spine have become increas-

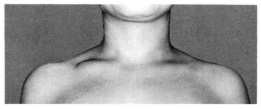

Figure 17.50. Clinical deformity caused by mal-union of the right clavicle of the young woman whose radiographs are shown in Figure 17.49. This permanent deformity, seen six months after injury, was a source of embarrassment to the patient.

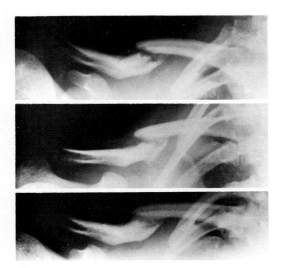

Figure 17.49. Fracture of the middle third of the right clavicle in a young woman who had sustained multiple injuries in an automobile accident. Note that the fracture is comminuted with an angulated middle segment and that the lateral fragment is displaced inferiorly and medially. *Top,* three weeks after injury. The patient stated that her shoulder had not been immobilized in any way during the preceding three weeks. The alignment of this fracture could have been improved initially and maintained by treatment. *Center,* three months after injury. New bone formation is apparent and although the fracture was clinically united at this time, bony union has been delayed. *Bottom,* six months after injury. The fracture is now radiographically united and, although there has been some remodeling at the fracture site, there is still an obvious deformity of mal-union.

ingly more common in the present age of high-speed travel, the majority being caused by automobile accidents. Although 80% of spinal injuries prove to be unaccompanied by serious complications, such as spinal cord injury, all spinal injuries must be considered initially to be potentially serious. Thus, the preliminary (first-aid) care and transporation of persons who have sustained such injuries, as discussed in Chapter 15, are extremely important.

In general, major injuries of the spinal column should be assessed in terms of their *stability. Stable injuries,* such as wedge compression fractures and even bursting compression fractures of vertebral bodies, are protected from significant displacement both initially and subsequently by intact posterior spinal ligaments; whereas *unstable injuries,* such as dislocations and fracture-dislocations, have been significantly displaced initially and may become further displaced because the posterior spinal ligaments have been torn. Assessment of stability sometimes requires that the radiographic examination be carried out with the injured part of the spine in varying degrees of flexion and extension—an example of stress radiography to detect occult joint instability—but always with the patient conscious and a physician or surgeon in control of the examination.

Initial and repeated neurological examination must be thoroughly conducted and recorded in all patients with spinal injury to determine the extent as well as the progress of complicating injuries to the spinal cord or nerve roots. *Traumatic paraplegia* has been discussed in Chapter 12.

Radiographic examination should always include a minimum of four projections (anteroposterior, lateral, right and left oblique) and sometimes special projections or even special techniques, such as tomography (laminography), myelography and computed tomography are required to elucidate the nature and extent of the injury.

INJURIES OF THE CERVICAL SPINE

The cervical segments, being the most mobile of the spinal column, are the most vulnerable to unstable injuries such as dislocations and fracture-dislocations; and furthermore, the spinal cord in the cervical region is particularly vulnerable to either compression or even transection. Indeed the most severe injuries of the upper part of the spinal cord are immediately fatal and the victim does not even reach a hospital.

Since many cervical spine injuries are associated with a severe blow on the head, all patients who have sustained a head injury should have a thorough clinical and radiographic examination of the cervical spine.

Fracture of the Atlas (C.1)

When an individual falls from a height and lands on the top of the head with the cervical spine straight, the occipital condyles of the base of the skull may split or burst the ring of the atlas. Provided there is no angulatory or rotatory injury, the displacement is not severe and the spinal cord is not injured. Radiographic examination should include an anteroposterior view through the open mouth.

Treatment. Since a bursting type fracture of the atlas is a stable injury the only treatment required—in the absence of spinal cord injury—is immobilization of the cervical spine in a plaster cast or carefully fitted cervical collar for approximately three months.

Displacements of the Atlantoaxial Joint (C.1–C.2)

The normal relationship between the atlas and axis is maintained to a large extent by the transverse ligament of the atlas that crosses behind the odontoid process (dens) of the axis.

Dislocation of the atlantoaxial joint as a result of trauma is seldom seen clinically because such a dislocation is likely to produce a fatal injury to the spinal cord. Gradual dislocation of this joint, however, may complicate inflammatory disorders such as rheumatoid arthritis as a result of softening and subsequent stretching of the transverse ligament. Local spinal fusion of the completely reduced atlantoaxial joint is indicated to protect the spinal cord.

Fracture-dislocation of the atlantoaxial joint includes a fracture of the base of the odontoid process and either anterior or posterior dislocation of the atlas, usually the former. Since the transverse ligament is intact, the odontoid process moves with the atlas and the spinal cord may not be compressed. The patient quite understandably feels that his head is "about to fall off" and anxiously supports it with his hands.

The treatment of undisplaced fractures of the base of the odontoid requires only immobilization of the cervical spine in a plaster cast or well molded plastic cervical collar. Reduction of *displaced fracture-dislocations of the atlantoaxial joint* is best accomplished by continuous skull traction through tongs (Fig. 17.51). After one month of skull traction the fracture is usually sufficiently stable that a plaster cast or a plastic collar can be

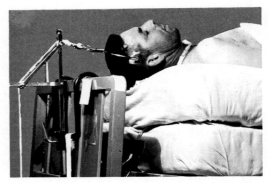

Figure 17.51. Continuous skeletal traction through tongs in the outer table of the skull for unstable fractures, dislocations and fracture-dislocation of the cervical spine.

applied to immobilize the cervical spine for an additional two months. Even a fibrous union of the fracture may provide adequate stability; if it does not, however, local spinal fusion is indicated.

Compression Fracture of a Cervical Vertebral Body

A flexion injury of the cervical spine without disruption of the posterior spinal ligaments may cause a compression, or crush type fracture of the cancellous bone of a vertebral body; the compression is most marked anteriorly so that the vertebral body becomes wedge-shaped. The spinal cord is not injured and the fracture is stable.

Treatment. Reduction of a wedge compression fracture of the cervical spine is neither necessary nor advisable. Support of the cervical spine in a plastic collar provides comfort for the patient during the six weeks required for bony healing (Fig. 17.52).

Flexion Subluxation of the Cervical Spine

When an individual's head moves forward suddenly and violently, as it does with the instant *deceleration* of a head-on collision or from a blow on the back of the head, one vertebral body in the lower half of the cervical spine may slide forward in relation to the subjacent vertebra. The posterior longitudinal ligaments are disrupted but provided the posterior facet joints do not override, the injury is classified as a *subluxation*. The subluxation may reduce spontaneously, however, so that initial radiographs may not reveal the true extent of the injury—hence the value of stress radiography to detect occult joint instability (Fig. 17.53a and b).

The spinal cord may be contused at the moment of injury but usually escapes serious injury unless the spinal canal has been narrowed by pre-existent osteophytes associated with degenerative joint disease of the cervical spine (cervical spondylosis).

Treatment. Passive extension of the cervical spine reduces the flexion type of subluxation and the reduction should be maintained by immobilization of the extended neck in a plaster collar for at least two months. If ligamentous healing is inadequate the resultant residual instability of the injured segment may cause symptoms of sufficient severity that local spine fusion becomes necessary (Fig. 17.53C).

Flexion Dislocation and Fracture-Dislocation of the Cervical Spine

In these injuries, which are more severe and much more serious than a flexion subluxation but which arise from the same mechanisms of injury, the posterior longitudinal ligaments are torn and the posterior facet joint on one or both sides has lost contact with its mate. The facet joints may be overriding and locked or they may be widely separated; there is usually a coexistent fracture of the anterior margin of the subjacent vertebra (Figs. 17.54 and 17.55).

This exceedingly unstable injury is frequently complicated by either complete transection or severe contusion of the spinal cord with resultant paraplegia.

Treatment. Reduction of a flexion dislocation or fracture-dislocation of the cervical spine may be difficult, particularly if the facet joints are locked in an overriding position. Powerful continuous skull traction under ra-

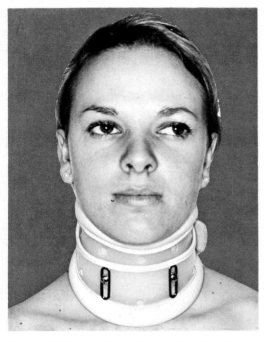

Figure 17.52. Adjustable plastic collar for the support of stable injuries of the cervical spine.

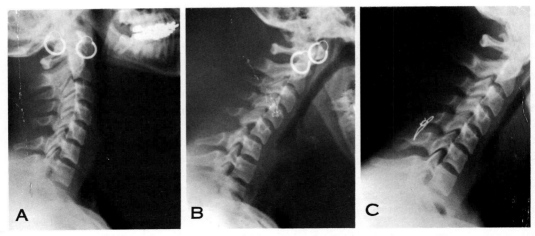

Figure 17.53. Flexion subluxation of the cervical spine at the C.5-C.6 level in a young woman who had been injured in a head-on automobile collision. *A*, the initial lateral radiograph does not reveal any frank evidence of a fracture or a dislocation but note the widening of the space between the spinous processes of C.5 and C.6 and also the soft tissue swelling between the trachea and the cervical spine at the C.5-C.6 level, both of which are clues that the cervical spine has been injured at this level. *B*, a lateral radiograph taken with the patient's neck in flexion (under the control of the surgeon and with the patient conscious) reveals a true flexion subluxation between C.5 and C.6. Note the gap between these two spinous processes indicating disruption of the posterior longitudinal ligaments. Note also that the posterior facet joints, although subluxated, have not overriden. These two radiographs serve as a good example of occult joint instability in the spine and emphasize the value of stress radiography. *C*, a lateral radiograph of the same woman's cervical spine after local posterior spinal fusion of C.5 to C.6. Fusion was necessitated by persistent segmental instability and pain.

diographic control is required—if necessary up to 40 pounds of traction—to distract the facet joints after which reduction is achieved by gradual extension of the neck and decreasing the amount of traction. The reduced dislocation or fracture-dislocation should then be immobilized in extension in a plaster cast of the Minerva type which incorporates the head, neck and chest for at least two months.

Failure to obtain a complete reduction by continuous traction is an indication for open reduction. Residual instability after the period of immobilization is an indication for local spinal fusion; indeed there is some justification for the opinion that local spinal fusion is indicated after every major dislocation or fracture-dislocation of the cervical spine for the purpose not only of preventing residual symptoms but also of preventing recurrent displacement from a subsequent injury.

Extension Sprains of the Cervical Spine

Whereas flexion injuries may produce a flexion subluxation, dislocation or fracture-dislocation as described above, *extension* injuries tend to produce extension *sprains*, some of which may represent *momentary subluxations*.

Mechanism of Injury. By far the commonest cause of significant extension injuries of the cervical spine in the present era is the rear-end collision. The mechanism of injury is as follows. An individual is sitting facing forward in a stopped automobile (for example at a traffic light), his back supported by the back of the seat but his head completely unsupported. At this moment his automobile is suddenly struck from the rear by a moving automobile; it is shot forward with considerable force and is thereby instantly *accelerated*. The body of the individual in the struck automobile is therefore instantly accelerated also; but his unsupported head is momentarily left behind with the result that his cervical spine is suddenly forced into extreme extension. Thus, the soft tissues on the anterior aspect of the neck are stretched and thereby sprained; the severity of the sprain depends on the rate of acceleration of the individual's body which, in turn depends on the force of impact and the rate of acceleration of his automobile when it was struck from the rear.

Terminology. These common injuries, which are best considered and described as

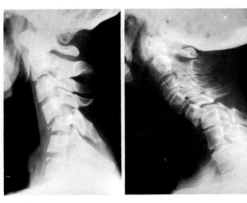

Figure 17.54 (*left*). Flexion fracture-dislocation of the cervical spine at the C.4–C.5 level in a young man who had dived into shallow water and had struck the back of his head on the bottom. He had an incomplete paraplegia. Note the forward displacement of C.4 on C.5, the fracture of the body of C.5, the locked posterior facet joints and the wide gap between the spinous processes of C.4 and C.5, indicating disruption of the posterior longitudinal ligaments.

Figure 17.55 (*right*). Flexion dislocation of the cervical spine at the C.5–C.6 level in a young woman who at the time of a head-on automobile accident was thrown from her car and landed on the back of her head. She was not wearing a seat belt! The initial radiographs were said to have been normal but three days after injury the patient became partially paraplegic—these radiographs reveal a complete dislocation. Note the forward displacement of C.5 on C.6, the complete loss of contact between the posterior facet joints and the wide gap between the spinous processes indicating complete disruption of the posterior longitudinal ligaments at this level. After gradual reduction of this extremely unstable dislocation by skull traction, a local posterior spinal fusion was performed and the patient's neurological lesion recovered.

acceleration extension sprains of the neck, are regrettably often referred to, especially in lay circles, as "whiplash injuries," a term that is both inaccurate and misleading (the head and neck are hardly comparable to the end of a whip). Moreover, the use of the emotional and dramatic term "whiplash" tends to exaggerate the seriousness of the injury and thereby leads to unrealistic litigation. The injury should be considered for what it is, namely a *sprain* of the neck, in the full realization that some sprains are understandably more severe than others and that some even represent momentary subluxation.

Clinical Features. The patient experiences pain that is not well localized in the front of the neck, and sometimes pain radiating into the upper limbs from nerve root irritation. As with other sprains, the pain may not be particularly severe at the time of injury but becomes more severe during the ensuing few days. Neck motion, especially extension, is guarded by muscle spasm. In the majority of patients with acceleration extension sprains of the neck, the symptoms are of relatively short duration but for others with more severe sprains the symptoms may persist for six months, a year or even longer. Those relatively few patients with particularly severe injuries may complain of symptoms that seem bizarre but that are explainable, since many different structures can be stretched at the time of injury. Thus, Macnab has suggested that blurring of vision and vertigo might be explained on the basis of injury to the cervical sympathetic nerves; difficulty in swallowing could be due to hemorrhage in the wall of the oral pharynx and esophagus; nystagmus and tinnitus might be due to vertebral artery spasm.

Radiographic Features. Despite the plethora of symptoms, there is a paucity of abnormal radiographic findings. The usual radiographic examination is negative although it is possible that stress radiography of the neck in extension might reveal evidence of occult segmental instability at one or more intervertebral disc spaces in the cervical spine.

Treatment. As with other sprains the initial treatment of acceleration extension sprains of the neck includes splinting and analgesics. Appropriate splinting can be provided by two, three or even four cervical ruffs (Fig. 17.56). If symptoms persist after the acute phase, a removable plastic cervical collar usually provides adequate splinting (Fig. 17.57). When the injury has been severe, the patient should lie in bed for a week or more—to take the weight off his neck. Persistent neck and arm pain can be relieved temporarily by intermittent cervical traction which can be readily applied by the patient at home (Fig. 17.58).

Patients who have sustained other significant injuries at the time of neck injury frequently complain of their neck long after symptoms have subsided from the other injuries. Thus, they should not be lightly dismissed as being "neurotic" or "litigation-minded." Such patients must be reassured that neck symptoms, though irritating and discouraging, will eventually subside. Only a small percentage of these patients ever require local spinal fusion for residual segmental instability.

Prevention. From your understanding of

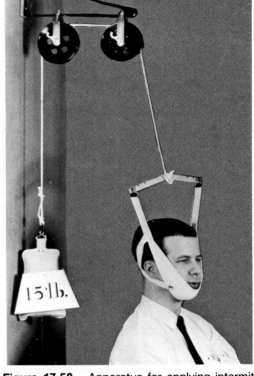

Figure 17.58. Apparatus for applying intermittent halter traction to the cervical spine. This form of treatment, which often provides temporary relief of pain, can be carried out in the patient's home.

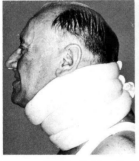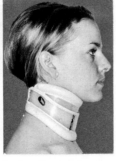

Figure 17.56 (*left*). Cervical ruffs made from stockinette filled with cotton wool. These three ruffs are supporting the head and providing relative immobilization of the cervical spine for this man who had sustained an extension acceleration sprain of his neck in a rear-end collision.
Figure 17.57 (*right*). Adjustable and removable plastic collar for the support of stable injuries, such as an extension acceleration sprain, of the cervical spine. The collar can be adjusted to provide immobilization in a more flexed position for an extension injury.

the mechanism of injury in acceleration extension injuries of the neck, you will appreciate that the most effective method of *prevention* is incorporation of head rests in the backs of automobile seats.

Fracture of the Seventh Cervical Spinous Process

The spinous process of the seventh cervical vertebra is longer than others in the cervical spine and to it are attached a multitude of muscles. As a result of sudden violent muscular contraction, this spinous process may be avulsed. The fracture is sometimes referred to as a "clay shoveler's fracture" since it is relatively common in workmen who are shoveling wet clay which unexpectedly sticks to the shovel at the end of the backward throw; the fracture may also occur during vigorous athletics.

pain and there is well localized tenderness. The diagnosis is readily confirmed radiographically (Fig. 17.59).

Treatment. Pain can usually be relieved by cervical ruffs which prevent flexion and extension of the cervical spine, but bed rest may be necessary for a few days. Occasionally surgical excision of the avulsed spinous process is required to relieve persistent pain.

INJURIES OF THE THORACIC AND LUMBAR SPINE

Fractures of the thoracic and lumbar spine are relatively common, particularly in the thoracolumbar region, and are usually the result of a fall on the buttocks or feet. The fractures are generally of the compression type, either *wedge compression* or *bursting compression*, and are *stable* injuries.

Less common but more serious are fracture-dislocations of the spine which are usually caused by automobile accidents. Since these are *unstable* injuries, either the spinal cord or the cauda equina is frequently damaged. The important topic of *traumatic paraplegia* is discussed in Chapter 12.

Wedge Compression Fractures

When the spine is in the flexed position, compression forces from below (as with a severe fall on the buttocks) or from above (as with a cave-in on a crouching miner) cause the spine to suddenly flex beyond its normal range. The compression is greatest on the concavity of the curve and hence on the anterior portions of the vertebral bodies.

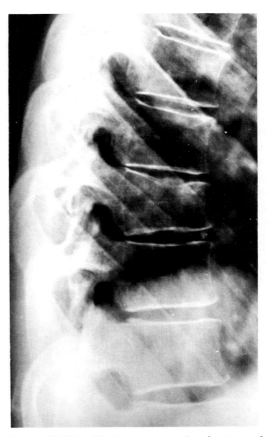

Figure 17.60. Wedge compression fracture of a vertebral body in the mid-thoracic region of a 35-year-old man who had slipped at the top of the stairs and had bounced down one flight on his buttocks. Note that the injured vertebral body has lost height and become wedge-shaped as a result of being compressed anteriorly. This is a stable injury.

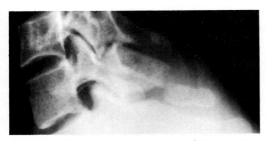

Figure 17.59. Avulsion fracture of the spinous process of C.7 (so-called "clay shoveler's fracture"). The patient, a professional wrestler, sustained this fracture as he attempted to throw his reluctant opponent out of the ring.

The posterior longitudinal ligaments remain intact and consequently one or more vertebral bodies are crushed anteriorly, the result being a *wedge compression fracture* with anterior impaction.

Clinically, the symptoms may be mild but there is local tenderness; the impaction is seen most readily in the lateral radiograph (Fig. 17.60).

Treatment. Since wedge compression fractures are stable injuries and since the spinal cord and cauda equina are not injured, relatively little treatment is required. For the young it may be reasonable to hyperextend the spine in an attempt to correct the slight kyphosis at the fracture site and then to apply a body cast. In general, however, it is wiser to allow the fracture to heal in its impacted state. If the symptoms are mild, a short period of bed rest followed by active exercises are all that is required. For more severe injuries the patient's pain can be relieved by wearing a body cast for four weeks during which time active exercises are performed. In the elderly, particularly with compression fractures through either osteoporotic bone or metastases, a spinal brace or reinforced surgical corset is more practical.

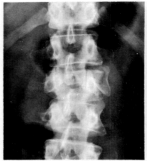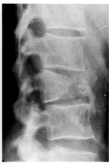

Figure 17.61. Bursting compression fracture of the second lumbar vertebra of a 41-year-old man who, on escaping from a prison at night with more haste than decorum, had jumped from a third-story window and landed on his feet in an upright position. Note that the adjacent intervertebral disc spaces are narrowed indicating that the discs have been driven into the vertebral body from above and below. The bursting nature of the comminuted fracture is more obvious in the lateral projection. Since the posterior longitudinal ligaments are intact, this is a stable injury. Despite this spinal injury and coexistent fractures of both os calci, the patient was able to get up and take off. Understandably, however, he was unable to keep ahead of his pursuers.

Bursting Compression Fractures

When the spine is relatively straight, (as with a fall from a height and landing on the feet) compression forces are vertical and the result is a bursting type of fracture of a vertebral body; the intervertebral disc is driven into the cancellous bone of the vertebral body and comminuted fracture fragments burst out in all directions. Nevertheless, the posterior spinal ligaments are intact and consequently the spinal column is stable. The spinal cord and cauda equina are seldom injured; only rarely is a posterior fragment driven backward sufficiently far to cause a neurological injury.

Clinically, the symptoms are more severe from a bursting compression fracture than from a simple wedge compression fracture. The patient's heels should be examined both clinically and radiographically; the aforementioned mechanism of injury explains the common coexistence of a fracture of the os calcis. Radiographs reveal the bursting nature of the fracture (Fig. 17.61).

Treatment. No reduction of the fracture is required. The patient is usually most comfortable lying in bed for the first few weeks after which he should wear a well fitted plaster body cast for eight weeks. Occasionally, residual segmental instability causes chronic low back pain of such severity that local spinal fusion is justified.

Fracture-Dislocations

Violent spinal injuries, such as may be sustained in automobile accidents, have a rotatory and sometimes a lateral force su-

perimposed upon a flexion force. The spine is literally torn apart; the posterior longitudinal ligaments are torn, the posterior facet joints may be fractured, the upper part of the involved vertebral body seems to be sheared off and the spinal column is dislocated and completely unstable. In the thoracic region the spinal cord is almost always injured and is frequently completely transected. In the lumbar region the cauda equina is usually damaged, but not necessarily transected.

Clinical features include shock from the severity of the injury. Some degree of neurological deficit is usually obvious. Complete neurological examination is essential, however, and must be repeated frequently during the first few days to detect any changes in the neurological picture. Radiographic examination depicts the gravity of the injury (Fig. 17.62).

Treatment. Management of an associated *traumatic paraplegia* (as discussed in Chapter 12), of course, takes precedence over treatment of the fracture-dislocation.

In the absence of paraplegia the fracture-dislocation must be reduced with care and the spine stabilized to prevent subsequent neurological damage. Open reduction, rigid internal fixation, and the addition of bone grafts are indicated.

Even in the presence of complete paraplegia, early open reduction, rigid internal fixation, and bone grafting reduce the risk of subsequent injury to nerve roots that may have been spared (Fig. 17.63). Moreover, this form of treatment greatly facilitates nursing care, diminishes the incidence of decubitus ulcers and renders the early phases of rehabilitation more effective.

Thorax

FRACTURES OF THE RIBS

The ribs, being flat bones (as opposed to long bones), are composed of cancellous bone surrounded by thin cortices. As you might expect, therefore, fractured ribs heal readily despite the continued movement of breathing; indeed, non-union is almost unknown.

Ribs are fractured by either striking or being struck by a hard object. Unless the

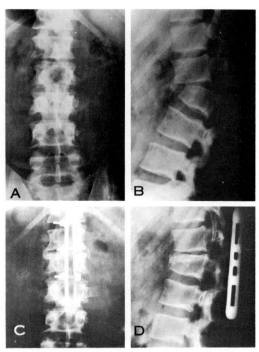

Figure 17.63. Severe fracture-dislocation of the lumbar spine at the L.3–L.4 level in a 38-year-old pilot of a small aircraft that crashed. This man sustained a severe cauda equina injury. *A* and *B*, initial radiographs revealing forward displacement of L.3 on L.4; the true extent of the injury is obvious only in the lateral projection. The posterior longitudinal ligaments were completely disrupted and the spine was completely unstable. *C* and *D*, radiographs of the same patient immediately after open reduction, internal fixation and bone grafting of the fracture-dislocation.

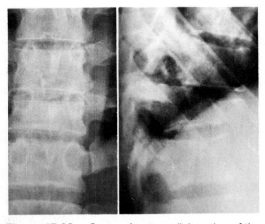

Figure 17.62. Severe fracture-dislocation of the thoracic spine at the T.9–T.10 level in a 24-year-old man whose speeding sports car went out of control and hit a tree. This man was rendered completely and permanently paraplegic. Note the forward displacement of T.9 and T.10 and the sheared off upper part of the body of T.10 in the lateral projection. The posterior longitudinal ligaments were completely disrupted and the spine was completely unstable.

injury is extremely severe, the fractured ends are seldom displaced because the ribs are firmly bound to one another by the intercostal muscles. Clinically there is local pain that is aggravated by deep breathing, coughing and sneezing. Local tenderness is readily detected and the pain is increased by anteroposterior compression of the chest (which "springs" the ribs outward). The fractures are usually, but not always readily visualized radiographically (Fig. 17.64).

Treatment

The chest wall cannot be completely immobilized. Circumferential strapping of the chest, however, does minimize movement and provides some relief of pain though the Clinically the patient experiences local

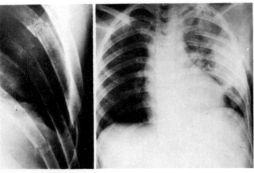

Figure 17.64 (*left*). Undisplaced fractures of the 7th, 8th and 9th left ribs in a 50-year-old-man who had slipped while getting out of the bathtub and had struck the left side of his chest on the edge of the tub.
Figure 17.65 (*right*). Contusion of the left lung in association with fractures of six ribs (2nd, 3rd, 4th, 5th, 6th, and 7th) in a 54-year-old-man who had been knocked down by an automobile. Note the diffuse radiographic density in the upper two-thirds of the left lung.

strapping may be irksome in itself. In the elderly, strapping of the chest is inadvisable because of the risk of hypostatic pneumonia. Injection of the regional intercostal nerves with a long-acting anesthetic agent often provides lasting comfort.

Complications of rib fractures include: (1) puncture of the pleura with a resultant hemothorax; (2) puncture of the lung with resultant pneumothorax; (3) contusion of the underlying lung (Fig. 17.65).

The Foot
FRACTURES OF THE METATARSALS

The metatarsals are most commonly fractured by either a heavy object dropping on the forefoot or a run-over injury with a metal wheel. Frequently more than one metatarsal is fractured, in which case the most significant aspects of the injury are not the fractures but the internal hemorrhage and impairment of circulation to the forefoot (Fig. 17.66).

Treatment

The metatarsal fragments should be sufficiently well aligned that no metatarsal head is left depressed into the sole (in which position it could cause a painful callus later). Pressure dressings and elastic bandages

must be avoided because of the impaired circulation; a well molded plaster cast is preferable. Occasionally Kirschner wire fixation is required to stabilize multiple fractures. After a period of at least four weeks of non-weight-bearing, a walking cast can be worn for an additional four weeks.

FRACTURES OF THE OS CALCIS (CALCANEUM)

The os calcis, which is composed principially of cancellous bone with a thin surrounding cortex, has a good blood supply and for these reasons fractures of this bone unite rapidly. The major problem related to these fractures is coexistent *intra-articular injury to the subtalar joint*.

The usual mechanism of injury is a fall from a considerable height on one or both heels. Thus, both heels should always be carefully examined. Moreover, there is a high incidence of associated compression fractures of the spine which should also be examined both clinically and radiographically in every patient who has sustained a fracture of the os calcis.

In the normal os calcis the superior surface of the tuberosity and that of the subtalar joint meet at an angle of approximately 40°—the *tuberosity-joint angle* or *salient angle* (Fig. 17.67A). When the os calcis is

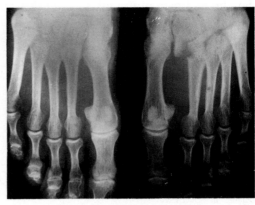

Figure 17.66. Displaced fractures at the base of the left 2nd, 3rd and 4th metatarsals and an undisplaced fracture of the base of the first metatarsal in a workman whose foot had been run over by one metal wheel of a heavy trolley. The foot was grossly swollen and the circulation to the toes was temporarily impaired.

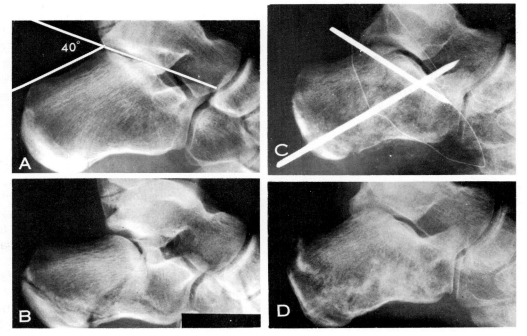

Figure 17.67.   Intra-articular fracture of the os calcis in a young man who, while on a psychedelic drug "trip" took an unplanned trip from a second-story balcony to the pavement and landed on his left heel. *A*, lateral radiograph of the patient's normal, uninjured heel showing the normal tuberosity-joint angle or salient angle of 40°. *B*, comminuted fracture of the patient's injured os calcis. The lateral portion of the subtalar joint is split off and depressed; the tuberosity-joint angle has been decreased to 20° as a result of compression of the os calcis. *C*, immediately after open reduction of the fractures, internal fixation with Kirschner wires and packing of the resultant defect on the lateral side with cancellous bone grafts. Note that the tuberosity-joint angle has been restored. *D*, three months after injury the fractures have united in satisfactory position.

crushed between the landing surface and the undersurface of the talus at the time of the fall, it is flattened somewhat and this angle is decreased or even reversed. The os calcis either splits into two or more major fragments or becomes severely comminuted into innumerable fragments. Since the subtalar joint is the most important structure in relation to fractures of the os calcis it is best to consider such fractures in two main groups—those that do not involve the joint (*extra-articular fractures*) and those that do (*intra-articular fractures*). Special radiographic projections are required to visualize the os calcis in three planes.

Extra-articular Fractures

Vertical split fractures of the tuberosity of the os calcis and horizontal "beak" fractures of the tuberosity are manifest by severe local pain and inability to bear weight; there is little swelling, however, and subtalar joint motion is not impaired.

Treatment. For *vertical split fractures*, the two major fragments should be manually compressed from side to side under anesthesia. The foot is kept elevated for one week after which a well molded plaster walking cast can be worn for six weeks. For the *horizontal "beak" type of fracture* the same period of elevation of the foot is required but the foot is held in equinus in the walking cast to prevent further displacement.

The results of treatment for extra-articular fractures are good.

Intra-articular Fractures

Fractures in which the lateral part of the subtalar joint is split off and severely comminuted crush fractures both involve the subtalar joint and are therefore much more serious than extra-articular fractures. In addition to the aforementioned symptoms, typical physical signs include marked swelling, broadening and loss of height of the heel and painfully restricted motion in the subtalar joint. Radiographs are essential in the differentiation of these two major types of intra-articular fracture (Figs. 17.67*B* and 17.68).

Treatment. The only fractures of the os calcis amenable to open reduction and internal fixation are those in which *the lateral portion of the subtalar joint is split off and depressed*. At open reduction the depressed portion of the joint surface is elevated and bone grafts are packed into the resultant defect (Fig. 17.67*C*). A plaster cast is worn for six weeks but no weight bearing is permitted until the fracture is united.

The *severely comminuted crush fractures* of the os calcis are not amenable to reduction (Fig. 17.68). *Non-operative* treatment of this severe injury involves elevation of the foot for at least one week and active exercises followed by gradually increasing weight bearing using crutches as soon as the acute pain has subsided. The results of this form of treatment are not good in that the heel remains broad, the subtalar joint is stiff (and often painful) and there is decreased calf muscle power (as a result of elevation of the tuberosity and consequent slackness in the muscle). Most patients do manage to walk about, however, with some residual symptoms within six months. An *operative* form of treatment for these severely comminuted crush fractures is delayed primary arthrodesis of the subtalar joint two or three weeks after injury. Weight bearing is not allowed for at least three months by which time the joint is usually fused. The results of such operative treatment, particularly for persons under 60 years of age, would seem to be somewhat better than the results of non-operative treatment; at least one source of residual pain—the subtalar joint—has been eliminated.

Regardless of the method of treatment, however, residual symptoms are likely to arise from the severely damaged fat pad under the os calcis.

FRACTURES OF THE NECK OF THE TALUS

The talus, like the carpal scaphoid, has no muscles attached to it, is largely covered by articular cartilage and has a precarious blood supply. It is not surprising, therefore, that fractures of the neck of the talus are associated with a high incidence of avascular necrosis of one fragment (the body) and nonunion.

The mechanism of injury is a severe dorsiflexion injury as may be incurred when the driver of an automobile has his foot pressed hard on the brake pedal at the moment of a head-on collision. If the injury is extremely severe the body of the talus may even be dislocated posteriorly.

Treatment

Closed reduction can usually be achieved by bringing the foot—and with it the head of the talus—into equinus (Fig. 17.69). The foot and ankle are then immobilized in this position in a below knee cast for at least eight weeks and no weightbearing is permitted during this time.

Complications

Avascular necrosis of the body of the talus complicates approximately half of all displaced fractures of the neck of the talus. The body becomes first relatively dense radiographically and eventually it becomes absolutely dense as revascularization takes

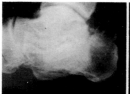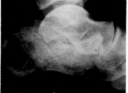

Figure 17.68. Severely comminuted fractures of both os calci of a 41-year-old fireman who fell 30 feet from a ladder and landed on his feet (he also sustained a bursting compression fracture of his lumbar spine). This man's subtalar joints are irreparably damaged. After two weeks of elevation of both feet, delayed primary arthrodesis of both subtalar joints was performed.

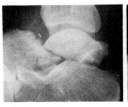
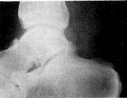

Figure 17.69. Displaced fracture of the neck of the talus in the right foot of a young man who had his foot pressed hard on the brake pedal at the moment of a head-on collision. *Left*, initial radiograph showing upward displacement and dorsiflexion of the foot through the fracture. *Right*, the post-reduction radiograph reveals satisfactory position of the fracture fragments.

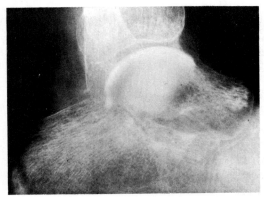

Figure 17.70. Avascular necrosis of the body of the talus as a complication of a fracture through the neck. In this radiograph, nine months after injury, the increased radiographic density in the body of the talus is both relative (to the surrounding living bone that has become osteoporotic from disuse) and absolute (in relation to the normal opposite talus since with revascularization, new bone has been laid down on dead trabeculae).

place and new bone is laid down on dead trabeculae (Fig. 17.70). Despite relief of weightbearing for many months, this complication almost inevitably leads to *degenerative joint disease of both the ankle and the subtalar joints*, necessitating arthrodesis of these joints. *Non-union* of the fractured neck of the talus is treated by bone grafting, provided the body of the talus is viable.

The Ankle

The normal ankle joint moves in one plane only—the plane of plantar flexion and dorsiflexion—and thus it is not surprising that the forces of abduction, adduction, external and internal rotation to which the ankle is so frequently subjected may tear ligaments or produce intra-articular fractures. Indeed, in adults, the ankle is the most frequently injured major joint in the body.

SPRAINS OF THE LATERAL LIGAMENT

The common "sprained ankle" is nearly always the result of an inversion injury. An individual steps on an uneven surface, his foot is forcibly inverted through the subtalar joint and adducted through the ankle joint. The lateral ligament is severely stretched and a few fibers may even be torn but the inherent stability of the ankle is not lost.

Clinically, the ankle is painful; localized tenderness and swelling can be detected inferior and anterior to the tip of the lateral malleolus. Radiographic examination is necessary to differentiate a simple sprain from an undisplaced fracture of the fibula, and, if the stability of the ankle is doubtful, stress radiography under local or general anesthesia is indicated to exclude a tear of the lateral ligament (Fig. 17.71).

Treatment

Simple sprains of the lateral ligament require only adhesive strapping of the ankle to provide external support for three weeks as discussed in Chapter 15 (Fig. 15.97). Weight bearing is permitted immediately and full recovery may be expected.

TEARS OF THE LATERAL LIGAMENT

The same mechanism of injury that produces a sprain of the lateral ligament may completely tear the ligament if the injury is sufficiently severe. In order for the ligament to be completely torn, the ankle joint must have been momentarily subluxated or even dislocated.

The clinical features are comparable to those of a sprain but the swelling is greater and the joint is unstable. Radiographic examination is necessary to exclude a fracture, and stress radiography under local or general anesthesia is essential to detect the degree of ankle instability (Fig. 17.71). The uninjured ankle should be similarly assessed for comparison.

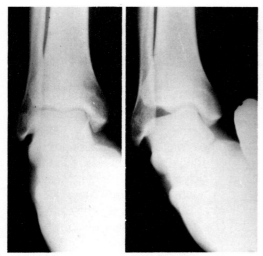

Figure 17.71. Occult joint instability. *Left*, anteroposterior radiograph of the ankle of a football player who, after an injury of his ankle, had pain, swelling and local tenderness over the lateral aspect of the joint. The radiographic examination of the joint is normal but this does not exclude occult joint instability. *Right*, anteroposterior radiograph of the same ankle while it is being stressed (stress radiograph) with the patient under general anesthesia. Note the marked opening up of the ankle joint (talar tilt) on the lateral side indicating joint instability associated with a complete tear of the lateral ligament of the ankle. The stress simulates the original injury.

Treatment

A complete tear of the lateral ligament of the ankle is a serious injury and can be more troublesome later than a fracture since bone heals more firmly than ligaments. The foot and ankle should be immobilized in a below-knee walking cast in a position of eversion and valgus for at least eight weeks; after the first week when the swelling has subsided the cast should be changed to obtain a better fit and better control of the ankle.

There is no evidence that surgical repair of this ligament offers any advantage over non-operative treatment.

Complications

If healing of the torn lateral ligament is inadequate, the patient will be plagued by *recurrent subluxation or even dislocation of the ankle*—particularly when walking on uneven ground. Simple measures such as an outflared heel and outside heel and sole

wedge in the shoe may control this problem but more often a new lateral ligament must be constructed surgically by means of a tenodesis using the tendon of the peroneus brevis muscle.

TOTAL RUPTURE OF THE ACHILLES TENDON

Sudden passive dorsiflexion of the ankle that is resisted by a powerful contraction of the calf muscle in an adult may result in a complete rupture of the Achilles' tendon (tendo achillis, calcaneal tendon). Most often the result of strenuous athletic activities, such ruptures can also occur from simple running or jumping, especially in middle-aged adults. Previous intratendinous injections of corticosteroid for tendinitis definitely cause local degenerative changes and predispose to rupture.

The patient, usually a male, experiences severe local pain and is unable to walk on his toes. Clinical examination reveals a gap in the tendon approximately 5 cm proximal to its insertion. Normally when an individual's calf is squeezed the ankle plantar flexes but not when the tendon is ruptured (Thompson's sign).

Some years ago non-operative treatment consisting of prolonged immobilization of the foot in a plantar flexed (equinus) position was advocated by many but in recent years the results of early operative repair have been proven to be definitely superior to those of non-operative treatment.

FRACTURES AND FRACTURE-DISLOCATIONS OF THE ANKLE

In adults the distal ends of the tibia and fibula (which are best considered as a unit) are fractured more often than any other bone with the exception of the distal end of the radius (Colles' fracture).

Mechanism of Injury

The wide variety of injuries can be more readily understood when you appreciate that the malleoli (medial malleolus, lateral malleolus and posterior margin of the tibia—sometimes referred to as "the third malleolus") can be either sheared off or avulsed. *Shearing injuries* fracture a malleolus at or above the joint line, the fragment having been pushed off by the talus. *Avulsion injuries* fracture a malleolus below the joint line, the fragment having been pulled off by the attached ligament. Thus, an abduction injury may produce a shearing fracture of the lateral malleolus and an avulsion fracture of the medial malleolus. A rotational injury, however, may shear off both malleoli, tear the distal tibiofibular ligament and even shear off "the third malleolus." If the distal tibiofibular joint is disrupted, the ankle mortice is too wide and there is always a lateral shift of the talus.

The term *"Pott's fracture-dislocation"* is often rather loosely used to include most fractures and fracture-dislocations involving the malleoli of the ankle. Thus, a *first degree injury* involves one malleolus, a *second degree injury* involves two malleoli (or the malleolus and one ligament) and a *third degree injury* includes all three malleoli (or two malleoli and one ligament).

Clinical Features

Ankle fractures and fracture-dislocations are particularly painful and the patient is unable to bear weight on the injured ankle. The swelling is variable but is often gross. The clinical deformity depends on the specific injury but, when both malleoli are fractured, the entire foot is displaced in relation to the leg (Fig. 17.72).

Radiographic Examination

Always include—in addition to the anteroposterior and lateral projections—two oblique projections lest the true extent of the injury escape detection.

Factors to Consider Concerning Treatment

Before discussion of the specific injuries, certain factors concerning treatment merit mention. The talus (which is still firmly attached to the foot) is the key to reduction of fractures and fracture-dislocations of the ankle since the malleoli are attached to the talus through their ligaments. Thus, in general, if the foot—and thereby the talus—is placed in proper relationship with the distal end of the tibia by reversing the mechanism of injury, the malleoli are guided back into

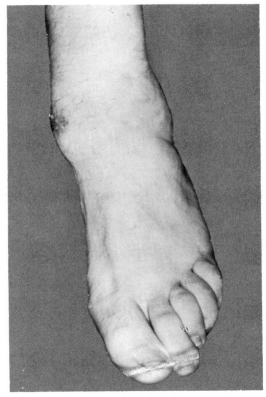

Figure 17.72. Clinical deformity of a fracture-dislocation of the ankle; this patient had sustained a second degree injury with fractures of both the medial and lateral malleoli. Note that the foot is displaced laterally and is rotated externally in relation to the leg.

reasonable position. Although reduction can usually be obtained, it may be difficult to maintain and hence internal fixation of one or more of the fractures may be required. Disruption of the distal tibiofibular joint must always be completely corrected, and such correction frequently necessitates internal fixation.

Various specific fractures and fracture-dislocations are discussed below.

Isolated Fractures of the Medial Malleolus

An abduction injury may avulse the medial malleolus below the joint line; an adduction or an external rotation injury may shear off the medial malleolus above the joint line. In either case, closed reduction is possible but the reduction is often unstable. Unless the reduction is perfect by closed means, open

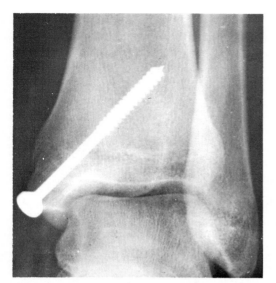

Figure 17.73. Post-reduction radiograph of the left ankle after open reduction of a displaced avulsion type fracture of the medial malleolus and internal fixation with a lag screw (which compresses the fracture). At operation a flap of periosteum was lifted out of the fracture site.

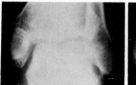 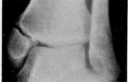

Figure 17.74. Non-union of a shearing type fracture of the medial malleolus in a 30-year-old man. Note the healed fracture of the shaft of the fibula. The non-union is more clearly seen in the oblique projection (*right*) than in the anteroposterior projection (left).

reduction and screw fixation are indicated since there is frequently a flap of torn periosteum interposed between the fracture fragments (Fig. 17.73). A below-knee cast should be worn for eight weeks and weight bearing may be permitted after the fourth week. A *complication* of medial malleolar fractures is *non-union* which necessitates bone grafting (Fig. 17.74).

Isolated Fractures of the Lateral Malleolus

In this, the commonest injury of the ankle joint, the lateral malleolus is sheared off above the joint line by either an abduction or an external rotation injury. Closed reduc-

tion is usually satisfactory since the reduction is stable and the only treatment required is immobilization of the ankle in a below-knee cast for six weeks. No weight-bearing is permitted for at least three weeks and often longer.

Fracture of the Lateral Malleolus and Tear of the Medial Ligament

In this common second degree injury, which is also the result of either abduction or external rotation, the lateral malleolus is sheared off and, in addition, the medial ligament of the ankle is torn so that the talus is displaced laterally. Radiographic examination reveals widening of the space between the talus and the medial malleolus (Fig. 17.75). Closed reduction of the fractured malleolus and of the lateral displacement of the talus is usually satisfactory but if the reduction is not perfect, open reduction and internal fixation of the fibula are indicated. A below-knee cast is worn for at least six weeks without weight bearing in order to allow firm healing of the ligament as well as of the fracture.

Fractures of Both Medial and Lateral Malleoli (Bimalleolar Fractures)

Severe injuries of either the abduction or external rotation type shear off the lateral

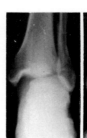 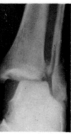 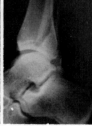

Figure 17.75. Shearing type fracture of the left lateral malleolus and lateral displacement of the talus in relation to the medial malleolus. *Left*, lateral displacement of the talus is most evident in the anteroposterior projection. *Center*, in this oblique projection the fibular fracture is seen to start below the distal tibio-fibular ligament, and hence there is no diastasis or separation. The lateral displacement of the talus is due to an associated tear of the medial ligament of the ankle. *Right*, in this lateral projection, what might be mistaken for a fracture of the posterior part of the tibia is the superimposed spiral fracture of the fibula.

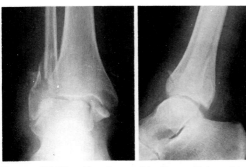

Figure 17.76. Fracture of both medial and lateral malleoli of the right ankle (bimalleolar fracture). The combination of abduction and external rotation has avulsed the medial malleolus but has sheared off the lateral malleolus. As a result of this second degree injury, the talus is displaced laterally in relation to the tibia.

malleolus above the joint line and avulse the medial malleolus below the joint line (Fig. 17.76). Although the malleoli can usually be reduced by closed means, the reduction is not always stable and may require open reduction and internal fixation of the medial malleolus and sometimes both malleoli. Immobilization in a below-knee cast is continued for at least three months.

Fractures of All Three Malleoli (Trimalleolar Fractures)

The addition of the posterior margin of the tibia as "the third malleolus" in this third degree injury is only an indication that external rotation has been of such severity that the talus has moved posteriorly to shear off part of the posterior margin. In other respects this injury is comparable to the bimalleolar fracture and is treated in the same way (Fig. 17.77). The fracture of the posterior margin of the tibia is usually small and seldom merits open reduction unless it involves a significant part of the weight-bearing surface.

Tibiofibular Separation

A severe abduction injury tears the tibiofibular ligament, and either avulses the medial malleolus or tears the medial ligament; in addition there is usually a fracture in the shaft of the fibula (Fig. 17.78). The talus is shifted laterally and reduction by closed means is usually unstable. A screw inserted across the tibiofibular joint is the most effec-

tive means of internal fixation. After a period of immobilization in a below-knee cast for eight weeks, the transfixion screw should be removed; otherwise it will eventually break as a result of subsequent motion at the tibiofibular joint.

Vertical Compression Fractures of the Tibia

These so-called "pylon" fractures are caused by landing on the feet from a considerable height and may either split or shatter the distal end of the tibia with complete disruption of the ankle joint. If there are only

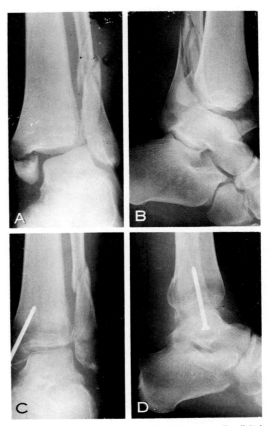

Figure 17.77. Fractures of all three malleoli (trimalleolar fracture) in the left ankle of a 36-year-old woman. *A*, note the avulsion type fracture of the medial malleolus, the lateral displacement of the talus and the comminuted spiral fracture of the shaft of the fibula. *B*, in this lateral projection the fracture of the posterior lip of the tibia ("the third malleolus") is apparent. *C* and *D*, anteroposterior and lateral radiographs after open reduction of the fractured medial malleolus and internal fixation with a screw. Note that the other two fractures have been thereby reduced and maintained in satisfactory position.

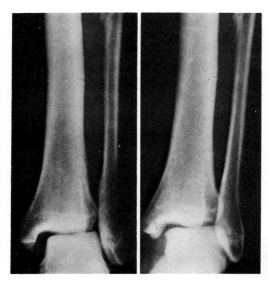

Figure 17.78. Tibiofibular separation of the left ankle in a 21-year-old skier who sustained an external rotation injury when his ankle harness failed to release. Note the lateral shift of the talus, which is more obvious in the anteroposterior projection (*left*) than in the oblique projection, (*right*), and which indicates that the medial ligament of the ankle has been torn. Note also the separation or diastasis of the tibiofibular joint. Did you also notice the spiral fracture of the mid-shaft of the fibula? This is a common site of fibular fracture in external rotation injuries; it may even be higher and emphasizes the importance of obtaining radiographs that include both the joint above and the joint below the fracture.

a few main fragments, open reduction and the AO system of rigid internal fixation may restore a reasonable joint surface (Fig. 17.79). The joint, however, may be irreparably damaged and the fracture too comminuted to secure by internal fixation; under these circumstances the most reasonable form of treatment is delayed primary arthrodesis of the ankle.

Complications of Ankle Joint Injuries

Ankle *joint stiffness* is a residual problem that follows many of the above described injuries. Active exercises help to regain motion and may have to be continued for as long as one year. Residual *swelling* of the soft tissues is almost inevitable and is difficult to prevent. After the period of immobilization, however, chronic swelling can be decreased, at least to some extent, by active exercises and by wearing an elastic stocking. *Non-union* is rare (except for the medial malleolus) but *malunion* is relatively common, usually as a result of loss of position of fragments after closed reduction.

Degenerative joint disease of the ankle is an almost inevitable sequel to malunion.

The Leg

FRACTURES OF THE SHAFTS OF THE TIBIA AND FIBULA

The shafts of the tibia and fibula are fractured more frequently than the shafts of any

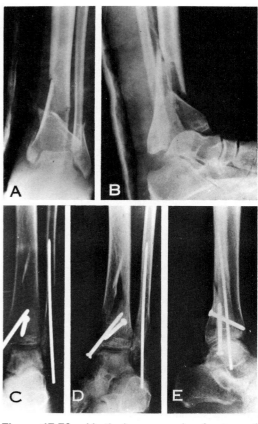

Figure 17.79. Vertical compression fracture of the left tibia of a 30-year-old steeplejack who fell 25 feet from a scaffold. *A* and *B*, initial radiographs with a temporary posterior plaster slab in place. Note the vertical fractures of the tibia and fibula with complete disruption of the ankle joint. *C* to *E*, postoperative radiographs after open reduction, internal fixation of the tibial fractures with screws and the fibular fracture with a thin intramedullary nail. Had the fractures been more comminuted, open reduction and internal fixation would not have been feasible.

of the other long bones. Furthermore, in adults the periosteum covering the tibia is thin, especially over its subcutaneous border, and consequently it is readily torn across with the result that tibial shaft fractures are often widely displaced. Understandably, the incidence of open fractures of the subcutaneous tibia is high. Moreover, the rate of union in tibial shaft fractures is slow, particularly when there has been severe disruption of the periosteum and surrounding soft tissues. Open reduction of severely displaced fractures of the tibial shaft is fraught with complications that are related to additional disturbance of blood supply to the bone ends, unsatisfactory skin healing in a tensely swollen leg, and postoperative infection. Thus, fractures of the shaft of the tibia present many serious problems.

Mechanism of Injury

The leg is particularly vulnerable to direct injury in automobile and motorcycle accidents. The forces are largely angulatory and the resultant fractures tend to be of the transverse or short oblique type—often with some comminution—the tibia and fibula being fractured at the same level. Rotational injuries of the tibia, which are common in skiers, tend to be oblique or spiral and may also be comminuted but the periosteum is usually intact.

Clinical Features

Swelling is a prominent feature of combined tibial and fibular fractures and, since the fascial compartments of the leg are relatively closed spaces, internal swelling frequently compresses vessels and thereby compromises the circulation to the foot. The skin may become so stretched by the swelling that areas of the epidermis lose their nutrition and become lifted up to form fracture blisters.

Radiographic Features

Unstable fractures of the tibia and fibular should always be temporarily splinted before the radiographic examination is conducted not only to prevent unnecessary pain but also to prevent further damage to the soft

tissues (Fig. 17.80). Four projections—anteroposterior, lateral and two obliques—provide the best indication of the extent of the injury and the relationship of the fracture fragments to one another.

Treatment

When both the tibia and fibula are fractured, treatment is aimed at reduction of the tibia. Even a slight amount of residual angulation or slight rotation at the fracture site results in obvious deformities and should therefore not be allowed to develop during treatment. Shortening under 2 cm is less serious since it can be well compensated by the patient while walking. The treatment of open fractures has been discussed in Chapter 15.

Stable transverse and oblique fractures of the tibia can usually be well managed by closed means using the principle of the intact periosteal hinge. When the mechanism of injury has been reversed and the fracture reduced, the intact periosteal hinge renders the reduction stable and prevents over-reduction. The plaster cast must then be applied in such a way that it holds the reduced fracture in the most stable position—just as the surgeon's hands were holding it. Therefore the cast should be applied first up to the knee (with the patient's leg hanging over the edge of a table) and then it should be carefully molded before it is extended to the top of the thigh with the knee flexed at least 30°. Inclusion of the partially flexed knee in the long leg cast helps to control rotation at the fracture site. Union is usually well advanced within three to four months (Fig. 17.81). An alternate form of treatment in-

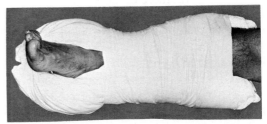

Figure 17.80.   Pillow splint for a fractured leg or ankle. There is less risk of circulatory disturbance and skin maceration with this type of splint than with an air splint.

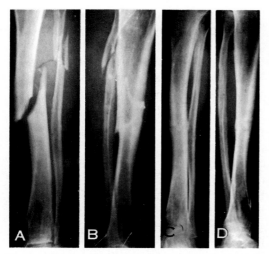

Figure 17.81. Oblique fracture of the mid-shaft of the tibia and a comminuted fracture of the fibula at a higher level—the result of a rotational injury. *A* and *B*, initial radiographs. Note the over-riding of the tibial fragments. *C* and *D*, four months after closed reduction and immobilization of the limb in a long leg cast. The fractures are firmly united in satisfactory position.

volves the use of a close fitting long leg walking cast in which the patient is encouraged to bear weight within a few days or more when the acute soreness has subsided. Even comminuted fractures of the tibia treated with early weight-bearing heal well, although there may be slight residual shortening (Fig. 17.82).

Incomplete correction of an angulatory deformity or subsequent loss of alignment in a cast after swelling has subsided can be corrected by appropriate wedging of the cast. Sometimes it is preferable to remove the cast completely, correct the residual deformity and apply a new, closely fitted cast.

For many fractures of the shaft of the tibia an acceptable alternative method of treatment is functional fracture-bracing after an initial period of up to six weeks of cast immobilization with the knee in extension.

Unstable oblique and spiral fractures of the tibia are prone to angulate and shorten after closed reduction. For this reason open reduction has often been performed using the AO system of internal fixation. Although used less frequently now than in the past

for fractures of the tibia, this is still a reasonable method of treatment provided it is restricted to carefully selected patients and their fractures as stated by Tile. (Fig. 17.83). Some of these fractures, however, can be more safely treated by non-operative means. As mentioned above, open reduction of tibial shaft fractures is fraught with *complications*, one of the most serious of which is postoperative infection with a resultant *infected non-union* (Fig. 17.84).

Unstable transverse and comminuted

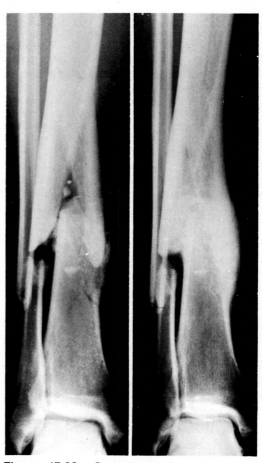

Figure 17.82. Comminuted fractures of the shafts of the tibia and fibula of a 22-year-old man who had been struck by an automobile while on his motorcycle. *Left*, the initial radiograph reveals shortening but satisfactory alignment. *Right*, the radiograph six months after closed treatment and early weight bearing in a long leg cast reveals firm union of the fractures with residual shortening of 2 cm. This amount of shortening is acceptable.

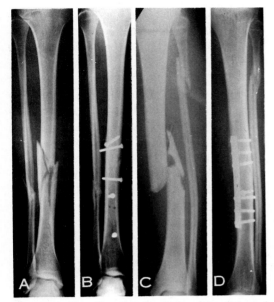

Figure 17.83. Unstable fractures of the tibia and fibula treated by open reduction and internal fixation. *A* and *B*, pre- and post-reduction radiographs of a comminuted fracture of the tibia and fibula in a 24-year-old woman as a result of a skiing injury. The fractures have been well maintained by screws. Nevertheless, this patient's fractures could have been treated equally well—and with greater safety—by closed means. *C* and *D*, initial radiograph and radiograph six months after a comminuted fracture of the mid-shaft of the tibia and of the fibula at a higher level. Note the large "butterfly" fragment. The tibial fracture has been treated by open reduction and internal fixation using a plate and screws. The result is satisfactory but could have been achieved more safely by closed means.

fractures of the tibial shaft are severe injuries which are associated with extensive soft tissue disruption; the latter accounts for their gross instability. While these fractures could certainly benefit from being stabilized, the risks of open reduction and internal fixation are particularly serious. These, the most serious of all fractures of the tibial shaft, many of them open fractures, should be treated with the least possible disturbance of the fracture site. The fracture can usually be aligned by light skeletal traction through a pin in the os calcis and counter-traction through a pin in the proximal end of the tibia, both pins being incorporated in a light plaster cast which rests on a Thomas splint (Fig. 17.85). Overdistraction of the fracture must be avoided. After six weeks, by which time the fracture is usually "sticky" (stable but still mobile), a long leg cast is applied.

An alternate method of treating completely unstable closed fractures of the midshaft of the tibia is closed ("blind") intramedullary nailing from the upper end of the tibia; the fracture site is not opened and the nail is driven across the reduced fracture site under radiographic control with an image intensifier.

Unstable segmental fractures of the tibial shaft are especially serious and can be difficult to control. Understandably these are often open fractures and are the result of an extremely severe injury. By means of external skeletal fixation "at a distance" these fractures can be stabilized while at the same time the associated soft tissue injuries are afforded the optimum opportunity to heal (Fig. 17.86).

Complications

Fractures of the soft shafts of the tibia and fibula are frequently complicated. *Ankle*

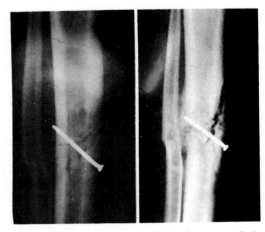

Figure 17.84. Closed oblique fracture of the tibia in a young adult. This simple fracture was treated (unnecessarily) by open reduction and internal fixation. *Left*, after operation a satisfactory reduction of the fracture. *Right*, four months later there is clear evidence of osteomyelitis, sequestra and an infected non-union. Unfortunately, the tibia is temptingly close to the skin but the temptation to operate upon it should be resisted on the basis of sound judgment.

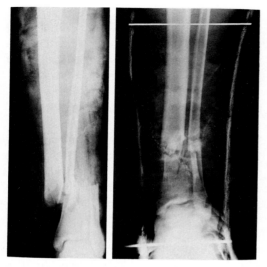

Figure 17.85. Unstable transverse comminuted fracture of the left tibia and fibula in a 30-year-old tree surgeon who, while treating a large tree, fell out of his patient! The 25-foot fall resulted in a severe fracture that was open from within. *Left*, this initial radiograph was obtained with a temporary posterior plaster splint in place. Note the comminution and also that the proximal fragment must be protruding through the skin on the medial aspect of the leg. The periosteum had been severely torn and consequently the fracture was extremely unstable. *Right*, after complete cleansing and debridement of the open wound, reduction of the fractures, wound closure and the insertion of two transfixion pins, one in the os calcis, the other in the proximal part of the tibia. Both pins have been incorporated in a light plaster cast to maintain the reduction by fixation "at a distance."

stiffness is common and may require vigorous exercises for one year or even longer. *Arterial injury*, a serious complication of high tibial fractures, must be recognized early and treated adequately to avoid gangrene. *Nerve injury* is common, particularly to the lateral popliteal nerve, with high fractures of the fibula—and occasionally from the local pressure of a plaster cast. *Persistent swelling* is almost inevitable but usually responds to active exercises and the use of an elastic stocking. *Delayed union* and *non-union* are common, particularly in severely displaced fractures; indeed if a tibial fracture is still mobile four months after injury, grafting with autogenous cancellous bone is indicated

(Fig. 17.87). *Mal-union*, which is nearly always preventable, produces not only an obvious deformity but may lead to degenerative joint disease in the malaligned knee or ankle joint.

Fractures of the tibia alone are not common. Being stabilized to some extent by the intact fibula, they are not severely displaced. Provided the fracture is reduced—by correcting angulation and rotation at the fracture site—the fibula does not hold the fragments apart. These fractures should be treated in the manner described above for stable transverse and oblique fractures.

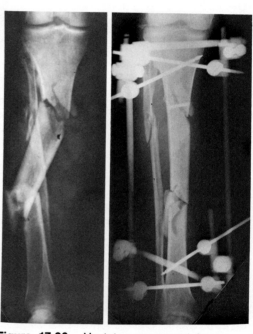

Figure 17.86. Unstable segmental fracture of the right tibia and fracture of the fibula in a 24-year-old man who had been involved in a motorcycle accident. The fracture was open from without; there was considerable skin loss and an associated arterial injury. *Left*, initial radiograph showing the large middle segment. Did you notice that this is an anteroposterior projection of the knee but a lateral projection of the ankle? This indicates a 90° external deformity through the fractures. *Right*, after complete cleansing and debridement of the open wound, reduction of the fractures, wound closure (which necessitated skin grafts) and the insertion of external skeletal fixation of the Roger-Anderson type. No cast was necessary and the fixation "at a distance" facilitated subsequent care of the soft tissues.

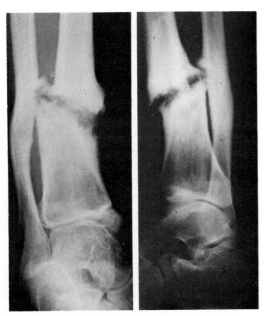

Figure 17.87. Non-union of an oblique fracture in the distal third of the right tibia. Note the broadening and sclerosis of the fracture ends, the varus deformity at the fracture site and the healed fracture of the fibula. Did you also notice the non-union of the medial malleolus?

Fractures of the fibula alone are relatively rare and you should always look for an associated fracture in the tibia or a fracture-dislocation at the ankle with disruption of the tibiofibular joint. Since the fibula is not a weight-bearing bone, isolated fibular shaft fractures require no immobilization and no restriction of weightbearing.

The Knee

FRACTURES OF THE PROXIMAL END OF THE TIBIA ("BUMPER FRACTURES")

The proximal end of the tibia, being composed almost entirely of cancellous bone and surrounded by a thin cortex, is susceptible to crushing injuries, particularly in persons over the age of 60 years in whom the cancellous bone tends to be relatively osteoporotic.

Mechanism of Injury

A severe abduction injury, usually a direct blow on the lateral aspect of the limb with the foot fixed on the ground, forces the knee into valgus and drives the femoral condyle into the lateral tibial plateau. The osteoporotic bone fractures before the medial ligament of the knee tears. The joint surface of the lateral tibial plateau may be crushed and depressed, the lateral condyle may be split off or both tibial condyles may be split off and associated with a transverse fracture. Frequently, the fractures are exceedingly comminuted. Clinically, the knee is acutely painful, and, since the fractures are intra-articular, there is always a tense hemarthrosis. Radiographic examination with at least four projections helps to access the extent of the comminution.

Treatment

While the knee joint may seem to be irreparably damaged, particularly with depressed lateral tibial plateau fractures, the intact lateral meniscus (which covers much of the articular surface of the lateral tibial plateau) provides a better gliding surface for the lateral femoral condyle than would be imagined from studying only the radiographs. This is fortunate since complete restoration of the tibial joint surface is often impossible by any means. Whatever form of treatment is used, the knee should be kept moving because residual knee joint stiffness is more disabling than residual deformity. In general, open reduction and internal fixation are more appropriate in relatively young adults than in the elderly. Treatment is best considered in relation to the various types of fractures.

Fractures of the lateral plateau with depression of the joint surface are usually severely comminuted (Fig. 17.88). In the elderly the most suitable form of treatment is closed reduction to shift the tibial plateau back into place followed by continuous balanced traction through a pin in the tibial shaft, the limb resting on the Pearson knee attachment of a Thomas splint. By this means, active motion can be initiated almost at once. The contour of the joint surface is disregarded but a valgus deformity is assiduously avoided. The traction is continued until the fracture is united, by which time the patient has a useful range of knee motion.

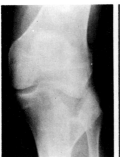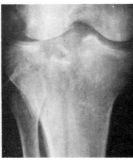

Figure 17.88. Fractures of the lateral plateau of the tibia. *Left,* severely comminuted fracture of the lateral plateau of the left tibia in a 75-year-old woman. The outer portion of the plateau has been split off and the lateral femoral condyle has been driven into the metaphysis of the tibia. Note the resultant valgus deformity of the knee. This elderly woman's fracture was treated by continuous traction through a pin in the tibia; her knee was kept mobile. *Right,* fracture of the lateral plateau of the right tibia in a 34-year-old man with depression of the joint surface. Note the lateral displacement of the lateral plateau in relation to the lateral femoral condyle. This young man's fracture was treated by open reduction and internal fixation of the vertical fracture, elevation of the joint surface through a "window" in the anterior cortex and packing of the resultant defect with cancellous bone grafts.

In younger persons the lateral condyle can be reduced at open operation and bolted to the medial condyle; at the same time the articular surface is elevated and the underlying defect is filled with autogenous cancellous bone grafts. The AO system of rigid internal fixation is particularly helpful in managing these fractures. After four weeks immobilization in an above-knee cast, the patient is encouraged to move the knee by active exercises, but weight-bearing is not permitted until the fracture is united.

Fractures of both tibial plateaus with marked comminution are best treated by means of continuous balanced traction and early knee motion as described above (Fig. 17.89). These fractures—which occur mostly in the elderly—are unsuitable for open reduction.

Fractures of the tibial plateaus with little comminution are seen more frequently in middle-aged adults and are grossly unsta-

ble. The most suitable form of treatment is frequently open reduction and internal fixation of the condyles (Fig. 17.90). The transverse element of the fracture can then be treated either in an above-knee cast or in continuous balanced traction.

Complications

The most serious complication of tibial plateau fractures is residual *knee stiffness* from both intra-articular and periarticular adhesions. Residual stiffness six months after injury is an indication for a gentle manipulation of the knee under anesthesia. *Injury to the lateral popliteal nerve* is common as a result of a local direct injury but can also be caused by local pressure from a plaster cast. *Degenerative joint disease* is less common than might be expected, partly because the most severely comminuted injuries occur in the elderly whose limited use of the knee and limited number of years in which to use it are such that significant degenerative changes may not develop. In younger persons degenerative joint disease limited to the lateral compartment of the knee can be effectively treated by means of a metallic hemi-arthroplasty of the MacIntosh type.

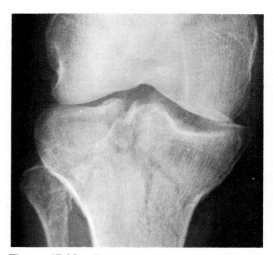

Figure 17.89. Fractures of both tibial plateaus with marked comminution in a 72-year-old woman. This elderly patient's fracture was treated by continuous skeletal traction through a pin in the tibia; her knee was kept mobile.

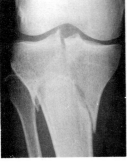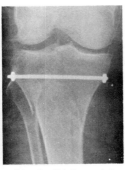

Figure 17.90. Fractures of both tibial condyles with little comminution in a 44-year-old woman. *Left*, initial radiograph which reveals separation of the two tibial plateaus. *Right*, after open reduction of the intra-articular part of the fracture and internal fixation with a transfixion bolt. Plaster immobilization was used to control the transverse element of the fracture.

INJURIES OF THE SEMILUNAR CARTILAGES (MENISCI)

The fibrocartilaginous menisci of the knee joint, although firmly attached to the tibia at their anterior and posterior ends, are only loosely attached peripherally and have a free tapered margin centrally. Thus, they are free to move slightly inward and outward during normal knee function. Under certain conditions described below, a meniscus may be ground between the joint surfaces with resultant splitting or tearing. The medial meniscus is much more vulnerable to such injuries than the lateral meniscus and consequently much of the discussion that follows pertains to tears of the medial meniscus.

Tears of the Medial Meniscus

The common injury of a torn medial meniscus occurs almost exclusively in young men, particularly those who engage in such sports as rugger, soccer, football and hockey and also those who work in a squatting position. Tears of the rather mobile medial meniscus are at least six times more common than those of the less mobile lateral meniscus; the difference in incidence may also be explained in part by the mechanism of their injury.

Mechanism of Injury. When an individual takes weight on his partially flexed knee and the tibia is externally rotated in relation to the femur, the medial meniscus is drawn toward the center of the joint; an abduction strain draws it in even farther. If, at this moment the normal ranges of external rotation and abduction are exceeded—as a result of either a fall or a blow on the lateral side of the knee—the medial meniscus may be trapped and then ground between the femoral condyle and the tibial plateau; it is thereby split along its long axis. In the aformentioned sports the lateral side of the lower limb is struck much more frequently than the medial side, and knee abduction injuries are more common than adduction injuries; this may explain the much higher incidence of medial meniscus tears.

Types of Tears of the Medial Meniscus. The commonest injury to a medial meniscus is the *bucket handle tear* (Fig. 17.91). Less common are the *posterior horn* and *anterior horn tears* (Fig. 17.92). Occasionally the peripheral soft tissue attachment of the meniscus is torn.

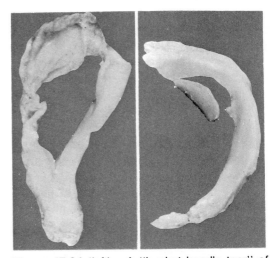

Figure 17.91 (*left*). A "bucket handle tear" of the left medial meniscus. The excised meniscus is seen from above; the inner portion of the meniscus had been displaced into the intercondylar notch.

Figure 17.92 (*right*). A tear of the posterior horn of the right medial meniscus. The excised meniscus is seen from above.

Clinical Features. The patient is usually able to relate a history of the typical injury as described above. He is usually unable to carry on and indeed may have to be carried off. If the tear has been of the *bucket handle type* with the inner portion dislocated into the intercondylar notch, the patient cannot fully extend the knee because of a mechanical block anteriorly. The term "locked knee" is often used to describe this phenomenon but the knee is still free to flex and is more precisely spoken of as being blocked rather than locked. Attempts to completely extend the knee passively are blocked by a springy resistance. Since the fibrocartilaginous menisci are avascular, there is no hemorrhage into the joint but a synovial effusion gradually develops over a few days. Even without treatment, the inner portion of the meniscus may slip back into place during the ensuing week or more—only to be displaced again as the result of a minor injury. In the patient's words he has "a trick knee." In between such episodes there may be little to find clinically other than measurable wasting of the quadriceps muscle.

A tear of the *posterior* or the *anterior horn* does not cause a block to extension although it may cause a "catching" sensation. The patient feels that his knee is unstable and likely to "give way" but he has difficultly localizing the problem to one side of the joint or the other. The patient experiences intermittent episodes of joint effusion and gradually the quadriceps muscle becomes somewhat atrophied.

Of considerable value in the clinical diagnosis of *posterior* or *anterior horn tears* is the McMurray test, which is conducted in the following way. With the patient's knee acutely flexed and one finger of the examiner's hand holding the foot, the tibia is alternately internally and externally rotated and then abducted and adducted. The free end of a posterior horn tear is thereby made to slip in and out between the joint surfaces with a palpable, and sometimes audible click. If no such sign is detected with the knee in acute flexion, the test is repeated in gradually increasing extension since it is only as the knee is partially extended that the click from the free end of an anterior horn tear will be palpated; indeed, the greater the extension of the knee at the time of the click the farther forward is the tear in the anterior horn.

Arthroscopy of the knee joint has proven to be of much value in the accurate diagnosis of tears of the menisci—both medial and lateral.

Radiographic Features. Plain radiographs provide no information concerning the state of the radiolucent menisci. Arthrography, by contrast, may prove extremely informative particularly when the clinical signs are equivocal (Fig. 17.93).

Treatment. When the diagnosis of a torn medial meniscus is established, the meniscus should be surgically excised (meniscectmony) since repeated episodes of displacement of the torn part of the meniscus are not only troublesome and temporarily disabling, they also lead inevitably to degenerative disease of the knee joint. Nevertheless, total meniscectomy may also lead

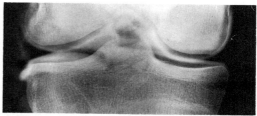
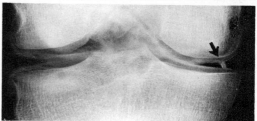

Figure 17.93. Arthrograms of the knee using a radio-opaque dye. *Top,* normal arthrogram of the right knee. Note the smooth wedge-shaped medial and lateral menisci clearly outlined by the dye in the joint. *Bottom,* arthrogram of the right knee revealing penetration of the dye into a vertical tear in the medial meniscus (*arrow*). By means of several oblique projections, the location and extent of the tear can be determined.

eventually to degenerative disease of the involved compartment of the knee.

For either bucket handle tears or flap tears of the menisci it is now considered preferable to excise only the "handle" or the "flaps," i.e. to perform only a partial meniscectomy, and this can be done either through an open arthrotomy or through the arthroscope (arthroscopic surgery).

Tears of the Lateral Meniscus

Because both the history and the physical signs are less definite, the relatively uncommon tears of the lateral meniscus are usually more difficult to diagnose clinically than those of the medial meniscus. The McMurray test may elicit a click from a torn posterior horn of the lateral meniscus when the flexed knee is gradually extended with the tibia adducted and internally rotated. Arthrography is often helpful in establishing the diagnosis as well as in detecting the presence of a congenital discoid cartilage (which is more prone to tear than a normal lateral meniscus).

Treatment. The only reasonable form of treatment for tears of the lateral meniscus is surgical excision of the entire meniscus (lateral meniscectomy).

LIGAMENTOUS INJURIES OF THE KNEE

The knee is basically a hinge joint through which occur flexion, extension and minor degrees of rotation. Its medial and lateral stability is provided by the strong medial and lateral ligaments while its anterior and posterior stability is provided by the anterior and posterior cruciate ligaments. Thus, these ligaments are vulnerable to any severe injury that forces the knee to move in an abnormal plane and such injuries are relatively common in sports such as football and hockey. A given ligament may be merely *sprained* (stretched with resultant tearing of a few fibers) or it may be *torn*, either partially or completely.

Tears of the Medial Ligament

Since the outer side of the knee is more exposed and hence more often struck than the inner aspect, the medial ligament is more often torn than any other ligament of the knee. A fierce tackle from the lateral side, for example, forces the ball carrier's knee into valgus and tends to open the knee joint on the medial side thereby spraining or even tearing the medial ligament. Indeed, if the injury is particularly severe, it may cause a tear not only of both portions (superficial and deep) of the medial ligament but also of the medial meniscus and the anterior cruciate ligament—"the unhappy triad" described by O'Donoghue.

Clinical Features. The patient usually feels "something give" in his knee at the moment of injury. The joint rapidly fills with blood and becomes acutely painful. Local tenderness is most marked over the course of the medial ligament, usually near its proximal attachment, and even gentle attempts to abduct the knee aggravate the pain. When a complete tear is suspected, examination should be repeated with the patient under general anesthesia to assess the stability of the knee.

Radiographic Features. Plain radiographs may show nothing more than soft tissue swelling. Stress radiographs, taken with the patient anesthetized, however, are extremely valuable in detecting occult joint instability (Fig. 17.94).

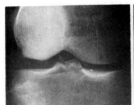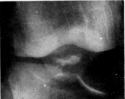

Figure 17.94. Occult joint instability of the right knee in a 21-year-old football player who had been tackled from the lateral side. *Left,* anteroposterior radiograph showing a normal relationship between the femur and tibia; this does not, however, exclude occult joint instability. Note the undisplaced fracture of the tibial spine. *Right,* anteroposterior radiograph of the same knee while it is being stressed in abduction with the patient under anesthesia. Note the marked opening up of the knee joint on the medial side which indicates a complete tear of both the superficial and deep portions of the medial ligament. Note also the displacement of the tibial spine fracture which indicates that the anterior cruciate ligament has been avulsed with its bony insertion.

Treatment. With *partial tears* of the medial ligament, the knee joint is stable even under anesthesia. The only treatment required, therefore, is aspiration of the hemarthrosis and immobilization of the extended knee in a cylindrical plaster cast for six weeks during which time the patient is allowed to walk and is encouraged to do isometric quadriceps exercises. With *complete tears* of the medial ligament, especially with associated tears of the anterior cruciate ligament, however, the knee joint is unstable. For middle-aged and elderly persons non-operative treatment by immobilization may be acceptable but for young persons—especially athletes—the ideal form of treatment is immediate exploration of the joint, surgical repair of the torn ligament or ligaments and capsule, and (if it is torn) excision of the medial meniscus. A delay of even a few days renders surgical repair much less satisfactory as the torn ends of the ligament become progressively more friable. Postoperative immobilization of the knee in a cylindrical cast for six weeks is necessary to permit sound healing of the ligament.

Tears of the Lateral Ligament

For reasons already mentioned, tears of the lateral ligament are less common than those of the medial ligament. The clinical and radiographic features as well as the treatment of lateral ligament tears are comparable to those of medial ligamentous tears with the sides reversed (Fig. 17.95). A unique complication of tears of the lateral ligament, however, is a traction injury of the lateral popliteal (peroneal) nerve which may even be irrecoverable.

Tears of the Cruciate Ligaments

The cruciate ligaments may be torn in association with tears of the medial or lateral ligaments but isolated tears of the cruciate ligament may also occur. Thus, if the tibia is driven forward on the femur (or the femur is driven backward on the tibia) or the knee joint is suddenly hyperextended, the *anterior* cruciate ligament may be torn. Examination reveals that the flexed knee is unstable when the tibia is pulled forward—the *"anterior drawer sign."*

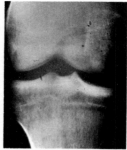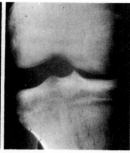

Figure 17.95. Occult joint instability of the right knee of a 20-year-old man who was knocked down by an automobile. *Left,* anteroposterior radiograph showing a normal relationship between the femur and the tibia; this does not, however, exclude joint instability. *Right,* anteroposterior radiograph of the same knee while it is being stressed in adduction with the patient under anesthesia. Note the marked opening up of the knee joint on the lateral side which indicates a complete tear of the lateral ligament. This patient also had a traction injury of his lateral popliteal (peroneal) nerve.

Another sign of anterior cruciate ligament insufficiency is the "lateral pivot shift" phenomenon described by Galway and MacIntosh. When the patient is completely relaxed and the involved knee is extended and the tibia is internally rotated, the lateral tibial plateau subluxates anteriorly in relation to the lateral femoral condyle. If a valgus strain is then applied to the knee and the joint is passively flexed, the subluxation is dramatically reduced as can be readily appreciated by both the examiner and the patient.

The reverse mechanism of injury may produce a tear of the *posterior* cruciate ligament in which case examination reveals that the flexed knee is unstable when the tibia is pushed backward—the *"posterior drawer sign."*

Treatment. Provided the medial and lateral ligaments of the knee are intact, strong quadriceps and hamstring muscles may effectively stabilize the knee even when one or other cruciate ligaments is torn. Operative repair is difficult and the most reasonable form of treatment for non-athletes is immobilization of the knee in a cylindrical cast. The patient is allowed to walk in the cast for six weeks and is encouraged to do quadriceps exercises, not only during the period of immobilization but also after.

For active athletic individuals who require good stability of the knee, currently available intra-articular and extra-articular methods of repair are reasonably effective.

Complications of Ligamentous Injuries of the Knee

The most troublesome complication of these injuries—especially for athletes—is residual *instability of the knee joint.* A knee brace is inadequate to provide stability and leads to disuse atrophy of surrounding muscles which aggravates the instability. Active exercises are indicated and help to develop strength in the muscles—particularly the quadriceps. Late repair of neglected ligamentous injuries may necessitate extensive reconstructive operations. Less frequently, residual *knee stiffness* is resistant to physiotherapy and requires a manipulation under an anesthetic. Occasionally *calcification* is seen at the site of avulsion of the proximal end of the medial ligament from the femoral condyle; this radiographic indication of a former injury at this site is sometimes referred to as *Pellegrini-Stieda's "disease."*

TRAUMATIC DISLOCATION OF THE KNEE

Extremely severe injuries to the knee, such as may be sustained in an automobile accident, tear all four major ligaments and result in a complete dislocation of the joint, an uncommon injury with understandably dramatic clinical and radiographic features (Fig. 17.96). The most serious immediate *complication* is a severe *injury to the popliteal artery*, which carries the risk of distal gangrene. The *medial popliteal nerve* may also suffer a serious injury. Treatment demands urgent reduction of the dislocation in the hope of minimizing the arterial and nerve injury, after which the major ligaments should be surgically repaired.

FRACTURES OF THE PATELLA

The patella is a sesamoid bone firmly embedded in the broad quadriceps expansion, and consequently the pull of the quadriceps muscle is not so much through the patella

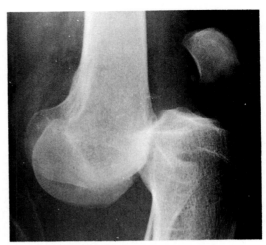

Figure 17.96. Traumatic anterior dislocation of the knee in a 28-year-old man who had sustained multiple injuries in an automobile accident. This amount of displacement indicates that all four major ligaments have been completely disrupted. This dislocation was complicated by an avulsion injury of the popliteal artery which necessitated surgical reconstruction with an arterial prosthesis.

as around it—through the aponeurotic expansion on the two sides and to a lesser extent in front. Thus, the patella is vulnerable to two entirely different types of injury; in the *indirect type*, tears of the quadriceps expansion at the level of the patella produce a transverse *avulsion fracture* of the patella whereas in the *direct type* (from a local blow) the patella is forcibly jammed against the lower end of the femur and sustains a *crush fracture* which is usually stellate and may be severely comminuted.

Avulsion Fractures

A sudden powerful contraction of the quadriceps muscle with the knee flexed, as may occur when an individual stubs his foot against something and tries to save himself from falling, may literally rip the entire quadriceps expansion transversely. Included in the tear is a transverse avulsion "tear" or fracture of the patella, the fragments of which are pulled far apart.

Clinically, the patient cannot actively extend the knee and since the fracture is intra-articular, a hemarthrosis is inevitable. The lateral radiographic projection depicts the nature of the fracture most clearly (Fig. 17.97).

Treatment. Avulsion fractures of the patella—at least in the young—require open reduction and internal fixation of the patella and medial and lateral quadriceps expansion. Kirschner wires crossing the fractures and a figure-eight wire (which passes around the ends of the Kirschner wires) provide the most effective type of internal fixation. A cylindrical walking cast is worn for three weeks, following which active exercises are encouraged; full flexion of the knee, however, is avoided for ten weeks. For the elderly, excision of the patella and repair of the expansion may be preferable.

Comminuted Crush Fractures

A direct fall on the flexed knee or a blow on the flexed knee from an object (such as the dashboard of an automobile at the time of a head-on collision) may produce a minor undisplaced crack of the patella or may

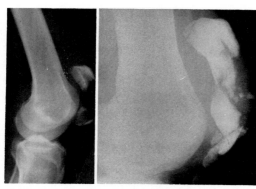

Figure 17.97 (*left*). Avulsion fracture of the patella in a 40-year-old man who, while running across a field, caught his foot in a groundhog hole. Note the wide separation of the fragments indicating a complete transverse tear of the entire quadriceps expansion. The patient was treated by internal fixation of the fractured patella and repair of the expansion.

Figure 17.98 (*right*). Comminuted crush fracture of the patella in a 42-year-old woman who was a passenger in the front seat of an automobile at the time of an accident. As she shot forward at the moment of impact, her patella was crushed and shattered by the dashboard. She was not wearing a seat belt. Treatment consisted of excision of the fragmented patella and reconstruction of the quadriceps expansion.

crush the patella so severely that it is literally shattered into many fragments.

Clinically, the patient is able to extend the knee since the medial and lateral quadriceps expansions are intact; a hemathrosis is inevitable and often excessive. The lateral radiographic projection is most useful in assessing the extent of the comminution (Fig. 17.98).

Treatment. Undisplaced crush fractures require aspiration of the hemarthrosis followed by three weeks of immobilization in a cylindrical walking cast; the fracture, if not displaced at the time of injury, will not become displaced subsequently. For the comminuted stellate fractures of the patella, it is clearly impossible to restore a smooth articular surface, and, consequently, the most appropriate method of treatment is total excision of all the patellar fragments and reconstruction of the quadriceps expansion. The functional results of such treatment are reasonably good provided the quadriceps muscle is actively exercised; even so, the patient may lose the ability to actively extend his knee through the last 5° or so ("extensor lag").

Complications of patellar fractures include *chondromalacia of the patella* and also *post-traumatic degenerative joint disease* of the patellofemoral component of the knee.

Traumatic Dislocation of the Patella

The mechanism of injury, clinical features and treatment of this injury in adults are comparable to those in older children and adolescents; they are discussed in Chapter 16.

INTERCONDYLAR FRACTURES OF THE FEMUR

The intercondylar type of fracture of the distal end of femur is comparable in many ways to that of the distal end of the humerus. Relatively uncommon, this severe fracture is usually the result of a fall on the flexed knee from a considerable height. The wedge-shaped articular surface of the patella is driven like a wedge between the two condyles and splits one or both from the shaft. Thus, the vertical component of the fracture is always intra-articular. Proximally there may be a transverse component in which case the comminuted fracture lines are T-shaped.

Clinically, the knee joint is grossly swollen by a tense hemarthrosis and there is usually evidence of abrasions or bruising over the front of the knee indicating the mechanism of injury; indeed the patella may also be fractured. Radiographic examination may require several projections to reveal the true extent of the injury since the comminution may be extreme (Fig. 17.99)

Treatment

The form of treatment depends primarily on the degree of comminution of the fracture. Of course the most important fracture to be completely reduced is the vertical fracture which extends into the knee joint. *Single fractures* which have split off only one condyle are best treated by open reduction and internal fixation with screws to restore the joint line. Widely displaced *double fractures*

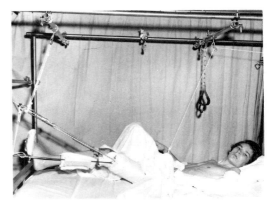

Figure 17.100. Continuous skeletal traction through a pin in the tibia. The thigh is resting in a Thomas splint and the leg is resting in a hinged Pearson knee attachment which permits knee motion.

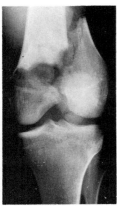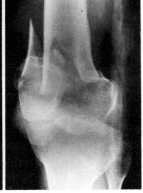

Figure 17.99. Comminuted intercondylar fracture of the left femur in a 20-year-old workman who fell 25 feet from a ladder and landed on his left knee. *Left*, anteroposterior radiograph revealing a T-shaped fracture, the vertical limb of which extends into the knee joint. Note the marked comminution. Did you also notice the undisplaced fracture of the patella? This is in keeping with the mechanism of injury, namely a fall on the flexed knee. *Right*, oblique radiograph revealing additional data concerning the displacement of the fragments and the extent of the comminution. This young man's fracture was treated by continuous skeletal traction through a pin in the tibia (Fig. 17.100).

with a transverse component may also be treated by open reduction and internal fixation of the vertical component; then the transverse fracture can be treated by continuous skeletal traction through a pin in the upper end of the tibia (Fig. 17.100). This method is preferable to prolonged operations in which an attempt is made to secure all the fragments since such surgical treatment usually leads to a permanent loss of knee motion.

Severely *comminuted fractures* in the intercondylar region defy internal fixation and are best treated by continuous skeletal traction which permits some knee motion as soon as the acute pain has subsided. Such motion somtimes helps to guide the articular fragments into acceptable position and diminishes the risk of permanent knee stiffness. In the *elderly* most intercondylar fractures of the femur are better treated by continuous skeletal traction than by open reduction.

Complications of these fractures include persistent *knee joint stiffness* and the late development of post-traumatic *degenerative joint disease of the knee.*

The Thigh
FRACTURES OF THE FEMORAL SHAFT

The femur is the largest bone in the body and its shaft is particularly strong in adults. Thus, a violent direct injury, such as may be sustained in an automobile accident, is required to produce a fracture of the femoral shaft; there is often extensive tearing of the periosteum and some degree of comminution with resultant instability of the fracture. Massive internal hemorrhage may lead to profound shock. Although union of the fracture can usually be achieved by closed treatment, it normally requires 20 weeks—and sometimes much longer.

Clinical Features

The patient's thigh is grossly swollen from internal hemorrhage; it is usually markedly deformed and completely unstable. The diagnosis is so obvious clinically that radiographic examination is best deferred until splinting of the fracture and rescusitative measures have been carried out.

Treatment

During the *emergency treatment* of patients who have sustained a displaced fracture of the femoral shaft, the limb should be immobilized in a temporary splint, not only to relieve pain but also to prevent further injury to the soft tissues (Fig. 17.101). Associated shock must be expeditiously treated.

Non-operative treatment carries fewer risks than operative treatment and is suitable for the majority of femoral shaft fractures; it does, however, require a considerably longer period in the hospital and a longer period of protection from the stresses of weight bearing. Continuous traction of either the fixed or balanced type is applied using a Thomas splint (Fig. 17.102). Whereas oblique, spiral and comminuted fractures require no prior reduction, trans-

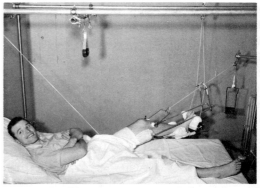

Figure 17.102. Continuous skeletal traction of the balanced type through a pin in the tibia. The thigh is resting in a Thomas splint and the leg is resting in a hinged Pearson knee attachment which permits knee motion.

verse fractures in adults should first be reduced under general anesthesia and then the traction device applied to maintain the reduction. Frequent radiographs are obtained to monitor the position of the fragments. Traction is continued for approximately 12 weeks during which time the patient is encouraged to exercise all muscles in the injured limb. When *clinical union* has been achieved, as evidenced by absence of local tenderness at the fracture site and absence of pain on applying angulatory forces, the traction device may be discarded (Fig. 17.103). Active exercises are continued but no weight bearing is permitted until there is evidence of *radiographic consolidation.*

An alternative method of treatment for fractures of the distal third of the femur is functional fracture-bracing after a period of approximately five weeks of traction.

Operative treatment including internal fixation with a large intramedullary nail is best suited for fractures of the middle third of the femoral shaft and is currently the favored method for such fractures. Although union of the fracture is not accelerated, the fracture is prevented from angulating or shortening pending consolidation (Fig. 17.104). Since there are considerable risks—particular infection—intramedullary nailing should not be undertaken lightly or merely for the "convenience" of either the patient or the surgeon. The following circumstances rep-

Figure 17.101. Thomas splint used for temporary immobilization of a displaced fracture of the femoral shaft during the emergency care of the patient.

resent clear-cut indications for intramedullary nailing of femoral shaft fractures: (1) failure to achieve an acceptable reduction by closed means; (2) associated multiple injuries (including head injury); (3) coexistent femoral artery injury requiring repair; (4) the elderly for whom prolonged bed rest is deleterious; (5) pathological fractures. The ideal

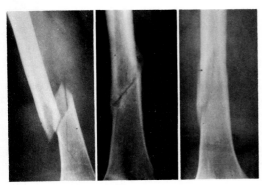

Figure 17.103. Spiral comminuted fracture of the distal third of the femur in a 45-year-old woman. *Left*, initial radiograph revealing displacement and comminution. *Center*, the position of the fragments obtained by continuous skeletal traction. *Right*, three months after injury, union is progressing satisfactorily.

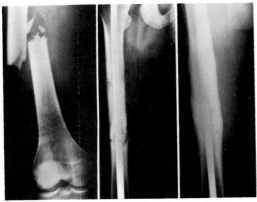

Figure 17.104. Comminuted transverse fracture of the middle third of the right femur in a 37-year-old physician who was injured in an automobile accident. *Left*, initial radiograph which reveals varus angulation and marked overriding of the fragments. Note also the comminution. *Center*, two months after closed reduction and closed ("blind") intramedullary nailing (Küntscher nail). Union is progressing at the usual rate. *Right*, one year after injury, complete radiographic consolidation of the fracture.

method of intramedullary nailing is the closed or "blind" technique in which the fracture site is not opened, the nail being inserted across the fracture site under radiographic control using an image intensifier. Even after intramedullary nailing of a fractured femoral shaft, however, immobilization in a hip spica cast for at least eight weeks is advisable. When the results of intramedullary nailing are good they are very good indeed—but when they are bad (as from infection) they are catastrophic!

Complications

Shock and *fat embolism* are early complications of fractured femoral shafts. The most troublesome late complication is *persistent knee stiffness* (which is to a large extent preventable through early and continued active exercises); either the quadriceps muscle or the patella may become adherent to the distal end of the femur and necessitate surgical release. *Non-union* in the absence of infection is rare but *delayed union* is an indication for autogenous cancellous bone grafting.

The Hip

TROCHANTERIC FRACTURES OF THE FEMUR

Fractures *between* the lesser and greater trochanters (*intertrochanteric fractures*) as well as those *through* the trochanters (*pertrochanteric fractures*) are best considered together as extracapsular or *trochanteric fractures* since their clinical manifestations and treatment are similar.

Trochanteric fractures are especially common in adults over the age of 60 years and occur more frequently in women than in men. Thus, these extracapsular fractures have the same age and sex incidence as intracapsular fractures of the neck of the femur and Colles' fractures of the distal end of the radius—and for the same reason, namely that they occur through bone that has become markedly weakened by a combination of senile and post-menopausal osteoporosis. Trochanteric fractures are often severely comminuted.

Clinical Features

The patient, usually an elderly woman, is either knocked down or falls down and is unable to get up, not only because of pain but also because of complete instability at the fracture site. Examination reveals that the entire lower limb lies in complete external rotation (Fig. 17.105). The limb usually appears short and the upper part of the thigh is swollen as a result of extracapsular bleeding into the soft tissues; indeed ecchymosis may appear in a few days. With intracapsular fractures of the femoral neck, by contrast, the bleeding is into the joint rather than into the groin or thigh. *Radiographic examination* clearly depicts the extent of the fracture.

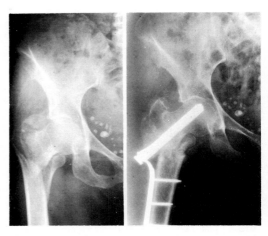

Figure 17.106. Unstable comminuted trochanteric fracture of the right femur in a 74-year-old woman. The fracture is extracapsular. *Left*, initial radiograph revealing marked comminution and a varus deformity. Note also the calcified phleboliths in the pelvic veins. *Right*, postoperative radiograph revealing that at the time of open reduction the femoral shaft has been displaced medially to provide more stability. A hip nail and plate with screws have been used for internal skeletal fixation.

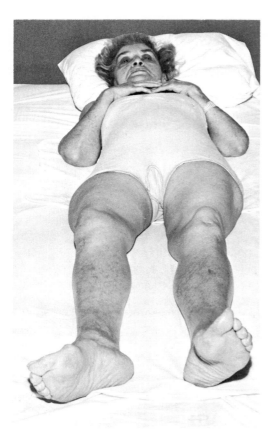

Figure 17.105. External rotation deformity of the entire right lower limb of an elderly woman. This deformity is seen with either a displaced trochanteric fracture or a displaced fracture of the femoral neck. It is usually more marked in the former.

Treatment

The blood supply in the cancellous bone of the trochanteric region is abundant and consequently trochanteric fractures virtually all unite. Thus, union can almost always be obtained by closed treatment using continuous traction. Nevertheless, union requires from 12 to 16 weeks and many elderly persons cannot tolerate such a prolonged period of bed rest even with the best possible nursing care. For this reason the preferred method of treatment is open reduction of the fracture and internal fixation with a combination of hip nail and plate with screws (Fig. 17.106). The distinct advantage of such internal fixation—particularly for the elderly—is that the patient is free to move about in bed immediately after operation, may be out of bed in a chair within a few days, and may be allowed to walk bearing partial weight on the injured limb with the help of crutches or a walker within a few weeks. For younger, more vigorous and more active persons who occasionally sustain a trochanteric fracture, it is safer to defer weight bearing until the fracture has clinically united, since the fixation device may break through metal failure if subjected to excessive stresses before the fracture is united.

In recent years, an alternative method of treatment for intertrochanteric fractures is the insertion—under radiographic control—of curved Enders nails from the medial side of the distal end of the femur; the nails are driven proximally to cross the fracture site.

Complications

Extracapsular or trochanteric fractures of the femur have relatively few complications in comparison with intracapsular fractures of the neck of the femur. Non-union and avascular necrosis almost never complicate trochanteric fractures; *mal-union* in the form of coxa vara is not uncommon, but the resultant shortening seldom exceeds 2 cm. This complication is of little significance in the elderly but should be avoided in younger patients by protecting the hip from weight bearing until the fracture is clinically united.

In the elderly, the mortality rate from intertrochanteric fractures of the femur is high—20% or higher.

FRACTURES OF THE FEMORAL NECK

Femoral neck fractures, whether they be *subcapital*, *transcervical* (mid-cervical) or *basilar* (base of the neck), may be considered together since they are all within the capsule of the hip joint (*intracapsular*) and both their clinical manifestations and their treatment are similar. Fraught with complications, femoral neck fractures are among the most troublesome and problematical of all fractures.

Garden's classification of intracapsular fractures of the femoral neck includes the following four types: Type I—incomplete; Type II—complete but undisplaced; Type III—partially displaced; Type IV—completely displaced. As you might expect, Types III and IV have a high incidence of avascular necrosis and non-union.

Fractures of the femoral neck, like trochanteric fractures and Colles' fractures of the distal end of the radius, are especially common in adults over the age of 60 years and occur more frequently in women than in men. The explanation is that these fractures occur through bone that has become markedly weakened by a combination of senile and post-menopausal osteoporosis.

Clinical Features of Displaced Fractures

The patient, most commonly an elderly woman, has a trivial mishap such as losing her footing on a slippery surface or tripping over an object; as she tries to "catch herself" she may suddenly put a torsional force on one hip, fracture the neck of the femur and *then* fall—so fragile is the femoral neck in the elderly. Under these circumstances the fracture is the *cause* of the fall rather than the result of it. If the fracture is displaced—as 95% are—the patient is unable to get up, not only because of pain but also because of complete instability at the fracture site. Examination reveals that the entire lower limb lies in external rotation, not usually so complete as that seen in patients with a trochanteric fracture (Fig. 17.105). The limb usually appears short but there is no obvious swelling since the hemorrhage from an intracapsular fracture is into the joint rather than into the soft tissues of the groin or thigh.

Radiographic Features

Since the distal fragment is always externally rotated and shifted proximally, the femoral neck appears short; upward displacement of an intracapsular fracture is somewhat limited by the hip joint capsule. Two projections at right angles to each other—an anteroposterior and a "cross-table lateral" projection—are essential to determine the relationship of the fragments to one another. In general the more nearly vertical the fracture line, the greater the shearing forces across it and the poorer the prognosis for healing. In 5% of femoral neck fractures the fragments, rather than being completely displaced, are *impacted* (as seen in both radiographic projections) and the fracture is therefore relatively stable.

Special Problems Related to Femoral Neck Fractures

The gross instability of the fracture site is aggravated by the long lever arm (the full length of the lower limb) distal to the fracture. Inability to control the proximal fragment necessitates internal fixation of the fracture and yet the osteoporotic bone is not well suited to hold metallic devices. Furthermore, the periosteum covering the intracapsular neck of the femur is exceedingly thin and has extremely limited powers of osteogenesis so that fracture healing in the femoral neck is almost entirely dependent upon endosteal callus formation. Added to all of these unfavorable conditions is the precarious blood supply to the femoral head through vessels that course along the femoral neck and are therefore vulnerable to disruption at the moment of fracture. Moreover, the development of a tense hemarthrosis may compress any uninjured vessels and further compromise the circulation to the femoral head. Thus, a displaced fracture of the femoral neck poses many serious problems, most of which are difficult to solve; indeed, it is often referred to as *"the unsolved fracture."*

Treatment of Displaced Fractures

In the years before the development of internal fixation, a fractured femoral neck in an elderly person usually triggered a series of deleterious events that led to the unfortunate victim's painful demise. From a humanitarian point of view alone, internal fixation of displaced fractures of the femoral neck is indicated; the elderly merit relief of pain no less than the young. Improvements in general anesthesia and general supportive measures for the frail and elderly have made early operation reasonably safe. Indeed such patients are usually much more likely to survive if they have an operation for their fractured femoral neck than if they do not.

Closed reduction and nailing of the fracture should be performed as soon as possible. Aspiration of the hemarthrosis at this time may minimize the risk of avascular necrosis. Reduction can usually be obtained by flexing, adducting and then internally rotating and extending the injured hip. Radiographic examination in two projections is used to assess the reduction (which must

be excellent), after which a flanged nail is driven across the reduced fracture under radiographic control—ideally with an image intensifier. Refinements of blind percutaneous nailing include exposure of the lateral aspect of the femur and the insertion of a combination nail and plate (Fig. 17.107). After satisfactory nailing of the fracture, the patient may be out of bed in a chair within a few days and may be allowed to walk bearing partial weight on the injured limb with the help of crutches or a walker within a few weeks.

Various techniques including the use of radio-opaque dyes and radioactive isotopes scintigraphy have been developed to assess the circulation of the femoral head at the time of operation. The results of these techniques serve as a useful guide to treatment, for, if the femoral head of an elderly patient is completely avascular, it is better excised and replaced by a metallic endoprosthesis

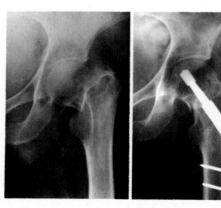

Figure 17.107. Transcervical fracture of the neck of the left femur in a 72-year-old woman. The fracture is intracapsular. *Left*, initial radiograph revealing varus deformity. The apparent shortening of the femoral neck is due to the marked external rotation of the distal fragment through the fracture site. *Right*, after closed reduction of the fracture and "blind" nailing of the fracture (which was not exposed). Note the improved neck-shaft angle. The lateral aspect of the trochanteric region was exposed, however, to apply the sliding (telescoping) nail and plate. Should any collapse occur at the fracture site or in the femoral head, the end of the nail can telescope into its sleeve and not penetrate the hip joint.

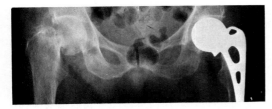

Figure 17.108. Transcervical fracture of the neck of the right femur in a frail 85-year-old woman. A similar fracture of the neck of the left femur had been treated one year previously by excision of the head and neck fragment followed by the insertion of a replacement prosthesis (Austin Moore type). This is a reasonable form of treatment for fresh fractures of the femoral neck in the very elderly.

immediately than reduced and nailed (Fig. 17.108). Prosthetic replacement is also indicated if a satisfactory closed reduction cannot be obtained or if the fracture is pathological due to a skeletal metastasis. The post-operative regimen of immediate mobilization and early walking is just as applicable after this type of treatment in the elderly as it is after nailing of the fracture.

Complications of Displaced Fractures

Only 50% of patients who have sustained a displaced femoral neck fracture obtain a satisfactory result from simple nailing of their fracture. The explanation for the unsatisfactory results in the remaining 50% of patients lies in the aforementioned inherent problems related to these fractures and in the resultant extremely high incidence of serious complications—by far the highest incidence of complications of any fracture in the body. The most significant of these complications are *avascular necrosis of the femoral head*, *non-union* and *degenerative joint disease of the hip.*

Avascular necrosis is an extremely common complication of femoral neck fractures because of the previously mentioned precarious blood supply to the femoral head. Radiographic evidence of this complication is not apparent immediately and may not become apparent for several months or even longer. You may find it helpful at this time to review the pathogenesis of avascular

necrosis of the adult femoral head, both the idiopathic and the post-traumatic type, in Chapter 13. Union of the fracture is delayed but not necessarily prevented; if the fracture unites, revascularization proceeds slowly up the neck but disintegration and collapse of the femoral head ensue before revascularization is complete and subsequent degenerative joint disease is inevitable (Fig. 17.109). The fracture may fail to unite, however, in which case revascularization of the femoral head cannot occur (Fig. 17.110). The treatment of avascular necrosis of the femoral head complicating femoral neck fractures—with or without non-union—is excision of the head and neck and replacement with a metallic prosthesis (Fig. 17.111).

Non-union develops in over 30% of dis-

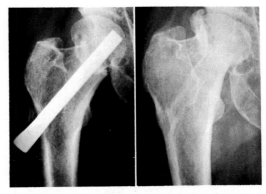

Figure 17.109. Post-traumatic avascular necrosis of the femoral head in a 65-year-old woman after fracture of the femoral neck. *Left*, the radiograph two months after internal fixation of the fracture with a Smith-Petersen nail reveals no significant change in the density of the femoral head. *Right*, the radiograph two years later reveals evidence of extensive avascular necrosis of the femoral head. The fracture of the neck of the femur has healed and the nail has been removed. Proximal to the original fracture site, however, is a larger segment of avascular necrosis. This triangular-shaped segment containing the weight bearing surface has collapsed resulting in marked joint incongruity. Note the evidence of bone deposition and bone resorption in the femoral head demarcating the necrotic fragment from the remainder of the head. Note also that this patient's hip is now adducted due to an adduction contracture. This patient's hip is irreparably destroyed.

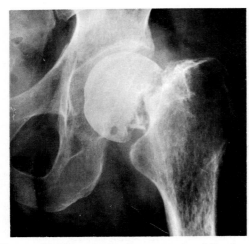

Figure 17.110. Avascular necrosis of the femoral head complicating a fracture of the femoral neck in a 40-year-old woman. The femoral head exhibits a relative increase in radiographic density (relative to the osteoporotic viable bone in the area). The fracture has failed to unite. Consequently, the femoral head has not been revascularized.

sis, the most reasonable form of treatment is excision of the ununited femoral head and neck and replacement with a metallic endoprosthesis. For younger patients whose femoral head is viable, however, reconstructive operations such as subtrochanteric femoral osteotomy or bone grafting are indicated since a united fracture and a viable femoral head are always superior to a metallic prosthesis (Fig. 17.113).

Post-traumatic degenerative joint disease develops slowly over the years as a result of either avascular necrosis with subsequent femoral head deformity or damage to the articular cartilage from the original injury or its treatment. Thus, in the elderly patient with a short life expectancy there may not be time for this complication to develop. In younger persons, however, post-traumatic degenerative joint disease of the hip is a serious complication which requires treat-

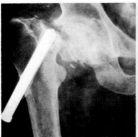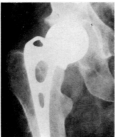

Figure 17.111. Avascular necrosis and non-union of a subcapital fracture of the neck of the right femur in a 60-year-old woman. *Left*, one year after injury, the nail has backed out, the fracture has redisplaced and there is an established non-union. The femoral head is radiographically dense relative to the surrounding bone and this indicates avascular necrosis of the head. *Right*, the same hip after excision of the head and neck fragment and replacement with a metallic endoprosthesis (Austin Moore type).

placed fractures and may be due in part to avascular necrosis but can also occur as the result of continued movement at the site of the fracture that has not been rigidly immobilized by the internal fixation device (Fig. 17.112). In the elderly and in all patients with non-union combined with avascular necro-

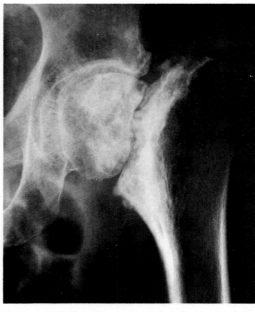

Figure 17.112. Non-union of a fracture of the femoral neck in an 85-year-old woman. The fracture had occurred five years previously and although there was no bony union, there was a firm fibrous union and the patient did not have pain. If pain had been a problem in this very elderly woman, a reasonable form of treatment would have been replacement of the proximal fragment with a metallic endoprosthesis.

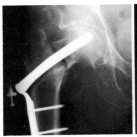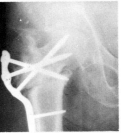

Figure 17.113. Non-union of a basilar fracture of the neck of the right femur in a 50-year-old man. The femoral head is viable. *Left*, one year after the fracture. Note that the fracture is ununited and the nail is beginning to bend (and soon would break from metal failure). The bolt of the nail plate junction has come loose and the rarefied area above and below the nail indicates that the nail has been moving up and down in the distal fragment. *Right*, three months after removal of the previous metal and subtrochanteric osteotomy of the femur with medial displacement of the femoral shaft. Both the fracture and the osteotomy are uniting satisfactorily.

ment by one or more methods as discussed in Chapter 11.

Impacted Fractures

In only 5% of patients is the femoral neck fracture truly impacted and therefore reasonably stable. Such a patient may actually walk around for several days on the impacted fracture before seeking medical attention. Physical signs are minimal and the involved hip may even be passively moved without causing pain. Radiographic examination in two planes reveals the impaction, the distal fragment nearly always being in abduction—hence the term *impacted abduction fracture*.

Treatment of impacted femoral neck fractures is somewhat controversial. If the fracture *remains* impacted it can be expected to heal within three months, without operation. Impacted fractures, however, may become *disimpacted* and therefore unstable; they then present all the serious problems associated with displaced fractures of the femoral neck. For completely cooperative and dependable patients in whom there is good clinical and radiographic evidence of firm impaction, non-operative treatment is reasonable; the patient is kept in bed for four

weeks and then allowed up on crutches with no weight bearing on the involved limb for at least eight weeks from the time of fracture. For less cooperative and less dependable patients and for those in whom the clinical and radiographic findings suggest that the fracture is not firmly impacted, the safest form of treatment is a simple form of internal fixation without disturbing the impaction (Fig. 17.114).

TRAUMATIC DISLOCATIONS AND FRACTURE-DISLOCATIONS OF THE HIP

The normal adult hip is one of the most stable joints in the body. Being a ball and socket joint, its stability is largely dependent on the shape of its articulating surfaces. Thus, severe violence is required to dislocate the hip. The hip may be dislocated *posteriorly* or *anteriorly* (with or without an associated fracture) or it may be dislocated *centrally* (in which case there is always an associated fracture).

Posterior Dislocations and Fracture-Dislocations

The normal hip joint is most vulnerable to dislocation when it is in a position of flexion and adduction. In this position a force transmitted along the shaft of the femur (as may

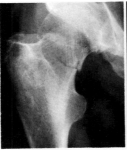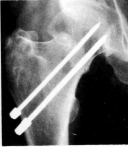

Figure 17.114. Impacted abduction fracture of the femoral neck in a 71-year-old woman who was an alcoholic. The clinical findings were minimal. *Left*, initial radiograph reveals impaction of the femoral neck into the head on the lateral side but no impaction on the medial side; there is a resultant abduction deformity at the fracture site. *Right*, the same hip after closed ("blind") pinning of the fracture with three threaded pins. Do you see only two pins? (The third pin is posterior to the inferior pin and superimposed upon it in this anteroposterior radiograph.)

occur from a dashboard injury or a fall on the flexed knee) may drive the femoral head posteriorly over the lip of the acetabulum to produce a posterior dislocation—much the commonest type. Since the femoral head escapes through a rent in the capsule, it is an extra-articular type of dislocation.

Clinical and Radiographic Features. The patient invariably lies with the injured hip in a position of flexion, adduction and internal rotation and the limb appears short; there is usually painful muscle spasm about the hip. Radiographic examination reveals that the femoral head lies well above the acetabulum; oblique projections reveal that it is also posterior (Fig. 17.115).

Treatment. As long as the hip is dislocated, the torn capsule and surrounding structures constrict the femoral neck vessels and thereby jeopardize the blood supply to the femoral head. For this reason posterior traumatic dislocation of the hip represents an emergency; the dislocation should be reduced as soon as possible to prevent the serious complication of avascular necrosis of the femoral head. Indeed, in adults whose hips are reduced within eight hours from the time of injury, the incidence of avascular necrosis is relatively low, whereas in those whose hips have remained unreduced for longer than eight hours, the incidence of this complication is high (approximately 40%).

Closed reduction is accomplished by applying upward traction on the flexed thigh in

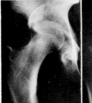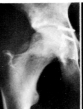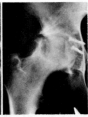

Figure 17.116. Posterior fracture-dislocation of the right hip in a 23-year-old bush pilot whose small aircraft had crashed. *Left,* initial radiograph revealing that the femoral head is lying above its normal position. Note the area of increased radiographic density above the lateral portion of the femoral head. This represents a widely displaced fracture of the posteromedial margin of the acetabulum. *Center,* complete reduction of the femoral head. The screws are holding the reduced posteromedial margin of the acetabulum in place. *Right,* one year later there is clear evidence of degenerative joint disease of the hip secondary to avascular necrosis of the femoral head.

external rotation and by forward pressure on the femoral head from behind. After reduction, which must be perfect both clinically and radiographically, the patient may be kept in bed with the limb in traction for eight weeks, but an even more effective form of treatment is immobilization of the reduced hip in a hip spica cast in its most stable position (extension, abduction and external rotation) for eight weeks to allow strong healing of the torn capsule.

Posterior Fracture-Dislocations

In approximately 50% of patients with posterior dislocations of the hip, a portion of the posterior lip of the acetabulum is fractured off at the moment of the dislocation. Small fragments are of little significance but a large fracture not only creates a significant defect in the acetabulum with resultant instability of the hip but also may be driven posteriorly to damage the sciatic nerve. If the fragment is small, it is usually pulled into place at the time of closed reduction; if it is large, however—and particularly if there is an associated sciatic nerve injury—the hip should be explored from behind, the fragment replaced and held with screws (Fig. 17.116). Less commonly a tangential frag-

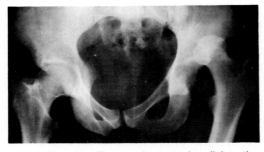

Figure 17.115. Traumatic posterior dislocation of the left hip in a 44-year-old man who had been involved in a head-on collision. Note that the femoral head is lying well above the acetabulum and that the femur is adducted.

ment of the anterior aspect of the femoral head is sheared off and needs to be removed.

Complications. Posterior dislocations and fracture-dislocations of the hip may be complicated by *avascular necrosis of the femoral head*, especially when there has been a delay in reduction as previously mentioned. A *sciatic nerve lesion*—usually a neuropraxia only—may complicate posterior fracture-dislocations.

Post-traumatic degenerative joint disease of the hip is an inevitable sequel to either avascular necrosis of the hip or residual incongruity of the joint surface at the site of a fracture-dislocation (Fig. 17.116).

Anterior Dislocations and Fracture-Dislocations

Much less common than posterior dislocation, anterior dislocations are caused by a violent injury which forces the hip into extension, abduction and external rotation—the position in which the hip is still lying when the patient is first seen. Radiographic examination depicts the femoral head below the acetabulum in the region of the obturator foramen; oblique projections reveal that it is anterior (Fig. 17.117).

Treatment. Closed reduction, which should be performed as soon as possible for reasons already mentioned, can be obtained by applying traction on the flexed thigh and then internally rotating and adducting the hip. After reduction, which must be perfect both clinically and radiographically, the pa-

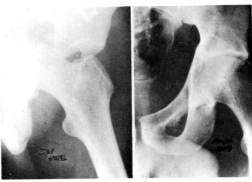

Figure 17.118. Central fracture-dislocation of the left hip of a 27-year-old man who was struck on the left side and then run over by a car. *Left*, the femoral head has been driven into the pelvis along with the medial wall of the acetabulum. The acetabular roof, however, is intact. *Right*, two years after closed reduction which had been accomplished by combined skeletal traction distally through the femoral shaft and laterally through the greater trochanter. The results are not always so satisfactory.

tient's hip should be immobilized in a hip spica cast in its most stable position (flexion, adduction and internal rotation). Anterior fracture-dislocations are rare, the fracture usually being of the femoral head rather than of the acetabulum.

Complications. Anterior dislocations and fracture-dislocations of the hip are seldom complicated by avascular necrosis of the femoral head or by nerve injuries. *Post-traumatic degenerative joint disease* of the hip may develop, particularly as a complication of a fracture-dislocation.

Central Fracture-Dislocations

A severe blow to the lateral aspect of the hip, especially when it is abducted (as may be sustained when an individual is struck from the side by an automobile or falls from a great height and lands on his hip), may drive the femoral head centrally through a comminuted fracture in the medial wall of the acetabulum. The amount of medial penetration of the femoral head into the pelvis varies from slight to extreme depending on the violence of the injury. The radiographic appearance is often striking (Fig. 17.118, *left*).

Treatment. Slight medial displacement of

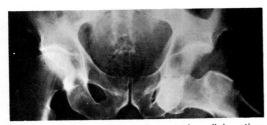

Figure 17.117. Traumatic anterior dislocation of the left hip of a 30-year-year old man who was struck by a truck. Note that the femoral head is below the acetabulum and medial to it and also that the femur is abducted. (Compare with Fig. 17.115.)

the femoral head can usually be reduced by longitudinal traction through a pin in the lower end of the femur combined with lateral traction through a pin in the greater trochanter. Continuous traction is maintained for eight weeks to allow healing of the fractures. Even extreme central dislocation of the femoral head can somtimes be reduced by such means (Fig. 17.118, *right*). If the comminution of the acetabular well is not extensive, open reduction of the fracture-dislocation and internal fixation of the fractures is indicated; but, if the comminution is extreme and there is no possibility of obtaining a stable joint, the central fracture-dislocation is sometimes left as it is, in the realization that the hip is irreparably damaged; joint motion is restricted but function is often better than might be expected.

Complications. An understandably common complication of central fracture-dislocation of the hip is *post-traumatic degenerative joint disease*, the severity of which depends on the amount of articular cartilage damage initially and the amount of residual incongruity of the joint surfaces.

The Pelvis

FRACTURES OF THE PELVIS

The adult pelvis, which includes the sacrum and the two innominate bones, is a strong, rather unyielding ring surrounding and surrounded by vital soft tissue structures including the pelvic viscera as well as the major blood vessels and nerves.

Violent injuries are required to fracture the adult pelvis and the most common of these are serious automobile accidents (which account for two-thirds of all pelvic fractures), falls from great heights, cave-ins and crushes. Thus, it is not surprising that more than half of the patients who have sustained a major pelvic fracture have sustained multiple injuries to other structures—some of which prove fatal—and many have significant complicatng soft tissue injuries in the pelvic region. Indeed, the most important aspects of fractures of the pelvis are not the fractures themselves but rather the associated *complications*—extensive internal hemorrhage from torn vessels and extravasation of urine from rupture of the bladder or urethra.

Clinical Features

The history of injury often provides a clue concerning the type of pelvic fracture as well as the complicating injuries that are likely to have been sustained. Shock, which may be profound, is a prominent feature in most patients because of the extensive internal hemorrhage. Physical examination reveals local swelling and tenderness; in unstable fractures there may also be deformity of the hips as well as instability of the pelvic ring.

Radiographic Features

Special radiographic projections are required to assess the precise nature of a pelvic fracture since the anteroposterior projection provides only a two-dimensional concept of the injury and the lateral projection, which would normally provide the third dimension, is unsatisfactory because of the overlap of the two innominate bones. Thus, in order to obtain a three-dimensional concept of the disturbed anatomy of the injury it is necessary to obtain: (1) an anteroposterior projection; (2) a tangential projection in the plane of the pelvic ring (with the tube directed upward 45°); (3) an inlet projection looking down into the pelvic ring (with the tube directed downward 45°).

In complex fractures of the pelvis, computed tomography is useful in detecting the precise site of the fracture(s) and the relationship between the fragments.

Emergency Treatment

A patient with a fractured pelvis requires emergency care centered on the two major *complications*—internal hemorrhage and extravasation of urine.

The pelvis is a particularly vascular anatomical area; consequently, displaced fractures of the pelvis may tear vessels (such as the large superior gluteal artery) with resultcant major internal hemorrhage and hence the patient may develop profound hemorrhagic shock.

While the patient's shock is being treated, a catheter should be inserted into the bladder to investigate the possibility of associated injury to the bladder or urethra. If there is blood in the urethra and a catheter cannot be passed, the urethra is almost certainly torn. Hence, a suprapubic cystotomy should be performed pending surgical repair of the urethra. If the catheter can be passed into the bladder and the urine contains blood, a cystogram should be carried out immediately to determine if the bladder has been ruptured, in which case it should be repaired as soon as possible (Fig. 17.119).

TREATMENT OF PELVIC FRACTURES

Since the bone of the pelvis is principally of the cancellous type and since its blood supply is abundant, fractures of the pelvis unite rapidly. Treatment of the various types of fractures is aimed at correcting significant fracture deformities in order to prevent malunion and resultant disturbance of function.

Types of Fractures

The wide variety of fracture patterns results from the equally wide variety of mechanisms of injury. Two major groups however merit separate consideration—those that are *stable* and those that are *unstable*. In each group there are individual fracture patterns, each with its specific mechanism of injury and method of treatment.

Stable Fractures of the Pelvis. Isolated

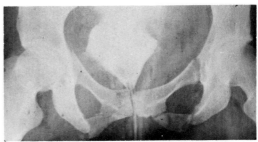

Figure 17.120. Cystogram in a 40-year-old woman who had sustained relatively undisplaced fractures of both pubic rami on both sides. The bladder (which was full at the time of injury) has ruptured through the dome as indicated by the dye that has extravasated into the peritoneal cavity. This type of rupture of the bladder is not due to a tear in the bladder wall from a sharp fracture fragment but is caused by a compressive blow on a full bladder—the same blow that fractures the pelvis.

fractures that do not transgress the pelvic ring do not interfere with stability of the pelvis in relation to weight bearing and hence do not require reduction.

Isolated fractures of the ilium from a direct injury, though painful, are of little significance and require only relief from weightbearing on the affected side until pain subsides within a few weeks.

Isolated fractures of the pubic rami result from a fall or a "straddle" type of injury. When both pubic rami are fractured, the most significant aspect of the injury is a commonly associated tear of the urethra or rupture of the bladder (Fig. 17.120).

Unstable Fractures of the Pelvis. Fractures that transgress and therefore disrupt the pelvic ring are serious injuries that interfere with stability of the pelvis in relation to weight bearing. Disruption of the ring at one fracture site in the pelvic ring can occur only if the ring is also disrupted (fractured, subluxated or dislocated) at a *second site*. Thus, both sites of disruption must be detected in order to appreciate not only what has happened but also what must be done to correct it. The lower limbs through their capsular attachment to the pelvis can be used to correct fracture deformities. The major types of unstable pubic fractures are best considered individually.

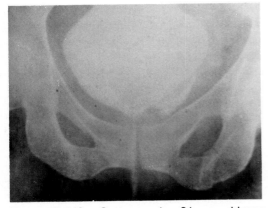

Figure 17.119. Cystogram in a 31-year-old man who had sustained an apparently undisplaced fracture of the left inferior and superior pubic rami. There must, however, have been some displacement of the fractures at the moment of impact since the left lateral wall of the bladder has been ruptured. Note the radio-opaque dye lying outside the bladder wall in the extraperitoneal tissues.

Anteroposterior compression fractures are the result of a severe crushing injury from front to back; the two innominate bones are forced apart anteriorly at the symphysis pubis (in a sense externally rotated) and both sacroiliac joints are spread open, although the sacroiliac disruption is difficult to detect radiographically (Fig. 17.121). The gap at the symphysis pubis can be closed by completely internally rotating both lower limbs (and in a sense internally rotating the two innominate bones); in addition, side-to-side compression is used to close the gap. A full hip spica cast is then applied with both lower limbs internally rotated and with side-to-side molding compression over the padded iliac crests. This is much more effective than a pelvic sling.

Lateral compression fractures are the result of a severe blow on one side or a crushing injury from side-to-side. The pubic rami are fractured and displaced on the *side* of impact and the second site of disruption is either through the sacrum or the sacroiliac joint on the *same* side. The mobile segment of the pelvic ring is hinged at its upper end and driven medially at its lower end (Fig. 17.122). This fracture is more likely than any other to rupture the bladder. Understandably, a pelvic sling or binder would increase

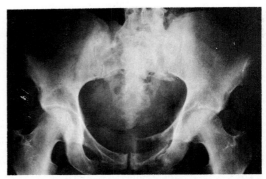

Figure 17.122. Lateral compression type of unstable fracture of the pelvis in a 21-year-old racing car driver whose car was sideswiped by another as he "spun out" on a tight corner. Note the displaced fractures of the left inferior and superior rami and also the disruption in the region of the sacroiliac joint on the same side (the site of the second break in the pelvic ring). The lower end of the mobile segment has been driven medially.

the displacement at the fracture site and should therefore be avoided. The fracture may reduce spontaneously when the patient is lying on a firm surface and for this reason an orthopaedic turning bed is useful in treatment, since the patient can be turned over without risk of lateral compression. Occasionally continuous traction on the abducted lower limb is required to obtain and maintain reduction.

Combined lateral compression and rotation fractures resemble a bucket handle in that the pubic rami are fractured on the side *opposite* the impact while either the sacrum or iliac wing is crushed and split on the *same* side as the impact. When the fracture is through the sacrum, the sacral plexus of nerves may be injured. The mobile segment, hinged above on one side and below on the other side, is usually forced upward, inward and over (in a sense internally rotated) (Fig. 17.123). The fracture deformity can usually be corrected by applying traction on the lower limb on the side of the displaced segment and then externally rotating the limb. A full hip spica cast is then applied with the lower limb in complete external rotation.

Vertical shear fractures occur as a result of falls from a great height or from certain types of industrial accidents. The pubic rami

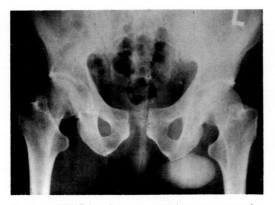

Figure 17.121. Anteroposterior compression type of unstable fracture of the pelvis in a 30-year-old auto mechanic who was pinned to the wall by a rolling automobile. Note the separation of the two innominate bones at the symphysis pubis. The innominate bones have swung outwards through the sacroiliac joints but this is not apparent radiographically.

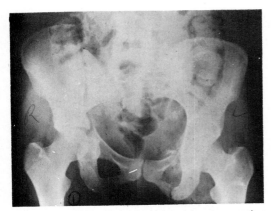

Figure 17.123. Combined lateral compression and rotation type of unstable fracture of the pelvis (bucket handle type) in a 44-year-old woman whose automobile had gone out of control and had rolled several times. Note the vertical fracture line lateral to the sacroiliac joint on the right side and the fractures of both pubic rami on the opposite side. There is also an undisplaced fracture of the acetabulum on the right side. The mobile segment, which in this patient has shifted upwards, is also free to swing forward and inward like a bucket handle.

and either the ilium or sacrum in the region of the sacroiliac joint are fractured on the *same* side by the upward thrust. Occasionally the upper site of disruption is through the sacroiliac joint. The mobile segment, which is confined to one half of the pelvis, is driven proximally and its lower end may be swung either forward or backward. The nerves of the sacral plexus are likely to be seriously injured. Vertical shear fractures are exceedingly unstable and require strong continuous skeletal traction through a pin in the femur in order not only to obtain but also to maintain reduction. If the lower end is swung forward, the traction is applied with the hip extended, whereas if the distal end is swung backward, the traction is applied with the hip flexed. Because of the risk of recurrent proximal displacement of the mobile segment in shear fractures, the traction must be maintained for approximately three months.

Under certain circumstances—such as an associated bladder injury or multiple injuries—an effective form of treatment for completely unstable fractures of the pelvis is

open reduction combined with external skeletal fixation of the Roger-Anderson type (Fig. 17.124).

After care for unstable pelvic fractures involves relief of weight bearing until the mobile segment is firmly stabilized by bony union. For most unstable fractures firm clinical union is usually achieved after two months. The shear-type fracture, however, is subjected to further shearing forces with weight bearing, and, consequently, as mentioned above, should be protected for three months.

Complications of Pelvic Fractures. *Internal hemorrhage* and resultant *shock* are the most common complications of unstable fractures. Either the *bladder* or the *urethra* is injured in approximately 15% of patients who have sustained a fracture of the pelvis. The bladder, which is particularly vulnerable when it is full, is injured almost twice as often as the urethra (Figs. 17.119, 120).

Injuries to the sacral plexus of nerves is a common and serious complication in association with fractures of the bucket handle and vertical shear type.

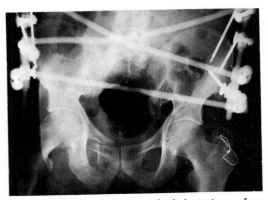

Figure 17.124. Severe vertical shear type of an unstable fracture of the pelvis that has been treated by open reduction and external skeletal fixation with the Roger-Anderson appliance. The patient had sustained multiple serious injuries including a ruptured bladder in a mine accident. The firm fixation "at a distance" facilitated his nursing care. The pubic rami are not completely reduced but the right sacroiliac joint, which had been dislocated, is in good position. Note also the wire loop in the region of the greater trochanter which had been avulsed at the time of injury to the pelvis.

THE CARE OF ATHLETES

From the beginning of time man has felt the need to excel in some type of physical activity and also to compete in such activities against others—as well as to compete against his own previous performances. Sports have become highly organized and have come to involve a large percentage of the young and not-so-young throughout the world.

For some, sports represent a pleasant recreational activity, whereas for others, sports represent a fiercely competitive vocation. Indeed, for the professional athlete, sport is synonymous with livelihood. Since all competitive athletic endeavors involve feats of strength, speed, endurance, skill and agility in varying proportions, it is understandable that physical injuries must be considered an inevitable part of the game for all who participate—nothing ventured, nothing sprained.

Physicians and surgeons have always had a responsibility for the care of injuries in athletes. Such care, however, is now well organized in that physicians or surgeons are provided for professional athletic teams and also for amateur teams in colleges and universities. There is a need to extend this care to the young athletes in secondary schools as well. Indeed, a relatively new specialty— sports medicine—has evolved; it is concerned with the etiology, diagnosis, treatment and prevention of disorders and injuries of trained athletes and also with the ideal methods of athletic training, optimum cardiorespiratory and muscle physiology as well as psychology of serious competition. Sports medicine is to athletes what pediatrics is to children and what geriatrics is to the elderly.

The establishment of sports medicine clinics in many centers has helped to improve the standard of orthopaedic care for both amateur and professional athletes.

The Etiology of Athletic Injuries and Their Prevention

With the increasing emphasis on physical fitness for all ages, it has been estimated that there are currently some 30 million recreational runner or "joggers" in North American alone. Of the serious runners, at least half will at some time develop one or more "over-use syndromes" that include (in order of decreasing frequency): painful chondromalacia of the patella ("patellofemoral pain syndrome"), tibial stress syndrome, Achilles peritendinitis, plantar fasciitis, patellar tendonitis, iliotibial band friction syndrome, tibial stress fracture, tibialis posterior tendonitis and peroneal tendonitis. The majority of these injuries or syndromes can be managed by the combination of reduction in running mileage, better training, local heat and nonsteroidal anti-inflammatory drugs.

Athletic injuries are either *intrinsic* or *extrinsic* in origin. *Intrinsic injuries* arise from the athlete's own physical activity, such as a violent muscular exertion or an awkward motion—the athlete "hurts himself." Such injuries are frequently due to inadequate physical condition or inadequate skill, both of which reflect inadequate athletic conditioning and training for the particular sport. Athletic conditioning and training, of course, are hard work but all play and no work makes the athlete a dull and vulnerable participant. Thus, the majority of intrinsic injuries are "over-use syndromes" and are to a large extent *preventable* through appropriate conditioning and training.

Extrinsic injuries are incurred by falls or blows from external forces—the athlete "gets hurt" by something or somebody other than himself. These injuries which are particularly common in body contact sports, are also to some extent *preventable* through adequate conditioning and training. Furthermore, they are at least partly preventable through the design and use of appropriate protective gear such as helmets and shoulder pads. Some extrinsic injuries can be prevented by the formulation and enforcement of safer rules and regulations in each particular sport. An analysis of the etiology and pathogenesis of athletic injuries by means of a review of movies taken during a game has already led to a better understanding of the specific activities that are especially dangerous in a given sport (such as "clipping" and "spearing" in North American football). Such activities can then be reasonably made illegal. Many serious injuries have been prevented by altering the surface on which the sport is performed; for example, artificial turf for football and the padded canvas "floor" for boxing.

Thus, physicians and surgeons share with athletes, trainers, coaches, referees and officials of athletic associations the important responsibility and obligation to prevent athletic injuries insofar as possible.

Terminology of Athletic Injuries

Musculoskeletal injuries incurred in sports are comparable to those incurred in other physical activities. Many athletic injuries, however, are quite understandably described by trainers, coaches, and the athletes themselves in colorful athletic jargon. Consequently, the following *glossary* of laymen's "locker-room terms" may be helpful in putting these injuries in professional perspective.

Baseball (or cricket) finger: avulsion of the extensor tendon of the distal interphalangeal joint; the injury may occur either through tendon or bone.

Blocker's arm (disease): either post-traumatic subperiosteal bone formation or myositis ossificans on the lateral aspect of the arm.

Bone bruise: a subperiosteal hematoma usually over the subcutaneous portion of either the tibia or the ulna.

Boxer's fracture: fracture of the neck of the fifth metacarpal.

Charley horse: a contusion and tearing of muscle fibers with resultant hematoma; the commonest muscle so injured is the quadriceps.

Footballer's (soccer player's) ankle: bony outgrowth from the anterior aspect of the distal end of the tibia and the superior surface of the neck of the talus, from repeated passive plantar flexion associated with kicking a ball.

Hip pointer: a contusion over the bony prominence of the iliac crest.

Jammed neck: a sprain of the joints of the cervical spine, usually from a lateral flexion injury.

Muscle cramp: sudden and severe pain associated with persistent spasm of a muscle, usually the gastrocnemius.

Pitcher's arm: medial epicondylitis of the elbow from chronic irritation of the common flexor origin.

Pulled groin: a strain of the adductor muscle origin.

Pulled hamstrings: a strain of the hamstring muscle origin.

Separated shoulder: either subluxation or dislocation of the acromioclavicular joint.

Shin splints: a painful condition in the region of the anterior tibial compartment of the leg from repetitive running on hard surfaces; there is inflammation and swelling in the musculotendinous portion of the muscles.

Shoulder pointer: a contusion over the bony prominence of the acromion.

Tennis elbow: lateral epicondylitis of the elbow from chronic irritation of the common extensor origin.

Tennis leg: partial rupture of the musculotendinous junction of the gastrocnemius muscle with or without rupture of the plantaris muscle.

Torn cartilage: torn meniscus of the knee joint.

The Athlete's Response to Injury

Athletes as a group are in a state of excellent physical health and are strongly motivated to make a speedy recovery from their injuries so that they may return to unrestrained athletic activity as soon as possible. To serious athletes—particularly professionals—who have trained themselves to compete in feats of strength, speed, endurance, skill and agility, even a relatively minor injury may make the dramatic difference between victory and defeat; more serious injuries may even threaten their entire athletic career and hence their livelihood.

It is not surprising, therefore, that while athletes are perfectly willing to risk injury during every competition, their psychological reaction to injury may *seem* to be unduly marked. It is hardly different, however, from the psychological reaction of a concert pianist who has injured his hand or an opera singer who has injured her vocal cords. Athletes, as a group, are sometimes considered to be "neurotic" but this is not really so. An athlete may *become* "neurotic" however, if his injury—or his concern about it—is not taken seriously by his physician or surgeon.

Aims of Treatment of Athletic Injuries

In addition to the aforementioned responsibility of *preventing* athletic injuries, the sports physician or surgeon must accept responsibility for the *treatment* of such injuries. The *principles* of musculoskeletal treatment discussed in Chapters 6 and 15 are as applicable to athletes as they are to any other individual. The following *aims* of treatment however, are particularly pertinent to athletes.

1. To base treatment on an accurate diagnosis of the precise nature and extent of the injury.

2. To initiate treatment immediately—at least within minutes of the injury.

3. To provide optimum definitive treatment that will restore function as completely as possible.

4. To minimize the inflammatory reaction to the injury. The repeated local injection of corticosteroids into a given site, however, should be avoided because of its deleterious effect on the tissues.

5. To accelerate the phases of tissue regeneration and repair.

6. To maintain and improve the function of surrounding muscles.

7. To advise the injured athlete (and his mentors) concerning the most appropriate time for return to unrestrained athletic activity. It is usually unwise to inject local anesthetic into a recently injured structure for the purpose of allowing the athlete to participate; the unhealed structure so injected, having lost the protection of pain, is particularly vulnerable to further injury. The interval of restraint should be as short as possible but as long as necessary in order to prevent the athlete from further injury during the healing phase.

8. To meet the psychological as well as the physical needs of the injured athlete.

Medical Aspects of Athletic Conditioning and Training

Until relatively recently the conditioning and training of athletes has been based on empiricism rather than on scientific knowledge. Through the application of a rapidly increasing body of pertinent scientific knowledge, sports physicians and surgeons have in recent years made many valuable contributions to these important aspects of an athlete's life.

Knowledge of muscle physiology has helped to develop the most effective methods for improving muscle strength and endurance. Likewise, recent advances in cardiorespiratory physiology have contributed greatly to the improvement in athletic performance and stamina. Certain conditioning exercises, once used extensively on an empirical basis, are now known to have harmful effects and are no longer recommended; for example, "deep knee bends" which stretch the ligaments of the knee joint and "sit ups" which frequently lead to troublesome low back pain.

Athletes will continue to break records in the pursuit of athletic excellence; the medical profession must strive to do likewise in relation to the care and prevention of athletic injuries.

THE CARE OF THE ELDERLY AND THEIR FRACTURES

As a result of man's increasing life span more persons are now reaching "old age," at which time decreasing coordination causes them to fall more frequently and senile weakening of their bones from osteoporosis renders them more susceptible to even minor injury. In this elderly age group, musculoskeletal injuries—particularly if treated by prolonged bed rest—may initiate a series of pathological processes that lead to the patient's progressive deterioration and even to his death.

In recent decades medical science, through the development of improved diagnostic, therapeutic and monitoring methods, has produced a significant increase in the *duration* or *quantity* of human life; more emphasis is required, however, on methods of improving the *quality* of human life during these additional years.

The Response of the Elderly to Injury

A significant musculoskeletal injury in an elderly person elicits a response that is greatly influenced by that patient's pre-existing physical and mental condition. Indeed, in this age group pre-existing degenerative and nutritional disturbances are exceedingly common; it has been estimated for example that at least 10% of elderly persons have some disturbance of their glucose metabolism alone. Thus, it is a combination of pre-existing complications and frequent super-imposed post-traumatic complications that account for *the high incidence of morbidity and mortality* after a significant fracture in the elderly.

Added to the purely *physical problems* of old age are the common pre-existing *psychological problems* of loneliness, insecurity and even feelings of being "no longer useful" or "no longer needed." Such psychological problems are accentuated by accidents; others—such as fear, confusion and even desperation—may be initiated by the unfamiliar setting of a hospital.

For all of these reasons the elderly person who has sustained a fracture needs and deserves alert medical care, realistic fracture treatment and kindly consideration. It is important not only to minimize *mortality* but also to minimize *morbidity*—both physical and mental. The specialty of geriatrics, concerned as it is with the care of the elderly, has contributed greatly to our understanding of the many problems associated with the care of musculoskeletal injuries in these patients.

Aims of Treatment for the Elderly

The *principles* of fracture treatment discussed in Chapter 15 are as applicable to the elderly as to the young. The *aims* of fracture treatment, however, are modified as necessary to fit the general needs of this group as well as the specific needs of each individual patient. General modifications of these aims merit consideration.

1. *To relieve pain.* The elderly withstand pain badly but they also tolerate usual adult doses of narcotics and sedatives badly, particularly if they have some degree of pre-existing cerebral arteriosclerosis. Immobilization of the fracture is still the most effective method of relieving pain arising from the soft tissues surrounding the fracture site.

2. *To obtain and maintain satisfactory position of the fracture fragments.* There is less need for perfect anatomical reduction of fractures in the elderly than in the young. For example, what might be considered satisfactory position after reduction of a Colles' fracture in an elderly person might not be at all satisfactory for a younger person who must not only use the healed wrist more and for many more years but also is more concerned about its appearance. Incomplete reduction of an intra-articular fracture can sometimes be considered satisfactory for an elderly person who is unlikely to develop degenerative joint disease during the relatively few remaining years of life. Fractures such as those of the femoral neck that require internal fixation, however, must be just as accurately reduced in the elderly as in the young.

3. *To allow, and if necessary, encourage union.* During adult life increasing age does not significantly affect the rate of fracture healing. Indeed, the period of immobilization of a given fracture can be somewhat reduced in the elderly who are unlikely to apply as much stress to their healing fractures as would a younger person. Moreover, persistent joint stiffness is much more frequent in the elderly than in the young and for this reason the period of immobilization should be as short as is consistent with achieving clinical union.

4. *To restore optimum function.* Rehabilitation of the elderly must begin from the time of initial treatment but the goals must be realistic. Rehabilitation of the elderly does

not mean rejuvenation; but the elderly who have sustained a fracture should be rehabilitated to at least their pre-injury state of physical and mental function.

The Treatment of Fractures in the Elderly

The treatment of specific fractures, dislocations and joint injuries is discussed in an earlier section of this Chapter and need not be reiterated. Much clinical judgment, both medical and surgical, is required, however, in determining the optimum form of treatment for a given elderly patient; consultation between physician and surgeon is essential.

Under some circumstances the risk of operation for a fracture in an elderly person is less than the risk of withholding operation—particularly if the non-operative alternative involves a long period of enforced bed rest as it would, for example, with a displaced trochanteric fracture of the femur.

The Prevention of Fractures in the Elderly

The most important predisposing factor in the high incidence of fractures among the elderly is the previously mentioned combination of *senile* and *postmenopausal osteoporosis*. The bones become slowly but progressively weaker and consequently may fracture as a result of even a trivial injury. Indeed, in a sense many fractures in the elderly are pathological fractures in that they occur through abnormal bone—bone that is pathological, weaker and hence more susceptible to fracture than normal bone.

One approach to *prevention* of the increasing problem of fractures in the elderly, therefore, is the prevention of the predisposing osteoporosis. You will recall from Chapter 3 and Chapter 11 that in *osteoporosis (osteopenia, too little bone)*, bone deposition is decreased because of decreased osteoblastic formation of matrix and, in addition, bone resorption is increased with the result that there is a marked diminution in the total amount of bone. This imbalance between bone deposition and bone resorption, an imbalance faced by astronauts in a weightless state, and moon walkers who are subjected to only one-sixth of the earth's force of gravity, is, at least under certain circumstances, reversible.

In the present era of scientific achievement—exemplified by man's conquest of space, the moon and beyond—the *prevention* of osteoporosis in the elderly *through scientific investigation* would seem a realistic goal. Science, like truth, is stranger than science-fiction—and more exciting!

Suggested Additional Reading

Allgower, M. and Spiegel, P. G.: Internal fixation of fractures. Evolution of concepts. Clin. Orthop. 138: 26–29, 1979.

Allman, F. L.: The non-operative technique for the treatment of acromio-clavicular injuries utilizing the Kenny Howard sling halter. In *Controversies in Orthopaedic Surgery*, edited by Leach, R. E., Hoaglund, F. T. and Riseborough, E. J. Philadelphia, W. B. Saunders, 1982.

Apley, A. G. and Solomon, L.: *Apley's System of Orthopaedics and Fractures*, 6th ed. London, Butterworth Scientific, 1982.

Bassett, C. A. L., Mitchell, S. N. and Gaston, S. R.: Treatment of ununited tibial diaphyseal fractures with pulsing electromagnetic fields. J. Bone Joint Surg. 63A: 511–523, 1981.

Bassett, C. A. L., Valdes, M. G. and Hernandez, E.: Modification of fracture repair with pulsing electromagnetic fields. J. Bone Joint Surg. 64A: 888–895, 1982.

Briggs, B. T. and Chao, E. Y. S.: The mechanical performance of the stand Hoffmann-Vidal external fixation apparatus. J. Bone Joint Surg. 64A: 566–573, 1982.

Brighton, C. T.: The treatment of non-unions with electricity. Current concepts review. J Bone Joint Surg. 63A: 847–851, 1981.

Brighton, C. T.: Present and future of electrically induced osteogenesis. In *Clinical Trends in Orthopaedics*, edited by Straub, L. R. and Wilson, P. D. Jr. New York, Thieme-Stratton, 1982.

Brooker, A. F. and Edwards, C. C.: *External Fixation—The Current State of the Art*. Baltimore, Williams & Wilkins, 1979.

Brown, P. W.: The nonoperative early weightbearing treatment of tibial shaft fractures. In *Controversies in Orthopaedic Surgery*, edited by Leach, R. E., Hoaglund, F. T. and Riseborough, E. J. Philadelphia, W. B. Saunders, 1982.

Charnley, J. *The Closed Treatment of Common Fractures*, 3rd ed. Edinburgh, Churchill-Livingstone, 1961.

Dandy, D. J.: Arthroscopic surgery of the knee. In *Current Problems in Orthopaedics Series*. Edinburgh, Churchill-Livingstone, 1981.

deHaas, W. G., Watson, J. and Morrison, D. M.: Non-invasive treatment of ununited fractures of the tibia using electrical stimulation. J. Bone Joint Surg. 62B: 465–470, 1980.

Dewar, F. P. and Barrington, T. W.: The treatment of chronic acromio-clavicular dislocation. J. Bone Joint Surg. 47B: 32–35, 1965.

Friedenberg, Z. B. and Brighton, C. T.: Bioelectricity

and fracture healing. Plast. Reconst. Surg. 68: 435–443, 1981.

Galway, H. R. and MacIntosh, D. L.: The lateral pivot shift: a symptom and sign of anterior cruciate ligament insufficiency. Clin. Orthop. 147: 45–50, 1980.

Gozna, E. R., Harrington, I. J. and Evans, D. C.: *Biomechanics of Musculoskeletal Injury.* Baltimore, Williams & Wilkins, 1982.

Grace, T. G. and Eversmann, W. W.: Forearm fractures: treatment by rigid fixation with early motion. J. Bone Joint Surg. 62A: 433–438, 1980.

Hansen, S. T. and Back, A. W.: Closed intramedullary nailing of the femur with reaming. In *Controversies in Orthopaedic Surgery* , edited by Leach, R. E., Hoaglund, F. T. and Riseborough, E. J. Philadelphia, W. B. Saunders, 1982.

Hastings, D. E.: The non-operative management of collateral ligament injuries of the knee joint. Clin. Orthop. 147: 22–28, 1980.

Heppenstall, R. B. (ed.): *Fracture Treatment and Healing.* Philadelphia, W. B. Saunders, 1980.

Hunter, G. A.: The results of operative treatment of trochanteric fractures of the femur. Injury 6: 202, 1975.

Hunter, G.: Treatment of fractures of the neck of the femur. Can. Med. Assoc. J. 117: 60–61, 1977.

Kennedy, J. C. (ed.). *The Injured Adolescent Knee,* Baltimore, Williams & Wilkins, 1979.

Inglis, A. E., Scott, N., Scalio, T. P. and Patterson, A. H.: Ruptures of the tendo achillis: objective assessment of surgical and nonsurgical treatment. J. Bone Joint Surg. 58A: 990–993, 1976.

Ireland, J. and Trickey, E. L.: MacIntosh tenodesis for anterolateral instability of the knee. J. Bone Joint Surg. 62B: 34–345, 1980.

Jackson, R. W. and Dandy, D. J.: *Arthroscopy of the Knee.* New York, Grune & Stratton, 1976.

McGinty, J. B.: Arthroscopy, a modality of diagnosis or treatment (Abraham Colles Lecture). J. Irish Coll. Phys. Surg. 11: No. 2, 1981.

McReynolds, I. S. The case for operative treatment for fractures of the os calcis. In *Controversies in Orthopaedic Surgery,* edited by Leach, R. E., Hoaglund, F. T. and Riseborough, E. J. Philadelphia, W. B. Saunders, 1982.

Mooney, V.: Nonoperative care using functional bracing for the fractured femur. In *Controversies in Orthopaedic Surgery,* edited by Leach, R. E., Hoaglund, F. T. and Riseborough, E. J. Philadelphia, W. B. Saunders, 1982.

Muller, M. E.: The role of internal and/or extraskeletal fixation: probable future refinements of techniques and their applications. In *Clinical Trends in Orthopaedics,* edited by Straub, L. R. and Wilson, P. D. Jr. New York, Thieme-Stratton, 1982.

Muller, M. E., Allgower, M., Schneider, R. and Willemeger, H.: *Manual of Internal Fixation—Techniques Recommended by the AO Group,* 2nd Ed. (translated by J. Schatzker) Berlin, Springer-Verlag, 1979.

Nelson, C. L., Weber, M., Bergman, B. and Gerdes, M.: Ender nailing of intertrochanteric fractures. In *Controversies in Orthopaedic Surgery,* edited by Leach, R. E., Hoaglund, F. T. and Riseborough, E. J. Philadelphia, W. B. Saunders, 1982.

Noble, J., Diamond, R., Walker, G. and Sykes, H.: The functional capacity of disordered menisci. J. R. Coll. Surg. Edinb. 27: 13–18, 1982.

O'Donoghue, D. H.: *Treatment of Injuries to Athletes.* Philadelphia, W. B. Saunders, 1962.

Parkes, J. C. II: The conservative method of treatment of fractures of the os calcis. In *Controversies in Orthopaedic Surgery,* edited by Leach, R. E., Hoaglund, F. T. and Riseborough, E. J. Philadelphia, W. B. Saunders, 1982.

Paterson, D. C., Lewis, G. N. and Cass, C. A.: Treatment of delayed union and nonunion with an implanted direct current stimulator. Clin. Orthop. 148: 117–128, 1980.

Pennal, G. F., Tile, M., Waddell, J. P. and Garside, H.: Pelvic disruption: assessment and classification. Clin. Orthop. 151: 12–21, 1980.

Rockwood, C. A. and Green, D. P.: *Fractures,* vols. 1 and 2. Philadelphia, J. B. Lippincott, 1975.

Ruedi, T. P. and Allgower, M.: The operative treatment of intra-articular fractures of the lower end of the tibia. Clin. Orthop. 138: 105–110, 1979.

Salter, R. B. and Harris, D. J.: The healing of intra-articular fractures with continuous passive motion. In American Academy of Orthopaedic Surgeons Lecture Series. St. Louis, C. V. Mosby, 1979, vol. 28, pp. 102–117.

Sarmiento, A.: The role of functional bracing and the likely further development of its technology. In *Clinical Trends in Orthopaedics,* edited by Straub, L. R. and Wilson, P. D. Jr. New York, Thieme-Stratton, 1982.

Sarmiento, A. and Latta, L. L.: *Closed Functional Treatment of Fractures.* Berlin, Springer-Verlag, 1981.

Sarmiento, A., Mullis, D. L. Latta, L. L., Tarr, R. R. and Alvarez, R.: A quantitative comparative analysis of fracture healing under the influence of compression plating vs. closed weight bearing treatment. Clin. Orthop. 149: 232–239, 1980.

Schatzker, J. and Lambert, D. C.: Supracondylar fracturs of the femur. Clin. Orthop. 138 77–83, 1979.

Schatzker, J., McBroom, R. and Bruce, D.: The tibial plateau fracture. The Toronto experience 1968–1975. Clin. Orthop. 138: 94–104, 1979.

Schatzker, J. and Tile, M.: The AO (ASIF) method of fracture care. In *American Academy of Orthopaedic Surgeons Instructional Course Lectures.* St. Louis, C. V. Mosby, 1980, vol. 29, pp. 41–50.

Smillie, I. S.: *Injuries of the Knee,* 5th ed. London, Churchill-Livingstone, 1978.

Taunton, J. E. and Clement, D. B.: Common injuries in runners: etiology and management. Mod. Med. Can. 36: 476–482, 1981.

Tile, M.: Indications for open reduction of tibial fractures. In *Controversies in Orthopaedic Surgery,* edited by Leach, R. E., Hoaglund, F. T. and Riseborough, E. J. Philadelphia, W. B. Saunders, 1982.

Tile, M. and Pennal, G. F.: Pelvic disruption: principles and management. Clin. Orthop. 151: 56–64, 1980.

Wilson, J. N. ed.: *Watson-Jones' Fractures and Joint Injuries,* 5th ed., Edinburgh, Churchill-Livingstone, 1976, vols. 1 and 2.

Uhthoff, H. (ed.): *Current Concepts of External Fixation of Fractures.* Berlin, Springer-Verlag, 1982.

PART 5

Research

"The practice of Medicine is an *art*—based on *science*."
—Sir William Osler

CHAPTER 18

The Philosophy and Nature of Medical Research*

Although a discussion of medical research may be considered by some to be "beyond undergraduate core curriculum," I am directing this chapter to *you* as a medical student because you have the *potential* to become a medical scientist or clinician-scientist—either part-time or full-time—and also because of my own personal conviction that research is essential to the continuing progress of all medical and surgical specialties.

My purpose is three-fold: first to help you to appreciate the importance and philosophy of medical research; second, to stimulate you to contemplate the possibility of your own personal involvement; and third, to share with you some thoughts concerning the *nature* of such research as well as some guidelines concerning the scientific method—thoughts and guidelines that I have found especially helpful during a 25-year period of consistent, part-time involvement in this fascinating and exciting facet of academic medicine.

For these purposes the terms "medical" and "medicine" are used in their broadest context in that they are meant to include all

medical and surgical specialties within the profession even though I write from my perspective as an orthopaedic surgeon-scientist.

A DEFINITION OF RESEARCH

The English noun *research* is derived from the French verb *rechercher*, which means simply to look again or to take a second look—in contradistinction to being satisfied with one superficial look. Thus, research involves taking a fresh and concentrated look at a given problem in an attempt to find a solution.

As the philosopher and critic John Ruskin wrote in 1853: "The work of science is to substitute facts for appearances and demonstrations for impressions."

From a distillation of definitions in various dictionaries, *research* could be defined as "an investigation or experimental study of some phenomenon directed to the discovery and interpretation of new data through the critical approach of the scientific method."

In Chapter 5, I referred to solving the mystery of a diagnosis as "the detective work of *clinical* medicine." In this sense, "medical research is the detective work of *scientific* medicine." Thus, the modern day *medical investigator* who is striving to solve a given biological mystery must bring to bear

* A modified version of the author's article entitled "The Philosophy and Nature of Surgical Research," published in the *Canadian Journal of Surgery*, vol. 23, pp. 349–354, 1980.

on the problem the same powers of astute observation, the same gathering of clues or data and the same processes of inductive and deductive reasoning used by the modern day detective or *criminal investigator*. As in detective work so also in research the magnifying glass of Sherlock Holmes has been replaced by the light microscope and even more sophisticated equipment such as transmission and scanning electron microscopes (Fig. 18.1).

THE VARIOUS TYPES OF RESEARCH

Medical research is usually divided, somewhat arbitrarily, into two major categories: *basic* research and *applied* research. While these two categories of medical research share the same demanding discipline of the scientific method, they differ in some respects.

Basic research, which is also called "pure research" or "fundamental research," is usually pursued for the sake of acquiring knowledge and understanding for their own sake, albeit with the hope that such acquisitions may prove to be relevant to health, even if indirectly and eventually. As the scientist John Polanyi has written, "The prime objective of basic science is to foster the discovery of new ideas and the applications will flow naturally from these discoveries."

Applied research, which is also known as "clinically oriented research," "mission-oriented research" or "targeted research," is usually pursued for the sake of solving a specific clinical problem in man in order that the resultant solution may be applied both directly and immediately. Such research may be conducted through *experimental investigations* in animals or through *clinical investigations* in human patients. Nevertheless, through applied or mission-oriented research basic or fundamental concepts may be discovered, just as through basic re-

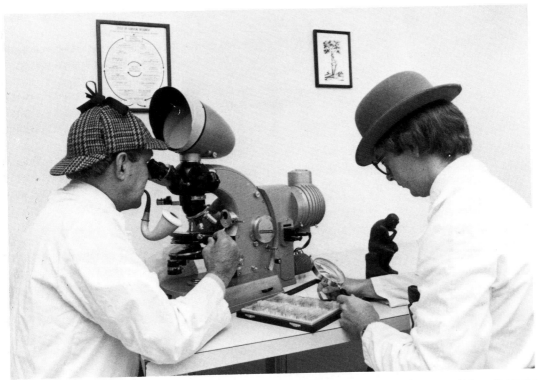

Figure 18.1. In order to solve a given biological mystery, the *medical investigator* and his colleagues must use the same processes of observation, data gathering and reasoning as the *criminal investigator* such as Sherlock Holmes and his colleague, Dr. Watson.

search practical applications of the research may be forthcoming.

While basic research and applied research are of equal importance, and indeed are often interdependent, it is understandable that in medical research the emphasis is on the applied or clinically oriented type of research, that is, as applied to the care of patients. However, the great French scientist Louis Pasteur has wisely said that "there are really no *applied* sciences—only the *application* of science, a very different matter."

THE IMAGE OF MEDICAL RESEARCH

As an undergraduate medical student of today, you may have been negatively influenced by the current trend among some of the young to harbor feelings of anti-establishment and anti-science. Added to this you will have heard much about the budgetary constraints on research funding through governments and also that there may be few opportunities for either full-time or part-time positions in medical research. Although such negative attitudes have often been exaggerated, they may explain—at least in part— why only approximately 5% of undergraduate medical students in North America are currently attracted to a career in medical research.

This negative image of research, although unjustified, is not new, for as the 19th century philosopher and critic John Ruskin wrote, "Science lives only in quiet places, and with odd people, mostly poor." But all of that has changed! Visit the medical or surgical research laboratories in your own university and you will find them not to be "quiet places" but rather hives of intellectual and physical activity; you may find the medical or surgical scientists unusual or uncommon individuals perhaps, but not "odd," and you will find that they are no longer "mostly poor."

THE GOALS AND IMPORTANCE OF RESEARCH

In the broad fields of medicine and surgery and their related basic sciences the primary goal of the various types of research is to achieve a more complete understanding of biological processes, both normal and abnormal, in order to make significant advances in the treatment of disorders and injuries in man through the development of more effective methods for their prevention, detection or treatment. In this sense, all medical research has a bearing on health— either directly or indirectly, either immediately or eventually.

In an academic setting, however, research has an additional goal, namely the enrichment of the *education*—as opposed to the mere *training*—of a clinician. In this context the term "education" implies the intelligent understanding of clinical teaching, while the term "training" implies uncritical acceptance of such teaching.

Research enhances the quality of medical education, both undergraduate and postgraduate, because the scientific atmosphere has a beneficial impact on all aspects of the educational program and, in addition, such an atmosphere is testimony to the fact that medicine as a science is dynamic, growing and constantly changing for the better. Furthermore, a lively and exciting program of medical research in a given university attracts the brightest young people as postgraduate students and new faculty members to that university.

Through your personal involvement in either clinical or experimental investigation as an undergraduate or postgraduate student you should acquire qualities such as intellectual curiosity, critical thinking, logic and discrimination that can be applied not only to your own work but also the work of your colleagues as expressed through both the spoken and the written word. Indeed, in any postgraduate surgical training program that does not include a significant amount of research activity, the potential clinician will receive more of a technical or trade school training than a true medical education in both the art and science of medicine.

In a given university the importance of medical research varies directly with the degree to which these two major goals are being achieved. Although much more emphasis on medical research is required throughout the world, such research has already gained a position of great importance in many of our major universities not only because of its intrinsic contributions to new knowledge but also for its contributions to medical education.

First-rate medical research within a university medical school invariably improves the quality of *patient care* in the affiliated teaching hospitals of that university—and indeed the quality of patient care in hospitals throughout the world—since new scientific knowledge is soon shared with fellow clinicians and scientists internationally through the media of scientific meetings and publications.

THE MOTIVATION FOR SEARCH AND RESEARCH

Search for knowledge that is both true and new has always challenged and motivated intelligent humans. In his famous 12th century prayer the physician-philosopher Maimonides expressed such motivation thusly: "Let the thought never arise that I have attained to enough knowledge."

The acknowledged "father" of surgical research is the 18th century surgeon John Hunter, whose insatiable curiosity concerning all biological phenomena combined with his brilliant logic led to innumerable experiments with highly significant results that were to change the course of surgical practice. Thus, he became one of the first surgeons in the world to apply the scientific method to surgical problems and to put surgery on a scientific, as opposed to an empirical, basis.

In a letter to Jenner concerning smallpox, Hunter wrote: "I think your solution is just; but why only think? Why not try the experiment?"

One of the world's leaders in the philosophy of science, Karl Popper, has stated that "it is not the possession of knowledge, or irrefutable truths, that constitute the man of science, but the incessant search for truth."

The underlying motivation of the scientist to become engaged in research—and indeed wedded to it—is a combination of intellectual curiosity and dissatisfaction with the current state of knowledge and understanding. As Voltaire has said: "Without the spirit of *constructive discontent* we would still be eating acorns and sleeping under the stars."

PERSONAL QUALITIES OF THE MEDICAL SCIENTIST

As a potential medical scientist you should consider the following eight personal qualities to be among those that are important, if not essential, for research. You must *have* integrity, intelligence, ingenuity and initiative and you must *be* inquisitive, innovative, industrious and incisive.

THE PHILOSOPHY OF MEDICAL RESEARCH

Inherent in the philosophy of research is the aforementioned "constructive discontent" with the existing state of knowledge and traditionally accepted—but unproven—concepts. And yet as an undergraduate medical student you will have acquired an incredible amount of cognitive information, at least some of which needs to be challenged. George Perkins, a distinguished British orthopaedic surgeon who dared to differ with his more traditional-minded contemporaries once stated that "the training of a medical doctor is such that it is difficult for him to break with tradition"—a sad commentary relevant to the difference between "training" and "education."

Although the success of research depends upon many factors, the pivotal and initiating factor is the scientific curiosity of the investigator, a curiosity that compels him or her to discover—or uncover—new data and new concepts through the application of the scientific method.

Understandably, the life of the clinician-scientist is not easy, but it can be very rewarding in terms of the quiet satisfaction that comes from achieving a scientific goal.

In a sense the clinician-scientist is a bridge-builder who constantly strives to bridge the gap between the practical art and theoretical science of medicine. To be effective in this role the medical scientist must merit the respect of both fellow clinicians and fellow scientists and this calls for exemplary performance in *both* fields. This important concept is epitomized by the motto of the Royal College of Physicians and Surgeons of Canada: *Mente Perspicua Manuque Apta*—"a keen mind and skillful hands."

THE NATURE OF MEDICAL RESEARCH—A CYCLE

Even the most inspired and idealistic of potential scientists must accept and work within the rigorous discipline of the scientific method, the essence of all research. Seemingly complex and formidable at first to the uninitiated or inexperienced, the scientific method is best understood if presented as a series of well planned phases or steps.

During many years of teaching and supervising both undergraduate and postgraduate research fellows, I have found the concept of what one might call the "cycle of medical research" to be most helpful in outlining and explaining the multiple phases of the time-honored scientific method (Fig. 18.2). The cycle consists of a series of guidelines that start with patients and come back to patients because medical research of the mission-oriented or targeted type is designed to find the solution to an unsolved clinical problem in patients and in due course, whenever appropriate, to apply the newly found knowledge to that problem.

In this cycle of medical research there are 16 phases, each of which merits your individual attention.

1. Recognize an Unsolved Clinical Problem

In order to find a solution to a given unsolved clinical problem it is essential that as a clinician-scientist you first *recognize* that problem or a component of it, and this involves being a keen and alert observer—a human biology watcher. Unfortunately a pure clinician may "have eyes but see not" and may miss the critical observation that would lead to recognizing an unsolved clini-cal problem and to its investigation. "In the field of observation," wrote Louis Pasteur, "chance favors the prepared mind."

2. Think

To *think* deeply, contemplatively and speculatively about an unsolved problem requires determination and self-discipline on your part since there are so many interruptions in the daily—and even nightly—life of a physician or surgeon. Furthermore, such thinking is more difficult and more taxing than, for instance, making a fairly obvious diagnosis, prescribing a routine medical regimen or performing a routine surgical operation. It may, however, bring its own rewards such as the intellectual exhilaration that results from successful problem-solving.

3. Review the Scientific Literature

Before embarking on any research project you will need to review the scientific background against which your work will stand. In medical research as in other forms of research there have been many examples of "rediscovering the round wheel" which could have been avoided had the investigator been aware of the historical background of the subject. Churchill and others have expressed the thought that those who do not read history are doomed to repeat the errors (and one might add, the experiments) of the past. Fortunately literature surveys have been tremendously facilitated by modern computerized library science. As you review the scientific literature relevant to the problem that you have recognized, you will not only be able to benefit from the labors of fellow scientists but you will also be stimulated to build upon such labors through your own original thinking and questioning.

4. Ask an Intelligent Question

Having read the historical background of the problem you then need to ask an intelligent question, and furthermore, a question that can be feasibly answered through research. In relation to a specific phenomenon under investigation the question frequently begins with, Why? How? What? or Which? Much time, effort and money will be wasted if an inappropriate question forms the un-

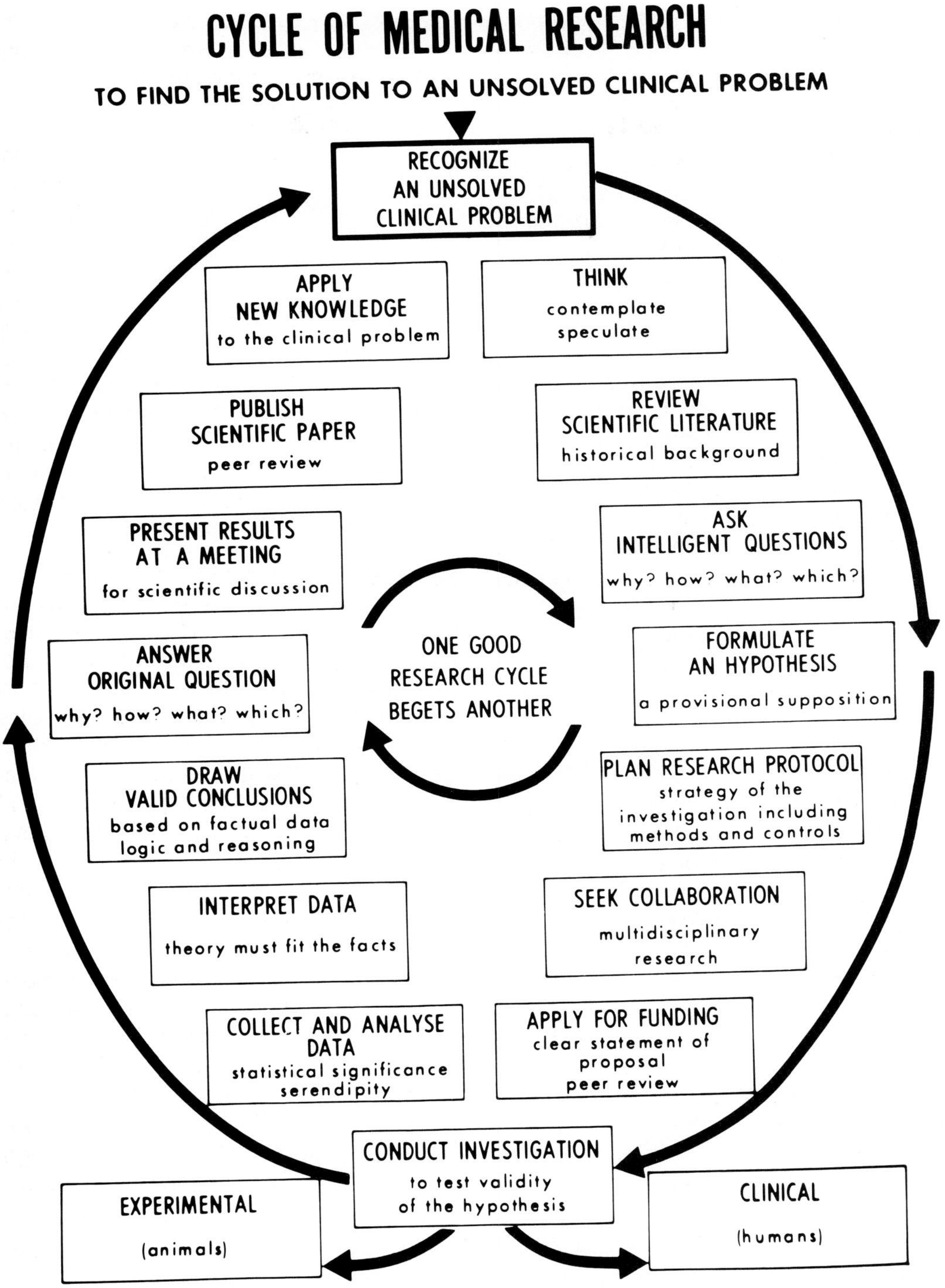

CYCLE OF MEDICAL RESEARCH

TO FIND THE SOLUTION TO AN UNSOLVED CLINICAL PROBLEM

Figure 18.2.   The "cycle of medical research," outlining 16 phases or stages of the scientific method relevant to *applied* research.

derlying basis for a research project, for as the scientist Sir Henry Tizard has emphasized, "The secret of success in science is to ask the right question."

5. Formulate a Hypothesis

As the first step toward answering your own question you should formulate a hypothesis (literally a subordinate thesis or a theoretical and provisional supposition which serves as a starting point for further investigation by which it may be proved or disproved). The working hypothesis is a carefully reasoned but as yet unproven answer to the question and should lend itself to the testing of its validity through the research project that is being planned.

6. Plan the Research Protocol

The next step in the *cycle of medical research* is to plan in detail the *protocol*, or stategy, of the investigation, that is, the experimental design, including the subjects of the investigation (either animals or human patients), the investigational methods, the equipment, the "controls" to deal with all possible variables and finally the proposed methods of analysis of the data including the determination of statistical significance. The protocol should be planned with the primary purpose of the investigation in mind, namely the testing of the validity of your hypothesis.

7. Seek Collaboration

As biomedical research becomes increasingly complex and sophisticated, you *must* be prepared to collaborate with scientists of other disciplines—such as physiology, biochemistry, microbiology, immunology, biophysics and biomedical engineering—in multidisciplinary research. Through such collaborative research one mind fertilizes another, and the scientific investigation grows in both depth and breadth. It was the importance of collaboration in research that Claude Bernard was extolling when he wrote: "Art is I; Science is We."

8. Apply for Funding

In this enlightened era of science which is intermittently darkened by the clouds of antiscience and the resultant constraints of research budgets from governments and other agencies, it should be encouraging for you, as a potential clinician-scientist, to realize that there *is still* money available to support well planned, clearly stated, exciting, significant and original research. The peer review system would still seem to be the most appropriate mechanism whereby your grant application may receive the fairest consideration and the highest possible standards of research may be maintained.

Two of the criteria by which your fellow scientists in the peer review system judge a given proposal are the scientific significance of the project in terms of new knowledge or understanding and also the likelihood of its success.

9. Conduct the Investigation

Through the scientific investigation you set out neither to prove nor to disprove your hypothesis but rather to test its validity with complete objectivity.

As a clinical physician or surgeon your inherent reverence for human life and human comfort will compel you to confine *experimental* investigations to animals and also to accept the principle that any proposed *clinical* investigations in humans must be morally and ethically acceptable to the review mechanisms of a university-based "human clinical investigation (or experimentation) committee" which includes clinician-scientists as well as members of other professions. Experimental investigations in animals must also be acceptable in that they must meet established government regulations to protect the comfort of the animals.

10. Collect and Analyze the Data

As you make observations and collect data during the progress of your investigation you should be alert to the possibility that an unexpected finding may have much significance—the phenomenon of *serendipity* (a word coined by Horace Walpole and based on the story of the Three Princes of Serendip who, during a long journey, never did reach their planned goal but who, unexpectedly and by chance, found many things of even greater interest and significance along the way). Indeed, many important discoveries have been made through serendipity: penicillin, polio vaccine, and cryoprecipitate to mention only three.

A serendipitous observation, of course, should stimulate another cycle of research.

But the scientist may fail to appreciate the significance of the unexpected, as Churchill pointed out when he wrote: "Man occasionally stumbles over the truth but he usually manages to pick himself up and continue on."

Provided that the protocol of your investigation has been well planned it should be possible for you to analyze your data accurately and to determine its statistical significance.

11. Interpret the Data

This phase of the cycle of medical research is one of the most important because you may have collected important data but unless your interpretation of these data is correct you may find yourself off your cycle and into the ditch of delusion.

In the interpretation of the data you must consider all of the data and not just those parts that seem to "fit" your hypothesis, because through the latter process you would, in fact, be deluding yourself, and others; you would be making the facts fit the theory rather than, as you should be, making the theory fit the facts. It may have been this type of intellectual dishonesty that George Bernard Shaw was contemplating when he wrote: "Beware of false knowledge—it is more dangerous than ignorance."

12. Draw Valid Conclusions

Through the application of sound logic and scientific reasoning you should draw valid conclusions—insofar as that is possible—on the basis of the factual data. This is another difficult phase of the cycle of medical research since the clinician-scientist may be tempted, subconsciously and unwittingly, to draw conclusions that are not justified by the factual data. When more than one interpretation of the data seems reasonable it may be necessary to initiate another cycle of research to clarify the matter.

13. Answer the Original Question

By the time you have reached this phase of the cycle you may well be able to answer the original question. You should not be disturbed if the answer is not that which you expected because, of course, you are seeking the truth rather than proof of a preconceived theoretical answer to the original question. The search for truth, however, is never-ending, because the more questions you answer the more questions you will raise to take their place. Each of these questions, in turn, will serve as the catalyst for the creation of another research cycle.

14. Present Results at a Meeting

Having completed the investigation it is important for you to present the results at a scientific meeting in order that you may benefit from the resultant discussion, both positive and negative. Indeed, constructive criticism of a given scientific investigation can only help you to improve upon its final presentation. It would be considered unprofessional for you as a medical scientist to share the results of your research with the general public through the lay media—press, radio or television—before these results have been either presented at a major scientific meeting or published in the scientific literature.

15. Publish a Scientific Paper

If your investigation has been worth doing it is worth publishing and you should seek publication in a reputable scientific journal which is critically refereed. Indeed, you have a moral obligation to publish a significant scientific investigation for, as Richard Bach has written in his book entitled *Jonathan Livingston Seagull*, "It is good to be a seeker but sooner or later you have to be a finder, and then it is well to give what you have found, a gift unto the world for whoever will accept it."

16. Apply the New Knowledge

As implied in the adjective "applied," this type of mission-oriented or targeted research frequently leads to new knowledge that can be applied to the unsolved clinical problem that initiated the cycle of medical research. The application may be relevant to an improved understanding of the etiology, pathology, pathogenesis, detection, treatment, or even prevention of the clinical problem under investigation. Such application is in keeping with Booker's law, which states that ''an ounce of application is worth a ton of abstraction.''

Thus the cycle of medical research is complete and you will have progressed from realistic research to clinical reality. It is hoped that you will have come to appreciate that it is better to move in the best circles of research than to walk the straight and narrow path of empiricism.

No matter how successful a scientist may be in solving problems, his or her ''spirit of constructive discontent,'' of which Voltaire wrote, is self-perpetuating, since one good idea begets another and one discovery leads to another.

In the final analysis, the success of any given medical research project will depend upon the intelligence and inquisitiveness of the individual scientist whose goal should be not to follow the established path of clinical empiricism but rather, through research, to explore where there is no path and leave a trail that leads into the future!

Index